MW01503912

Blackwell's Primary Care Essentials: The Complete Guide

Fourth Edition

Blackwell's Primary Care Essentials Series

Blackwell's Primary Care Essentials: The Complete Guide

Fourth Edition

Daniel K. Onion, MD, MPH, FACP

Professor of Community and Family Medicine
Dartmouth Medical School
Director Emeritus, Maine-Dartmouth Family Practice
*   Residency Program*
Augusta, Maine

Blackwell
Publishing

© 2003 by Blackwell Science
a Blackwell Publishing company

Blackwell Publishing, Inc., 350 Main Street, Malden, Massachusetts 02148-5018, USA
Blackwell Science Ltd., Osney Mead, Oxford OX2 0EL, UK
Blackwell Science Asia Pty Ltd, 550 Swanston Street, Carlton, Victoria 3053, Australia
Blackwell Verlag GmbH, Kurfürstendamm 57, 10707 Berlin, Germany

02 03 04 05 5 4 3 2 1

ISBN: 0-632-04633-3

Library of Congress Cataloging-in-Publication Data
Onion, Daniel K.
  Blackwell's primary care essentials. The complete guide / by Daniel
K. Onion.—4th ed.
     p. ; cm.—(Blackwell's primary care essentials series)
Rev. ed. of: The little black book of primary care. 1999.
Includes index.
  ISBN 0-632-04633-3 (pbk.)
  1. Primary care (Medicine)—Handbooks, manuals, etc.
  [DNLM: 1. Primary Health Care—Handbooks. WB 39 O58b 2002]
I. Title: Complete guide. II. Title: Primary care essentials. III. Onion,
Daniel K. Little black book of primary care. IV. Title. V. Series.
RC55 .O65   2002
616—dc21   2001008675

A catalogue record for this title is available from the British Library

Acquisitions: Nancy Duffy
Development: Julia Casson
Production: Debra Lally
Cover design: Leslie Haimes
Typesetter: TechBooks in York, PA
Printed and bound by Edwards Brothers in Ann Arbor, MI

For further information on Blackwell Publishing, visit our website:
www.blackwellscience.com

Notice: The indications and dosages of all drugs in this book have been recommended in the
medical literature and conform to the practices of the general community. The medications
described and treatment prescriptions suggested do not necessarily have specific approval
by the Food and Drug Administration for use in the diseases and dosages for which they are
recommended. The package insert for each drug should be consulted for use and dosage as
approved by the FDA. Because standards for usage change, it is advisable to keep abreast
of revised recommendations, particularly those concerning new drugs.

Table of Contents

Preface

Frontline doctors are the primary care physicians who still practice medicine the way it has been practiced through the millennia. They are the first and usually the only professional healer to see a person who decides he or she needs one. There is no filter, no screening. It is exhilarating and scary work. Exhilarating to fit the puzzle of a patient's problem and personality into the medical model and provide relief; scary because it is impossible to fit it always correctly, efficiently, and in a way that is satisfying to the patient. The knowledge and wisdom expected of a "real doc" seem impossibly infinite. Primary care is a humbling calling.

Nearly all physicians, as medical students or residents, start a "little black book" system of relevant medical facts and opinions sometime during their early training to try to encapsulate, master, and/or summarize that infinite and ever changing sea of medical knowledge. Most abandon their attempts, either as they subspecialize, or as volume overwhelms their systems for organizing and integrating new with older information.

This book is intended as a starter notebook that students or residents in primary care may add to and modify as they encounter new information. It is NOT a comprehensive compilation of facts, for nobody's notebook could be; rather, it offers a framework for organizing clinical information from a variety of sources including lectures (place or person and date noted), journals (journal abbreviation, volume, and page or issue number noted), and texts (name and edition date noted). Thus it contains both "pearls" and literature-debated issues, most with very specific references to each bit of information, which makes the text unique among medical texts. Disease processes about which there is little current controversy or new information are treated briefly; the book assumes the user already knows the basics. Its 6000+ fact-specific references for virtually every aspect of clinical primary care are unique for a medical manual.

Clinicians may use this book both for references and for noting new data themselves. Most journal articles and many talks convey only a small bit of truly new information to the practitioner; hence a word or two plus the source reference is all the reader need note to update and personalize that section. Since not all articles, even in the best clinical journals, carry new information relevant to the practicing primary care physician, the size of my book has remained relatively constant over 25 years. My practice is to look for the kernel of relevant articles and talks and not to attempt to transcribe monographs.

The book is organized in alphabetical order by medical specialty, with the exception of Emergency Medicine, which is placed first for quick and easy access. I group diseases in related clusters to allow browsing among related diseases; where no obvious cluster exists, I have alphabetized them; for instance, the gi sections are organized mouth to anus. The danger of alphabetizing is that the reader and I may not use the same key word. I hope the index, which I have tried to make very complete, will put us on the same page. Most chapters have a miscellaneous section at the end for unclassifiable information in that area, brief comments about less important diseases, and for differential diagnoses not unique to one disease. When drugs are used for many diseases in a given section, relevant drug summaries appear at the beginning of chapters; otherwise, drugs specific to one or two diseases are discussed under those diseases. Liberal abbreviations ("doc talk") (see page xviii) are used to save space and mimic clinical conversation; most should be familiar to American clinicians. Differential diagnoses of various signs, symptoms, and lab results are outlined in those (Sx, Si, Lab) sections, or under complications, as rule outs (r/o).

The book consists primarily of references and information about technical medicine and thereby de-emphasizes ideas and compilations focused on psychosocial issues, although such paradigms are obviously crucial to the application of technical knowledge. Some sections are less extensive than others, partly a reflection of my own training and experience, and partly because in some areas, like pediatrics, subjects which can be related to another specialty appear there rather than under pediatrics.

This fourth edition is being published both electronically by Skyscape for personal digital assistants under its original title *The Little Black Book for Primary Care,* and in print by Blackwell as part of its new primary care series, which previous editions of this book inspired, under the title *The Complete Guide*. It is being produced to accompany 9 other books using my original disease page format and aimed at primary care physicians and midlevel clinicians. Since the whole series is now called *Primary Care Essentials,* the print text has been renamed and both print and electronic versions have been updated substantially from the 3rd edition 4 years ago. The 4th edition incorporates many suggestions made by readers and reviewers as well as new references. Much clinical medicine is learned "on the hoof", so portability is essential. In response to consistent requests to make the book truly small enough to fit in a white coat pocket, Skyscape has produced it in a Palm Pilot electronic format, and I have reduced the Blackwell print version by cutting some of the more esoteric and rarer disease sections. Elimination of the previous spiral binding should also help make it smaller still.

I welcome readers/users suggestions and corrections.

Daniel K. Onion
Maine-Dartmouth Family Practice Residency
15 E. Chestnut St.
Augusta, Maine 04330
*email:*DanielKOnion@dartmouth.edu
November, 2001

Acknowledgments

Several physicians kindly reviewed and critiqued the various sections of this book; I have not always followed their advice as I made judgements about what a primary care physician might want to know, so the residual errors are mine. For their help, I am grateful. They include:

Emergency Medicine
Steve E. Diaz M.D.
MaineGeneral Medical Center
Waterville, Maine

Cardiology
John Sutherland, M.D., F.A.C.C.
Arizona Heart Institute
Phoenix, Arizona

Dermatology
Eleanor E. Sahn, M.D.(coauthor)
Clinical Associate Professor of Dermatology and Pediatrics
Medical University of
    South Carolina
Charleston, South Carolina

Ear, Nose, and Throat
William H. Maxwell, M.D.
Assistant Clinical Professor
    of Otolaryngology
University of Vermont
Portland, Maine

Endocrinology
Thomas Bigos, M.D.
Professor of Medicine
University of Vermont
Portland, Maine

Endrocrinology: Lipids
Leonard Keilson, M.D., M.P.H.
Associate Professor of Medicine
University of Vermont
Portland, Maine

Gastroenterology
David W. Hay, M.D.
Adjunct Assistant Professor of
    Community and Family
    Medicine
Dartmouth Medical School
MaineGeneral Medical Center
Waterville, Maine

Geriatrics
Karen Gershman, M.D.
    (coauthor)
Assistant Professor of Community
    and Family Medicine
Dartmouth Medical School
MaineGeneral Medical Center
Augusta, Maine

Hematology/oncology
Donald Magioncalda, M.D.,
Adjunct Assistant Professor of
    Community and Family
    Medicine
Dartmouth Medical School
MaineGeneral Medical Center
Augusta, Maine

Infectious Disease
Stephen D. Sears, M.D., M.P.H.,
    (coauthor)
Adjunct Assistant Professor of
    Community and Family
    Medicine
Dartmouth Medical School
MaineGeneral Medical Center
Augusta, Maine

Nephrology
Charles Jacobs, M.D.
Adjunct Assistant Professor of
    Community and Family
    Medicine
Dartmouth Medical School
MaineGeneral Medical Center
Waterville, Maine

Neurology
Alexander McPhedran, M.D.
Associate Professor of Community
    and Family Medicine (Emeritus)
Dartmouth Medical School
MaineGeneral Medical Center
Augusta, Maine

Obstetrics & Gynecology
Russell N. DeJong, Jr., M.D.,
    (coauthor)
Assistant Professor of Community
    and Family Medicine
Dartmouth Medical School
MaineGeneral Medical Center
Waterville, Maine

Ophthalmology
Maroulla Gleaton, M.D.
Adjunct Assistant Professor of
    Community and Family
Dartmouth Medical School
MaineGeneral Medical Center
Augusta, Maine

Orthopedics
Anthony R. Mancini, M.D.
MaineGeneral Medical Center
Augusta, Maine

Pediatrics
James MacMahon, M.D.
Associate Professor of Pediatrics
University of Vermont
Maine Medical Center
Portland, Maine

Psychiatry
David Moore, M.D.
Associate Clinical Professor
Department of Psychiatry
University of Louisville School
    of Medicine
Louisville, Kentucky

Pulmonary
Edward Ringel, M.D
Adjunct Assistant Professor of
    Community and Family
    Medicine
Dartmouth Medical School
MaineGeneral Medical Center
Waterville, Maine

Rheumatology
Margaret A. Duston, M.D.
Adjunct Assistant Professor of
    Community and Family
    Medicine
Dartmouth Medical School
MaineGeneral Medical Center
Waterville, Maine

Urology
Pamela Ellsworth, M.D.
Assistant Professor of Surgery
Dartmouth Medical School
Hanover, New Hampshire

Surgery
Cameron McKee, M.D.
Adjunct Assistant Professor of
    Community and Family
    Medicine
Dartmouth Medical School
MaineGeneral Medical Center
Augusta, Maine

I thank Malcolm. W. (Kip) MacKenzie, M.D., who, as a Dartmouth Medical student doing book reviews for Norton, connected me with medical publishers. Many other medical students, residents, and colleagues with whom I have had the pleasure of working over the last 30 years have made multiple other good suggestions including many for this fourth edition. And finally, I am grateful to Debbie DeVoe who has tirelessly helped me prepare this edition for publication.

Abbreviations

MEDICAL ABBREVIATONS

AA	Alcoholics anonymous
A_2	Aortic (first) component of S_2
ab	Antibodies
ABGs	Arterial blood gases
ac	Before meals
ACE	Angiotensin convertine enzyme
ACEI	ACE imhibitor
Ach	Acetylcholine
ACLS	Advanced cardiac life support
ACOG	American College of Obstetrics and Gynecology
ACTH	Adrenocorticotropic hormone
AD	Right ear
ADH	Antidiuretic hormone
ADHD	Attention deficit hyperactivity disorder
ADLs	Activities of daily living
AF	Atrial fibrillation
AFB	Acid-fast bacillus
Afib	Atrial fibrillation
AFP	Alpha fetoprotein
Aflut	Atrial flutter
ag	Antigen
AGN	Acute glomerular nephritis
AI	Aortic insufficiency
aka	Also known as
Al	Aluminum

ALA	☐ levulinic acid
ALS	Amyotrophic lateral sclerosis
ALL	Acute lymphocytic leukemia
ALT	SGPT; alanine transferase
AMI	Anterior myocardial infarction
AML	Acute myelogenous leukemia
ANA	Antinuclear antibody
ANCA	Antineutrophil cytoplasmic autoantibodies
AODM	Adult onset diabetes mellitus
AP	Anterior-posterior
AR	Aldose reductase
ARA	Angiotensin receptor antagonist
ARDS	Adult respiratory distress syndrome
AS	Aortic stenosis, or left ear
ASA	Aspirin
asap	As soon as possible
ASCVD	Arteriosclerotic cardio-vascular disease
ASD	Atrial septal defect
ASHD	Arteriosclerotic heart disease
ASLO	Antistreptolysin O titer
ASO	Antistreptolysin O titer

AST	SGOT; aspartate transferase	cc	Cubic centimeter
asx	Asymptomatic	CEA	Carcinoembryonic antigen
atm	Atmospheres		
ATN	Acute tubular necrosis	cf	Compare
AU	Both ears	CF	Complement fixation antibodies
AV	Arteriovenous; or atrial-ventricular		
		CHD	Congenital heart disease
avg	Average		
AVM	Ateriovenous malformation	chem	Chemistries
Ba	Barium	chemoRx	Chemotherapy
bact	Bacteriology	CHF	Congestive heart failure
BAL	British anti-Lewisite		
bc	Birth control	CI	Cardiac index
bcp's	Birth control pills	CIN	Cervical intraepithelial neoplasia
BCG	Bacille Calmette-GuŽrin		
BCLS	Basic cardiac life support	CIS	Carcinoma in situ
BE	Barium enema	Cl	Chloride
bid	twice a day	CLL	Chronic lymphocytic leukemia
BiPAP	Bi (2)-positive airway pressures		
		CMF	Cytoxan, methotrexate, 5-FU
biw	twice a week		
BJ	Bence Jones	CML	Chronic myelocytic leukemia
bm	bowel movement		
BM	Basement membrane	cmplc	Complications
BP	Blood pressure	CMV	Cystomegalovirus
BPH	Benign prostatic hypertrophy	CN	Cranial nerve; or cyanide
BS	Blood sugar	CNS	Central nervous system
BSE	Breast self exam		
BSOO	Bilateral salpingo-oophorectomy	CO	Cardiac output
		c/o	Complaining of
BUN	Blood urea nitrogen	col	Colonies
bx	Biopsy	COPD	Chronic obstructive lung disease
C′	Complement		
Ca	Calcium, or cancer depending on context	cp	Cerebellar-pontine
		CP	Cerebral palsy
CABG	Coronary artery bypass graft	CPAP	Continuous positive airway pressure
CAD	Coronary artery disease		
cAMP	Cyclic AMP	CPC	Clinical/pathologic conference
cath	Catheterization		
CBC	Complete blood count	CPG	Coproporphyrinogen

CPK	Creatine phophokinase	DKA	Diabetic ketoacidosis
CPR	Cardiopulmonary resuscitation	DMSA	Dimercaptosuccinic acid
		DNA	Deoxyribonucleic acid
cps	Cycles per second	d/o	Disorder
CREST	Calcinosis, Raynaud's, esophageal reflux, sclerodactyly, telangiectasias	DOE	Dyspnea on exertion
		DPG	Diphosphoglycerate
		DPI	Dry powder inhaler
		DPN	Diphosphopyridine nucleotide
CRH	Corticotropin releasing hormone.	DPNH	Reduced DPN
crit	Hematocrit	DPT	Diphtheria, pertussus, tetanus vaccine
CRP	C reactive protein		
crs	Course	DS	Double strength
c + s	Culture and sensitivity	dT	Diphtheria tetanus adult vaccine
C/S	Cesarian section		
CSF	Cerebrospinal fluid	DTaP	Diphtheria, tetanus, acellular pertussis vaccine
CT	Computerized tomography		
Cu	Copper	DTRs	Deep tendon reflexes
CVA	Cerebrovascular accident	DTs	Delerium tremens
		DU	Duodenal ulcer
CVP	Central venous pressure	DVT	Deep venous thrombosis
d	Day/s	dx	Diagnosis or diagnostic
dB	Decibel	EACA	□-aminocaproic acid
DAT	Dementia, Alzheimer's type	EBV	Ebstein-Barr virus
		ECM	Erythema chronicum marginatum
DBCT	Double blind controlled trial		
		EF	Ejection fraction
D + C	Dilatation and curettage	eg	for example
D + E	Dilatation and evacuation (suction)	EGD	Esophagogastroduodenoscopy
DES	Diethyl stilbesterol	EKG	Electrocardiogram
DHS	Delayed hypersensitivity	ELISA	Enzyme-linked immunosorbent assay
DI	Diabetes insipidus		
dias	Diastolic	E/M	Erythroid/myeloid
DIC	Disseminated intravascular coagulation	EM	Electron microscopy
		EMG	Electromyogram
dig	Digoxin	EMT	Emergency Medical Technician
dip	Distal interphalangeal joint		
		Endo	Endoscopy
DJD	Degenerative joint disease	Epidem	Epidemiology

ER	Estrogen receptors; or emergency room	GHRH	Growth hormone releasing hormone
ERCP	Endoscopic retrograde cholangio-pancreatography	gi	Gastrointestinal
		glu	glucose
		glut	Glutamine
ERT	Estrogen replacement therapy	gm	Gram
		GN	Glomerulonephritis
ESR	Erythrocyte sedimentation rate	GnRH	Gonadotropin releasing hormone
et	Endotracheal	GTT	Glucose tolerance test
et al.	and others	gtts	Drops
etc	And so forth	gu	Genitourinary
ETOH	Ethanol	GVHD	Graft vs. host disease
ETT	Exercise tolerance test	HBIG	Hepatitis B immune globulin
F	Female; or Fahrenheit		
FA	Fluorescent antibody, or folic acid	HCG	Human chorionic gonadotropin
FBS	Fasting blood sugar	HCGrH	HCG releasing hormone
Fe	Iron		
FEV$_1$	Forced expiratory vital capacity in 1 sec	HCl	Hydrochloric acid
		HCO$_3$	Bicarbonate
FFA	Free fatty acids	hct	Hematocrit
FIGLU	Formiminoglutamic acid	HDL	High density lipoprotein
fl	Femtoliter		
FMF	Familial Mediterrranean fever	H & E	Hematoxylin and eosin
		hem	Hematology
freq	Frequency	hep	Hepatitis
FSH	Follicle stimulating hormone	H. flu	Hemophilus influenza
		Hg	Mercury
FTA	Fluorescent treponemal antibody	hgb	Hemoglobin
		HgbA$_1$C	Hemoglobin A$_1$C level
FTT	Failure to thrive	HGH	Human growth hormone
f/u	Follow up		
FUO	Fever of unknown origin	5-HIAA	5-Hydroxy indole acedic acid
FVC	Forced vital capacity	Hib	Hemophilus influenza B vaccine
fx	Fracture		
g	Guage	his	Histidine
GABA	□-Aminobutyric acid	HIV	Human immunodeficiency virus
gc	Gonorrhea		
GE	Gastroesophageal	HLA	Human leukocyte antigens
GFR	Glomerular filtration rate		

HMG-COA	Hydroxymethylglutaryl-coenzyme A	incr	Increased
h/o	History of	INH	Isoniazid
H + P	History and physical	INR	International normalized ratio (protimes)
hpf	High power field	IP	Interphalangeal
HPV	Human papilloma virus	IPG	Impedance plethysmography
hr	Hour/s		
HRIG	Human rabies immune globulin	IPPB	Intermittent positive pressure breathing
hs	At bedtime	IPPD	Intermediate purified protein derivative
HSP	Henoch-Schonlein purpura	IQ	Intelligence quotient
HSV	Herpes simplex virus	ITP	Idiopathic thrombocyto-penic purpura
HT	Hypertension		
5HT	5-Hydroxytryptophan	IU	International units
HUS	Hemolytic uremic syndrome	IUD	Intrauterine device
		IUGR	Intrauterine growth retardation
HVA	Homovanillic acid		
hx	History	iv	Intravenous
I or I_2	Iodine	IVC	Inferior vena cava
IADLs	Instumental activities of daily living	IVP	Intravenous pyleogram
		IWMI	Inferior wall myocardial infarction
IBD	Inflammatory bowel disease		
		J	Joule
ibid	Same reference as last reference above	JODM	Juvenile onset diabetes mellitus
ICU	Intensive care unit	JRA	Juvenile rheumatoid arthritis
I + D	Incision and drainage		
IDDM	Insulin dependent diabetes melitus	JVD	Jugular venous distension
		JVP	Jugular venous pressure/pulse
ie	in other words		
IEP	Immunoelectrophoresis	K	Potassium
IF	Intrinsic factor	kg	Kilogram
IFA	Immunofluorescent antibody	KOH	Potassium hydroxide
		KS	Kaposi's sarcoma
IgA	Immunoglobulin A	KUB	Abdominal xray ("kidneys, ureters, bladder")
IgE	Immunoglobulin E		
IgG	Immunoglobulin G		
IgM	Immunoglobulin M	L	Liter; or left
IHSS	Idiopathic hypertrophic-subaortic stenosis	LA	Left atrium; or long acting if after a drug
im	Intramuscular		

LAP	Leukocyte alkaline phosphatase	MIC	Minimum inhibitory concentration
LATS	Long acting thyroid stimulating protein	min	Minute
		MMR	Measles, mumps, rubella
LBBB	Left bundle branch block	mOsm	Milliosmole/s
LDH	Lactate dehydrogenase	mp	Metocarpal phalangeal
LDL	Low density lipoproteins	6MP	6-mercaptopurine
LES	Lower esophageal sphincter	MR	Mitral regurgitation
		MRA	Magnetic resonance angiography
LFTs	Liver function tests	MRFIT	Multiple risk factor intervention trial
LH	Luteinizing hormone		
LHRH	LH releasing hormone	MRI	Magnetic resonance imaging
LMW	Low molecular weight		
LP	Lumbar puncture	MRSA	Methicillin resistant staph aureus
LS	Lumbosacral		
LV	Left ventricle	MS	Multiple sclerosis; or mitral stenosis
LVH	Left ventricular hypertrophy		
		MSH	Melanocyte stimulating hormone
lytes	Electrolytes		
m	Meter/s	mtx	Methotrexate
M	Male	Multip	Multiparous pt
MAI	Mycobacterium avium intracellulare	μ	Micron
		μgm	Microgram
MAO	Monamine oxidase	Na	Sodium
mcp	Metacarpal-phalangeal joint(s)	NAD	Nicotinamide adenine dinucleotide
MD	Muscular dystrophy; or physician	NADH	Reduced form of NAD
		NCI	National Cancer Institute
MDI	Metered dose inhaler		
meds	Medications	ncnc	normochromic normo-cytic
MEN	Multiple endocrine neoplasias		
		NCV	Nerve conduction velocities
mEq	Millieqivalent		
mets	Metastases	neb	nebulizer
METS	Metabolic equivalents	neg	negative
mg	Milligram	NG	Nasogastric
Mg	Magnesium	NH	Nursing home
MHC	Major histocompatibility locus	NH$_3$	Ammonia
		NICU	Newborn intensive care unit
MI	Myocardial infarction/ or mitral insufficiency		

NIDDM	Noninsulin-dependent diabetes mellitus	P_2	Pulmonary (2nd) component of S_2
nl	Normal	PA	Pernicious anemia; or pulmonary artery
nL	Nanoliter		
nm	Nanometer	PABA	Paraminobenzoic acid
NMRI	Nuclear magnetic resonance imaging	PAC	Premature atrial contraction
NNH	Number needed to harm	PAF	Paroxysmal atrial fibrillation
NNT	Number needed to treat		
noninv	Noninvasive laboratory	PAN	Polyarteritis nodosa
NPH	Normal pressure hydrocephalus	Pap	Papanicolaou
		PAP	Pulmonary artery pressure
npo	Nothing by mouth		
no.	Number	par	Parenteral
NS	Normal saline	PAS	p-Amino salicylic acid
NSAID	Nonsteroidal anti-inflammatory drug	PAT	Paroxysmal atrial tachycardia
NSR	Normal sinus rythmn	Patho-phys	Pathophysiology
NST	Nonstress test		
Nullip	Nulliparous pt	Pb	Lead
NV + D	Nausea, vomiting and diarrhea	PBG	Porphobilinogen
		pc	After meals
NYC	New York City	PCP	Pneumocystis pneumonia
O_2	Oxygen		
OB	Obstetrics	PCTA	Percutaneous transluminal angioplasty
OCD	Obsessive compulsive disorder		
		PCR	Polymerase chain reaction
OD	Overdose; or right eye		
OGTT	Oral glucose tolerance test	PCWP	Pulmonary capillary wedge pressure
OH	Hydroxy-	PDA	Patent ductus arteriosus
OM	Otitis media	PEG	Percutaneous endoscopic gastrostomy
op	Operative or out patient		
O + P	Ova and parasites	PEP	Protein electrophoresis
OPD	Outpatient department	PERRLA	Pupils equal round reactive to light and accomodation
OPV	Oral polio vaccine		
OS	Left eye		
osm	Osmoles	PFTs	Pulmonary function tests
OTC	Over the counter		
OU	Both eyes	PG	Prostaglandin
oz	Ounce	PHLA	Post heparin lipolytic activity
P	Pulse		

phos	Phosphatase	PTH	Parathormone
PI	Pulmonic insufficiency	PTT	Partial thromboplastin time
PID	Pelvic inflammatory disease	PUD	Peptic ulcer disease
		PUVA	Psoralen + UVA light
PIH	Pregnancy induced hypertension	PVC	Premature ventricular tachycardia
pip	Proximal interphalangeal joint	q	Every
		qd	Daily
PMI	Point of maximal impulse of heart	qid	4 times a day
		qod	Every other day
PMNLs	Polymorphonuclear leukocytes	qow	Every other week
		qt	Quart
PMR	Polymyalgia rheumatica	R	Right, or respirations
PND	Paroxysmal nocturnal dyspnea	RA	Rheumatoid arthritis
		RAIU	Radioactive iodine uptake
PNH	Paroxysmal hemoglobinuria	RAST	Radioallergosorbent test
po	By mouth	RBBB	Right bundle branch block
PO₄	Phosphate	rbc	Red blood cell
polys	Polymorphonuclear leukocytes	RCT	Randomized controlled trial
pos	Positive	RDS	Respiratory distress syndrome
PP	Protoporphyrin		
ppd	Pack per day	re	About
PPD	Tuberculin skin test	rehab	Rehabilitation
PPG	Protoporphyrinogen	REM	Rapid eye movement
pr	By rectum	RES	Reticuloendothelial system
pRBBB	Partial right bundle branch block	retic	Reticulocyte/s
		Rh	Rhesus factor
pre-op	Pre-operative	RHD	Rheumatic heart disease
prep	Preparation	RIA	Radioimmunoassay
primip	Primiparous pt	RIBA	Radio-immuno blot assay
prn	As needed	RMSF	Rocky mountain spotted fever
PROM	Premature rupture of membranes		
		ROM	Range of motion
PS	Pulmonic stenosis	ROS	Review of systems
PSA	Prostate specific antigen	RNA	Ribonucleic acid
PSVT	Paroxysmal supraventricular tachycardia	RNP	Ribonucleoprotein
		r/o	Rule out
PT	Protime	RSV	Respiratory syncytial virus
pt (s)	Patient (s)		

Note on PO₄: PO_4

RTA	Renal tubular acidosis	SRS	Slow reacting substance
rv	Review	SS	Sickle cell disease
RV	Right ventricle	SSKI	Saturated solution of potassium iodide
RVH	Right ventricular hypertrophy	SSRI	Selective serotonin reuptake inhibitor
rx	Treatment	SSS	Sick sinus syndrome
S_1	First heart sound	Staph	Staphylococcus
S_2	Second heart sound	STD	Sexually transmitted disease
S_3	Third heart sound, gallop	STS	Serologic test for syphilis
S_4	Fourth heart sound, gallop	SVC	Superior vena cava
SAB	Spontaneous abortion	SVT	Supraventricular tachycardia
SAH	Subarachnoid hemorrhage	sx	Symptom/s
Sb	Antimony	sys	Systolic
SBE	Subacute bacterial endocarditis	T_i	Fever/temperature
sc	Subcutaneous	T_3	Triiodothyronine
SD	Standard deviation	T_4	Thyroxin
sens	Sensitivity	TA	Temporal arteritis
SER	Smooth endoplasmic reticulum	T + A	Tonsillectomy and adenoidectomy
serol	Serology/ies	tab	Tablet
SGA	Small for gestational age	TAH	Total abdominal hysterectomy
si	Signs	tbc	Tuberculosis
SI	Sacroiliac	TCAs	Tricyclic antidepressants
SIADH	Syndrome of inappropriate ADH	TBG	Thyroid binding globulin
SIDS	Sudden infant death syndrome	tcn	Tetracycline
		Td	Tetanus/diphtheria, adult type
SKSD	Streptokinase, streptodornase	TEE	Transesophageal echo-cardiogram
sl	Sublingual		
SLE	Systemic lupus erythematosis	TENS	Transcutaneious electrical nerve stimulation
SNF	Skilled nursing facility	Tfx	Transfusion
soln	Solution	THC	Tetrahydro-cannabinol
s/p	Status post	TI	Tricuspid insufficiency
specif	Specificity	TIA	Transient ischemic attack
SPEP	Serum protein electrophoresis	TIBC	Total iron binding capacity
SR	Slow release	tid	3 times a day

TIPS	Transjugular intrahepatic porto-systemic shunt	VDRL	Serologic test for syphilis ("Venereal Disease Research Lab")
tiw	Three times a week		
TM	Tympanic membrane	VF or	
Tm	Trimethoprim	Vfib	Ventricular fibrillation
Tm/S	Trimethoprim/sulfa	VIP	Vasoactive intestinal peptide
TNF	Tumor necrosis factor		
TNG	Nitroglycerine	vit	Vitamin
TNM	Tumor, nodes, metastases	VLDL	Very low density lipoprotein
TPA	Tissue plasminogen activator	VMA	Vanillymandelic acid
		vol	Volume
TPN	Total parental nutrition	V/Q	Ventilation/perfusion
TPNH	Triphosphopyridine reduced	vs	versus
		VSD	Ventricular septal defect
TRH	Thyroid releasing hormone		
		VT or	
TS	Tricuspid stenosis	Vtach	Ventricular tachycardia
TSH	Thyroid stimulating hormone	V-ZIG	Varicella-zoster immune globulin
tsp	Teaspoon	w	With
TTP	Thrombotic thrombo-cytopenic purpura	W/s	Watt/seconds
		w/u	Work up
TURP	Transurethral resection of prostate	wbc	White blood cells or white blood count
U	Units	wgt	Weight
UA	Urinanalysis	wk	Week/s
UBO	Unidentified bright object	WNL	Within normal limits
		WPW	Wolff-Parkinson-White Syndrome (short PR interval)
UGI	Upper gastrointestinal		
UGIS	Upper GI series		
URI	Upper respiratory illness	xmatch	Crossmatch
US	Ultrasound	yr	Year/s
USPTF	US preventive task force	ZE	Zollinger-Ellison syndrome
UTI	Urinary tract infection		
UV	Ultraviolet	Zn	Zinc
UVA	Ultraviolet A	>	More than
UVB	Ultraviolet B	>>	Much more than
UUB	Urine urobilinogen	<	Less than
vag	vaginally	<<	Much less than
val	Valine	→	Leads to (eg, in a chemical reaction)
VCUG	Vesico-urethrogram		

JOURNAL ABBREVIATIONS

Acta Obgyn	Acta Obstetricia et Gynecologica Scandinavia
ACP J Club	American College of Physicians Journal Club supplement to Annals of Internal Medicine
Age Aging	Age and Aging
Am Fam Phys	American Family Physician
Am Hrt J	American Heart Journal
Am J Clin Path	American Journal of Clinical Pathology
Am J Dis Child	American J of Diseases of Childhood
Am J Med	American Journal of Medicine
Am J Obgyn	American Journal of Obstetrics and Gynecology
Am J Psych	American Journal of Psychiatry
Am J Pub Hlth	American Journal of Public Health
Ann EM	Annals of Emergency Medicine
AnnIM	Annals of Internal Medicine
Ann Neurol	Annals of Neurology
Ann Rv Public Health	Annual Review of Public Health
Arch Derm	Archives of Dermatology
Arch IM	Archives of Internal Medicine
Arch Phys Med Rehab	Archives of Physical Medicine and Rehabilitation
Arthritis Rheum	Arthritis and Rheumatism
BMJ	British Medical Journal
Brit J Rheum	British Journal of Rheumatology
Bull Rheum Dis	Bulletin of Rheumatic Diseases
Can Med Assoc J	Canadian Medical Association Journal
Circ	Circulation
Cleve Clin J Med	Cleveland Clinic Journal of Medicine
Clin Exp Rheum	Clinical and Experimental Rheumatology
Clin Ger Med	Clinics in Geriatric Medicine
Clin Orthop	Clinical Orthopedics
Clin Perinatol	Clinical Perinatolgoy
Contraceptive Tech	Contraceptive Technology
Crit Care Med	Critical Care Medicine
Curr Concepts Cerebro Dis	Current Concepts of Cerbrovascular Disease
Diab Care	Diabetes Care
Diab Res Clin Pract	Diabetes Research and Clinical Practice
Emerg Med Clin N Am	Emergency Medical Clinics of North America
Epidem Rev	Epidemiology Review
FDA Bul	Federal Drug Administration Bulletin

Fam Pract Recert	Family Practice Recertification
Fam Pract Survey	Family Practice Survey
Fertil Steril	Fertility and Sterility
GE	Gastroenterology
Ger Med Today	Geriatric Medicine Today
Gerontol	Gerontologist
Ger Rv Syllabus	Geri_atric Review Syllabus
HT	Hypertension
Inf Contr Hosp Epidem	Infection Control and Hospital Epidemiology
Inf Dis Clin NA	Infectious Disease Clinics of North America
Jama	Journal of the American Medical Association
J Am Acad Derm	Journal of the American Academy of Dermatology
J Am Coll Cardiol	Journal of the American College of Cardiology
J Am Ger Soc	Journal of the American Geriatric Association
J Cardiovasc Pharmacol	Journal of Cardiovascular Pharmacology
J Chronic Dis	Journal of Chronic Disease
J Clin Epidem	Journal of Clinical Epidemiology
J Clin Immunol	Journal of Clinical Immunology
J Fam Pract	Journal of Family Practice
J Gen Intern Med	Journal of General Internal Medicine
J Gerontol	Journal of Gerontology
J Ger Psych Neurol	Journal of Geriatric Psychiatry and Neurology
J Infect Dis	Journal of Infectious Disease
J Intern Med	Journal of Internal Medicine
J Investig Derm	Journal of Investigative Dermatology
J Lab Clin Med	Journal of Laboratory and Clinical Medicine
J Peds	Journal of Pediatrics
J Pharm Experim Ther	Journal of Pharmocology and Experimental Therapy
Mccvd	Modern Concepts of Cardiovascular Disease
Md State Med Assoc J	Maryland State Medical Association Journal
Med	Medicine
Med Aud Dig	Internal Medicine Audio Digest
Med Care	Medical Care
Millbank Q	Millbank Quarterly
MKSAP	American College of Physicians Medical Knowledge Self Assessment Test.
Mmwr	CDC Morbidity and Mortality Weelky Review
Mod Med	Modern Medicine
Nejm	New England Journal of Medicine
Neurol	Neurology
Obgyn	Obstetrics and Gyecology

Obgyn Cl N Am	Obstetrics and Gynecology Clinics of North America
Ophthalm	Ophthalmology
Ped Derm	Pediatric Dermatology
Ped Infect Dis J	Pediatric Infectious Disease Journal
Ped Rv	Pediatric Review
Peds	Pediatrics
Post Grad Med J	Postgraduate Medicine Journal
Psych Ann	Psychiatric Annals
Rev Inf Dis	Review of Infectious Disease
Rx Let	Prescribers Letter
Scand J Gastroenterol	Scandanavian Journal of Gastroenterology
Semin Arth Rheum	Seminars in Arthritis and Rheumatology
Sci Am Text Med	Scientific American Textbook of Medicine
West J Med	Western Journal of Medicine

Page Format

Below is outlined the uniform format of all disease pages:

SYSTEM/SPECIALTY

DISEASE NAME (Other Names)

General references, reviews

Cause: Agent, if relevant; mechanism of dissemination, if relevant

Epidem: Epidemiologic information

Pathophys: Pathophysiology

Sx: Symptoms

Si: Signs

Crs: Course of disease

Cmplc: Complications, including differential diagnoses of diseases with similar presentations

Lab: Tests and interpretation of their results, eg, pathology, chemistries, hematologies, etc., with sensitivity and specificity data if available

Xray: Radiologic and other studies usually performed by radiology departments

Rx: Treatments:
  Preventive if relevant
  Therapeutic of existing disease, further divided into medical vs surgical if appropriate and of complications

Chapter 1
Emergencies

D. K. Onion

1.1 GENERAL ISSUES

Definition: Diagnosis and treatment too urgent to allow time to look things up; all diagnostic findings (hx, sx, and si), w/u, and rx must be memorized

Medication Routes: Can give epinephrine, atropine, lidocaine, diazepam (Valium), and naloxone (Narcan) via ET at 2–2.5 × the iv dose, chase w 10 cc sterile water

Pediatric Special Cases:

- Endotracheal tube sizes (internal diameter) = 3 mm for newborn, 3.5 mm for 6 mo, 4 mm for 18 mo, size thereafter = 4 + (age/4) in mm (Nejm 1991;324:1477) or width of 5th fingernail (Ann EM 1993;22:530)
- Nasogastric and Foley tube sizes = 2 × ET size
- Fluid resuscitation: intraosseous infusions, eg, of proximal tibia very effective and fast if <5 yr old (technique—Nejm 1990;322:1579); 20-g needle w 300 mm Hg pressure can infuse 1500 cc/hr (Ann EM 1987;16:305)
- Weight estimates: weight in kg = 2 × age + 8; blood volume = 80 cc/kg of weight (Nejm 1991;324:1477)

• Normal vital signs by age:

Table 1.1.1

Age	Systolic BP*	Pulse	Respirations
Newborn	60–90	94–145	30–60
Infant	74–100	124–170	30–60
Toddler	80–112	98–160	24–40
Preschool	82–110	65–132	22–34
School age	84–120	70–110	18–30
Adolescent	94–140	55–105	12–16

*Or calculate lower limit (5th percentile) of normal = 70 + 2 × (age in yrs) (Nejm 1991; 324:1477).

1.2 EMERGENCY PROTOCOLS

CARDIAC ARREST AND ARRHYTHMIAS

CARDIAC ARREST
(ACLS, Am Hrt Assoc 1994; Nejm 1992;327:1075)

Si: No effective pulse or respiration (don't be fooled by agonal respirations); unconscious

Procedures: Chest thump, debatably (only if defibrillator not available) CPR, first if >4+ min post arrest (Jama 1999;281:1182), perhaps with interposed abdominal counterpulsation by open hands (Jama 1992;267:379), or active (suction) decompression/compression (improved outcomes—Nejm 1999;341:569). Chest compressions alone w/o ventilation is adequate and may be better than full CPR in 1st 5–10 min of arrest, esp if doing solo (Seattle—Nejm 2000;342:1546). If circulation not restored within 20–25 min of adequate CPR and patient is normothermic (>86°F [>30°C]), stop, since no survivors beyond that (Nejm 1996;335:1473). NEVER QUIT CPR whether EMD, VFib, or asystole, UNTIL NORMOTHERMIC.

If **electromechanical dissociation** (pulseless electrical activity), then r/o or rx hypothermia, hypovolemia, tamponade, tension pneumothorax, hypoxemia, acidosis, hyperkalemia, drug OD (especially cardiac meds), and pulmonary embolus

Meds:

- Epinephrine 1 mg of 1:10,000 iv or ET (in children, 10 μgm/kg, ie, 0.1 cc/kg of 1:10,000 iv or ET); higher doses show no benefit (Nejm 1992;327:1045,1051).
- NaHCO$_3$ no help, worsens by hyperosmolarity and paradoxical CNS acidosis (Ann EM 1990;19:1; Med Let 1992;34:30)
- CaCl$_2$ not helpful (Ann IM 1986;105:603) unless pt has hyperkalemia (Med Let 1992;34:30)

if **asystole:**

- Atropine 1 mg, repeat × 1 (in children, 0.03 mg/kg, 0.1 mg minimum dose)
- Epinephrine 1 mg, repeat × 1 (in children, 10 μgm/kg, ie, 0.1 cc/kg of 1:10,000 iv or ET)

Then rx-specific conditions found (eg, Vtach, heart block, etc.)

HEART BLOCK

Hx: Loss of consciousness or weakness

Procedures: Pacemaker, external or temporary, although in-the-field use of external pacer doesn't increase survival (Nejm 1993;328:1377)

Meds:

- Atropine 0.5 mg iv, repeat once if no response (in children, 0.01 mg/kg iv or ET but 0.1 mg is minimum dose no matter the weight)
- Dopamine 5–20 μgm/kg/min drip
- Epinephrine 2–10 μgm/kg/min drip
- Isoproterenol 1 mg in 500 cc drip (in children, 0.02 μgm/kg/min drip, titrate up)

SUPRAVENTRICULAR TACHYCARDIAS (PAT, AV nodal reentrant and AV reentrant tachycardias, atrial flutter, atrial fibrillation)

Hx: Dizzy, "fluttering"

Si: Narrow complexes on EKG; IF WIDE, RX AS Vtach

Procedures: Carotid sinus massage; cardioversion at 30–100 W/s
synchronized; overdrive external pacing at 120 mA, at rate faster
than SVT rate in 3–5 beat pulses (Ann EM 1993;22:1993)

Meds:

- Adenosine analog (Adenocard) 12 mg (6 mg in small people)
iv push 5 min later if did not convert w 6 mg (Ann IM 1991;114:
513; 1990;113:104; Nejm 1991;325:1621) or in children 0.1
mg/kg, repeat w 0.2–0.3 mg/kg (Ann EM 1992;21:1499); 10 sec
half-life; for PAT and A-V reentrant types only, not Afib or Aflut
(Med Let 1990;32:63), especially since it can cause enhanced A-V
conduction, ie, Aflut at 2:1 or 3:1 can be converted to 1:1
conduction (Nejm 1994;330:288) though becoming controversial;
most pts have angina-like chest pain w rx; ok in pregnancy (Am J
EM 1992;10:54), avoid in asthma
- Verapamil 2.5–5 mg, repeat in 20 min at 5–10 mg iv (0.1 mg/kg in
children)
- Sotalol (Betapace) 1 mg/kg iv bolus (Nejm 1994;331:31), other
β blocker
- Digoxin 0.5 mg iv, then 0.25 mg iv q 4 h to 1.5 mg total in 24 h;
becoming less popular

VENTRICULAR TACHYCARDIA

Hx: Loss of consciousness usually but not always
Si: Wide complexes
Procedures: Chest thump; cardioversion with 200 W/s synchronized;
sedate if awake (in children, defibrillate at 2 J/kg, double if needed)
Meds:

- 1st: Amiodarone (Rx Let 1999;6:70) 150–300 mg iv over 10 min,
then 1 mg/min drip; or
- 2nd: Procainamide up to 1 gm over 20 min or until response, then
2–4 mg/min drip; or
- 3rd: Magnesium sulfate 1–2 gm iv push (2–4 cc of 50% soln) in
50–100 cc D5W; or
- 4th: Lidocaine 75–150 mg iv bolus, then 2–4 mg/min drip (in
children, 1 mg/kg bolus iv or ET, then 0.03–0.04 mg/kg/min drip);
or

- 5th: Bretylium 5 mg/kg iv over 10 min, repeat 10 mg/kg, then 2 mg/min drip, but out of favor; or
- 6th: Sotalol 100 mg iv over 5 min, may be better than lidocaine (Lancet 1994;344:18)

VENTRICULAR FIBRILLATION

Hx: Loss of consciousness
Procedures: Chest thump; defibrillation with 2–300 W/s
Meds:
- Epinephrine 1 mg of 1:10,000 iv or ET (in children, 10 μgm/kg, ie, 0.1 cc/kg of 1:10,000 iv or ET); or
- Vasopressin (Pitressin) 40 U iv × 1; then more defibrillations, and consider:
- Amiodarone (Nejm 1999;341:871) 150–300 mg iv; can drip 1 mg/min to hold in NSR
- Procainamide as above, or
- Magnesium sulfate 1–2 gm iv, especially if looks like torsades de pointes
- Lidocaine as above, or
- Bretylium as above

COMA/CONFUSION/SEIZURE

SEIZURE (p 542)

Hx: By observers of tonic-clonic activity, and postictal gradual recovery; possible past h/o seizures
Si: Unconscious, lateral tongue bites, r/o cardiac arrest by checking pulses and respiration; procedures: place prone, iv, oral airway; last resort, general anesthesia
Meds: (Jama 1993;270:854) (see p 542)
None at first. Wait; if doesn't resolve, may be status epilepticus; give iv thiamine + glucose, plus:
- Diazepam (Valium) 5–10 mg iv, may repeat (in children, 0.1 mg/kg, up to 0.5 iv, pr, or ET); or lorazepam (Ativan) 1–2 mg iv;

or midazolam (Versed) 0.2 mg/kg (Crit Care Med 1992;20:483), used especially in children

- Phenytoin 15–20 mg/kg at 50 mg/min iv in rapid flow saline (no glucose) (in children, 10 mg/kg slowly × 1 or × 2 up to 30 mg/kg iv); or fosphenytoin (Cerebyx), new iv form, comes in phenytoin equivalents, can give much faster and safer iv, eg, 100–150 mg/min
- Phenobarbital 750–1500 mg iv slowly (in children, 5 mg/kg/dose up to 20 mg/kg total over 1 h iv or im)
- Lidocaine iv as for PVCs

of **status epilepticus:** (Nejm 1998;338:970; 1982;306:1337)
65% successful for overt status, 25% for occult type (obtunded + positive EEG)

- 1st: IV thiamine 100 mg + glucose, or
- 1st: Lorazepam (Ativan) (best—Nejm 2001;345:631) 2 mg/min iv to 0.1 mg/kg; or diazepam (Valium) up to 20 mg iv, or as rectal gel 5 mg/cc in syringes for home use w repetitive sz's (Nejm 1998;338:1869); or midazolam (Versed) 0.2 mg/kg
- 2nd: Fosphenytoin 20 mg/kg iv over 10 min (can use phenytoin 1–1.5 gm over 30 min), repeat 10 mg/kg if still seizing
- 3rd: Phenobarbital 15 mg/kg at 100 mg/min iv (may need to intubate), or
- 3rd: Lidocaine 100 mg bolus, 2 mg/min drip
- 4th: General anesthesia

HYPOGLYCEMIA

Hx: Insulin use or alcoholism
Si: Intoxication, coma
W/u: Draw blood sugar
Procedures: 25 gm (50 cc of 50% soln) glucose stat iv with 100 mg of thiamine (see below); may repeat × 1; in children, 2 cc of a 50% soln or 4 cc of a 25% soln (ie, 1 gm) per kg iv

ALCOHOLISM

Si: Intoxication, coma
W/u: Blood alcohol, r/o other ODs w hx and levels

Meds:
- Thiamine 100 mg iv/im (Jama 1995;274:562) to avoid precipitating Wernicke's, continue × 3 d
- MgSO$_4$ 2 gm iv or im and continue 8–10 gm qd × 3 d if renal function ok

INTRACRANIAL MASS/BLEED

Hx: Trauma
Si: Eye si's including lateral gaze palsies, pupillary inequalities
W/u: CT or MRI; neurosurgical consult
Procedures: Burr hole, if deteriorating, on side of dilated pupil; elevate head of bed to 45°
Meds:
- Mannitol 1.5–2 gm/kg as 20–25% soln over 30–60 min
- Dexamethasone 5–10 mg iv push, efficacy unknown

MENINGITIS OR ENCEPHALITIS

W/u: Lumbar puncture asap
Meds:
- Ceftriaxone or cefotaxime 2 gm iv (adult) or 50–75 mg/kg (child), plus vancomycin 1gm iv (adult) or 10–15 mg/kg (child) to cover penicillin-resistant pneumococci, plus ampicillin at age extremes to cover *Listeria*

Plus, in children, dexamethasone 0.15 mg/kg repeated × 3 q 6 h

DYSPNEA

ANAPHYLAXIS (p 17)

Hx: Bee sting, penicillin et al. exposure less than 2 h previously
Si: Shock, wheezes, with or without rash and hives
Procedures: Tourniquet if practical and sc or im source, iv, O$_2$

Meds:
- Epinephrine 0.5–1 mg im, or sc (in children, 10 μgm/kg, ie, 0.01 cc/kg of 1:1000 sc), repeat q 30 min
- Diphenhydramine (Benadryl) 25–50 mg (in children, 1 mg/kg) iv/im; + cimetidine 300 mg iv
- Hydrocortisone 200–400 mg iv, or methylprednisolone 60–80 mg iv followed by prednisone 60 mg po qd × 2–3 d
- Aminophylline 9 mg/kg load, 0.7 mg/kg/h perhaps if bronchospasm

ASTHMA/COPD (p 710, 717)

Hx: Often presents w empty inhaler; usually long h/o similar problems
Si: Speaks in less than whole sentences, papilledema, wheezing but may be diminished as worsen, asterixis, accessory muscle use, P >100, pulsus paradoxicus
W/u: Chest xray, ABGs or O_2 saturation, PFTs
Procedures: IV, D5W if age >50, otherwise D5S to repair usually depleted state; O_2; intubation
Meds:
Primary meds:
- Albuterol 5 cc of 0.5% soln by neb q 15–20 min × 3–4 or continuous (half dose in children <5 yr), plus
- Ipratropium 500 μgm (250 in children <5 yr); plus
- Hydrocortisone 200–400 mg iv bolus or methylprednisolone (Solu-Medrol) 60–100 mg, or equivalent (in children, methylprednisolone 0.5 mg/kg iv)

Other meds to consider:
- Terbutaline, in children 0.01 mg/kg sc up to 0.3 mg maximum; in adults, 1 mg sc or in neb
- Epinephrine (if age <35) 0.5 mg sc or 1 mg in 500 D5S (in children 10 μgm/kg, ie, 0.01 cc/kg of 1:1000 sc up to 0.3 cc)
- Aminophylline load (if not on it already) and drip as above (in children, 6 mg/kg iv over 20 min then 1 mg/kg/h)
- Heliox (helium-oxygen gas mixture) which decr turbulence
- Morphine 2–4 mg iv

CROUP, SEVERE (p 656)

Meds:
- Racemic epinephrine 0.5 cc in 4 cc water via aerosol; admit if recurs within 30 min
- Dexamethasone (Decadron) 0.6 mg/kg iv or im

EPIGLOTTITIS (p 172)

Hx: Rapid onset
Si: Drooling, leaning forward, dysphagia; airway obstruction especially if stressed, eg, by looking in throat with tongue blade
W/u: Lateral neck xray
Procedures: Consider/prepare for intubation or tracheostomy
Meds:
- Ceftriaxone, or ampicillin 50 mg/kg (200 mg/kg/d) and chloramphenicol 25 mg/kg (100 mg/kg/d) iv
- Racemic epinephrine + dexamethasone (Decadron) as above

PULMONARY EDEMA

Sx: PND, DOE
Si: Orthopnea, rales, edema, S_3, JVD, P >100
W/u: EKG, chest xray
Procedures: D5W iv; O_2; phlebotomy/tourniquets; Foley; non-invasive positive pressure respiration (Chest 1998;114:1185) w BiPAP (Nejm 1991;325:1825), CPAP, or endotracheal intubation
Meds:
- Morphine 2–5 mg iv
- TNG 0.4 mg sl or 10–20 μgm/min iv
- Furosemide 20–40 mg iv; or dobutamine 2.5–15 μgm/kg/min iv (250 mg amps) + nitroprusside 1–5 μgm/kg/min (50 mg amps)
- Aminophylline iv, 5–10 mg/kg load, then 0.3–0.5 mg/kg/h
- Captopril 12.5–25 mg po chewed and swallowed
- Digoxin, consider later

PULMONARY EMBOLUS (p 12)

TENSION PNEUMOTHORAX

Hx: Chest trauma or sudden onset with past history of pneumothorax
Si: Increased resonance, decr breath sounds, cyanosis, tracheal deviation
W/u: Chest xray later
Procedures: Tap upper anterior chest in 2nd intercostal space, midclavicular line with over-the-needle catheter (Nejm 1991;324: 1479); f/u chest tube

FRACTURES

MIDFEMORAL FRACTURE

Hx: Fall, trauma
Si: External rotation, deformity, distal pulses may be compromised
W/u: Xray (later); type and xmatch
Procedures: Thomas (traction) splint; saline iv

CERVICAL FRACTURE

Hx: Diving, fall from pickup tailgate, or any headfirst fall; consider in any head injury
Si: Pain, paresthesias, weakness
W/u: Xrays after immobilized; must include all of C7, may require swimmer's view; or CT. Films unnecessary if: (1) no midline cervical tenderness; (2) no focal neurol deficit; (3) normal alertness; (4) no intoxication; and (5) no other distracting significant injury (Nejm 2000;342:94, 138); or Canadian Cervical Spine rules (Jama 2001; 286:1841) which require above plus ability to rotate neck 45° to each side
Procedures: Splint and in-line immobilization of neck before xrays
Meds: Methylprednisolone 30 mg/kg iv over 15 min w 5.4 mg/kg/h iv × 24 h for spinal cord injury (Nejm 1990;322:1405)

FLAIL CHEST

Hx: Steering wheel injury
Si: Paradoxical motion
W/u: Xray later
Procedures: Bag breathe, then respirator; epidural block for pain control

PELVIC FRACTURE

Hx: Crush injury usually, male unable to void
Si: Rectal to look for high-riding prostate
W/u: Urethrogram; pelvic xray. Crit; type and xmatch
Procedures: MAST for transport; DO NOT CATHETERIZE bladder until
  urethrogram; 2 large-bore iv's

SHOCK WITH CHEST PAIN

ANAPHYLAXIS (p 17)

AORTIC DISSECTION

Hx: Back and/or neck pain; h/o hypertension
Si: Transiently absent pulses, bruits; BP differences between extremities
W/u: Chest xray, CT of chest; arteriogram
Meds:

- Nitroprusside iv (p 43) to BP <100 systolic, and
- Metoprolol 5 mg iv, or
- Propranolol 1–2 mg iv or esmolol 50–200 μgm/min

MYOCARDIAL INFARCTION
  (Nejm 1996;335:1660)

Hx: Chest pain, substernal radiation in distribution of a tree, worse supine

Si: Gray cadaveric skin, often middle-aged man, shock with relative bradycardia

W/u: EKG, chest xray

Procedures: IV, O_2; consider emergent angioplasty

Meds:

- Thrombolysis if sx <6 h old (possibly up to 12 h), pain, and ST elevations
- ASA 80–160 mg po
- Dopamine 2–10 μgm/kg/min (200 mg amp) and/or dobutamine (p 38) if shock
- Nitroprusside (p 43) if low cardiac output and BP allows
- Morphine, enough to decrease pain, up to 20 mg iv in divided doses
- Metoprolol (Lopressor) 5 mg iv × 3 within 24 h unless heart block, hypotension, or severe bradycardia
- ACE inhibitor within 24 h and for at least 6 wk
- Perhaps TNG 50 mg iv q 3–5 min or 10^+ μgm/min drip (3 mg in 20 cc = 0.15 mg/cc)
- Perhaps referral for PCTA if available

PERICARDIAL TAMPONADE

Hx: Steering wheel trauma; or possible acute inflammatory pericarditis

Si: Shock, although BP may be elevated in 1/3 of pts (Nejm 1992;327: 463); paradoxical pulse of >20 mm Hg; JVP elevation

Procedures: Pericardiocentesis w 18-g spinal needle

PULMONARY EMBOLUS

Hx: Bedridden, long trip, leg trauma, or positive family hx; cough, dyspnea

Si: No orthopnea or increased pain supine unlike MI

W/u: ABGs, chest xray, EKG, V/Q scan, IPG or Doppler ultrasound, PT, PTT, platelets, guaiac, crit

Procedures: IV, O_2

Meds:
- Heparin 5000 U bolus, 1000-h drip, adjust q 12–24 h; or weight-adjusted to 80 U/kg bolus and 18 U/kg/h
- Perhaps thrombolysis if severe sx

SEPSIS/SEPTIC SHOCK

Hx: Post-surgery, Foley, other predisposers
Si: BP decr but relative bradycardia, fever sometimes, decr urine output
W/u: Blood and other cultures; Gram stain buffy coat
Procedures: Saline or Ringer's based on CVP; in children, 20 cc/kg boluses until hemodynamically stable, may take 3–5
Meds:
- Antibiotics: ceftriaxone or ceftazidime 1 gm iv q 12 h + gentamicin 5 mg/kg/24 h iv in divided doses
- Pressors: norepinephrine 0.05–0.25 μgm/kg/min titrated to BP is better than dopamine (Jama 1994;272:1354)

VOLUME LOSS/BLEEDING (including anaphylaxis, toxic shock, bleeding, spinal cord shock)

Hx: Postural sx sometimes (dizzy when stands)
Si: Systolic BP decreases by ≥25 mm; P increases >100 or ≥20/min when standing from supine position; in children especially: delayed capillary refill, altered consciousness, increased pulse and respirations before BP decreases
W/u: Type and xmatch; clotting studies; lytes; guaiacs
Procedures: 2 large-bore iv's to transfuse blood and saline maximally, use fluid warmer if possible; in children, 20 cc/kg saline, Ringer's, or fresh frozen plasma, may bolus up to 70 cc/kg in 1st hour (Jama 1991;266:1242); MAST (warmed); 10 cc/kg packed rbc's, 20-g needle + 300 mmHg pressure allows 70 cc/min of packed rbc infusion if diluted 1:1 w saline
Meds: Dopamine 10 μgm/kg/min drip, titrate up to BP or 25 μgm/kg/min

HISTAMINE TRANSFUSION REACTIONS (Anaphylaxis)

Hx: Pruritus, dyspnea
Si: Hives/rash, wheezing, fever
W/u: ABGs and/or central venous gases (Nejm 1989;320:1312)
Procedures: Stop transfusion; MAST if shocky
Meds:
- Diphenhydramine (Benadryl) 25–50 mg iv or im
- Epinephrine 0.5–1 mg iv or sc
- Hydrocortisone 200–400 mg iv
- H_2 blockers (eg, cimetidine 300 mg iv)

FEBRILE TRANSFUSION REACTIONS

Cause: Many or most due to interleukins in plasma which increase w age of the unit, not white cell antigens; more common (10–30%) w platelet transfusions than w rbc transfusions (Nejm 1994;331:625), r/o infected unit
Hx: Malaise, nausea
Si: Fever, chills, rigors
W/u: Culture bag and perhaps patient
Procedures: Stop transfusion or remove supernatant plasma
Meds: Diphenhydramine (Benadryl) as above or in bag

HEMOLYTIC TRANSFUSION REACTIONS (with renal shut-down)

Hx: Back pain
Cmplc: ATN with hemolysis
W/u: UA, repeat xmatch, look at serum for free hgb
Meds:
- Mannitol (1 amp) +
- $NaHCO_3$ (1 amp) in 1000 cc D5W

DROWNING

Nejm 1992;328:53

Cause: Water inhalation/immersion

Epidem: 7000 drowning deaths/yr in US; majority are freshwater; 1/4 are teenagers

Pathophys: Pulmonary edema, metabolic acidosis, and hypoxia with very rapid changes in V/Q ratios and lung elasticity. Freshwater may enter the circulation and cause hypervolemia and hemodilution with red cell lysis, which in turn causes hyperkalemia leading to ventricular fibrillation and death, or hemoglobinemia/uria leading to renal damage; lung cells also lysed. Salt water pulls plasma into alveoli and causes hypovolemia and hemoconcentration leading to pulmonary edema, anoxia, and death. Surfactant changes cause decreases in lung compliance

Sx:

Si: Drowning: ARDS with decr lung compliance and consequent blood gas changes

Crs: If comatose, 40–50% recover, 10–20% die, and 30–50% survive w brain damage

Cmplc: Hypothermia (p 16); ATN from hypotension and myoglobinuria; anoxic neurologic damage; diminished platelet numbers and/or function; DIC within hours in freshwater drowning (Ann IM 1977;87:60); ARDS; Vfib; hypoglycemia; hyperkalemia; impaired drug clearance

Lab:

Chem: If K^+ >2 × normal, universally fatal

Hem: Crit decreases over the first 1–2 h

Path: At postmortem in freshwater drowning, lungs show intra-alveolar and interstitial edema as well as altered surface tension. In salt water drowning, major finding is pulmonary edema and only slight changes in surface tension

Rx: CPR, CPAP/PEEP, rx pH <7.1 w bicarb; avoid too high O_2 concentrations, which can further decrease surfactant; treat hypothermia (p 16); antibiotics only w gastric or dirty water aspiration. Initial abdominal thrust no use unless airway obstruction suspected

HYPOTHERMIA

Nejm 1994;331:1756; Postgrad Med 1990;88:55; Ann IM 1985; 102:153

Cause: Drowning, outdoor exposure, often associated with alcohol/drugs/overdoses, bacteremia in the aged, CVA, DKA, pancreatitis, hypothyroidism, hypoadrenalism

Epidem:

Pathophys: "Cold diuresis" occurs because of peripheral vasoconstriction and/or renal inability to resorb water. Hypoxic damage as hgb dissociation curve shifted to left, releasing less O_2 to tissues

Sx: Decr cold perception

Si: Must use special thermometer that can register <95°F (<35°C)

Mild = 95–90°F (35–32.2°C); moderate = 90–82.4°F (32.2°–28°C); severe = <82.4°F (<28°C)

<95°F (<35°C) causes ataxia, slowed reflexes, sinus bradycardia (don't do CPR as long as you can feel a pulse even if very slow), hypotension; <82.4°F (<28°C) unconciousness occurs, fixed and dilated pupils

Crs:

Cmplc: DIC within hours; Vfib; hypoglycemia; hyperkalemia; impaired drug clearance. Late cardiomyopathy due to multiple micro infarcts

Lab:

Chem: Screens for above causes; if K^+ >2 × normal, universally fatal

Noninv: EKG shows Osborn J waves (wide, upright slur in terminal QRS) (Nejm 1994;330:680) which are pathognomonic for hypothermia, occur at <80°F (27°C); general QRS widening follows and predicts ventricular fibrillation

Rx: (Med Let 1994;36:116)

Rewarm core first

If 85–90°F (34–36°C) and cardiovascularly stable, use warmed blankets, warmed D5S, and O_2/air (104°F [41.6°C])

If <85°F (<34°C) (Vfib risk) and/or unstable, then use warm lavages via Foley catheter, NG tubes, rectal tubes; intraperitoneal lavage (can raise by 36°F [2.2°C] per h); pleural continuous warm lavage (Ann Emerg Med 1990;19:204) can raise by 68°F (20°C) per h; or extracorporeal cardiopulmonary bypass, which is very effective (Nejm 1997;337:1500), consider transferring to get it

If in Vfib or standstill, rewarm to 90°F (32.2°C) before cardioverting or quitting; beware of impaired lidocaine metabolism

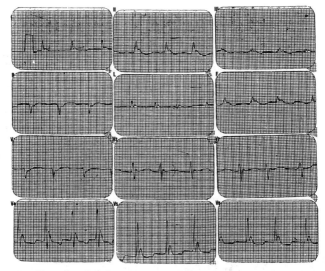

Figure 1.2.1 Hypothermic Osborn waves. Wide, upright slurs in terminal QRS.

Antibiotics pending culture workup

Avoid heating blankets which can rewarm periphery before core and cause shock and hyperkalemia, although active rewarming of trunk alone may be ok

Avoid insulin for hyperglycemia since insulin resistance occurs at hypothermic temperatures but will resolve later, causing hypoglycemia (L. Baggott 1/93)

1.3 OVERDOSES, STINGS, AND POISONINGS

ANAPHYLAXIS

Cause: Aspiration, ingestion (Nejm 1992;327:380), or parenteral use of drugs and other haptens, eg, penicillin, anesthetics, radiocontrast agents, ACE inhibitors, NSAIDs (Nejm 1994;331:1282); foreign antigens, eg, insect stings (Nejm 1994;331:523) including fire ants (Ann IM 1999;131:424), desensitization shots, semen (Ann IM 1981;94:459); polysaccharides, eg, dextran

Epidem: Increased incidence in atopic persons

Pathophys: Respiratory distress due to both upper tract edema and lower tract bronchospasm perhaps due to leukotrienes (Ann IM 1997;127: 472), previously called slow reacting substance (SRS). Hypotension due to histamine, kinins, and perhaps leukotriene release. Diarrhea and gi sx may be due to serotonin. Several drug-induced types of reactions are not IgE mediated, eg, those by radiocontrast agents, ACE inhibitors, and NSAIDs (Nejm 1994;331:1282)

Sx: Respiratory distress; vascular collapse; cutaneous rash/itch; gi nausea, vomiting, diarrhea, and pain especially if antigen taken po

Si: Upper or lower airway obstruction; vascular collapse; rash

Crs: Onset in 0.5–3 min, pts die in 15–120 min if they're going to; recurs in 28% if rechallenged (Ann IM 1993;118:161)

Cmplc: Respiratory or vascular collapse, death

Lab:

Chem: Serum tryptase levels increased, helps to distinguish from other causes of shock (Nejm 1987;316:1622)

Serol: RAST testing, 20% false neg compared to skin testing

Skin tests: Pos test is very specific at 0.1–1 μgm/cc if anaphylaxis truly present (Nejm 1994;331:523); whole insect preparations no use, pure venom very specific. Passive transfer: patient's serum sc to animal or volunteer, challenge at 24 h

Histamine release from basophils in vitro very specific, 20% false neg, expose to 0.1 μgm/cc venom

Rx: Emergent:
- Tourniquet if practical and sc or im source; ice packs
- Support vital signs w iv fluids, O_2, neb
- Epinephrine 0.5–1 mg iv, im, or sc (in children, 10 μgm/kg, ie, 0.01 cc/kg of 1:1000 sc) or smaller iv doses, repeat q 30 min
- Diphenhydramine (Benadryl) 25–50 mg (in children, 1 mg/kg) iv/im + cimetidine 300 mg iv
- Hydrocortisone 200–400 mg iv, or methylprednisolone 60–80 mg iv followed by prednisone 60 mg po qd × 2–3 d
- Aminophylline 9 mg/kg load, 0.7 mg/kg/h perhaps, if bronchospasm

Preventive options:
- Epipen home sc epinephrine kit
- Desensitize with venom (Med Let 1993;35:63) 95% effective × 3–5 yr then stop; better than whole-body extracts (Nejm 1990;

323:1627). Probably worth doing in adults in whom half will have a systemic (not just large local) reaction after a first if stung again; but in children if reaction is just urticarial, none will have a worse reaction if stung again and thus not worth doing (Nejm 1990; 323:1601)

- Steroids: for IVP dye reaction (not true anaphylaxis since doesn't always recur after previous episode), 150 mg prednisone divided q 24 h beginning 18 h before and continuing 12 h after procedure helps (Ann IM 1975;83:159); or methylprednisolone 32 mg po 12 h and 2 h before dye exposure, helps some but not all (Nejm 1987;317:845); or diphenhydramine 50 mg im × 1 (Ann IM 1975;83:277). New hyperosmolar agents 20 × as expensive but less vagal and cardiac depression and perhaps less anaphylactoid (rv—Nejm 1992;326:425, 431)

For idiopathic anaphylaxis, prednisone 60 mg qd × 1 wk, then qod and decrease to 5–10 mg qod; plus hydroxyzine 25 mg tid helps decrease frequency and severity (Ann IM 1991;114:133)

OVERDOSES/POISONINGS

General rx: (Jama 1999;282:1113; in children—Nejm 2000;342:186)
Call poison control center
Activated charcoal 1–2 gm/kg up to 75–100 gm po or via NG tube q 2 h × 3 doses w cathartic eg, sorbitol; contraindicated if no bowel sounds, or if patient stuporous and not intubated; ineffective for boric acid, alcohols, alkalis, cyanide, heavy metals, and mineral acids
If altered or unconscious, give naloxone 2 mg iv + amp (50 cc) of 50% glucose iv + thiamine 100 mg iv/im
If pinpoint pupils give naloxone 2 mg iv, and r/o hypothermia. Empty stomach, unless ingestions of corrosives, high viscosity or <2 cc/kg of low viscosity petroleum distillates, with:
Gastric lavage with large-bore Ewald tube in L lateral Trendelenberg position
Ipecac po, 30 cc for adults, 15 cc for children age 1–12, or 10 cc age 6 mo–1 yr; rarely used even as prehospital rx in US w incr popularity of charcoal, since emesis may result in inability to give charcoal soon; but completely empties stomach 70% of the time unlike lavage which does so 12% of the time (J Roy Soc Med 1991; 84:35)

• **Acetaminophen (Tylenol) OD** (p 25)

• **Aspirin OD** (p 27)

• **β-Blocker OD**
Rx: Glucagon 5–10 mg iv w saline, not supplied diluent (phenol); titrate
  to normal vital si's; 2–10 mg/h maintenance

• **Barbiturate OD**
Sx: Bullae on hands (Nejm 1970;283:409)
Rx: IV fluids; HCO_3 to alkalinize urine especially with phenobarb (a
  weak acid); activated charcoal decreases half-life from 110 h to 45 h
  (Nejm 1982;307:676, 692), po 50–100 gm × 1 then 20–60 gm q
  4–12 h

• **Bee Sting** (p 17)

• **Benzodiazepine OD**
Rx: Supportive care
  Flumazenil (Romazicon) 1 mg iv over 3 min (an antagonist) q 1 h (BMJ
    1990;301:1308), may not reverse the respiratory depression and
    may precipitate seizures (Med Let 1992;34:66) especially in mixed
    ODs w cocaine or cyclic antidepressants

• **Butanediol** purported dietary supplement for weight loss, muscle
  building, and sexual enhancement; mutiple lethal and near-lethal
  responses reported (Nejm 2001;344:87)

• **Chloroquine Toxicity/OD**
Sx: >5 gm fatal without rx
Rx: Ventilation, diazepam (Valium), and epinephrine produce >90%
    survival (Nejm 1988;318:1)
  Cardiac monitor × 6^+ h
  No ipecac

• **Cocaine Use** (Med Let 1996;38:43, Nejm 1996;334:965, 1995;
    333:1267)
Sx: Used nasally or iv, or smoked as "free-base" or "crack"

Pathyophys: Overt and silent CNS (Jama 1998;279:376) and cardiac (Nejm 2001;345:351) vasoconstriction

Cmplc: Neurologic: delirium, seizures, ischemic and hemorrhagic CVAs (Nejm 1990;323:699) Cardiac: MIs and arrhythmias (Nejm 1986:315:1438, 1495), premature atherosclerosis, silent ST elevations on Holter even 3 wk after discontinuation (Ann IM 1989;111:876), false pos CPK-MB elevations, EKG changes of MI only in 36% when actually present

Rx: of agitation: iv benzodiazepines

of chest pain: nitrates plus O_2 and ASA; if not enough, use phentolamine, verapamil, or thrombolytics; avoid lidocaine (Med Let 1990;32:93) and labetolol as well as other β blockers which can result in unopposed α-stimulationt

• Digitalis Toxicity/OD

Rx: Fab fragments (Digibind) 40 mg iv per 0.6 mg of digoxin or digitoxin taken (Nejm 1992;326:1739; Med Let 1986;28:87); $MgSO_4$ 2 gm iv while waiting

• Ethylene Glycol Antifreeze Ingestion (Nejm 1981;304:21)

Pathophys: Alcohol dehydrogenase converts to glycolic acid, which causes acidosis and is metabolized into oxalate; this produces high osmolar gap

Lab: High osmolar gap = measured osmoles - calculated osmoles (calculated = $2 \times Na$ + glucose/18 + BUN/2.8); r/o methanol and/or ethanol ingestion

Rx: Ethanol po or iv continuous to levels of 100–125 mg%; to inhibit alcohol dehydrogenase

Fomepizole (Antizol) (Nejm 1999;340:832) 15 mg/kg iv load, then 10 mg/kg q 12 h × 48 h, then 15 mg/kg q 12 h until ethylene glycol level <20 mg%; cost: $4000/rx

Hemodialysis especially if large ingestion, acidotic, level >50 mg%, or renal failure

Thiamine 100 mg iv + pyridoxine 2–5 gm

• Iron OD (p 29)

• Isoniazid (INH) OD

Rx: Pyridoxine gm for gm; if unknown amount, start with 5 gm iv

• **Kerosene/Gasoline/Camphor Ingestion**

Rx: Remove clothing soaked w substance and wash skin to decr dermal absorption

Avoid emesis/lavage if possible because of aspiration risk

Gastric aspiration or lavage if >2 cc/kg because CNS, liver, and renal damage possible at that level; charcoal

• **Lithium OD** (p 694)

Rx: Na polystyrene SO_4 (Kayexalate) absorbs Li and other cations like K^+

• **Lye Ingestion**

Rx: Do not induce emesis or place NG tube; steroids do not prevent strictures (Nejm 1990;323:637); charcoal not useful; dilution controversial

• **Marine Sting Injuries** (Ann IM 1994;120:665; Nejm 1992;326:486)

Cause: Man-o-War, jellyfish, anemones, and corals (all coelenterates); sting ray; stone, lion, and scorpion fish

Pathophys: Nematocysts inject polypeptide toxin-coated threads

Sx + Si: Local inflammation, vesicles

Cmplc: Anaphylaxis, acute renal and/or hepatic failure, persistent reactions, mononeuritis multiplex

Rx: Warm water (T° ≤113°F [≤45°C]) irrigation × 30–90 min to denature the venom

• **Methanol Ingestion**

Pathophys: Converted by alcohol dehydrogenase to formic acid, which causes brain and optic nerve toxicity and acidosis

Lab: Methanol level >20 mg%; high osmolar gap (see ethylene glycol above), r/o ethylene glycol and/or alcohol ingestion

Rx:

- Alcohol dehydrogenase inhibition w: ethanol iv, or fomepizole (Antizol) (Nejm 2001;344:424) 15 mg/kg iv over 30 min, then 10 mg/kg q 12 h × 4 doses, then 15 mg/kg q 12 hr
- Bicarb and supportive rx
- Folate 1 mg/kg iv q 4 h × 6
- Hemodialysis for large ingestions, levels >50 mg%, acidosis (pH <7.1), sx

- **Neurotoxic Shellfish Poisoning** (Am J Pub Hlth 1991;81:471)

Cause: Ingestion of shellfish contaminated with dinoflagellate (red tide) neurotoxin; when from fish, called ciguatera poisoning (see scombroid below)

Epidem: Occurs in epidemics

Sx: Cooking does not prevent; onset in 1/2–10 h. Paresthesias (81%); reversal of hot-cold sensations (17%); vertigo (60%); myalgias; abdominal pain (48%); nausea (44%); rectal burning; headache (15%)

Si: Ataxia (27%); bradycardia; dilated pupils

Crs: 8–48 h

Rx: Charcoal, respiratory support; mannitol 1–2 gm/kg; possibly calcium channel blockers, lidocaine

- **Organophosphate Poisoning** (eg, malathion, Diazinon, parathion, and "nerve gas") (Med Let 1995;37:43)

Pathophys: Acetylcholinesterase inhibitors

Sx: H/o pesticide acute exposure

Si: Increased bronchial nasopharyngeal and gi secretions, muscle twitching and weakness, seizures, garlic breath (r/o arsenic)

Rx:

- Atropine 2–6 mg iv/im, then more q 5 min until secretions decrease, may take 15–20$^+$ mg
- Pralidoxime HCl 1 gm iv over 15–30 min, may repeat × 1 in 1 h, or iv infusion of 500 mg/h
- Diazepam 5–10 mg iv if seizures likely

- **Pennyroyal Herb Poisoning** (Ann IM 1996;124:726)

Sx: Used as an abortion inducer; nausea and vomiting within 1 h of ingestion

Si: Shock, metabolic acidosis

Cmplc: Hepatic necrosis, DIC, hypoglycemia

Rx: Lavage

- **Psychedelic Drug Use/OD** (Med Let 1996;38:43; Ann IM 1979;90:361)

Amphetamines; rx sx with diazepam (Valium) (Med Let 1990;32:93), hydration; avoid phenothiazines, which decrease seizure threshold

Cocaine use (p 20)

LSD and other hallucinogens; rx by decr sensory stimulation (dark, quiet room), companion, benzodiazepams prn

Marijuana (Nejm 1972;287:310)
Glue sniffing; ATN and hepatitis with hydrocarbon inhalation (Ann IM 1970;73:713)

• **Salt (NaCl) OD**
Rx: Dialysis preferable; if can't, use D5W with 100 mg furosemide (Lasix) q 1 h and watch Ca^{2+} and pH

• **Scombroid Fish Poisoning** (Nejm 1991;324:716)
Cause: Ingestion usually of spoiled tuna, mackerel, bonito, bluefish, mahi mahi, et al.
Epidem: Most common type of fish poisoning in US
Sx + Si: Peppery metallic flavor to fish; headache, flushing, diarrhea within 10–30 min of ingestion; cooking does not prevent
Crs: 3 h without rx; faster with rx
Cmplc: r/o **ciguatera (fish) poisoning** (Ann IM 1995;122:113) from dinoflagellate ingestion by fish; cooking does not prevent; sx of diarrhea, neuralgias, "loose teeth," dysphagia, loss of temperature sensation, et al., may last mos–yrs; rx like red tide poisoning (see above)
Rx: Diphenhydramine (Benadryl) 50 mg iv, im, or po

• **Theophylline Toxicity/OD** (Ann IM 1984;101:457)
Si + Sx: Seizures (15%), Vtach (20%) in all >60 μgm/cc, low K^+ (100%), elevated glucose (98%), low PO_4 (80%), low Mg^{2+} (75%)
Lab: Toxicity with levels >35 μgm/cc
Rx: Charcoal; hemoperfusion over charcoal if level >100 μgm/cc in acute, >40–60 μgm/cc in chronic toxicity, one of few indications for hemoperfusion (Med Let 1986;28:80); dialysis if hemoperfusion not available
  of tachycardia, hypotension, and ventricular arrhythmias: esmolol; or low dose propranolol, eg, 0.5 mg iv in adults (0.01 mg/kg to max of 1 mg/dose in children), repeat in 5–10 min if BP and P don't decr; complete β blockade occurs at 0.2 mg/kg

• **Tri- and Tetracyclic Antidepressant OD**
Pathophys: Anticholinergic effects and fast channel blockade

Lab: Monitoring EKG × 24 h adequate (Jama 1985;254:1772); drug levels not predictive of cmplc (Nejm 1985;313:474); seizures predicted (in 34%) by QRS >0.10 sec and Vtach/fib predicted (in 50%) by QRS >0.16 sec (Nejm 1985;313:474) or R_{aVR} >3 mm has best predictive (43%) value for seizure or ventricular arrhythmias (Ann Emerg Med 1995;26:195)

Rx: Supportive usually is adequate; rx arrhythmias or wide QRS w bicarb 1–2 mM/kg iv if heart block or ventricular arrhythmia (B. Higgins, ME Med Ctr 10/92)

• **Vacor Rat Poison Ingestion** (Nejm 1980;302:73)

Pathophys: Induces a diabetic ketoacidosis in normal person; also produces peripheral, autonomic, and CNS neuropathies which are usually fatal

Rx: IV nicotinamide within minutes may help

ACETAMINOPHEN (Tylenol) OD

Nejm 1988;319:1557

Cause: Acetaminophen po

Epidem: Common overdose and common co-ingested drug

Pathophys: Toxic metabolite causes liver failure; can occur at "nontoxic" levels in alcoholics (Ann IM 1986;104:398) and be inadvertant (Nejm 1997;337:1112)

Sx: H/o OD >10 gm (>140 mg/kg), usually ≥15 gm (4 gm/d is maximal therapeutic dose) within 24 h but can occur at just 4 gm/d in alcoholics (Med Let 1996;38:55). May have no sx for 72 h

Si: None

Crs: Most hepatitis is transient, but it can be fatal

Cmplc: Hepatitis more common if fasting and/or w concomitant ethanol ingestion (Jama 1994;272:1845), and/or w hepatic enzyme inducing drugs like seizure medications

Lab:

Chem: Acetaminophen level initially on all drug ODs and, if positive, at 4, 8, and 12 h after OD and plot on nomogram (Nejm 1988;319:1558); if 4-h level >200 μgm/cc or 12-h level >50, hepatic toxicity likely; if half-life >4 h then hepatitis likely, if >12 h then encephalopathy likely

Rx: Acetylcysteine 140 mg/kg load, then 70 mg/kg × 17 doses q 4 h po or
via NG tube; or 300 mg iv over 20 h, iv probably not as good as po.
Treat levels of >150 μgm/cc at 4 h, >50 at 8 h (see FIG. 1.3.1
nomogram). Works regardless of level, probably by increasing
tissue O_2 delivery (Nejm 1991;324:1852). Best result if start within
4–8 h but still worth doing up to 24 h postingestion. Activated
charcoal binds acetylcysteine but one dose ok since have 12 h to

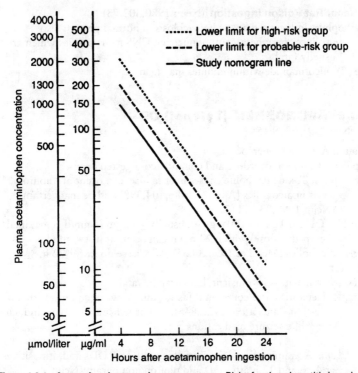

Figure 1.3.1 Acetaminophen overdose nomogram. Risk of serious hepatitis based on
plasma Tylenol levels. (Reproduced with permission from Smilkstein MJ, et al. Efficacy
of oral N-acetylcysteine in the treatment of acetaminophen overdose, analysis of the
national multicenter study (1976 to 1985) Nejm 1988;319:1558, Copyright 1988, Mass.
Medical Society.)

start acetylcysteine and one dose may help adsorb some of the acetaminophen and other drugs taken concomitantly; if did get charcoal, consider increasing initial acetylcysteine dose by 20–40%. Odansetron 4 mg iv can help nauseated pts tolerate

ASPIRIN (Salicylate) OD
Ann IM 1976;85:745

Cause: ASA ingestion of >10 gm (120 mg/kg), >500 mg/kg usually fatal, acute or chronic build up

Epidem: Common in children, adult suicides, and the elderly treating various medical illnesses with ASA (insidious, high morbidity and mortality)

Pathophys: Respiratory stimulation via respiration centers and chemoreceptors; oxidative metabolism uncoupling. Direct CNS stimulation; gastric irritant

Sx: Dizziness; can be precipitated by steroid withdrawal; nausea, tinnitus, emesis

Si: Fever and hypermetabolism; respiratory alkalosis then metabolic acidosis; confusion evolving into convulsions

Crs:

Cmplc: CNS damage with seizures, from anoxia; coma; shock
Pulmonary edema even as ASA level decreasing due to increased capillary permeability, especially in smokers (Ann IM 1981; 95:405)

Lab:
Chem: Salicylate level initially and 6 h postingestion; >70 mg % (indicates 10–30 gm ingested); therapeutic levels in RA ≤30 mg %; lytes show respiratory alkalosis evolving into metabolic acidosis or a combination of both
Hem: PT increased
Urine: 10% $FeCl_3$ to 1 cc of urine shows a purple color

Xray: KUB may show size of pill bolus in gi tract

Rx: Respiratory alkalosis alone usually requires no rx
Glucose iv to avoid ASA-induced hypoglycemia (Nejm 1973;288:1110)
of metabolic acidosis: supportive care and respirator; correct lyte imbalances, eg, acidosis; dialyze soon; $NaHCO_3$ 1 mM/kg w 20 mEq KCl diluted in 500 D5(1/2)S at 2–3 cc/kg/h iv to alkalinize urine or as iv push without increasing fluids probably best (BMJ 1982;285:1383)

Vit K for PT prolongation
Hemodialysis if initial salicylate level >120 mg % or 6-h level
>100 mg %, or renal failure, hypoxia, CHF, pulmonary edema, or
persistent CNS changes (seizures, coma, confusion)

CARBON MONOXIDE POISONING
Nejm 1998;339:1603

Cause: Carbon monoxide: $O=C \leftrightarrow O^- = C^+$
Epidem: Oxidation of fuels in presence of insufficient O_2 forms
carboxyhemoglobin, eg, car exhaust, fire smoke, gas appliances in
campers and enclosed-cabin pleasure boats (Jama 1995;274:1615)
especially at high altitudes (Sci Am Text Med 1982). Rarely from
methylene chloride, absorbed cutaneously from paint thinner and
metabolized to CO in liver
600 accidental and 3000–6000 suicidal deaths/yr in US
Pathophys: $C=O$ binds with the same 2 electrons in Fe^{2+}, as O_2 does, to
bring its total electron complement to a stable 36.
Carboxyhemoglobin has a high association rate but a slow
dissociation rate (200 times oxygen's hgb binding affinity), ie, it
shifts the hgb dissociation curve to the left (increased affinity) and
thus decreases hgb's carrying capacity despite normal pO_2. Because
CO also greatly increases the other 3 hemes' affinity for O_2, even
one CO per hgb reduces O_2 dissociation. Also poisons
mitochondrial cytochrome cellular respiration system.
Children physiologically more susceptible to injury.
Sx: If >10% of hgb is carboxyhemoglobin, sx include headache and
dizziness; get level in pts with these sx if others in house have
similar sx and home heating system would be compatible with CO
poisoning (Ann IM 1987;107:174)
If 30–40% carboxyhemoglobin: severe headache, easy fatiguability. If
40–60% carboxyhemoglobin: unconscious
Si: Retinal hemorrhages, flame-shaped (Sci Am Text Med 1982); pink skin
and mucous membranes
Crs: Recovery may take months
Cmplc: CNS damage including permanent memory loss and seizures, and
peripheral neuritis from the anoxia, hyperthermia from sweat gland
necrosis; precipitation of ischemic heart disease (Nejm 1995;

332:48). Delayed (3–240 days) neuropsych sx and si, including personality changes, dementia, incontinence, psychosis, all w 50–75% 1 yr recovery

R/o cyanide poisoning from combustible plastics in burn patients w oxygen refractory acidosis

Lab:

ABGs: Normal pO_2; depressed O_2 saturation, but not pulse oximetry, which is falsely high (Ann Emerg Med 1994;24:252); metabolic acidosis if severe

Chem: Carboxyhemoglobin level, >10–15%; can also be up to 15% in smokers

Rx: Prevent w home CO detectors (Jama 1998;279:685)

Support oxygenation with 100% O_2 as soon as suspect, 1 atm pressure allows 2 vol % O_2 to be carried in plasma alone

Hyperbaric chamber (Nejm 1996;334:1642 vs no help—Med J Austr 1999;170:203) if available and practical but O_2 at 3 atm results in plasma carrying 6 vol%; higher pressure with <50% O_2 is better with less toxicity and lung collapse; consider especially if levels >25%, pregnant, angina, unconscious or other mental status changes

Exchange transfusion?

IRON OVERDOSE, ACUTE

J Peds 1964;64:218

Cause: Ferric (Fe^{3+}) or ferrous (Fe^{2+}) iron; sx if >20 mg/kg, serious if >40 mg/kg, potentially lethal if >60 mg/kg

Epidem: Accidental or suicidal poisoning; most common accidental poisoning in children

Pathophys: Direct corrosive effect on gi mucosa causes markedly increased absorption of hepatotoxic iron salts; subsequently iron and ferritin are released from periportal cells leading to vasodepressor effect and shock

Sx: Nausea, vomiting, abdominal pain, diarrhea. Seizures, then 2–3 h respite, then fatal seizures

Si: GI bleeding

Crs:

Stage 1 (1/2–6 h postingestion): Nausea, vomiting

Stage 2 (6–24 h): Latent, though may be absent in severe OD

Stage 3 (4–40 h): Systemic toxicity including shock, seizures, and death

Stage 4 (2–5 wk): Late cmplc, eg, gi strictures/obstruction

Cmplc: Gastric perforation, later strictures, intestinal obstruction; shock, coma, coagulopathy, hepatic failure, acidosis

Lab:

Chem: Serum iron level 4–6 hr after ingestion, not later because redistribution falsely depress levels, then at 10 hr in case of delayed absorption; within 1–2 hr if chewable or liquid forms ingested; >300 μgm% causes mild toxicity; >500 μgm% causes serious toxicity; >1000 μgm% often fatal

Glucose often >150 mg %

Hem: WBC often >15,000; TIBC no help

Urine: Deferoxamine challenge test occasionally used, urine may be rose-colored if serum-free iron is present

Xray: KUB, iron tablets often seen unless ingested liquid, chewable, or multivitamin preparations

Rx: Perhaps ipecac prehospital; lavage stomach w saline, although there is danger of perforating an already eroded stomach, or lavage whole bowel w PEG; fluids for shock. No charcoal

Deferoxamine 1 gm stat, 0.5 gm q 4–12 h up to 6 gm qd im, or iv if in shock, at 10–15 mg/kg/h (higher doses precipitate shock) up to 6 gm qd total; cannot use via gastric lavage; may have cytoprotective effects independent of chelation

Maybe someday L_1, an oral iron chelator, 1st choice (Clin Pharmacol Ther 1991;50:294)

LEAD POISONING, CHRONIC

CDC, Preventing Lead Poisoning in Young Children [Oct. 1991]

Cause: An acquired porphyria due to elemental Pb ingestion; paint ingestion esp in children (Nejm 1974;290:245), battery fumes, moonshine (Nejm 1969;280:1199), pottery glazes commercial and homemade (Nejm 1970;283:669), air contamination from smelter (Nejm 1975;292:123), indoor firing range users (Am J Pub Hlth 1989;79:1029), and radiator repair mechanics (Nejm 1987; 317:214). Tetra-ethyl Pb from gas results in encephalopathy, without porphyria or blood changes

Epidem: Common in young children; adult exposures usually occupational, eg rehab'ing old buildings. Inversely correlated w vit C intake (Jama 1999;281:2289)

Pathophys: Pb inhibits by chelating sulfhydryl (SH) groups of ALA dehydrogenase (ALA → PBG), ferrochelatase (PP → heme), and possibly ALA synthetase. In adults, gout and gouty nephropathy; latter always associated with overt or silent Pb intoxication (Nejm 1981;304:520)

Sx: In severe poisoning, abdominal colic, relieved by palpation! h/o family pet illness, eg, dog (Am J Pub Hlth 1990;80:1183)

Si: In severe poisoning, anemia, gingival margin lead line, motor peripheral neuropathy, eg, wrist drop, neuroses, and psychoses

Crs: Progressive, si and sx roughly correlate w blood lead levels; cognition deficits only partially reverse w long term rx (Jama 1998;280:1915)

Cmplc:

- Antisocial/delinquent behaviors long term (Jama 1996;275:363)
- Renal impairment (Ann IM 1999;130:7; Jama 1996;275:1177)
- Gout and gouty nephropathy
- Encephalopathy, mortality without rx is 50%, with rx is 3%
- Mental deficiencies and neurologic abnormalities even at blood levels <50 μgm % (Nejm 1988;319:468; Jama 1979;222:462) and long term in children with elevated Pb in teeth representing old exposure (Nejm 1990;322:83) or with umbilical cord Pb levels ≥10 μgm/cc (Nejm 1987;316:1037). Measurable behavioral problems at levels ≥15–50 μgm % (Am J Pub Hlth 1992;82:1356); before age 3, eventual IQ impaired even at average blood levels <10 μgm % (Nejm 1992;327:1279)
- Hypertension, many who are called "essential hypertensives" with creatinine >1.5 mg% (Am J Pub Hlth 1999;89:330; Jama 1996;275:1171; and Nejm 1983;309:17 vs. Jama 1996;275:1563)
- Dental caries (Jama 1999;281:2294)

Lab:

Chem: Whole blood Pb levels; tooth levels (deciduum) can be used for epidemiologic studies (Nejm 1974;290:245)

Hem: Rbc stippling (RNA and mitochondria), siderocytes. Free erythrocyte protoporphyrin no longer used as screening test because only sensitive down to 30–40 μgm % and levels lag weeks

Urine: Increased coproporphyrins and protoporphyrins, no PBG elevations; Pb levels elevated; EDTA mobilization tests

Xray: KUB may show Pb opacities in gut; bones show lead lines at metaphyseal calcification line in children due to increased calcium laid down at zone of provisional calcification in rapidly growing bones, not in adults

Rx: (Med Let 1991;33:78)

Screen all children with serum lead levels at 6–12 mo and q 6–12 mo to age 24 mo, screen older children only if high risk

Table 1.3.1

Level	Plan
<10 μgm %	Repeat per above schedule
10–25 μgm %	Repeat, improve environment, give po Fe, which decreases Pb absorption
25–45 μgm %	Aggressive rx of environment, po Fe; chelation not effective (Nejm 2001;344:1421,1470)
45+ μgm %	Refer for chelation w succimer

Chelation w (none have been shown to improve neurologic function aside from seizures)
- Succimer (DMSA, dimercaptosuccinate) po (Jama 1991;265:1802) if no gi toxicity or encephalopathy, or
- BAL (dimercaprol) im if level >100 μgm/cc and/or sx; contraindicated in peanut allergy; followed not sooner than 4 hr (to avoid encephalopathy) by
- EDTA iv
- Vitamin C perhaps (Jama 1999;281:2289,2340)

NARCOTIC ADDICTION, WITHDRAWAL, OD, HEROIN OD

OD—Ann IM 1999;130:584

Cause: Opium derivatives and synthetic opioids including propoxyphene (Darvon)

Epidem: Increased prevalence in urban areas, physicians (Nejm 1970; 282:365)

Pathophys: Psychic dependence much greater problem than the very real though less common physical dependence (Nejm 1983;308:1096)

Sx: Of withdrawal, in first 48 h restless, yawning, chills, increased pilomotor activity ("cold turkey"), progresses over 24 h to cramps, diarrhea, sweating, vomiting, tachycardia, hyperventilation, hypertension, seizures (neonates)

Si: Of OD: small pupils, somnolence, and hypoventilation (if all 3 present, 92% sens, 76% specif); needle tracks

Of withdrawal: jerky respirations leading to muscle twitching

Crs:

Cmplc: Of addiction: hepatitis B; false-positive serologic tests for Q fever and/or VDRL (Ann IM 1968;69:739); pulmonary edema (Ann IM 1972;77:29); endocarditis especially right-sided (Ann IM 1973; 78:25); nephrotic syndrome and renal failure (Nejm 1974;290:19)

Of OD: hypostatic pneumonia, pulmonary edema

Lab: Urine: opiate screens; may be falsely positive w/ quinolone antibiotics (Jama 2001;286:3115)

Rx: (Ann IM 1999;130:584)

of OD: observe, rx depressed respirations w naloxone (Narcan) 0.4 mg challenge test if addiction suspected, if no withdrawal then 2 mg iv (or sc/im), then 2 mg iv q 2–3 min up to 10 (in children, 0.01 mg/kg iv or ET; repeat q 3 min until respond, then q 20 min); or more expensive nalmefene (Revex) (Med Let 1995;37:95) 0.5 mg iv then 1 mg 2–5 min later, use 0.1 mg challenge dose first if suspect addiction

of withdrawal sx: clonidine 0.1 mg b-qid helps gi NV+D and cramps (Ann IM 1984;101:331), but methadone 1st choice (Med Let 1985;27:77) at 40–100 mg po qd (Jama 1999;281:1000)

of addiction (Nejm 2000;343:1290) (available through addiction treatment clinics):

- Methadone 80–120 mg qd po results in less severe withdrawal sx; helps up to 50% come off, decreases crime rates (Nejm 1971;285:320), better than rehab (Jama 2000;283:1303,1337, 1343); 50 mg po qd may be enough for maintenance (Ann IM 1993;119:23); beware of phenytoin (Dilantin) po which increases metabolism and precipitates withdrawal (Ann IM 1981;94:349)
- Levomethadyl acetate maintenance (LAAM) (Jama 1997; 278:1945), <100 mg qod or Mon, Wed, Fri as effective as methadone, more dangerous if abused iv since delayed reaction (Jama 1972;222:437)
- Naltrexone 100–150 mg tiw, $2/50 mg, Antabuse approach, blocks narcotic effect (Med Let 1985;27:11); or iv × 8 hr w general anesthesia then discharge w sc naltrexone pellet being done in for-profit detox clinics (Jama 1998;279:229; 1997;277:363)
- Buprenorphine 16–32 mg po tiw; or 3 mg sl qd × 3, then clonidine 0.1–0.2 mg po q 4 hr prn sx, plus naltrexone 25 mg po qd × 2; 80% successful OP detox at 1 week (Ann Im 1998;127:526)

EMERGENCIES

Chapter 2
Cardiology

D. K. Onion

2.1 MEDICATIONS

ANTICOAGULANTS

Antiplatelet drugs:
- Acetylsalicylic acid (aspirin, ASA) (Nejm 1994;330:1287) 80–325 mg po qd (Med Let 1998;40:59; 1995;37:14) vs 10–30 mg po qd doses (Ann IM 1994;120:184); inhibits platelet stickiness; can be used safely w warfarin (Nejm 1993;329:530); cheap. Adverse effects: gastric intolerance only at doses ≥30 mg qd (Ann IM 1994;120:184), asthma, incr bleeding time for 2 d, platelet dysfunction for 7–10 d
- Clopidogrel (Plavix) (Med Let 1998;40:59; Rx Let 1997;4:71) 75 mg po qd for anticoagulation alone or w ASA for TIAs, 300 mg po load then 75 mg qd × 3–12 mo w ASA + heparin marginally better for unstable angina (Nejm 2001;345:494; 1998; 338:1488,1498,1539; Ann IM 1998;129:394); as good as ASA or ticlopidine without neutropenia of latter; takes days to take full effect, hepatic metabolism; rare gi bleeding, rare TTP (Nejm 2000; 342:1773); $87/mo
- Ticlopidine (Ticlid) (Med Let 1998;40:59) 250 mg po bid; antiplatelet effect different from aspirin's; can be used if aspirin-intolerant or w aspirin if need extra antiplatelet effect as w coronary stents × 1 mo (Nejm 1996;334:1084), decreases restenosis rates after peripheral revascularizations (Nejm 1997; 337:1726) or for TIAs (Med Let 1992;34:65). Adverse effects: agranulocytosis (1%), reversible, occurs in first 3 mo; marrow

aplasia; cholestasis, TTP (Ann IM 1998;128:541) in 0.02% (Jama 1999;281:806). $114/mo

Platelet Glycoprotein IIb/IIIa Receptor Antagonists (Med Let 1998; 40:89); all useful in unstable coronary syndromes and peri-stenting (Nejm 2001;344:1879,1888,1895,1937); all cost ~$2000/crs
- Tirofiban (Aggrastat) (Nejm 1998;338:1488,1498,1539) as part of triple rx of unstable angina; effects last <4 hr
- Eptifibatide (Integrilin) (Nejm 1998;339:436); effects last <4 hr
- Abciximab (ReoPro); effects last <48 hr; used w coronary artery stenting (Nejm 1999;341:319)

Heparins:
- Low molecular weight heparins (Am J Med 1999;106:660; Nejm 1997;337:688, Med Let 1997;39:94, 1993;35:75):
  - Enoxaparin (Lovenox) (Nejm 1996;334:677) 30 mg or 1 mg/kg or 3000 anti-Xa U sc bid; or
  - Tinzaparin (Innohep) (Med Let 2001;43:14; Nejm 1997;337: 657,663) 175 U sc qd
  - Dalteparin (Fragmin) 2500 anti-Xa U sc qd; or European types, eg,
  - Reviparix sc bid (Nejm 1997;337:663)

New types approved for DVT prophylaxis only; can be used to anticoagulate pts w heparin-induced thrombocytopenia (Med Let 2001;43:12):
  - Ardeparin (Normiflo) 50 anti-Xa U/kg q 12 hr
  - Danaparoid (Orgaran) 750 anti-Xa U bid;

Despite costs, LMW heparins are clearly better with less bleeding (5%—Ann IM 1994;121:81) for rx of acute pulmonary emboli and acute DVT (Arch IM 2000;160:229; Nejm 1997;337:657,663, 1996;334:672,682,724), overlap w coumadin × 5 d or 2 d of PT INR >2 to prevent paradoxical thrombosis; and better DVT/PE prevention at 40+ mg sc qd over 6 d (Nejm 1999;341:793; 1996; 335:701; 1992;326:975; Ann IM 1992;117:353); also work for unstable angina and may be better @ 1mg/kg q 12 hr (Rx Let 1998; 5:32); much less thrombocytopenia (Med Let 2001;43:11), and less osteoporosis than unfractionated heparin. $23/d
- Heparin (Nejm 1991;324:1565) prophylactic regimen = 5000 U iv q 12 h (Am Hrt J 1980;99:574) or sc (Mod Concepts Cardiovasc Dis 1976;45:105), therapeutic regimen = 5000 U load then 1200 U iv/h (Nejm 1986;315:1109) continuous infusion (or 80 U/kg bolus and 18 U/kg/h—Ann IM 1993;119:874) checking q 6 h PTT until stable at 1.5–2 × control. Circadian increases in PTT

of 50% in the evening complicate adjusting dose more often than daily (Arch IM 1992;152:1589; BMJ 1985;290:341); PTTs also vary by lot and manufacturer by 50% (Ann IM 1993;119:104). Reversible with protamine at 1 mg per 100 U of heparin given in the past 4 h (Ann IM 1989;111:1015). Strong organic acid which binds activated factor II (prothrombin) and blocks fibrin formation and factor XI activation of factor IX; also inhibits activated prothrombin-platelet interaction; renal excretion, half-life = 105 min; works for venous and arterial thrombosis; can use in pregnancy because does not cross placenta. Adverse effects: bleeding especially when given with probenecid or in renal failure, excessive prothrombin prolongation, immune platelet clumping leading to thrombosis and thrombocytopenia w iv or sc prophylactic rx in 1% after 5 d, reversible (Nejm 2001;344:1286; 1995;332:1330; 1987;316:581; Ann IM 1984;100:535) but 60% have ischemic damage and 25% mortality despite early cessation (Am J Med 1999;106:629) and f/u warfarin rx may precipitate limb gangrene (Ann IM 1997;127:804)

Coumarins:

- Warfarin (Coumadin) (Nejm 1991;324:1865) prophylaxis w 1 mg po qd prevents venous thrombosis without increasing the PT, eg, with indwelling catheters (Ann IM 1990;112:423); usual therapeutic dose = 7.5–15 mg po qd to a PT INR of 2–3 for routine anticoagulation, 3–4 for artificial valves (J Am Coll Cardiol 1998;32:1486; ACP J Club 1994;120[suppl 2]:52; seconds prolongation or ratio to control is inadequately precise—Nejm 1993;329:696), then maintain with 2.5–7.5 mg qd. Overlap prolonged PT 2–5 d with heparin as switchover (Nejm 1996;335:1822; 1984;311:645) because it inhibits liver synthesis of factors X (3-d half-life), IX (1.25 d), VII (7 h), and II (4 d); PT measures factor VII because it has the shortest half-life, thus takes at least 2 d after PT is in range, for factor II to come down and the hypercoaguable state w low protein C induced by warfarin to reverse (Nejm 1996;335:1822).

   Adverse effects: rare cholesterol emboli with blue toes (Circ 1967;35:946); or perhaps related skin necrosis especially in pts w protein C heterozygous state, requires emergent vit K, heparin + protein C rx (Nejm 1994;331:1282); bleeding especially due to drug interactions, risk of serious bleeding rx (Ann IM 1996;124:970) ≈ 2%/yr in therapeutic range (4.5%/yr over age 80), correlates w higher PTs and 1st 3 mo of rx, not age or gender (Ann IM 1993;118:511); risk of intracranial bleed ≈ 2%/yr w PT 2 × control, much higher if PT higher (Ann IM 1994;120:897)

Potentiated by foods and drugs (Ann IM 1994;121:676) that either displace from carrier protein or compete for degradation enzyme, including acetaminophen (Tylenol) (Jama 1998;279:657), allopurinol (Nejm 1970;283:1484), amiodarone, disulfiram (Antabuse), ASA, cimetidine (Ann IM 1979;90:993), clofibrate, COX 2 NSAIDs (Rx Let 1999;6:32), erythromycin, ethacrynic acid, flu shots peaking at 1 week (Nejm 1981;305:1262), fluconazole, glucagon (Ann IM 1970;73:331), indomethacin, INH, metronidazole (Nejm 1976;295:355), miconazole, nalidixic acid, nortriptyline (Nejm 1970;283:1484), omeprazole, phenylbutazone, phenytoin, piroxicam (Feldene), propranolol, quinidine (Ann IM 1968;68:511), sulfa drugs (Med Let 1977; 19:7), vitamin E, desiccated thyroid, tolbutamide, trimethoprim/ sulfa (Ann IM 1979;91:321)

Counteracted by avocados, barbiturates, carbamazepine, chlordiazepoxide (Librium), cholestyramine, ethanol, glutethimide, griseofulvin, sucralfate, vitamin K (1 mg reverses >50% in 16 hr—Lancet 2000;356:1551), and locally with dental surgery by tranexamic acid mouthwash (Nejm 1989;320:840)

Perioperatively hold × 4 doses until INR <1.5, resume day after surgery; rarely need heparin coverage (Nejm 1997;336: 1506); no need to hold prior to dental surgery if in therapeutic range (Rx Let 1998;5:57)

Hirudins:
- Argatroban (Med Let 2001;43:11) 2 μgm/kg/min, incr or decr on PTTs; hepatically metabolized, used if heparin-induced thrombocytopenia, a little cheaper than lepirudin.
- Bivalirudin (Angiomax) (Med Let 2001;43:37) used in unstable angina instead of heparin when angioplasty planned
- Desirudin (Revasc), a recombinant hirudin 15 mg sc bid; direct inactivator of thrombin; no antidote to reverse; better than LMW heparin as DVT prophylaxis post hip replacement (Nejm 1997;337:1329,1383); perhaps in future for acute coronary syndrome (Nejm 1996;335:775)

- Lepirudin (Refludan) (Med Let 1998;40:94) 0.4 mg/kg bolus then 0.15 mg/kg/hr iv; use when can't use heparin because of thrombocytopenia; $3900/wk

ANTIARRHYTHMICS
(Ann IM 1995;122:705; Med Let 1991;33:55; 1989;31:35; all may increase sudden death—Nejm 1983;309:1302)

Transient vasoconstrictors:
- Adenosine (Adenocard) 6 then 12 mg iv for SVT (not Aflutter or Afib), converts 91% (Ann IM 1990;113:104) to 99% (Ann IM 1997;127:417), effect gone in 10 sec; theophylline inhibits effect. Adverse effects: Afib in 12% which could be dangerous if WPW present resulting in ventricular response >240/min
- Ibutilide (Corvert) (Med Let 1996;38:38) 1 mg iv over 10 min, repeat × 1 if necessary; converts 20–40% of Afib and 40–70% of Aflut to NSR. Adverse effects: long QT torsade de pointes syndrome

Class IA (all cause torsades de pointes Vtach)
- Disopyramide (Norpace CR) (Ann IM 1982;96:337) 150–300 mg bid; renal excretion. Adverse effects: strongly negative inotrope causes CHF (Nejm 1980;302:614), is an anticholinergic and so causes urinary retention
- Procainamide (Pronestyl) 0.5–2 gm SR po t-qid, or 100 mg iv push q 5 min up to 1 gm, then 2–4 mg/min drip; used for ventricular arrhythmias; renal excretion. Adverse effects: ANA-positive in 50–80% at 6 mo, clinical SLE in 10–20%; 21% Coombs-positive, 3% with clinical hemolytic anemia (Nejm 1984;311:809), thrombocytopenia
- Quinidine (Nejm 1998;338:35) 400–1600 mg po, or 100 mg iv q 3–6 h; rarely need now, for SVTs primarily, but ventricular antiarrhythmic effect as well; decreases conduction velocity, which increases depolarization time, which in turn increases the QT and QRS intervals (if >150% of baseline, stop); renal excretion, need stomach acid to absorb. Adverse effects: increases digoxin levels (Nejm 1979;300:1238), diarrhea, long QT syndrome w sudden death

Class IB:
- Moricizine (Ethmozine) (Nejm 1992;327:227; Ann IM 1992;116:375,382; Med Let 1990;32:99) suppresses PVCs but increases sudden death

- Phenytoin (Dilantin) 100 mg iv q 5 min up to 1 gm load, then 400 mg/d iv or po; good vs ventricular and supraventricular arrhythmias, especially in digoxin toxic state since it causes no further prolongation of A-V conduction; hepatic metabolism. Adverse effects: folate deficiency, potentiates warfarin and vice versa via competition for hepatic metabolism, inhibits insulin release (Nejm 1972;286:339), vitamin D antagonism (Nejm 1972;286:1316), hypotension when given iv because of strongly basic diluent
- Lidocaine 100–150 mg iv then 1–4 mg/min drip (Nejm 1967;277:1215); depresses pNa in all heart tissue, decreasing automaticity, excitability, and conduction velocity (no help), and increasing refractory period unrelated to membrane potentials; for ventricular arrhythmias mainly; hepatic metabolism; no cross-allergy with procaine; 1.5 h half-life, incr to 3.5 h after 24 h; levels incr by cimetidine (Ann IM 1983;98:174), and propranolol from decreased hepatic blood flow (Nejm 1980;303:373). Adverse effects: mildly negative inotrope, hypotension, seizures and confusion, occasional increase in A-V block
- Mexiletine (Mexitil) (Med Let 1986;28:65; Nejm 1987;316:29) 100–400 mg po q 8 h; like lidocaine, used for PVCs, but can worsen them; hepatic metabolism. Adverse effects like lidocaine; ~$40/mo
- Tocainide (Tonocard) (Nejm 1986;315:41; Ann IM 1985;103:387; Med Let 1985;27:9) 400–600 mg po tid; used for PVCs, lidocaine analog, no incr PR, QRS, or QT. Adverse effects: nausea and vomiting, abdominal pain, confusion, psychoses, nightmares, agranulocytosis; ~$50/mo

Class IC (all prolong QT at standard doses (Am J Cardiol 1984;53 [suppl #3])

- Flecainide (Tambocor) and encainide (withdrawn in 1994); shown to increase sudden death by increasing Vtach, Vfib, and post-MI shock (Nejm 1991;324:781), especially in the face of depressed LV function (Ann IM 1990;113:671); may be useful for paroxysmal SVT and PAF if other drugs fail (Med Let 1992;34:71)
- Propafenone (Rythmol) (Nejm 1990;322:518; Med Let 1990;32:37) 2 mg/kg iv push, 150–300 mg po tid; for PAT, Afib (Ann IM 1997;126:621), and other SVTs including reentrant types like WPW (Ann IM 1986;105:655) and ventricular arrhythmias (Ann IM 1991;114:539)

Class II—β blockers: (Med Let 2001;43:9—generic price $1.50/mo, rest all about the same, $15–30/mo; Nejm 1982;306:1456). Lipid solubility (see * below) causes fatigue, nightmares, worsens triglycerides but may help LDL/HDL ratios (Ann IM 1995; 122:133). Increases drug interactions

Non ß-1 (cardiac) selective:

- Carteolol* (Cartrol) similar to pindolol but half the price
- Naldolol (Corgard) (Nejm 1981;305:678) 40–160 mg po qd single dose; 70% renal excretion, so decrease dose in renal failure
- Penbutolol* (Levatol) similar to pindolol but half the price
- Pindolol* (Visken) (Med Let 1989;31:69; Nejm 1983;308:940) 20 mg po bid; some sympathomimetic effect, hence less bradycardia. Adverse effects: can increase angina (BMJ 1984;289:951) and perhaps cardiac mortality (ACP J Club 1992;116[suppl 2]:1) so not protective post-MI; $42/mo
- Propranolol* (Inderal) 20–600+ mg po divided b-qid or 1–5 mg iv. Adverse effects: half-life prolonged by cimetidine (Nejm 1981; 304:692); CHF, asthma, hyperkalemia (Nejm 1980;302:431), rebound PVCs and other malignant arrhythmias with abrupt cessation, prolongs lidocaine half-life, suicide (Am J Psych 1982; 139:92)
- Sotalol (Betapace) (Med Let 1993;35:27) 80–160 mg po bid or 1 mg/kg bolus; class IIB and III effects; useful in SVTs, Vtach where may be better than lidocaine (Lancet 1994;344:18), can be used to prevent Vtach and decrease automatic defib discharge frequency (Nejm 1999;340:1853); no negative inotropism. Adverse effects: prolonged QT, hence torsades de pointes (Nejm 1994;331:31), increases mortality in LV dysfunction (Lancet 1996;348:7)
- Timolol* (Blocadren) 10–20 mg po bid

ß-1 selective: (Use, if must, in smokers, Raynaud's, diabetes; avoid in migraine, CHF (Med Aud Dig 1982;29:19)

- Atenolol (Tenormin) 50–100+ mg po qd single dose; renal excretion
- Betaxolol (Kerlone) (Med Let 1990;32:61) 5–10 mg po qd
- Bisoprolol (Zebeta) (Med Let 1994;36:23) 1.25–10 mg po qd-bid; $24/mo
- Esmolol (Brevibloc) (Med Let 1987;29:57) 0.5 mg/kg iv; like propranolol but shorter, 10–20 min half-life; used especially for rapid rx of Afib

- Metoprolol* (Lopressor) (Med Let 1978;20:97; Nejm 1979; 301:698) 10–400 mg po qd divided b-tid, or as CR/XL qd (Jama 2000;283:1295); β-1 selective at doses <100 mg qd

Non β-1 (cardiac) selective w α blocking: (Most useful in CHF) (Cir 2000;101:558)

- Bucindolol
- Carvedilol (Coreg) (Nejm 1998;339:1759; 1996;334:1349; Med Let 1997;39:89; Rx Let 1997;4:31) 3.125–25 mg po bid; has β blocker and α blocker vasodilatory effect, used in CHF; adverse effects: dizziness, bradycardia, edema, diarrhea, blurred vision; many drug interactions, eg, w digoxin, cimetidine, SSRIs
- Labetalol (Normodyne) (Med Let 1984;26:83) 100–600$^+$ mg po; helps cardiac output w α blockade. Adverse effects: postural hypotension, rare hepatotoxicity (Ann IM 1990;113:210), and the worst sexual dysfunction of all the β blockers

Class III: (Prolong repolarization; all can cause long QT and torsade, especially in pts w low EF)

- Amiodarone (Cordarone) (Ann IM 1995;122:689; Nejm 1981;305:539; Ann IM 1984;101:462; Med Let 1995;37:114 [iv], 1986;28:49 [po]) 150 mg iv bolus in 10 min then 1 mg/min × 6 h then 1/2 mg/min × 18 h then d/c, repeat bolus if Vfib/Vtach recurs; or 800–1600 mg po qd × 1–3 wk, then decrease to 400 mg po qd; 35-d half-life; for life-threatening Vfib and Vtach resistant to other rx or post-MI for a year (Ann IM 1994;121:529; Circ 1993;87:309), 75% effective by survivals and does not worsen arrhythmias, also used for Afib and PAT (Ann IM 1992;116:1017) in lower doses like 200 mg qd (J. Love 10/94), may help CHF and arrythmias prophylactically post-MI (Lancet 1997;1417; Circ 1997;96:2823); weeks-long half-life, and drug interactions (Nejm 1987;316:455). Adverse effects: sun-induced blue skin (Nejm 2001;345:1464), severe hepatotoxicity (Nejm 1984;311:167), hypo- (22%) or hyperthyroidism (10%) (monitor w TSH and T_4 q 3 mo —Ann IM 1997;126:63); elevated cholesterols independent of the TSH effect (Ann IM 1991;114:128); constipation and anorexia; insomnia; ataxia; pulmonary fibrosis in 2% (Ann IM 1982;97:839); incr digoxin levels; irreversible shock with anesthesia sometimes (Mod Concepts Cardiovasc Dis 1983;52:31); reversible and irreversible visual loss (Rx Let 1997;4:45); iv doses can cause

hypotension, bradyarrhythmias, and occasionally long QT syndrome
- Bretylium (Ann IM 1979;91:229; Nejm 1979;300:473; Med Let 1978;20:105) 5–10 mg/kg iv, then 1–2 mg/min drip; sympathetic blocker, for resistant Vtach and Vfib, contraindicated in digoxin toxicity and aortic stenosis
- Dofetilide (Tikosyn) (Med Let 2000;42:41; Nejm 1999;341:858) 250–500 μgm po bid; for Afib conversion or maintenance, especially in CHF; renal clearance; interacts w long QT drugs, cimetidine, ketoconazole, trimethoprim, Compazine, megestrol, etc, but not digoxin or warfarin. Adverse effects: long QT and torsade in 3% so start in hospital
- Ibutilide (Corvert) (Nejm 1999;340:1849); 1 mg iv; sometimes converts but always facilitates electrical cardioversion of Vfib and Afib. Adverse effects: long QT
- Sotalol (Betapace) (p 40)

Class IV—Calcium channel blockers: (Nejm 1999;341:1447; Med Let 1999;41:23; 1997;39:13,103). Adverse effects: all slow AV conduction and decr myocardial contractility; metabolism of many inhibited by grapefruit (Med Let 1995;37:73); incr MIs, sudden death, and atherosclerosis w short-acting types (Jama 1996;275; 785,829) and/or in diabetics; all about $1/d at similar doses (Med Let 1991;34:99) except generic verapamil which is $4/mo, or $12/mo as slow release
- Diltiazem (Cardizem) (Med Let 1983;25:17) 0.25 mg/kg iv bolus then 5–10 mg/h; or 120–480 mg po qd as long acting form; use for rapid Afib, Prinzmetal's angina although all calcium blockers work; 4–8 h half-life; less AV block than verapamil; less peripheral vasodilatation than nifedipine; most expensive po; precipitates CHF more often the lower the ejection fraction is (Circ 1991; 83:52)
- Verapamil (Calan) (Med Let 1987;29:37) 5–10 mg iv over 1–2 min, repeat in 30 min, 4–6 h half-life; long-acting 120–480 mg qd to bid; for SVTs, angina, IHSS, hypertensive crisis. Adverse effects: incr digoxin levels, heart blocks, avoid in WPW (Med Let 1982; 24:56; Ann IM 1982;96:409), decreased insulin secretion and glucose tolerance, negative cardiac inotrope (decreases cardiac output), hypotension when given after quinidine (Nejm 1985; 312:167), constipation, incr effect and decreased clearance in elderly (Ann IM 1986;105:329)

Dihydropyridines: (Potent vasodilators; cause reflex tachycardia, peripheral edema)
- Amlodipine (Norvasc) 5–10 mg po qd; may be ok for pts w CHF (Nejm 1996;335:1107)
- Bepridil (Vascor) 200–400 mg po qd. Adverse effects: long QT and torsades de pointes
- Felodipine (Plendil) (Med Let 1991;33:115) 5–20 mg po qd; good for hypertension, first-pass metabolism so levels incr by liver disease, cimetidine, and grapefruit juice. Adverse effects: like other dihydropyridines, including gingival hyperplasia. Cheapest
- Isradipine (DynaCore) 2.5–5 mg po bid (Med Let 1991;33:51)
- Nicardipine (Cardene) (Med Let 1989;31:41) 20+ mg timed release bid; good for angina and hypertension, very like nifedipine, but little negative inotropic effect. Adverse effects: gum hypertrophy and gingival hyperplasia. Cheaper than diltiazem
- Nifedipine (Procardia) 10–40 mg po t-qid, or 30–120 mg XL qd; least variable pharmacokinetics compared to diltiazem and verapamil over time (Med Let 1982;24:39), minimal negative inotropic effect, no A-V block effect, use for angina, hypertension (not crisis). Adverse effects: peripheral edema, hypotension, flushing, and dizziness from peripheral venodilatation; possibly incr rate of MIs, esp w higher doses and short-acting formulations (Jama 1996;275:423) as w other dihydropyridines (Jama 1995; 244:360,654)
- Nisoldipine (Sular)(Med Let 1996;38:13) 20–60 mg po qd; for HT. Adverse effects: headache, edema, dizziness; toxicity incr by cimetidine, fatty meals, and grapefruit juice (Med Let 1995;37:73)

DIURETICS
(Nejm 1998;339:387; Med Let 1999;41:23; 1995;37:45)

Thiazides: NSAIDs decrease effectiveness (Med Let 1987;29:1), worsen LDL/HDL ratios (Ann IM 1995;122:133); many different kinds, but most commonly used:
- Chlorothiazide; chlorthalidone; trichlormethiazide
- Hydrochlorothiazide 12.5–25 mg po qd. Adverse effects: hypokalemia especially with steroids but use w K-sparing diuretics prevents MRFIT study-type hypo-K and hypo-Mg mortality (Nejm 1994;330:1852), pancreatitis, rashes, elevated levels of lithium, LDL cholesterol, uric acid, calcium, and blood sugar

CARDIOLOGY

- Indapamide (Lozol) 1.25–2.5 mg po qd; perhaps less-adverse lipid effect than hydrochlorothiazide, works even in renal failure; $0.50/pill, not worth it (Med Let 1990;31:103)

Potassium-sparing distal diuretics: Beware of hyperkalemia with po KCl, IDDM, renal failure, salt substitutes, and ACE inhibitors
- Amiloride (Midamor) (BMJ 1983;286:2015; Med Let 1981; 23:109) 5–20 mg po qd; K^+ sparer, but also not an aldosterone antagonist; does have an antihypertensive effect, causes low uric acid. Adverse effects: potentiates warfarin; causes elevated BUN when used w triamterine
- Spironolactone (Aldactone) 50–100 mg po qd; aldosterone antagonist. Adverse effects: hyperkalemia, gynecomastia, and impotence due to incr testosterone metabolism into estrogens (Ann IM 1977;87:398)
- Triamterene (Dyrenium) 25–50 mg bid po; a K^+ sparer but not an aldosterone antagonist and no antihypertensive effect

Loop diuretics:
- Bumetanide (Bumex) (Med Let 1983;25:61) 1–5 mg po iv or im, 1 mg comparable to 40 mg of furosemide. Adverse effects: like furosemide
- Ethacrynic acid (Edecrin) 25–100 mg po iv, rarely used now
- Furosemide (Lasix) 20–320 mg po iv or im as single dose or divided; works even in renal failure when resistant to thiazides, rapid onset, short half-life. Adverse effects: causes hypokalemia, severe volume depletions possible, direct and indirect decreases in preload, elevates uric acid, blood sugar, and pH; for 40 mg qd, $2/mo generic, $6.50/mo as Lasix
- Metolazone (Zaroxolyn) 2.5–10 mg po qd or qod; works even in renal failure, long-acting, some proximal tubule effect too. Adverse effects: severe electrolyte imbalances
- Torsemide (Demadex) (Med Let 1994;36:73) 2.5–20 mg po/iv; lower doses as good as thiazides for HT; half-life twice that of furosemide; no drug interactions. Adverse effects: same as furosemide. $14/mo for 10 mg qd

VASODILATORS

Nitrates: (Nejm 1998;338:520; Med Let 1994;36:111)
- Nitroglycerine 0.3–0.4 mg sl or spray (Med Let 1986;28:59) prn pain, or isosorbide dinitrate (Isordil) 5–20 mg po tid, or isosorbide

5-mononitrate (Ismo or Monoket) 20 mg po bid at 8 am and 3 pm (Ann IM 1994;120:353) ($40/mo); or as long-acting (Imdur) 30–120 mg po qd ($20+/mo), or as patch or 2% paste; decreases preload and causes coronary artery dilatation, tolerance and tachyphylaxis if used 24 h/day, thus nights off necessary for continued effect (Med Let 1994;36:13; Ann IM 1991;114:667; Nejm 1987;316:1635,1440)

- Nitroprusside (Nipride) 0.5–8 μgm/kg/min iv; mixed pre- and afterload reduction; use for hypertensive crises, acute mitral regurgitation and VSDs, pulmonary edema with hypertension, normotension, or even mild shock. Adverse effects: thiocyanate toxicity after 48 h, especially if renal failure

Angiotensin-converting enzyme inhibitors (ACEIs): (Med Let 1996; 38:104; 1995;37:45,58); all may show slowly progressive renal disease (Ann IM 1989;111:503) even w early renal failure (BMJ 1994;309:833); less effective in blacks (Nejm 2001;344:1351), but still much better than Ca channel blockers (Jama 2001;285:2719); avoid in pregnancy because of potentially fatal effects in 2nd and 3rd trimesters (Jama 1997;277:1193; Med Let 1997;39:44); can cause rare severe angioedema (Jama 1997;278:232)

- Benazepril (Lotensin) 10–40 mg po in 1–2 doses qd
- Captopril (Capoten) (Nejm 1988;319:1517; Med Let 1982;24:89) 12.5–100 mg po bid, ineffective if creatinine >2.8 mg% (Ann IM 1986;104:147); mixed pre- and afterload reduction, positive effects on quality of life in contrast to enalapril, α-methyldopa, and propranolol (Nejm 1993;328:907). Adverse effects: hypotension, especially if on diuretics (decrease dose of latter before starting); renal failure (20%) if systolic BP <90 especially in summer and/or w renal artery stenosis, usually reversible (Ann IM 1991;115:513; 1987;106:346); hyperkalemia, especially in diabetics; cough (5–20%), often prominent and disabling (Ann IM 1992;117:234), treatable with indomethacin 50 mg po bid or nifedipine XL 30 mg po bid (J Cardiovasc Pharmacol 1992;19:670); nephrotic syndrome (1%); agranulocytosis; loss of taste; rash (Med Let 1980;22:39); cholestatic jaundice (Ann IM 1985;102:56); $106/mo for 50 mg tid
- Enalapril (Vasotec) (Med Let 1986;28:53) 2.5–40 mg po qd or bid, same doses in CHF (Nejm 1987;316:1429); similar to captopril but more hypotensive, activated in liver, excreted in

CARDIOLOGY

kidney, 24-h effect. Adverse effects: hyperkalemia and elevated creatinine (Nejm 1986;315:847); $40/mo for 20 mg qd
- Fosinopril (Monopril) 10–40 mg po qd in 1–2 doses qd
- Lisinopril (Zestril or Prinivil) (Med Let 1988;30:41) 10–40 mg po qd; similar in most respects to captopril; $23/mo for 5 mg bid
- Moexipril (Univasc) 7.5–30 mg po qd; $15/mo for 7.5 mg qd
- Peridopril (Aceon) (Med Let 1999;41:105; Rx Let 1999;6:56) 4–8 mg po qd or split bid; similar to all the others
- Quinapril (Accupril) 5–80 mg po qd or divided bid; $27/mo for 20 mg qd
- Ramipril (Altace) 2.5–10 mg po bid; $21/mo for 2.5 mg po qd
- Trandolapril (Mavik) 1–4 mg po qd; $18/mo

Angiotensin receptor antagonists (ARAs): (Med Let 1999;41:105): Cardiac and renal protective effects like ACEIs (Nejm 245:851, 861,870,910); try when intolerant of ACEIs, eg, cough or angioedema; less effective in blacks, avoid in pregnancy because of 2nd and 3rd trimester fetal damage (ACP J Club 1996;124:10, HT 1995;25:1345); all $40/mo for minimal dose (Med Let 1999;41:105), $5–$10/mo more than ACEIs (Rx Let 1997;4:63)
- Candesartan (Atacand) (Med Let 1998;40:109; Rx Let 1998;5:62) 16–32 mg po qd, less if volume depleted and/or on other antihypertensives
- Losartan (Cozaar) (Med Let 1995;37:57) 25–50 mg po qd-bid or w 12.5 mg of hydrochlorothiazide (Hyzaar) i po qd-bid
- Valsartan (Diovan) (Med Let 1997;39:44) 80–320 mg po qd; $34 per 30 d
- Irbesartan (Avapro) (Rx Let 1997;4:63) 150–300 mg po qd
- Telmisartan (Micardis) (Rx Let 1999;6:2) 40–80 mg po qd

Vasopeptidase inhibitors (VPIs):
- Omapatrilat (Vanlev) (Rx Let 2000;7:18); ACE and enopeptidase inhibition which cause vasodilation and natiuresis; FDA approval pending

Direct vasodilators: (Med Let 1995;37:45)
- Diazoxide (Hyperstat) (Curr Concepts Cerebro Dis 1982;17:5; Nejm 1976;294:1271) 300 mg iv push over 10–20 sec for hypertensive crisis but no longer first choice (nitroprusside w propranolol instead), effects last 3 h; give with furosemide; protein-bound; get other drugs in soon. Adverse effects: rarely can cause hypotension, but can cause CNS infarcts

- Hydralazine (Apresoline) 25–50 mg qid po or iv; afterload reduction, used often w isosorbide chronically to get combined pre- and afterload reduction. Adverse effects: SLE, especially in women at >200 mg qd, occurs in 5% of males and 20% of women after 3 yr at 200 mg qd (BMJ 1984;289:410); reflex tachycardia
- Minoxidil (Loniten) (Med Let 1980;22:21; Nejm 1980;303:922) 5–20 mg po bid; afterload reduction, "an oral nitroprusside"; adverse effect: hirsutism
- Morphine 2–5 mg iv; pre- and afterload reductions
- Dihydropyridine Calcium Channel Blockers (p 42)

α-Adrenergic receptor blockers: (Med Let 1999;41:23; 1995;37:45)
- Prazosin (Minipress) (Ann IM 1982;97:67; Nejm 1979;300:232) 1–30 mg po qd divided b-tid; mixed pre- and afterload reduction, like nitroprusside, no reflex tachycardia, used for hypertension, CHF, and Raynaud's; first dose often causes hypotension; tachyphylaxis w CHF but not in hypertension (Nejm 1986; 314:1547); $2/mo generic
- Doxazosin (Cardura) 1–16 mg po qd hs (Med Let 1991;33:15); not as good as thiazides (Jama 2000;283:1967); $30/mo
- Terazosin (Hytrin) (Med Let 1987;29:112) 1–20 mg po qd; similar to prazosin; $52/mo

OTHER ANTIHYPERTENSIVES
(Med Let 1995;37:45; 1991;33:33)

- α-Methyldopa (Aldomet) 0.5–3 gm po qd divided; central sympathetic action. Adverse effects: sedation, hemolytic anemia, impotence, hepatitis, incr haloperidol (Haldol) and lithium toxicities
- Clonidine (Catapres) (Med Let 1985;27:95; Nejm 1975;293:1179) 0.1[+] mg po bid ($13/mo) or patch q 1 wk ($25/mo); central sympathetic block. Adverse effects: severe rebound hypertension when stopped; sedation, dry mouth, retinopathy, blocked by tricyclics, patch causes skin reactions
- Fenoldopam (Corlopam) (Med Let 1998;40:57) 0.1–1.6 μgm/kg/min; dopamine-1 receptor antagonist; useful for rx of HT crisis, as good as nitroprusside, can increase intraocular pressures
- Guanethidine (Ismelin) 10–300 mg po qd; half-life is 5 d. Adverse effects: diarrhea, asthma, inability to ejaculate, potentiation of hypoglycemics, inhibition by phenothiazines and tricyclics
- Guanfacine (Tenex) (Med Let 1987;29:49) 1–3 mg po qd; like clonidine

- Reserpine 0.1–0.25 mg po qd; acts via peripheral sympathetic blockade. Adverse effects: depression, acid peptic disease

INOTROPES

- Amrinone (Inocor) (Nejm 1986;314:350) 0.75 mg/kg bolus and drip at 5–10 µgm/kg/min; a vasodilator and an inotrope, no better than dobutamine and digoxin, may be worse (Ann IM 1985;102:399). Adverse effects: depressed platelets, fever, hypotension
- Digoxin (Mod Concepts Cardiovasc Dis 1990;59:67; Nejm 1988; 318:358); daily maintenance dose 0.25–0.5 mg po, or 0.125–0.25 mg iv; digitalizing dose is 2–3 mg po, or 1–2 mg iv over 24 h; major effects are A-V block and positive inotropy without increasing O_2 demand; ~80% gi absorption; 60% renal excretion so decrease dose in renal failure; therapeutic blood level = 0.5–2 µgm %, which is incr by quinidine (Nejm 1981;305:209), verapamil, amiodarone, nifedipine, all NSAIDs including ASA (Mod Concepts Cardiovasc Dis 1986;55:26), antibiotics via incr absorption (Nejm 1981;305:327); decreased effect or levels with hypocalcemia (Nejm 1977;296:917), decreased absorption because of antacids especially Mg trisilicates, Kaopectate, Dilantin (Nejm 1976; 295:1034); misleadingly low levels in achlorhydrics and pts on omeprazole because higher % of active drug is absorbed (Ann IM 1991;115:540); digoxin overdose toxicity treatable with Fab fragments (Nejm 1982;307:1357), not dialyzable. Adverse effects: neurologic including nausea and vomiting, visual distortions even at therapeutic levels (Ann IM 1995;123:676), confusion, gynecomastia, cardiac including PVCs, A-V and other exit blocks, PAT with block, junctional tachycardia, bidirectional A-V tachycardias
- Dobutamine (Dobutrex) (Ann IM 1983;99:490) 2–15 µgm/kg/min; predominantly an inotrope; especially used in cardiovascular shock when the pulse rate is already maximal; better than digoxin and diuretics in immediate post-MI CHF (Nejm 1980;303:846)
- Dopamine 2–10 µgm/kg/min; ino- and chronotropic, renal blood flow sparing at these doses; used for shock

THROMBOLYTICS

- Anistreplase (Eminase) (Med Let 1989;31:15), similar to streptokinase
- Streptokinase 1.5 million U iv over 30 min + ASA 100–160 mg po qd + iv β blocker (Ann IM 1991;115:34); like urokinase, causes plasmin

activation; used for MIs and in higher longer doses for pulmonary emboli and DVT. Adverse effects: more allergic reactions than urokinase with repeat administrations so can't reuse at least within 6 mo; <10% bleed, stroke rate <1% but much higher if diastolic BP >110 at time of administration (Nejm 1992;327:1); $200/treatment

- Tissue plasminogen activator (TPA) (Nejm 1997;337:118; 1993;329: 673,1615; Ann IM 1991;114:417); all followed by or coincident w continuous iv heparin for at least 1 d + ASA 100–160 mg po qd + iv β blocker (Ann IM 1991;115:34). Adverse effects: bleeding <10%, stroke rate <2%, but 0.4% more than for streptokinase (Nejm 1992;327:1); $2750/treatment, may be worth it especially in anterior MIs and the elderly (Nejm 1995;332:1418)
  - Reteplase (Retavase) 10 U bolus q 30 min × 2; recombinant mutant TPA, cleared more slowly than natural TPA (alteplase), hence can give as bolus
  - Alteplase, 100 mg iv over 1.5 h, 2/3 in 1st 30 min; double bolus method doesn't work (Nejm 1997;337:1124)
  - Tenecteplase (TNKase) (Med Let 2000;42:106) 30–50 mg (based on wgt, 30 mg if <60 kg, 50 if >90 kg) iv bolus over 5 sec, half-life = 25 min
- Urokinase 4400 U/kg load in 10 min, then same/h x 24 h; $50/100,000 U

CARDIOLOGY

2.2 ARTERIOSCLEROTIC HEART DISEASE

ATHEROSCLEROSIS

Nejm 1993;329:247 [women]

Cause: Multiple, including elevated cholesterol (Nejm 1981;304:65); smoking, passive (Nejm 1999;340:920) and active, correlates most w pack-years not w quitting (Jama 1998;279:119); hypertension; lack of estrogen (Ann IM 1976;85:447); genetic, especially in women. Possibly induced by *Chlamydia pneumoniae* endovascular infection (Jama 1999;281:427,461; Lancet 1997;350:404; Ann IM 1996;125:979; 1992;116:273) or other causes of inflammation indicated by elevated C-reactive protein levels (Jama 1999; 282:2131,2169; Circ 1998;98:731; 97:425); but no correlation between chlamydial IgG titers and ASHD found in women (Ann IM 1999;131:573)

Atherosclerosis, continued

Epidem: Incr incidence in Western countries although it has decreased in last 25 yr, half due to decrease in risk factors and half due to medical rx (Nejm 1996;334:884) w improving post-MI survival (Nejm 1998;339:861)

Incr in diabetes, hypertension, obesity (Nejm 1990;322:882), pseudoxanthoma elasticum, myotonic dystrophy, alkaptonuria and ochronosis; homocystinuria (p 239) and other causes of mild homocystinuria like B_{12}, folate and pyridoxine deficiencies, prevent w vitamin supplements (Nejm 1995;332:286) although unclear if mildly elevated homocysteine levels are cause or effect of ASCVD (Jama 1995;274:1526); hyperlipidemias (p 204) especially LDL elevations often associated w apolipoprotein ε4 allele (Jama 1994; 272:1666), and w elevated lipoprotein (α) (Jama 1996;276:544); sleep disorders (Am J Med 2000;108:396)

Weak (ACP J Club 1998;129(2):50) or no association w triglyceride elevations alone, although they are markers for other risk factors (Nejm 1993;328:1220). Risk factors increase prevalence in aorta and coronaries in young people at trauma autopsy (Nejm 1998; 338:1650)

Decreased in moderate (7–20 drinks/wk) alcohol drinkers (Jama 1999; 282:239; Nejm 1997;337:1705, Ann IM 1997;126:372, Nejm 1995; 332:1245; 1993;329:1829), via incr TPA as well as HDL (Jama 1994;272:929) and flavins in red wine which appears to decr cancer mortality also (Ann IM 2000;133:411); in runners (Nejm 1980;303: 1159), and otherwise regularly exercising men (Nejm 1998;338:94; 1993;328:533,538,574; 1993;329:1829) and women (Jama 2001; 285:1447) via protective elevations of HDL cholesterol component; with high fiber diets (20+ gm qd) (Jama 1999;281:1995) like those high in fruits and vegetables (Ann IM 2001;134:1106); with incr fish intake perhaps via thromboxane A effect (Nejm 1986;314:937); in women who take po postmenopausal estrogens? (p 624)

Pathophys: (Nejm 1999;340:115)

Wall stress causes fibrous plaques which later infiltrate with cholesterol; impaired fibrinolysis may also play a role in genesis. Onset by age 18 yr (Nejm 1986;314:138). Hemorrhage into plaque causes sudden occlusions

Endothelin, a peptide, elevated in pts w ASCVD so possible cause (Nejm 1991;325:997)

Sx: Claudication, angina, MI, sudden death, TIA/CVA, abdominal angina

Si: Renal hypertension; bruits, absent peripheral pulses; CVAs; arcus senilis in whites <50 yr (Nejm 1974;291:1323) is a risk factor independent even of cholesterol levels (Am J Pub Hlth 1990; 80:1200); retinal fundal vessel plaques

Crs: Reversible with rx (Ann IM 1994;121:348 vs Mod Concepts Cardiovasc Dis 1978;47:79; 1977;46:27; Ann IM 1977;86:139)

Cmplc: All of above

Lab:

Chem: Cholesterol (p 206). Apolipoprotein A_2 (Nejm 2000;343:1149) or A_1 (Nejm 1983;309:385) (components of HDL) may be better predictors

Path: Lipid in foam macrophages and smooth muscle; free cholesterol crystals between intima and media

Xray: Electron beam CT screening of unproven value (Nejm 1998; 339:1964,1972,2014,2018)

Rx: Prevent (rv of all in women—Nejm 1995;332:1758) w
- School education programs (Nejm 1988;318:1093)
- Stopping smoking
- Rx of elevated cholesterol (p 204) to get LDL < 100 mg% (Nejm 1997;336:153; Circ 1994;89:1329) at least in pts w ASHD; helps both by decreasing plaques and by preventing coronary artery spasm (Nejm 1995;332:481,488); low saturated rather than total fat diet, ie, "Mediterranean diet" may be best (Jama 1997;278: 2145, 2185)
- Exercise (Jama 2001;285:1447; 1998;279:440) moderate (2–3 mph) walking 1–2 hr/wk; total more important than intensity; increases fibrinolysis (Nejm 1980;302:987)
- Rx of diabetes and hypertension
- ASA 80–320 mg po qd decr MIs and CVAs (Lancet 2001;357:89) especially if CRP chronically elevated (Nejm 1996;336:973,1014)
- Folic acid (Jama 2001;286:936) $1/2$-1 mg po qd; now "in the flour" (Nejm 1999;340:1449), or other anti-homocystinemia meds (p 239) to keep levels <10 μM/L (Rx Let 1999;6:8) like pyridoxine or betaine, esp for pts w established ASHD
- ACE inhibitors in pts w diabetes or vascular disease and other risk factors decr MI, sudden death, and CVAs, even if normal EF, NNT-4 = 14 (Nejm 2000;342:454)
- Alcohol at 2–3 drinks qd decreases mortality by 25% (Am J Pub Hlth 1993;83:805)

- Omega 3 or N₃ fatty acids, as qd capsule (Lancet 1999;354:447) or 1 fatty fish meal/mo decreases incidence of cardiac arrest by 50% (Nejm 1997;336:1046; Jama 1995;274:1363) vs 5 meals/wk (ACP J Club 2000;132:6) which also decr stroke risk by 50% (Jama 2001;285:304)
- Perhaps: medroxyprogesterone to increase HDL cholesterol in postmenopausal females (Nejm 1981;304:560); or statins if elevated CRP levels (Nejm 2001;344:1959)
- No help from:
- Vit E, antioxidant, prevents LDL oxidation but DBCTs show no effect (Nejm 2000;342:154; Jama 1996;275:693). No stroke reduction either (Ann IM 1999;13:963)
- EDTA chelation of various heavy metals (Med Let 1994;36:48)
- β-carotene (Nejm 1996;334:1145,1150,1189; Jama 1996;275: 693,699)

Of disease, various tertiary maneuvers to fix damage especially surgery, eg, CABG, femoral-popliteal bypass, etc.; plus dietary measures, eg, "Mediterranean diet" reduces subsequent mortality from 5% to 1% (Arch IM 1998;158:1181; Lancet 1994;343:1454) and can reverse ASHD vessel diameter narrowing (Jama 1998;280:2001)

ANGINA

Cause: Atherosclerotic heart disease; "microvascular angina" caused by impaired vasodilatation capabilities in all arterioles seen in hypertension patients, causes 10–20% of angina (Nejm 1988;319: 1302; 1987;317:1366); rarely amyloidosis (Ann IM 1999;131:838) which looks like microvascular angina because angiography normal, progresses to CHF. Chronic, asymptomatic CMV infection may increase rate of progression (Nejm 1996;335:624)

Epidem: 80% of ischemic events are asx, hence angina is the tip of the ischemic iceberg (Mod Concepts Cardiovasc Dis 1987;56:2; rv of silent isch w/u and rx—Nejm 1988;318:1038); mental stress is as good an inducer of angina as exercise (Nejm 1988;318:1005)

Pathophys: Spasm may occur even when there is no fixed lesion if vessel wall mast cell nests are present (Nejm 1985;313:1138). Unstable angina usually due to a platelet thrombus (unlike red thrombus of

MI—Nejm 1992;326:287) or fracture of a plaque at the site (Nejm 1986;315:913). Paradoxical vasoconstriction with stress may occur because plaque prevents normal endothelial cell induction of coronary dilatation (Nejm 1991;325:1551)

Sx: Onset with first exercise after rest, more frequently in unfamiliar settings, worse supine, worse outdoors (B. Lown, 1985). Relieved by Valsalva, carotid sinus pressure, and TNG promptly (r/o esophogeal spasm pain)

Si: S_4; mitral regurgitant murmur during pain

Crs: ST depressions of >1 mm especially those lasting >60 min at rest or asx are associated with an MI within 6 mo in 15% of the cases (Nejm 1986;314:1214) even when medically rx'd

Cmplc: MI

r/o esophageal reflux, which can clinically mimic exactly (Ann IM 1992; 117:824), but value of dx studies questionable once ischemia is r/o (Ann IM 1996;124:959); carbon monoxide induction if onset at home in winter (Nejm 1995;322:48); syndrome X: anginal/ischemic sounding chest pain and ST depressions w normal coronaries usually in women (Nejm 2000;342:829, 885), responsive (50%) to imipramine 50 mg po hs (Jama 1995;273:883; Nejm 1994;330:1411; 1993;328:1659,1706), prognosis is good (Nejm 1977;297:916)

Lab:

Chem: CPK-MB may elevate mildly, but subsequent mortality is incr by any elevation above upper limit of normal (Jama 2000;283:247); troponin T levels elevated >0.06 µgm/L (Nejm 2000;343:1139; 1992;327:146)

Hem: CRP levels >1.55 mg/L, associated w 10 × higher 14 d mortality (J Am Coll Cardiol 1998;31:1460)

Noninv: EKG normal in 50% when asx, 30% when sx (B. Lown, 1985); Wellens Syndrome (Am Hrt J 1982;103:730): evolving anterior T inversions w/o enzyme or Q wave changes, assoc w severe LAD lesions

Exercise testing (Nejm 2001;344:1840; 1999;340:340; ACC/AHA guidelines—J Am Coll Cardiol 1997;30:260; Mayo Clin Proc 1996;71:43). Contraindicated in CHF, aortic stenosis, IHSS, unstable angina; can't interpret ST changes in face of LBBB, WPW, digoxin, pacing, resting ST depressions >1mm, LVH, or lack of changes w submaximal test (<85% maximal pulse achieved). Use

CARDIOLOGY

1$^+$ mm ST depressions if downsloping or horizontal at 0.06 sec after J point, or 1.5 mm ST depressions if upsloping at 0.08 sec after J point; or if ST depression at rest, positive if STs depress ≥2 mm more; severity worse if depressions go from 0.5 mm to >2 mm and start in first 3 min, or last 8 or more minutes (Nejm 1979;301:230), and/or hypotension during ETT. Sensitivity 66% but sens/specif depend on pretest probability (Nejm 1979;300:1350); scoring system predicts 5-yr survival and annual mortality (Nejm 1991;325:849). ST depression not predictive of anatomic site, rarer ST elevations are (Ann IM 1987;106:53). If induce paired PVCs or PVCs are >10% of all beats, 10 yr mortality incr 10% over baseline (Nejm 2000;343:826)

Nuclear (sestamibi and/or thallium) scan at peak exercise compared to resting, about 75% sens/specif (Nejm 2001;344:1840); a better predictor of long-term outcome than ETT or Holter (Jama 1996; 277:318; Ann IM 1990;113:575); incr lung uptake predicts poor 5-yr outcome (Nejm 1987;317:1485). Non-exertional testing w dipyridamole (Persantine), dobutamine, arbutamine (Med Let 1998; 40:19), or adenosine (Jama 1991;265:633) iv thallium test as good as ETT; theophylline blocks and reverses effect of dipyridamole (Med Let 1991;33:87); used when pt cannot walk on treadmill

Echocardiogram w dobutamine stress (Am J Cardiol 1993;72:605); about same sens/specif as Persantine thallium; done w progressive 5–40 μgm/kg/min dobutamine infusion; can also distinguish whether a reversible perfusion defect is also associated w a reversible contraction abnormality, often an issue w reversible thallium defects next to an old infarct

Rx: Stopping smoking decreases mortality × 2.8 (Nejm 1984;310:951; BMJ 1983;287:324)

Maximize 1 drug before adding a second (Nejm 1989;320:709)

ASA 75–325 mg po qd prevents MIs but causes mild increase in stroke (Lancet 1992;340:1421; Ann IM 1991;114:835)

Aggressive lipid lowering in chronic stable angina w normal EFs w atoravastatin 80 mg qd as or more effective than angioplasty (Nejm 1999;341:70)

Anti-anginal meds (Med Let 1994;36:111):
- Nitrates to dilate spasms, increase collaterals, and decrease platelet adhesion; po, sl, buccal, or paste tid; tolerance develops so

avoid hs or 24 h rx (Nejm 1987;316:1635), also helpfully decr gi
bleeding if on NSAIDs (Nejm 2000;343:834). Adverse effects:
hypotension, especially if recent sildenafil (Viagra) rx. Costs (Med
Let 1987;29:39)
- β-blockers decrease pulse, BP, platelet adhesion; avoid in
  Prinzmetal type because can increase spasm
- Calcium channel blockers dilate spasm and decrease afterload but
  are 2nd choices after above

Of unstable angina (Nejm 2000;342:101; Am J Med 2000;108:41):
ASA 75–325 mg po qd (Nejm 1992;327:175) w TNG (Nejm
1988;319:1105) and LMW heparin, eg, enoxaparin 1 mg/kg sc bid
(J Am Coll Cardiol 1995;26:313) better than plain heparin (Circ
1998;97:1702; Nejm 1997;337:447); possibly w glycoprotein
IIb/IIIa inhibitors (Jama 2000;284:1549) like: tirofiban (Aggrastat)
iv (Nejm 1998;338:1488,1539) or eptifibatide (Integrilin) iv
(NNT = 75) (Nejm 1998;339;436), or abciximab (reoPro) (Med Let
1998;40:89) iv; thrombolysis no help (Circ 1994;89:1545)

Surgical:
- Angioplasty (Nejm 1994;331:1037,1044; 1994;330:981) w or
  w/o stenting (Nejm 1997;336:817); works for stable and unstable
  angina as well (Nejm 1985;313:342), in elderly even age >80 yr
  (Ann IM 1990;113:423); also useful for single vessel disease but
  more complications than medical rx (Nejm 1992;326:10);
  outcome similar to CABG except more re-operations (Lancet
  1995;346:1179,1184); but when combined w stent placement
  (Nejm 1999;341:1949,1957,2005; 1998;339:1672; 1996;
  334:1084) and ticlopidine/ASA × 1 mo (Nejm 1998;339:1665),
  restenosis rate much less but costly (Nejm 1998;339:1702; Lancet
  1998;352:87); avoid in diabetics and pts w multivessel disease
  who should get CABG
- CABG increases survival significantly (Lancet 1994;344:563) in
  left main disease, patients with abnormal ETT, and 3-vessel
  disease in patients with ejection fx >30% (Nejm 1988;319:332;
  1987;316:981), and perhaps older pts; minimal incr survival in
  other pts with stable angina or asx post MI with bypassable
  lesions (Lancet 1994;344:563; ACP J Club 1995; 122(2):29).
  2/3 develop significant disease in grafts in 10 yr (Nejm 1984;
  311:1329). Significant cognitive decline in 50% at hosp d/c, 24%
  at 6 mo, but 42% at 5 yr (Nejm 2001;344;395, 451)

CARDIOLOGY

- Atherectomy (Nejm 1993;339:221, 228, 273) for eccentric lesions of unstable angina
- Experimental transmyocadial laser revascularization? (Nejm 1999;341:1021; Lancet 1999;354:885)

MYOCARDIAL INFARCTION

Cause: Atherosclerotic (85%) including spasm (Nejm 1983;309:220) with superimposed thrombus in 90% of those; emboli (15%—Ann IM 1978;88:155); and now occasionally cocaine-induced spasm when used as anesthesia or as recreational drug (Nejm 1989;321:1557)

Epidem: Incr incidence with h/o:
- Concurrent BCP use, ×2 (Nejm 2001;345:1787)
- Carbon monoxide acute exposures, eg, firefighters; and chronic CS_2 exposures, eg, disulfiram (Antabuse) use, rayon manufacturing (Med Aud Dig 1984;31:7)
- Cholesterol elevations of total and/or LDL, often with cholecystitis hx (Nejm 1981;304:1396), presence of an arcus senilis (Nejm 1974;291:1382), or birth control pill use (Nejm 1977;296:1166)
- Cocaine use or withdrawal (Ann IM 1989;111:876; Nejm 1986; 315:1438,1495)
- Coffee, high decaffeinated but not regular coffee intake (Nejm 1990;323:1026); later study finds no incr incidence w either (Jama 1996;275:458)
- Exercise test showing ischemia (Nejm 1983;309:1085)
- Family h/o MIs prematurely (age <55 or 65 yr) (Nejm 1994; 330:1041)
- Homocysteine levels >15 μM/L correlate w worse prognosis (Nejm 1997;337:230)
- Hypertension
- Menopause if surgical and pts not placed on estrogen; but no sharp increase in natural menopause or in BSOO pts put on estrogen (Nejm 1987;316:1105)
- Sedentary work; in longshoremen, MIs but not CVAs incr, thus not a general ASCVD effect (Nejm 1975;292:545)
- Sexual activity incr risk slightly but not at all if regular, eg, 3 ×/wk exercise (Jama 1996;275:1405)

- Smoking increases risk × 3, but risk decreases to normal over 2 yr after stop (Nejm 1985;313:1511), increases risk × 5 if >1 ppd, ×2 if 1–4 cigarettes qd in women (Nejm 1987;317:1303)
- Stress, day to day (Jama 1997;277:1521) but not type A personality? (Nejm 1988;318:65, 110)
- Viral URI in past 2 wk (Ann IM 1985;102:699), or chronic *Chlamydia pneumoniae* infections? (Ann IM 1996;125:979, 1992;116:273)

Decr incidence with: exercise, >6 METS >2 h/wk divided tiwqiw (Nejm 1994;330:1549); fish intake 1–4/mo (Jama 1995;274:1363; Nejm 1995;332:977; 1985;312:1205,1254); 2–3 alcoholic drinks qd (Nejm 1993;329:1829; Ann IM 1991;114:967) in men, vs 2–3/wk in women (Nejm 1995;332:1246); better control of hypertension, cholesterol, etc, in US (Nejm 1985;312:1005, 1053)

Pathophys: Platelet aggregations and thrombi (Nejm 1990;322:1549) on plaque fissures cause thrombosis w or without spasm (Nejm 1991;324:688; 1984;310:1137); or paradoxical vasoconstriction w stress because plaque prevents normal endothelial cell induction of coronary dilatation (Nejm 1991;325:1551)

Sx: Chest pain, substernal, in "distribution of a tree," worse supine; diaphoresis, dyspnea; associated with heavy exertion 5–40 × more frequently depending on conditioning state (Nejm 1984;311:874); CNS sx are the presenting sx in 50% of patients over age 60 yr. No recognizable sx ("silent") ± 25% (Ann IM 2001;135:801), and even in women w h/o ASHD 5% still silent (Ann IM 2001;134:1043)

Si: Pericardial rub on day 2^+, usually without ST changes (Nejm 1984; 311:1211); S_4 gallop; fever <103°F (<39.4°C); transient S_2 paradoxical split

Right ventricular infarct syndrome (Nejm 1998;338:978; 1994;330: 1211): acute inferior MI, Kussmaul's si (paradoxical increases in JVP with inspiration) (Ann IM 1983;99:608), high CVP with low PAPs and PCWPs so all nearly equal, like pericardial tamponade (J. Love 3/95, Nejm 1983;309:39,551), low cardiac output; occurs in 50% of IWMI pts (Nejm 1993;328:982) but clinically significant in 30% (Nejm 1988;338:978) and nearly 100% of those w CPK levels >2000 IU (J. Sutherland 1/96); reversible w reperfusion rx (Nejm 1998;338:933)

Rectal exam important for guaiac and detection of BPH (Nejm 1969; 281:238; 1970;282:167)

CARDIOLOGY

Crs: 33% are "silent" and unrecognized (Ann IM 1995;122:96) vs 25% are unrecognized, half of these are asx, yet prognosis just as bad (Framingham—Nejm 1984;311:1144); 15% in hospital mortality before thrombolytics, now 7–10%; 10% of survivors get severe pump failure, another 10% get persistent angina, 10% "flunk" discharge mini-ETT, another 10% "flunk" maximal ETT at 6 wk; remaining 50% do fine (Nejm 1986;314:161)

Prognosis is similar for Q-wave and non-Q-wave infarcts (Am J Med 2000;108:381) although non-Q-wave MIs are followed by more infarcts and angina but are associated w less CHF (Jama 1992;268:1545); is not affected by 1st-degree heart block, PVCs, or Vtach (Ann IM 1992;117:31), RBBB (Ann IM 1972;77:677), or type A personality (Nejm 1985;312:737); better prognosis if preinfarction angina preceded (Nejm 1996;334:7)

Age-adjusted 6 mo survival for women under age 75 is 15% worse than for men (Nejm 1999;341:217; 1998;338:8; Jama 1998; 280:1405) primarily because have worse MIs

Concomitant RV infarct increases IWMI mortality from 6% to 30% (Nejm 1993;328:982); mitral regurgitation, when severe, is associated w a 50% 1-yr mortality despite all interventions (Ann IM 1992;117:18)

Cardiac arrest survival is 45% if bystanders start CPR (Ann IM 1979; 90:737), 11% otherwise (Nejm 1972;286:976)

In elderly, aggressive invasive study and rx does not improve mortality (US vs. Canadian 65+ yr olds—Nejm 1997;336:1500)

Cmplc:
- Altered binding proteins change meaning of measured levels of quinidine (Ann IM 1987;107:48), cholesterol, etc.
- Aneurysm of left ventricular, occurs in 40% with anterior MI, develops in first 48 h, leads to emboli, CHF, and PVCs, 60% 1-yr mortality (Nejm 1984;311:100), although rate may be lower now w thrombolysis
- Anxiety neurosis (Mod Concepts Cardiovasc Dis 1975;44:59), impotence (Ann IM 1980;92:514)
- Arrhythmias esp. PVCs and Vtach
- CHF
- Dressler's syndrome (Arch IM 1959;103:38)

- Heart block (p 73) (Mod Concepts Cardiovasc Dis 1976;45:129) occurs in 5% of inferior MIs, 3% of anterior MIs, and in 100% with anterior MI + RBBB causing 75% mortality
- Mural thrombi without aneurysm in 11% of acute MIs, 2% of others (J Am Coll Cardiol 1993;22:1004)
- Papillary muscle rupture causes CHF with a normal sized left atrium by TEE, occurs most often with inferior MIs (Nejm 1969;281:1458), rx with nitrites (Ann IM 1975;83:313, 422), and surgery (Ann IM 1979;90:149)
- Pericardial tamponade from inflammation (r/o RV infarct—Nejm 1983;309:39,551) since both functionally acutely constrict pericardial space by fluid or dilated RV (J. Love 3/95)
- Rupture of septal wall, usually day 3–5, to create a VSD (Circ 2000;101:27; Nejm 1972;287:1064), or rupture into pericardial sack causing tamponade (Nejm 1996;334:319)
- Shock (7.5%—Nejm 1991;325:1117); immediate revascularization improves survival (Jama 2001;285:190)
- Stroke, esp if EF <28% post MI (Nejm 1997;336:251), prevent w warfarin anticoagulation

Lab:

Chem: Enzymes (Ann IM 1986;105:221):

CPK and fractions up in 12 h, peak at 2 d, last 4 d; CPK-MB subfractions MB2 and MB1 in 1st 6 h after onset of pain have 95% sens/specif and may be used to send home from ER (Nejm 1994;331:561,607); total CPK correlates with MI size; may double in MI but still be less than upper limit of normal (Am J Cardiol 1983;51:24); MB band is incr also by incr death and regeneration of skeletal muscle (Ann IM 1981;94:341) and by decreased clearance in myxedema; MM is incr by hypothyroidism, myopathy; BB band is incr by CNS and/or smooth muscle damage (Bull Rheum Dis 1983;33[2]:1)

LDH and fx's: isoenzymes 4 and 5 (rapidly migrating) incr, r/o renal and red cell source

AST (SGOT) up in 24 h, peaks at 2–4 d, lasts up to 7 d

Malondialdehyde (MDA)-modified LDL >0.85 mg% (Jama 1999; 281:1718), 95% sens and specif for unstable angina or MI; combined w troponin I, is 99% sens and specif

Troponin I and T levels elevate over first 8 hr (84–96% sens, 80–95% specif)(J Fam Pract 2000;49:550) and stay up for 7–10 d; "false pos" levels really represent ischemia (Nejm 1997;337:1648,1687);

levels correlate w worse outcomes (Nejm 1996;335:1333,1342, 1388); also useful perioperatively when surgery may increase CPK (Nejm 1994;330:670)

Noninv Lab: (Ann IM 1989;110:470; Nejm 1983;309:90)

Echo for mitral regurgitation, aneurysm, ejection fraction estimation, and mural thrombi with 77% sens and 93% specif (Nejm 1982;306:1509)

EKG (p 123) may show ST elevations (50% sens), duration of elevation correlates with extent of injury (Nejm 1969;280:123), T inversions much less specif (r/o acute cholecystitis—Ann IM 1992;116:218). In RV infarct, ST elevations present in V_1, or $V_{3-6}R$, especially V_4R w 80^+% sens/specif (Nejm 1993;328:981). See Fig. 2.2.1

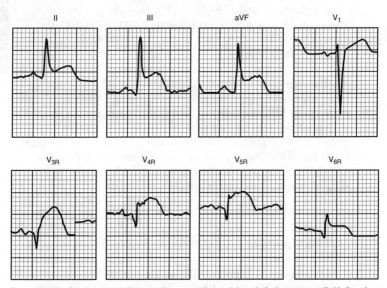

Figure 2.2.1   An electrocardiogram from a patient with an inferior myocardial infarction and right ventricular infarction.   ST-segment elevation is evident in leads II, III, and aVF, with the associated right ventricular myocardial infarction indicated by Q waves and ST-segment elevation in the right precordial leads (V_{3R} through V_{6R}). (Reproduced with permission from Kinch J. Ryan T. Current Concepts - Right ventricular Infarction, Nejm 1994;330:1214, Copyright Mass. Medical Society.)

New RBBB or LBBB indicate occlusion of anterior descending proximal to 1st septal branch (Nejm 1993;328:1036), both worsen prognosis (Ann IM 1998;129:690)

ETT (Circ 1996;94:2341): if angina or CHF in the hospital, do a submax ETT to 5 METS or 70% predicted at 4–6d post MI on therapy, estimates prognosis (Nejm 1979;301:341), perhaps with thallium (85% sens/specif—Ann IM 1990;113:684,703); if asx, full ETT with or without thallium at 10–14 d or if did submax then at 2–3 wk, predicts 5-yr survival (Ann IM 1987;106:793)

Holter monitor at 4–7 d post MI for ST depressions possibly better than submax ETT (Nejm 1996;334:65); or at 1–3 mo after MI, better than ETT? (Nejm 1981;304:376)

Xray: Ventriculogram with technetium scan; eject fraction, if <40%, 1-yr mortality climbs steeply from 5% (Nejm 1983;309:331)

Rx:

Preventive interventions:

- ASA tab qod (Nejm 1992;327:175; 1989;321:129) or qd 75–325 mg (Ann IM 1996;124:292; Med Let 1995;37:14) after angina or MI, or as part of rx of HT (Lancet 1998;351:1755)
- Dietary interventions like lowering cholesterol helps by meta-analysis (Nejm 1990;323:1112) as does American Heart Association diet (BMJ 1992;304:1015) and "Mediterranean diet" (p 52). As primary prevention, NNT-5 = 53; as secondary prevention, NNT-5 = 16 (J Fam Pract 1996;42:577)
- Estrogen replacement rx (p 624) may help
- Perioperative β blockers like atenolol 5–10 mg iv per and post op + 50 mg po bid during hospitalization decr risk of cardiac morbidity/mortality by 11% (Nejm 1996;335:1713,1761)
- Smoking cessation decreases risk to baseline in 3 yr (Nejm 1990; 322:213); probably ok to use nicotine patch post MI (Nejm 1996; 335:1792)

Post-MI preventive interventions: above, plus

- β blocker within 24 h of MI and cont'd indefinitely (Bmj 1999; 318:1730; Jama 1998;280:623), improves survival even if elderly, low EF, non-Q wave MI, or have COPD (NNT-2 = 10) (Nejm 1998;339:489—but not an RCT); like metoprolol 5 mg iv q 5 min × 3 then 50 mg po bid × 1 d then 100 mg bid, or atenolol 50–100 mg po qd if no contraindications, helps prevent recurrent MIs (Circ 1994;90:762; TIMI study—Nejm 1989;320:618); and fatal ventricular arrhythmias; use in elderly as well (Jama 1997;

277:115) in post-Q-wave MI, increases survival for 6$^+$ yr (timolol—Nejm 1985;313:1055), all work (Med Let 1982;24:44)

- ACE inhibitors within 24 h of MI (Circ 1998;97:2202) especially if anterior MI, CHF, elevated pulse; and for 6 wk (Lancet 1994; 343:1115); cont'd indefinitely if EF <40% (J Am Coll Cardiol 1996;27:337; Ann IM 1994;121:750; Nejm 1992;327:669, 1992;327:629, 685); like captopril 50 mg tid, increases ETT performance and decreases LV size (Nejm 1988;319:80), or ramipril 2.5–5 mg po bid (Lancet 1997;349:1493); especially in anterior MIs (Nejm 1995;332:80); prolong life after MI even if no sx (Med Let 1994;36:69)
- Statin (HMG CoA) lipid rx post-MI reduces further MIs and mortality (NNT-5 = 30–33—Nejm 1996;335:1001, Lancet 1994; 344:1383; or better, NNT-1 = 25—Jama 2001;285:430)); rx LDL to <100 mg% (Jama 1997;277:1281; Nejm 1997;336:153); helps in elderly age 65–75 too (Ann IM 1998;129:681)
- Fibrate rx of HDL <40 mg%, eg, w gemfibrosil (Nejm 1999; 341:410); for MI, NNT-5 = 23 (ACP J Club 2000;132:44)
- Anticoagulation with warfarin helps post-MI for years (Nejm 1990;323:147), controversial
- In all diabetics, continuous iv insulin × 24 h then qid sc × yrs, improves survival, NNT-1 = 13 (J Am Coll Cardiol 1995;26:57)

Of acute MI (Nejm 1997;336:847; Circ 1996;94:2341):

- ASA 325 mg po stat helps survival dramatically (Nejm 1997; 336:847)
- Thrombolysis w streptokinase, TPA, etc. (p 48) (Nejm 1993; 329:703,723,1650; Ann IM 1990;112:529; 1990;113:907,949, 961; Mod Concepts Cardiovasc Dis 1991;60:19,25; 1990;59:7, 13); perhaps by ambulance crews (Nejm 1993;329:383); helps all pts including those over age 75 yr (Nejm 1992;327:7) although intracranial bleeding risk increases from <1/2% under 65, to 2.5% over 75 (Ann IM 1998;129:597), hence still unclear if should use over age 75 (Circ 2000;101:2239); if sys BP ≥175 or dias ≥100, bleeding risk is double (Ann IM 1996;125:891); use if pain is <6 h duration, or if 6–12 h and STs still elevated (Lancet 1996;348:771, 1993;342:759,767) or LBBB and good story (Jama 1999;281:714; Ann IM 1998;129:690); does not help ST depressions which should be rx'd w TNG, ASA, and heparin. Give

concomitantly or follow either with heparin iv × 1⁺ d (Nejm 1990;323:1433) + ASA 160 mg po qd + β blocker (Ann IM 1991;115:34). CPK-MB and troponin T levels should rise 5 × at 60 min and 5–10 × at 90 min to indicate reperfusion (90% sens, ~65% specif) (J Am Coll Cardiol 1998;31:1499)

- β blocker and ACEI rx as above
- Nitroglycerin, as patch or iv if volume ok especially if cont'd pain, perhaps even if no pain; especially helpful if any element of CHF or if large anterior MI; avoid if recent sildenafil (Viagra) use
- MgSO₄ (J Am Coll Cardiol 1996;28:1328; Circ 1996;94:2341) 1–2 gm bolus over 5 min, then drip over 24 h; if long QT or Mg low, perhaps for all but esp if elderly; improves survival (incr only from 89% to 92%) (Lancet 1992;339:1553) vs no help in ISIS-4 (Lancet 1995;345:669)
- Insulin iv then sc qid x mos in all? diabetics, decr mortality at 1⁺ yr, NNT-1 = 15, NNT-3 = 10 (Bmj 1997;314:1512)
- CCU care; can move out within 24 h if no couplets and EKG and CPK negative (Nejm 1980;302:943).
- Rehab programs probably help (ACP J Club 1999;131:41) over 3 mo if 3 wk post-MI ETT achieves <8 METS (Ann IM 1988; 109:650,671). Get 3-wk post-MI ETT and return to work at 4 wk unless severe ischemia (Ann IM 1992;117:383; Nejm 1992; 327:227)
- Angioplasty (PCTA) (Nejm 1994;330:981), standard now for acute MI in high volume centers; or do after thrombolysis if sx or ischemia on discharge submaximal ETT or 3 wk maximal ETT, no advantage sooner (Nejm 1987;317:581) or if no ischemia, ie, "ischemia guided rx" (Nejm 1998;338;1785,1838; Circ 1992; 86:1400; TIMI—Nejm 1989;320:618); better success in high volume centers (Nejm 2000;342:1573)

Possibility of using as acute primary, rx w stenting and abciximab, of evolving acute MI rather than thrombolysis, looks promising if available (Nejm 2000;343:385; 1999;341:1413; ACP J Club 1998;129(3):64; even in elderly—Jama 1999;282:341)

- CABG after angiography if low eject fraction (21–49%) and multivessel disease, or left main disease; can do it 1 mo post-MI (Nejm 1982;307:1065). For all non-Q-wave MIs, angiography and invasive rx if ETT 1 mo post-MI is severely abnormal (Nejm 1990;322:943); diltiazem 90 mg po q 6 h until then

CARDIOLOGY

Of complications:

- Bradyarrhythmias: rx in IWMI only if pain, PVCs, CHF, or pulse <45/min and unstable, then pace (Nejm 1975;292:572); in anterior MI, pace to prevent 20–40% evolving to complete heart block if anterior MI + RBBB, RBBB + left anterior hemiblock, RBBB + left posterior hemiblock, or LBBB; bifascicular block evolving into trifascicular block during MI needs permanent pacer even if returns to normal later (Mod Concepts Cardiovasc Dis 1976;45:129)
- CHF/shock: dobutamine (Nejm 1980;303:846) + nitroprusside acutely; or perhaps early revascularization to improve on 60% mortality (Nejm 1999;341:625); ACE inhibitors as above
- Mural thrombi in anterior MI, prevent with heparin to PTTs ~48 s for 10 d, sc not enough (Nejm 1989;320:352)
- Papillary muscle rupture acutely, surgery sooner not later (Nejm 1996;335:1417)
- Pericarditis should not be rx'd with indomethacin, which can cause spasm (Nejm 1981;305:1171); other NSAIDs better
- RV infarct, increase preload w iv saline, avoid nitrates and diuretics (lower preload), dobutamine drip, nitroprusside drip, sequential pacing, isoproterenol to unload RV (Nejm 1993;328:982)
- Ventricular arrhythmias: lidocaine; later amiodarone or implantable defibrillator for sudden death survivors (Circ 1995; 91:2195)
- Wall rupture or VSD development, surgery if slow (Nejm 1983; 309:539)

CONGESTIVE HEART FAILURE

Jama 1997;277:1712 (clinical correlates), Mod Concepts Cardiovasc Dis 1990;59:43,49,63

Cause: ASHD, dilated (systolic dysfunction), or hypertensive (diastolic dysfunction) cardiomyopathy; occasionally valve disease; and more rarely A-V malformations, Paget's disease, hyperthyroidism, beriberi, severe anemia as with pernicious anemia, multiple myeloma rarely (Nejm 1988;319:1652), tocolytic rx of premature labor (Ann IM 1989;110:714), NSAIDs in elderly (Rx Let 2000;7:25)

Epidem: Associated with hypertension in 40% of men and 60% of women (Jama 1996;275:1557), systolic BP >160 just as significant as a diastolic >95. In US, incidence is 400,000/yr

Pathophys: (Ann IM 1994;121:363; Nejm 1990;322:100)

Most CHF is due to systolic dysfunction, but 10–30% is due to diastolic dysfunction (Nejm 2001;344:1756), eg, chronic systemic hypertension, mitral stenosis, constrictive pericarditis, IHSS, etc., conditions which prevent normal diastolic filling. Hypertrophy in response to load creates dysfunctional myocardial cells (Ann IM 1994;121:363). ACE inhibitors, β blockers, and calcium channel blockers may help relax hypertrophic myocardium as well as decrease afterload (Ann IM 1992;117:502; Nejm 1991;325:1557). Inadequate production of endogenous atrial natriuretic peptide, an atrial hormone that promotes diuresis (Nejm 1998;339:321; 1986;315:533). Cardiac asthma is due to bronchial edema and hyperresponsiveness (Nejm 1989;320:1317)

Sx: Dyspnea on exertion, orthopnea, paroxysmal nocturnal dyspnea, ankle edema, bowel bloating and sense of fullness pc, nocturia

NY Heart Association Classification:

I. No dyspnea on moderate exertion
II. Dyspnea w moderate exertion; 25% 4 yr mortality
III. Dyspnea w mild exertion; 50% 4 yr mortality
IV. Dsypnea at rest; 50%/yr mortality

Si: JVD, S_3 gallop (techniques—Nejm 2001;345:612); both correlate w worse prognosis (Nejm 2001;345:574)

Pulse >100 (pulse > dias BP = 53% sens, 80% specif—Bmj 2000; 320:220); displaced point of maximal impulse, dullness in L 5th intercostal space ≥10.5 cm from sternum (Am J Med 1991; 91:328); pleural effusions R > L (Nejm 1983;308:696).

Central apnea in 45%, especially Cheyne-Stokes respirations from incr sens to pCO_2 (Nejm 1999;341:949,985), rx w theophylline 250 mg po bid (Nejm 1996;335:562)

Crs: 70$^+$% 5-yr mortality if due to hypertension (Framingham—Jama 1996;275:1557), 50% 1-yr mortality after start medications; over age 70, 70% 2-yr mortality after pulmonary edema (Ann IM 1971;75:332)

Cmplc: Sleep apnea (Ann IM 1995;122:487)

Lab:

Chem: Hyponatremia due to inappropriate ADH (Nejm 1981;305: 263); N-atrial natriuretic peptide level >0.8 nM/L, 43% sens, 90% specif (Bmj 2000;320:220)

CARDIOLOGY

Hem: ESR low when acute and severe, correlates with fibrinogen levels (Nejm 1991;324:353)

Inv monitoring: Swan-Ganz monitoring now discouraged because of incr morb and mort (Jama 2001;286:309), use only when cardiac output and/or wedge data will change rx; in and out as quickly as possible (Ann IM 1985;103:445) since cmplc are pulmonary infarction, pulmonary artery rupture, knotting, endocardial thrombosis (50%), subsequent endocarditis (8%) (Nejm 1984; 311:1152)

Urine: Proteinuria, why? (Nejm 1982;306:1031)

Xray: Chest shows redistribution of blood to apices on upright, perihilar "haze," Kerley B lines, incr heart size, pleural effusions R > L (Nejm 1983;308:696) possibly because thoracic duct provides a "pop-off valve" to L pulmonary vasculature, ie, better lymphatic drainage (J. Sutherland 6/95)

Rx: (Nejm 1996;335:490; Ann IM 1994;121:363)

Acute:

- O_2 at 2–3 L/min (Ann IM 1989;111:777) w CPAP (Nejm 1991; 325:1825)
- Dobutamine iv acutely best choice immediately post-MI, better than dig or diuretics, no arrhythmias, short half-life (Nejm 1980; 303:846)
- Nitrates, eg, nitroprusside iv or nitroglycerine iv drip
- Experimental atrial natriuretic peptide, nesiritide iv (Nejm 2000; 343:246)

Chronic: (see medication section p 34 for dosing) (Med Let 1999; 41:12; Nejm 1998;339:1848). Generally use ACE inhibitors and other vasodilators, diuretics, + digitalis (Nejm 1993;329:1; Mod Concepts Cardiovasc Dis 1990;59:49)

- Exercise training helps (Jama 2000;283:3095; Circ 1999;99:1173; Ann IM 1996;125:1051)
- Avoid NSAIDs (Rx Let 2000;7:25), especially if hyponatremia (Nejm 1984;310:347), and most calcium channel blockers (Nejm 1996;335:1107)
- ACE inhibitors alone increase survival from 50% to 73% at 6 mo (Jama 1995;273:1450; Med Let 1994;36:69; Nejm 1987;316: 1429) to doses of enalapril 20 mg qd, or lisinopril 30 mg qd (Circ 1999;100:2312), or captopril 150 mg qd (Rx Let 1999;6:13); may

need to decrease diuretic doses to avoid hypotension; less effective in blacks (Nejm 2001;344:1351). Or ARA like losartan (Cozaar) 12.5–50 mg po qd or valsartan 80 mg qd–160 bid if cough or angioedema prevent ACEI use, may also improve mortality (Lancet 2000;355:1582; 1997;349:747)

- β blockers (Med Let 2000;42:54) to reduce sympathetic tone, improve survival even in severe CHF if can tolerate (Nejm 2001; 344:1651,1659,1711; Jama 2000;283:1295; Lancet 1999;353:9; Can J Cardiol 1998;14:1045; Nejm 1998;339:1759; 1996;334: 1349; Med Let 1996;38:93)
  - Metoprolol 12.5–25 mg of CR/XL type or in tid doses titrated up to 100–200 mg po qd, or
  - Bisoprolol (Zebeta) 1.25–10 mg po qd, or
  - Carvedilol (Coreg) 3.125–25 mg po bid
- Spironolactone (Med Let 1999;41:81) 12.5–25 mg po qd, if creat <2.5 mg%, used w ACEI and digoxin improves survival and hospitalization by 30% (Nejm 1999;341:709, 753)
- Diuretics like thiazides, furosemide, and occasionally metolazone (Zaroxolyn), always use with ACEIs; decreased po absorption with incr CHF (Ann IM 1985;102:314); transient CHF worsening for 20 min via renin-angiotensin system (Ann IM 1985;103:1)
- Nitrates, eg, nitroprusside acutely, or TNG paste 1–5 in. q 3–6 h, or isosorbide up to 40 mg po t-qid also clearly shown to prolong life
- Inotropes like digitalis glycosides, especially if S_3 gallop (Ann IM 1984;101:113; Nejm 1982;306:699) and/or EF <35% (Nejm 1993;329:1), decreases admission for CHF but doesn't decr mortality (Nejm 1997;336:525); amrinone ok acutely but decreases platelets chronically po, no increase in survival (Lancet 1994;344:493 vs ACP J Club 1995;122(2):33)
  - Vasodilators such as hydralazine especially w nitrates when ACEI intolerant
  - Co-enzyme Q10 (Clin Investig 1993;71:S134) 50 mg po b-tid, incr mitochondrial ATPase and decr CHF cmplc; experimental
if IVCD (QRS >0.15 sec), atriobiventricular pacing improves sx and function (Nejm 2001;344:873)

Surgical: heart transplant, 3500/yr in US, 65% 5 yr survival (Jama 1998;280:1692)

of Cheyne-Stokes breathing: O_2 or CPAP improves survival (Nejm 1999;341:985)

2.3 ARRHYTHMIAS

PAROXYSMAL SUPRAVENTRICULAR TACHYCARDIAS

Cause: Aberrant conduction pathways with different conduction rates within the AV node **(AV nodal reentrant tachycardia)** (AVNRT), or outside the AV node **(AV rentrant tachycardia, Wolff-Parkinson-White syndrome)** (AVRT, WPW) (p 72) allowing setup of circus movement continous stimulation when the aberrant or usual pathway conducts retrograde; or ectopic irritable atrial focus **(paroxysmal atrial tachycardia)** (PAT), often associated with digoxin toxicity especially if manifest w associated block, eg, 2:1 or 3:1

Epidem: AVNRT and AVRT of about equal prevalence and each represent about 45% of all PSVTs; PAT constitutes 9%, and rare other syndromes like **permanent junctional reentrant tachycardia** (PJRT), the last 1%

Pathophys: Re-entrant tachycardias occur w things that increase excitability, decrease refractory period, and increase conduction velocity. See Fig. 2.3.1

Sx: Paroxysmal episodes of palpitations often associated with dizziness, nausea; precipitated by caffeine, alcohol, nicotine, hyperthyroid states, ephedrine in diet supplements, etc.; often relieved by Valsalva maneuver by patient. Neck pounding in AVNRT types but not accessory pathway (WPW or AVRT) SVT because nearly coincident atrial and ventricular contraction in AVNRT cause cannon waves in neck, which can be felt (Nejm 1992;327:772)

Si: Tachycardia 150–210/min

Crs: Recurrent from teenage years on

Cmplc: Rare permanent junctional reentrant tachycardia variant associated with myocardiopathy stays in arrhythmia a long time, reversible if rx'd

Post-PAT T-wave inversions may last days–weeks (Nejm 1995;332:161)

Lab: EKG shows SVT w narrow complexes; AVNRT usually has no apparent P waves, AVRT has Ps closer to the last QRS than to the next one, and PAT and PJRT have Ps closer to the next QRS and beyond the T wave. PSVT is very regular, even when aberrant and wide, unlike Vtach; QRS aberrancy always <0.14 sec whereas Vtach often (>50%) >0.14 sec, axis is −30° to +120° unlike the

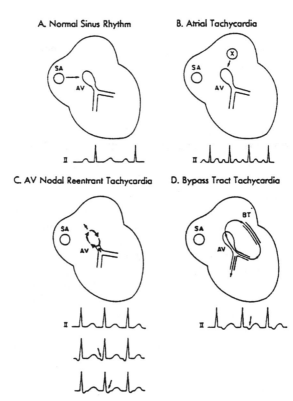

Figure 2.3.1 Major types of paroxysmal supraventricular tachycardia (PSVT). (Reproduced with permission from Goldberger AL, Goldberger E, eds. Supraventricular arrhythmias. In: Clinical electrocardiography. 5th ed. St. Louis: Mosby, 1994:159.)

LAD with Vtach 60% of time (J. Love 9/85) (see Brugada criteria p 56)

Rx: Carotid sinus pressure

Adenosine 6–12 mg iv, gone in 10 sec, potentiated by dipyridamole and carbamazepine, inhibited by theophyllines (Med Let 1990;32:63); or verapamil 5–10 mg iv; perhaps propranolol iv 1–5 mg

Electrical cardioversion with sync if meds fail or if unstable, ok to do even if dig on board as long as levels therapeutic and not toxic, and K+ ok (Ann IM 1981;95:676); in resistant cases, implanted atrial burst pacers (Ann IM 1987;107:144) or catheter ablation of atrial slow pathway works 95% of the time (Med Let 1996;38:40; Nejm 1994;330:1481).

For chronic prevention: avoid stimulants; β blockers; maybe verapamil or digoxin though both can worsen some

ATRIAL FIBRILLATION (Afib)(Nejm 2001;344:1066), FLUTTER (Aflut) AND RELATED TACHYCARDIAS
[including **WAP, MFAT** (Nejm 1990;322:1713), and **SSS** (Mod Concepts Cardiovasc Dis 1980;49:61, 67)]

Cause: Associated with: normal variations, idiopathic, CHF, and rheumatic heart disease (Framingham—Nejm 1982;306:1018), atrial dilatation (eg, in mitral stenosis or regurgitation), pericarditis, COPD especially with hypoxia and bronchodilators (Nejm 1968; 279:344), ASHD; w hyperthyroidism especially in the elderly as measured by low TSH, which has a 30% 10-yr incidence in contrast to 10% 10-yr incidence w normal TSH (Nejm 1994;331:1252) and w toxic multinodular goiter; w alcoholic myocardiopathy

Aflut and MFAT often (60%) from pulmonary disease including pulmonary emboli

Epidem: Common; supraventricular prematures are not associated with ASHD or sudden death (Ann IM 1969;70:1159)

Pathophys:

Sx: Polyuria, palpitations, faintness

Si:

Crs:

Cmplc: Chronic Afib causes embolic CVA in 20% if recent CHF, HT, or previous embolus (Ann IM 1992;116:1) but <1%/yr if none of those and no increase in LA size or LV dyskinesis on echo (Ann IM 1992;116:6); likewise others find rate only 1.3% after 15 yr where no other disease and under age 60 (Nejm 1987;317:699); embolic CVA incr × 5 in ASHD type compared to age-matched controls, ×17 in rheumatic (Neurol 1978;28:973).

In SSS, 16% develop arterial emboli (Nejm 1976;295:190)

r/o hyperthyroidism, silent mitral stenosis, alcoholic myocardiopathy, and pulm embolism

Lab:

Chem: TSH

Noninv: EKG: SSS is diagnosed by SVTs alternating w some heart block, and suggested by P <90 after 1–2 mg atropine, or asystole >3 sec after carotid sinus massage.

MFAT, P >100, and ≥3 different PR intervals and P-wave morphologies; looks superficially like AF but digoxin won't help it; WAP is same thing but rate <100

Holter to find, when intermittent; or better, event monitor (Ann IM 1996;124:16)

Echo, TEE is 99% specific, 100% sens for LA thrombus (Ann IM 1995;123:817).

Rx: (Med Let 1991;33:55); in pregnancy (Ann IM 1983;98:487); all but β blockers may prolong or cause ventricular arrhythmias (Ann IM 1992;117:141)

• Afib: (Nejm 2001;344:1067)

Perioperative prevention post CABG w amiodarone (Nejm 1997;337:1785)

Rate control: iv verapamil, diltiazem, β blocker like esmolol, or digoxin but latter's rate is easily overridden by catechol/exercise stimulation (Ann IM 1991;114:573)

Conversion: especially if LA size is <50 mm, use cardioversion (Mod Concepts Cardiovasc Dis 1989;58:61); embolic risk post conversion in 1st 48 h ≤1% but if >48 h is 5–7% (Ann IM 1997;126:65), but if unknown onset and TEE negative, can start warfarin × 4 wk and procede w immediate cardioversion w/o incr embolic risk (Nejm 2001;344:1411; Ann IM 1997;126:200 vs Ann IM 1995;123:882)

Medical conversion w: amiodarone 30 mg/kg po × 1 converts 87% (NNT = 2) (Am J Cardiol 2000;85:462; Ann IM 1992;116:1017); propafenone (Rythmol) 300 mg po, converts 75% w/i 8 hr safely (Ann IM 1997;126:621), not yet FDA approved; or ibutilide (Corvert) 1 mg iv over 10 min, repeat × 1 (Med Let 1996;38:38); perhaps w procainamide, dofetilide 500 mg po bid (Med Let 2000;42:41), or clonidine 0.075 mg po repeat in 2 h by decreasing sympathetic tone (Ann IM 1992;116:388); digoxin alone is no better than placebo (Ann IM 1987;106:503)

Electrical cardioversion with sync and w transthoracic or esophageal-transthoracic paddles (R. Fletcher 1/00) if unstable or eventually if meds fail, ok to do even if dig on board as long as levels therapeutic and not toxic, and K^+ ok (Ann IM 1981;95:676); start at 300 J not lower (Am J Cardiol 2000;86:348);

Maintenance rx: amiodarone 200 mg po qd (Arch IM 1998;158:1669; Ann IM 1992;116:1017) cheapest and best (Heart 2000;84:251); sotalol or other β blocker; verapamil; or digoxin, which controls resting but not exercise rate; quinidine? (Nejm 1998;338:37) po which holds in NSR better but death rate is 3× placebo (Circ 1990;82:1106), or procainamide; possibly dofetilide esp if in CHF (Med Let 2000;42:41; Nejm 1999;341:857,910); or flecainide but tricky (p 39)

Anticoagulate chronic (Ann IM 1999;131:688; Jama 1999;281:182; Nejm 1992;327:1451) or intermittent AF if can clinically with warfarin (Nejm 1990;322:863) to INR >2 but <4 best balances risk and benefits (Lancet 1996;348:633; Nejm 1996;335:540,587, 1995;333:5) which reduces risk of CVA from 7% to 1–2% at any age (NNT-1.5 = 25) (Circ 1991;84:527; Nejm 1990;323:1505) especially in SSS variant (Nejm 1976;295:190). Annual bleeding risk ~2.5% (Ann IM 1992;116:6); chronic AF anticoagulation benefit very small (NNT = 200) (Ann IM 1999;131:492) to nonexistent (Ann IM 1994;121:41,54) if very low risk: age <60 yr, no h/o TIA, no valve disease, normal echo, and no hypertension. Use ASA if can't use warfarin (Ann IM 1999;131:492; Nejm 1990;323:1505) or low risk (Jama 2001;285:2864)

Radioablation of ectopic foci which are often in pulmonary veins (Nejm 1998;339:659); or maze creation surgery (R. Fletcher 1/00)

Ablation of AV node w permanent pacer (Nejm 2001;344:1043)

- Aflut: carotid sinus pressure trial, then rx as Afib above; radioablation much more clearly helpful
- MFAT: rx the primary disease, usually COPD or sepsis; verapamil iv with pretreatment with iv $CaCl_2$ (Ann IM 1987;107:623) or po for chronic; Mg iv, especially if low; β blockers if no COPD
- SSS: permanent pacer preferably w atrial pacing to reduce emboli (Lancet 1994;344:1523), then medications to control tachycardias

WOLFF-PARKINSON-WHITE (WPW) SYNDROME

Mod Concepts Cardiovasc Dis 1989;58:43

Cause: Aberrant conduction pathways around the AV node; sometimes are inherited as autosomal dominant single amino acid substitution in a protein kinase gene on chromosome #7 (Nejm 2001;344:1823), and sometimes are developmental (Nejm 1987;317:65)

Epidem: Common

Pathophys: Circus movements set up between the atria and ventricle via the aberrant pathway antegrade and/or retrograde causing the recurrent tachycardias

Sx: Recurrent tachycardias, feel like "butterflies" in the chest. Often precipitated by alcohol, coffee, smoking, and other stimulants

Si: When asx, none; when in PAT, pulse = 180; or less commonly in Afib, pulse is irregular and fast

Crs: (Ann IM 1992;116:456)

Recurrent tachycardias over years in 1/2 found in asx phase; rarely limiting or fatal, 0/20 deaths in Manitoba heart study; disappears over several years in many cases

Cmplc: Sudden death; fatigue

Lab:

Noninv: EKG has a short PR interval (<0.12 sec, usually <0.10) with delta wave; type A, most common, has large R in V_1 from an accessory pathway in left lateral atrium (Am J Cardiol 1987;59: 1093). r/o **Lown-Ganong-Levine syndrome,** similar but no delta wave, ie, no antegrade conduction; Fabry's disease (Nejm 1973;289: 357). See Fig. 2.3.2

Rx: of PSVT, electrical cardioversion w synchronizer on if unstable acutely, otherwise procainamide (Med Let 1996;38:75) or propranolol iv (Mod Concepts Cardiovasc Dis 1989;58:43); or adenosine 3–12 mg iv (Nejm 1991;325:1621) if not in Afib (p 3); digoxin or verapamil iv/po work but dangerous if in Afib with aberrancy (wide irregular QRS) present because can cause Vfib (Mod Concepts Cardiovasc Dis 1989;58:43; Nejm 1979;301:1080)

Cath lab ablation of accessory pathway (Nejm 1999;340:534; 1991;324:1605,1612) if sx

BRADYARRHYTHMIAS AND HEART BLOCKS

Nejm 2000;342:703

Cause: Digoxin, ASHD, congenital, granulomatous disease, metastatic calcification (Nejm 1971;284:1252)

Epidem: Rarely associated w HLA-B27 and aortic insufficiency (Ann IM 1997;127:621)

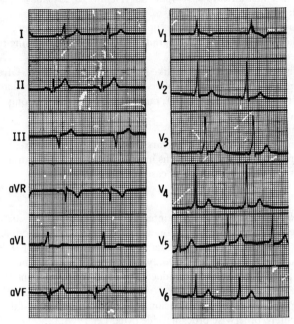

Figure 2.3.2 Wolff-Parkinson-White syndrome. (Reprinted with permission from Chung EK. Pocket guide to ECG diagnosis. Cambridge, MA: Blackwell Science, 1996:355.)

Pathophys: Congenital is associated w maternal autoantibody disease (SLE, Sjögren's, etc.), w anti-SSA (Ro antibodies) (Ann IM 1994;13:544)

Sx: 1st degree heart block usually causes no sx
2nd degree may cause dizziness or dyspnea
3rd degree may cause syncope, especially on standing

Si: 1st degree heart block = PR >0.22 sec
2nd degree = some unconducted P waves
3rd degree = no relationship between Ps and QRSs

Crs: 1st degree heart block usually benign if not associated with organic disease (Nejm 1986;315:1183)

Cmplc: r/o: Lyme disease if from endemic area, even if no other sx, w serology, rx with antibiotics and temporary not permanent pacer (Ann IM 1989;110:339)

Athletes' arrhythmias (Sports Med 1998;25:139), eg, 1st and 2nd degree (Mobitz I) heart blocks, sinus bradycardia, junctional rhythms; all from incr vagal tone, all go away w exercise and deconditioning

Lab:

Noninv: EKG; Holter monitor may still miss a majority of intermittent heart blocks (Nejm 1989;321:1703)

Mobitz I (Wenkebach) heart block; intranodal; progressively incr PR, then dropped beat w progressively shortening R-R; usually in A-V node, especially w digoxin or inferior MI/ischemia, but can occur in SA node (detect by closer and closer R-Rs), or in distal system if BBB conduction pattern

Mobitz II heart block, infranodal; fixed PR and dropped beats; R-R intervals of drop are exactly 2× the normal R-R interval, unlike Mobitz I; if several in a row, may have distal escape rythmn; usually going to need permanent pacing; r/o hyperkalemia and rarely meds (procainamide, quinidine, amiodareone) as causes

Rx: 1st degree may not need rx; 2nd and 3rd degree: isoproterenol iv or sl, atropine iv, theophylline 100 mg/min iv up to 250 mg (Ann IM 1995;123:509), or external pacer, until can get transvenous pacemaker

Transvenous pacemaker, temporary first, then permanent unless inferior MI, which will usually reverse spontaneously. Prophylactic pacers in bifascicular blocks only if 2 or more syncopes and even then questionable (Nejm 1982;307:137, 180). Placement with EKG guidance, sample leads (Nejm 1972;287:651). Coronary sinus placement ok for temporary; tip is seen posteriorly on lateral chest xray

Permanent pacemaker (rv—Ann IM 2001;134:1130; Nejm 1996;334:89; Mod Concepts Cardiovasc Dis 1991;60:31): dual-chamber "physiologic" types more expensive, use when need atrial kick (Ann IM 1986;105:264), mainly in pts w SSS (Nejm 1998;338:1097); use may decr later Afib incidence (Nejm 2000;342:1385). See Table 2.3.1

Thus a VVI pacer paces the ventricle, and senses ventricular beats by inhibiting the next paced beat.

Ventricular pacer cmplc: "pacer syndrome," coincident atrial and ventricular contractions from retrograde atrial activation cause low cardiac output sx (Ann IM 1985;103:420), tachyarrhythmias due to "endless loop" of PVC causing a retrograde P which is sensed,

CARDIOLOGY

Table 2.3.1 Pacer Nomenclature

Chamber Paced	Chamber Sensed	Sensing Mode of Response
Ventricle	V	Triggered
Atrium	A	Inhibited
Dual	D	D
	0 (none)	0 (none)

R added to designation if rate-adaptive capability present.

causing a V pace, causing a retrograde P which is sensed, etc, can occur with any sensing pacer. Cellular phone interference is minimal unless phone is put over pacer (Nejm 1997;336:1473)

PREMATURE VENTRICULAR CONTRACTIONS, VENTRICULAR TACHYCARDIA, AND SUDDEN DEATH

(Mod Concepts Cardiovasc Dis 1991;60:55; Nejm 1981;304:1004)

Cause: Idiopathic, scar from myocardiopathy (Nejm 1988;318:129) including alcoholic "holiday heart" (Ann IM 1983;98:135), or MI with re-entry, CHF, mitral prolapse syndrome, torsades de pointes (p 80)

In children, young adults (Nejm 1996;334:1039) and athletes (Jama 1996;276:199) most common causes are IHSS (36%), cardiomyopathies, congenital heart disease esp tetralogy of Fallot and pulmonic stenosis, long QT syndrome, mitral valve prolapse, cocaine, Marfan's w aortic dissection, anomalous coronary arteries (13%), Kawasaki's induced coronary aneurysms; rarely Vfib induced by "commotio cordis" blow to chest, eg, baseball at ascent of T wave (Nejm 1998;338:1805)

Epidem: Incr with tobacco, caffeine (not so!—Ann IM 1991;114:147), carbon monoxide levels >100 ppm (Ann IM 1990;113:343), alcohol (Nejm 1979;301:1049,1060), and subtle ST-T wave electrical alternans (Nejm 1994;330:235). Decreased 50% w weekly fish consumption (Jama 1998;279:23)

Pathophys: Incr sympathetic tone? (Nejm 1991;325:618)

Sx: Syncope which may progress to sudden death

Si: Vtach is mildly irregular by EKG, unlike very regular PSVT and Aflut with 2:1 block

Crs: Of sudden death: 47% 2-yr mortality after first episode; 86% if no MI, 16% if transmural MI (J. Love 2/86; Nejm 1982;306:1341; 1975;293: 259); if asx, prognosis very good even if complex arrhythmias or Vtach (Nejm 1985;312:193) even in pts w CHF (Circ 2000;101:40)

Of PVCs in asx men: 2x incidence of later MI or other cardiac event (Ann IM 1992;117:990)

Cmplc: r/o digoxin toxicity; mitral valve prolapse (p 96); "slow ventricular tachycardia" is a benign regular accelerated idioventricular rhythm <100/min and asx, seen often (30%) in inferior MIs;

Lab:

Noninv: EKG;

Vtach: unlike supraventricular tachycardias with aberrancy, Vtach QRSs are wide (85% >0.14 sec—0% false positives, 30% false negatives—J. Love 7/86), and are not as regular; however, 5% are ≥0.11 s because they originate close to the conduction system (Ann IM 1991;114:460).

Brugada criteria (98% overall sensitivity) indicating Vtach rather than SVT w aberrancy (Circ 1991;83:1649):
1. No precordial RS complex, ie, all pos or all neg (20% sens), or
2. Beginning of any precordial R to S nadir >0.10 sec (52% sens), or
3. AV dissociation present, or
4. RBBB pattern, LAD, R/S < 1 in V_6 and only positive R forces in V_1; or LBBB pattern + Q in V_6; and R in V_1 or V_2 >0.04, or beginning of R to S nadir in V_1 or V_2 >0.07, or notching of S down stroke in V_1 or V_2.

Holter monitor w exercise (Nejm 1993;329:445)

Rx: (Med Let 1991;33:55) (rv of w/u and rx of sudden death survivors—Mod Concepts Cardiovasc Dis 1986;55:61). See Fig. 2.3.3

Field defibrillation with external automatic defibrillator by BCLS personnel increases number of pts alive at hospital discharge from 20% to 30% (Seattle—Nejm 1988;319:661), 4% to 5.2% (Ontario—Jama 1999;281:1175) or as high as 75% if provided w/i 3 min (Nejm 2000;343:1206,1210,1259); in elderly >age 70 yr CPR success so low not worth it? (Ann IM 1989;111:199 vs Jama 1990;264:2109). If field trial unsuccessful, not worth continuing in ER (Nejm 1991;325:1393). Antiarrhythmic drug-induced type has the highest incidence within the 1st 3 d, so start drug rx in hospital (Nejm 1988;319:257)

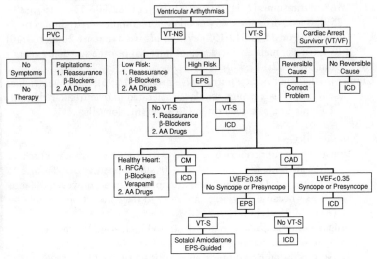

Figure 2.3.3 Treatment algorithm for patients with ventricular arrhythmias. (Reprinted with permission, Journal of the American Medical Association, 1999;281:176. Copyright 1999, American Medical Associaton.)

Acutely, if sustained, 1st chest thump; then cardioversion with 200–360 J; lidocaine, bretylium, procainamide, amiodarone, or sotalol (may be better when occurs w MI—Lancet 1994;334:18)

Chronic (Nejm 1994;331:785; Ann IM 1991;114:499): no clear evidence yet that rx increases survival but β blockers esp sotalol, and amiodarone used (Nejm 1998;338:35; Ann IM 1994;121:529); huge natural variability day to day and month to month (Nejm 1985;313:1444)

After sudden death episode, immediate angiography (Nejm 1997; 336:1629) and try stopping all drugs; then:

  • Implantable defibrillator (Nejm 2000;133:901; Med Let 1994;36:86), after EP studies, 1st choice over antiarrhythmics in post-sudden death survivors (Nejm 1997;337:1577; Circ 1995; 91:2195), and in post-MI pts w EF <35–40% and documented asx runs of Vtach, this approach decreases the 30% 2 yr mortality

by 50–75% (Nejm 1999;341:1882; 1996;335:1933) vs no better
than amiodarone rx? (Circ 2000;101:1297)

- Antiarrhythmics, debatably (Nejm 1999;341:1882) like β blockers
  even if CHF, RAD, DM, elevated lipids (Ann IM 1995;123:358),
  eg, metoprolol bid (Nejm 1992;327:987), or sotalol (Nejm 1994;
  331:31), or amiodarone if CHF present (Nejm 1995;333:77); then
  trials using programmed stimulation (Nejm 1987;317:1681) and
  Holter monitor (Nejm 1986;315:391) often in combination w procainamide, propranolol, quinidine, phenytoin (Dilantin), digoxin.

When driving allowed?: no consensus but most states require 6–12 asx
  months (Ann IM 1991;115:560), but most pts on rx resume sooner
  and accident rate lower than gen'l population (Nejm 2001;345:391)
Surgical aneurysmectomy

LONG QT SYNDROME
Nejm 2000;343:352; Ann IM 1995;122:701; Nejm 1992;327:846

Cause:

Primary types: most are autosomal dominant; 4 mutations affect
  cardiac ion channels (Nejm 1998;339:960); some are autosomal
  recessive (Romao-Ward syndrome—Nejm 1997;336:1562), or with
  associated deafness (Jervell and Lange-Nielsen syndromes); or
  sporadic

Secondary type: from quinidine, procainamide, disopyramide (IA
  antiarrhythmics), sotalol, indapamide (Lozol); hypokalemia,
  hypocalcemia, and hypomagnesemia; arsenic poisoning; nonsedating
  antihistamines like astemizole (FDA Bull 1992;22[2]:2); macrolides
  (p 338), moxifoxacin, or ketoconazole-like antibiotics (Jama 1996;
  275:1339); phenothiazines especially thioridazine (Mellaril) and
  haloperidol (Haldol) (Ann IM 1993;119:391), tricyclics, lithium,
  and atypical antipsychotics (p 689) esp ziprasidone (Geodon) (Rx
  Let 2001;8:15); CVAs, and other CNS trauma; alcoholism;
  abnormal liver function tests; liquid protein diet (Ann IM 1985;
  102:121); anorexia nervosa; vagotomy or endarterectomy; acute
  MI, myocarditis; mitral valve prolapse; pheochromocytoma

Epidem:

Pathophys: Abnormal K^+ outward or Na^+/Ca^{2+} inward repolarizing
  currents making susceptible to β adrenergic-induced instability
  (Ann IM 1995;122:701; Nejm 1995;333:384). Secondary causes
  can bring out a primary type. Perhaps due to defective *ras* gene

proteins which normally modulate K pumps in cell membrane (Sci 1991;252:704)

Sx: Often precipitated by fever. Syncope (63%) and sudden death (5%), often swimming (Nejm 1999;341:1121) by hx in autosomal dominant type; deafness in autosomal recessive type. SIDS in children (Nejm 2000;343:262)

Si: Torsades de pointes Vtach (Mod Concepts Cardiovasc Dis 1982;51:103)

Crs: 78% mortality without rx (over what time?) is reducible to 6% with β blocker rx (Mod Concepts Cardiovasc Dis 1985;54:45)

Cmplc: Sudden death

r/o pheochromocytoma, which can produce the syndrome

Lab:

Chem: PCR analysis to find gene defect in pt and family (Nejm 1999; 341:1121)

Noninv: EKG may show torsades de pointes Vtach; between attacks of Vtach, shows QTc >0.44 sec; in pts w positive family hx, specif 87% in men and 64% in women, sens 95% in men and 100% in women; >0.47 sec, in men is 100% specif but only 60% sens, in women 98% specif and 90% sens. Holter monitor for arrhythmia detection. See Fig. 2.3.4

Rx: If sx or documented Vtach by Holter, stop all drugs and be sure potassium is ok; 1st choice rx = β blockers (Circ 2000;101:616)

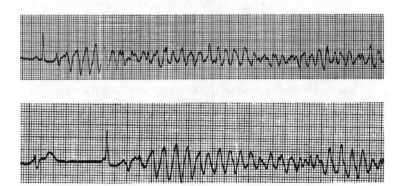

Figure 2.3.4 "Torsades de pointes" ventricular tachycardia. (Reprinted with permission from Chung EK. Pocket guide to ECG diagnosis. Malden, MA: Blackwell Science, 1996:267.)

especially propranolol; also used but now less often are phenytoin (Dilantin)/tocainide; pacemaker; left-sided cervicothoracic sympathectomy; automatic defibrillator

of torsades: 1st choice $MgSO_4$ iv even if not low (Med Let 1991;33:55; Circ 1988;77:392); fix K^+; defibrillate; iv isoproterenol if not congenital type and if no ischemic heart disease; overdrive pacer (Ann IM 1983;99:651)

2.4 HYPERTENSION

ESSENTIAL HYPERTENSION

Cause: Low calcium, and/or potassium intakes? (Ann IM 1985;103:825; Sci 1984;224:1392). Genetic by defective angiotensin gene on chromosome #1 (Nejm 1994;330:1629); elevated insulin levels? (Arch IM 1992;152:1649); possibly chronic low-level lead exposure (Am J Pub Hlth 1999;89:330)

Epidem: Incr prevalence in blacks, perhaps due to G6PD deficiencies (Nejm 1970;282:1001); in sleep apnea, especially in older men, is this cause or effect? (Nejm 2000;342:1377; Ann IM 1985;103:190); with >2 drinks of alcohol qd (Ann IM 1986;105:124); with insulin resistance (Nejm 1991;324:723)

Both systolic and diastolic pressures are significant in the elderly (Ann IM 1989;110:901; Mod Concepts Cardiovasc Dis 1980;49:49). More benign in premenopausal women than men of same age (Ann IM 1987;107:158)

Pathophys: Renally secreted prostaglandins protect; renin-aldosterone-angiotensin worsen. Elevated ADH does not increase BP. Calcium and sodium intakes modulate BP via parathyroid hormones and the renin-angiotensin system (Ann IM 1987;107:919), but long-held postulates that HT prevalence in populations is proportionate to their average Na intake much debated (Sci 1998;281:898, 933). Alcohol induces via CRH release (Nejm 1995;332:1733)

Sx: None usually; occasionally epistaxis, headache

Si: Correct BP-taking technique (Jama 1995;273:1211); mild HT if diastolics 90–105 mmHg and/or systolics 140–160; moderate, diastolics 105–120 and/or systolics >160; severe, systolic $\geq$210, diastolics 120^+. Use correct cuff size (Lancet 7/3/82:33); systolic false increase in elderly due to lead pipe arteries, tell by "Osler's maneuver" (feel artery when occluded above by BP cuff—Nejm 1985;312:1548); r/o white coat HT present in 20% (Jama 1997;278:1065)

Crs: In elderly, LVH decreases over 6 mo and function improves if rx'd with verapamil, atenolol, or thiazides (Jama 1998;279:778; Nejm 1990;3322:1350) or better w ACEIs as 1st choice, then calcium channel blockers, then β blockers and diuretics (Jama 1996;275: 1507). Rx of isolated systolic HT (>160) reduces CVAs by 1/3 (NNT-5 = 33) (Jama 1991;265:3255), stroke mortality by 36%, and cardiac mortality by 25% (Ann IM 1994;121:355), as does rx of systolic and diastolic HT up to age 85 (NNT-1 = 75 in preventing death) (Lancet 1995;345:825; 1991;338:1281).

Isolated moderate systolic HT still associated w incr cardiovascular risks of 1.5 × (Nejm 1993;329:1912)

Cmplc: Hypertensive crisis (Nejm 1995;332:1029): papilledema, obtundation and seizures, renal failure; encephalopathy (Curr Concepts Cerebro Dis 1982;17:5) with stroke (much less frequent in low-renin type—Ann IM 1977;86:7)

Chronic renal failure

Cardiovascular including LVH which, when present, increases risk of MI, CVA, Vtach, death, and sudden death 3–4x more than hypertension alone (Nejm 1992;327:998; 1987;317:787; Ann IM 1986;105:173); CHF, which has bad prognosis, 25–30% 5 yr survival (Jama 1996;275:1557)

Diabetes via hypertension-induced insulin resistance (Nejm 1987;317: 350);

r/o secondary types of HT (Nejm 1992;327:543): sleep apnea (present in 30%!?) (Nejm 2000;342:1377; Ann IM 1994;120:382; 1985;103:190), alcohol and other drug/medicine use, primary renal disease, renovascular causes including coarctation of the aorta (check coincident radial and femoral pulses, rarely need check temporal and radial in proximal type—Nejm 1973;288:899), pheochromocytoma, Cushing's, Conn's, toxemia of pregnancy and BCPs, lead-induced renal disease (most "essential hypertensives with creatinine >1.5 mg %"—Nejm 1983;309:17), acromegaly

Lab: Routine initial w/u: urine analysis, K^+, BUN/creatinine, EKG (3–8% sens) or echo (100% sens, unknown specif) for LVH

Noninv: Ambulatory monitoring of questionable value (Ann IM 1993;119:867,889)

Rx:

Nondrug regimens, various (BMJ 1994;309:436; Ann IM 1985;102:359)

- Increase K^+ intake, natural or supplemental (J Hypertens 1991; 9:465; Ann IM 1991;115:753; Nejm 1987;316:235; 1985;312: 746, 785), especially if on a diuretic, to avoid paradoxical elevation of BP from hypokalemia (Ann IM 1991;115:77)
- Lose weight if obese (Ann IM 2001;134:1), better than Na restriction because fewer adverse sx (Ann IM 1998;128:81; 1991;114:613; HT 1991;17:210); helps in the elderly as well (Jama 1998;279:839)
- Regular aerobic exercise (Nejm 1995;333:1462), although benefit debatable (Jama 1991;266:2098)
- Decrease alcohol (Ann IM 1986;105:124)
- Incr fruit/vegetable fiber and decreased saturated-to-polyunsaturated fat ratio (Nejm 2000;344:3,53; 1997;336:1117)
- Lessen sodium intake to <3gm Na qd; helps in elderly as well (Arch Intern Med 2001;161:685; Nejm 2001;344:3,53; Jama 1998;279:839)
- Incr calcium intake, eg, 1 gm po qd (Ann IM 1985;103:825) at least if deficient (Jama 1996;275:1016) but the effect, though positive, is inconsequential (Ann IM 1996;124:825)
- Perhaps supplemental Mg^{2+}
- Avoid or stop NSAIDs (Jama 1994;272:781; Ann IM 1994;121: 289) especially indomethacin (Indocin), piroxicam (Feldene), and ibuprofen (Ann IM 1987;107:628)
- Behavior modification of minimal help (Ann IM 1993;118:964)

Drug regimens (p 38; Circ 2000;101:450; Med Let 1995;37:45). "Go low, go slow" drug rx should follow several month attempt at nondrug rx if diastolic 90–100 (Ann IM 1992;116:686) but drug rx clearly helpful if persists (Arch IM 1997;157:638)

Stepped care (start with one and maximize dose; then add a second and later a third from different drug groups sequentially), one drug alone controls 50–66% (Nejm 1993;328:914), two drugs control 90% (Nejm 1992;327:543)

Thiazide diuretics and/or β blockers, the only 2 types shown to help in long term trials (Arch IM 1997;157:2413; Jama 1997;278:

CARDIOLOGY

1745), but others probably helpful (Jama 1997;277:739; 1996; 275:1577)

If appear resistant, first r/o pseudoresistance with home BPs and an echo for LVH (Ann IM 1990;112:278). Overtreatment below diastolic of 85 increases cardiac events and no help for CNS events (Jama 1991;265:489), debatable (Nejm 1992;326:251)

1st:
- Thiazides usually first choice (Can Med Assoc J 1999;161:25) especially in elderly >60 (Jama 1998;279:1903; Rx Let 1998;5:43), and even in diabetics (Jama 1996;276:1886); in mild hypertension, may increase mortality perhaps from hypokalemia, hypomagnesemia, or hyperlipidemia (MRFIT—Jama 1997:277: 582; 1983;249:366); erectile dysfunction more common than with ACEIs or β blockers (Ann IM 1991;114:613); eg, hydrochlorothiazide 25 mg po qd, or w K^+ sparer like amiloride 5–10 mg po qd, better than β blocker in elderly (BMJ 1992;304: 405) or as Dyazide (hydrochlorothiazide 25 mg + triamterene 50 mg) avoids all the MRFIT mortality risks (Ann IM 1995; 122:223; Nejm 1994;330:1852)
- β blockers; all about same (Med Let 1982;24:44); no significant side effects (DBCT—Am J Med 2000;108:359) although may slightly incr subsequent type 2 diabetes (Nejm 2000;342:905)

2nd:
- ACE inhibitors: eg, captopril 25–50 mg po bid (Med Let 1985;27: 103). Not as good as diuretics or β blockers (Lancet 1999;353: 611). May best preserve renal function even w early renal failure, eg, enalapril 5 mg po qd-qid (NNT = 4) (BMJ 1994;309:833); clearly best (fewer MIs, CVAs and sudden deaths) in NIDDM pts (Nejm 1998;338:645; Rx Let 1998;5:44). Angiotensin II receptor blockers (ARAs) equally good (Nejm 2001;345:851,861,870,910) alone though more expensive, or used w ACEIs (Bmj 2000; 321:1440)

3rd:
- Calcium channel blockers, long acting types only, eg, diltiazem SR 60–180 bid (Ann IM 1987;107:150) or long-acting nifedipine (Ann IM 1986;105:714) although some studies suggest produces more cognitive impairment than atenolol (Ann IM 1992;116:615)

4th:
- Direct vasodilators like hydralazine or minoxidil; or adrenergic inhibitors like clonidine, α-methyldopa; or α receptor blockers like prazosin 2–10 mg po bid, or doxazosin but less good than thiazides (Jama 2000;283:1967)

Experimental
- Endothelin receptor antagonists like bosentan (Nejm 1998;338:784) 500 mg po qd

In pregnancy, propranolol ok (Nejm 1981;305:1323); so are hydralazine, α-methyldopa, clonidine; avoid teratogenic ACEIs

In elderly age 65–80, thiazides best monoRx choice (Jama 1998;279:1903), rx w thiazide or β blockers clearly helpful so long as no other complicating contraindications, NNT-5 = 18 to prevent MI/CVA (Jama 1994;272:1932); NNT-5 = 10 if diabetic; and rx of isolated systolic HT halves rate of CHF development, NNT-4.5 = 15 (Jama 1996;276:1886) and CVAs over age 60 (Jama 2000;284:465). Over 80, esp if frail, rx may do more harm than good (ACP J Club 1999;131:29; Lancet 1991;338:1281; 1986;2:589)

In diabetes, diastolic goal should be 80 mm rather than 85–90 as in other HT pts (Lancet 1998;351:1755; ACP J Club 1998;129(3):59)

of HT crisis (Nejm 1990;323:1178; Med Let 1989;31:32): 1st nitroprusside drip or fenolopam (corlopam) (Nejm 2001;345:1548) drip, 2nd line drugs: propranolol 1–3 mg bolus q 5–10 min iv or other β blocker best; labetalol 20–80 mg over 20 sec up to 300 mg q 10 min iv; diazoxide 50–150 mg iv q 5 min with propranolol 3 mg/h and/or diuretic; hydralazine 10–20 mg iv × 1; nicardipine iv drip. Then, po nifedipine, clonidine, or captopril etc. Nifedipine 10–20 mg sl with pinholed capsule used in the past but no studies to show helpful and definite substantial complications (Jama 1996;276:1328)

RENOVASCULAR HYPERTENSION

Nejm 2001;344:431

Cause: Atherosclerosis of renal arteries w renal artery stenosis (90%), renal artery fibromuscular hyperplasia (10%), coarctation of aorta, other intrinsic renal disease

Epidem: 0.2–4% of all hypertensives (Can Med Assoc J 1973;117:492)

Pathophys: Decr flow to the renal juxtaglomerular apparatus causes renin production leading to angiotensin II (8-peptide), which causes arterial constriction, which increases aldosterone

Sx: None usually unless hypertension severe; then headache, CHF sx, epistaxis

Si: Coarctation lacks coincident radial and femoral pulses, rarely need to check temporal and radial in proximal type (Nejm 1973;288:899).

Hemorrhages and exudates in fundi; 30% of patients with them have renovascular hypertension (Nejm 1979;301:1273).

Abdominal bruit present in 60% (40% false neg), but 28% of all hypertensives have, so specif ≤35% (65% false positive rate) (Nejm 1967;276:1175); others find higher specif (90%), and if restrict to continuous bruits, sens = 40%, specif = 99% (Jama 1995;274:1299)

Crs:

Cmplc: Like essential hypertension

Lab: (Ann IM 1992;117:845)

Chem: Peripheral plasma renin (50–80% sens, 85% specif) with coincident urine Na^+ (Mod Concepts Cardiovasc Dis 1979;48:49) most useful if low since can then stop w/u; or renin levels before and after po captopril challenge show an increase to above 12 μgm/L/h; if creatinine <1.5 mg%, sens ≥75%, specif ≥90%. Uric acid elevated (Ann IM 1980;93:817). Hypokalemia; urinary K^+ <60 mEq/24 h after 3 d of 4^+ gm Na diet (G. Aagaard, 1969)

Xray: Renal scan (scintigraphy) before and after captopril 50 mg po shows decreased flow in affected kidney, 90% sens/specif (Ann IM 1992;117:845; Jama 1992;268:3353) vs 72% sens, 90% specif (Ann IM 1998;129:705)

Duplex ultrasound if hard to control HT and azotemia and/or peripheral vascular disease, 98% sens/specif (Ann IM 1995;122:883); can also use to calculate a renal artery resistance index to decide between angioplastic or surgical repair (Nejm 2001;344:410)

Angiography

Rx:

Medical rx as good or better than angioplasty or perhaps even surgery (Nejm 2000;342:1007) when cause is atherosclerosis, unlike fibromuscular hyperplasia

Percutaneous transluminal angioplasty (Nejm 1997;336:459) w stenting

Surgical correction even in face of diminished renal function may help both BP and function (Nejm 1984;311:1070). In coarctation, pretreat with propranolol to prevent postop hypertension (Nejm 1985;312:1224)

PHEOCHROMOCYTOMA
Ann IM 2001;134:315; Nejm 1992;327:1009

Cause: Neoplasia of adrenal or extraadrenal autonomic ganglia (Nejm 1969;281:805); genetic transmission often as an autosomal dominant

Epidem: 95% are isolated cases; 5% are associated with autosomal dominant detectable oncogenetic defects causing (Nejm 1996; 335:943, Jama 1995;274:1149) MEN type IIa (Sipple's syndrome), which includes medullary carcinoma of the thyroid, bilateral pheochromocytomas, parathyroid adenomas (10%), and mucosal neuromas (10%); rarely are associated with MEA type IIb (pheochromocytoma, gi ganglioneuromatosis, and Marfanoid habitus), or von Recklinghausen's disease, or von Hippel-Lindau disease (retinal angiomas, CNS hemangiomas, renal cysts, and cancer) where 19% have pheo (Nejm 1993;329:1530)

Pathophys: Epinephrine and norepinephrine are released, as well as precursors in malignant types. Rule of 10s: 10% are familial; 10% are bilateral; 10% are extraadrenal (D. Oppenheim 2/91)

Sx: Pheo triad: paroxysmal (lasts minutes to hours; in 50%) palpitations, perspiration, and pain (headache, chest, and abdominal); 55/76 pheo's had at least 2/3; 3/76 had none. Weight loss, anxiety, tremor, diarrhea (Nejm 1975;293:155), nausea and vomiting, weakness; only 9% have no sx at all

Si: Orthostatic systolic BP drop (already maximally constricted); hypertension (60% chronically; 40% have only with attacks); circumoral pallor

Crs:

Cmplc: Myocarditis and cardiomyopathy, diabetes, CVA, malignant degeneration in 10%

r/o baroreflex failure w episodic hypertensive spells if h/o neck surgery (Nejm 1993;329:1449,1494)

Lab:

Chem: Plasma catechols >2000 pgm/cc, supine 30 min after needle placed; best test, 5–10% false negatives, no false positives. Clonidine suppression test if plasma catechols 1000–2000: 0.3 mg po with plasma norepinephrine level before and at 3 h; all normals suppress to <300 pg/cc (Nejm 1981;305:623). Plasma metanephrines and normetanephrins as good or better? (Nejm 1999; 340:1872; Ann IM 1995;123:101,150)

Table 2.4.1 Sensitivity and Specificity of Biochemical Tests for Diagnosis of Pheochromocytoma*

Biochemical Test	Sensitivity (%)	Specificity (%)	Sensitivity at 100% Specificity
Plasma metanephrine level	99	89	82
Plasma catecholamine level	85	80	38
Urinary catecholamine level	83	88	64
Urinary metanephrine level	76	94	53
Urinary vanillylmandelic acid level	63	94	43

*The sensitivities of tests of plasma metanephrines or plasma and urinary catecholamines were determined, respectively, as the percentage of patients with pheochromocytoma who had positive test results for normetanephrine or metanephrine or for norepinephrine or epinephrine. The specificities of tests of plasma metanephrines or plasma and urinary catecholamines were determined as the percentage of patients without pheochromocytoma who had negative test results for both normetanephrine and metanephrine or for both norepinephrine and epinephrine. The sensitivities and specificities of tests of urinary metanephrines reflect tests of urinary total metanephrines (that is, the combined sum of free plus conjugated normetanephrine and metanephrine). The sensitivities at 100% specificity indicate the percentage of patients with pheochromocytoma in whom test results are so high that they unequivocally confirm the presence of a pheochromocytoma. These sensitivities were determined by increasing the upper reference limits for each test to levels at which no patient without pheochromocytoma had a positive test result. Sensitivity was determined for tests in 151 patients, and specificity was determined for tests in 349 patients. (Ann Im 2001;134:318)

24-h urine metanephrines, 5% false pos, 2% false neg, 50% pos predictive value, or as metnephrine/creatinine ratio >0.354 is even better (Ann IM 1996;125:300)

VMA, 20–60% false neg; catechols, especially free norepinephrines, 80–100% sens, 98% specif (Nejm 1988;319:136). See Table 2.4.1

Xray: CT of adrenals picks up if >1 cc in size (92% sens, 80% specif)

MRI may better distinguish malignant from benign pheos

Rx: Volume replete the usually huge deficits, eg, 10$^+$ L

Meds:

- Phentolamine 5 mg iv gives a short effect
- Nitroprusside drip for rapid control or during surgery
- Phenoxybenzamine 40–100 mg po qd, beware of lowered insulin requirements

- Prazosin 2–5 mg po bid, then propranolol
- Metyrosine 0.25–1 gm po in qid doses (Med Let 1980;22:28)

Surgical removal under a blockade, eg, with phenoxybenzamine or prazosin and with huge volume replacement

of malignant pheo: combination chemotherapy (Ann IM 1988;109:267)

2.5 ENDO/PERI/MYOCARDITIS

ENDOCARDITIS, SUBACUTE AND ACUTE BACTERIAL

Ann IM 1981;94:505; Nejm 2001;345:1318

Cause: *Streptococcus viridans and pneumonia; Staphylococcus aureus* (usually acute bacterial endocarditis); enterococcus; coag-neg staph, nonenterococcal group D strep often misidentified as enterococcus (Ann IM 1974;81:588); and rarely anaerobes, fungi, gram negatives, lactobacillus, psittacosis organism (Nejm 1992;326: 1192), and other unusual organisms (Nejm 1992;326:1215) like *Bartonella sp.* (Ann IM 1996;125:646)

Epidem: 4000–8000 cases/yr in US; 75% in pts w abnormal or prosthetic valves. Incr in patients with mitral valve prolapse syndrome, congenital (VSD, PDA, tetralogy of Fallot) heart disease, especially aortic stenosis both repaired and unrepaired (1.5–20% at 30 yr) (Jama 1998;279:599), and rheumatic heart disease even when given SBE prophylaxis before dental work and surgical procedures (Jama 1983;250:2318)

Pathophys: <5% are right-sided; higher in iv drug users. Renal damage: diffuse vasculitis, focal "embolic" glomerulonephritis, and renal infarction

Sx: Fever (98%), hematuria (29%), weight loss

Si: Murmur (85% at presentation, 99% eventually; 66% in right-sided type); splenomegaly and/or infarction (25–50%); mucosal petechiae and splinter hemorrhages in nails (29%); clubbing (13%); Roth spots in fundi (2%); Osler's nodes in fingers

Crs: 100% die without rx; 80% 10-yr survival w rx (Ann IM 1992;117: 567)

Cmplc: CHF (25%) due to chordae rupture and myocarditis; peripheral systemic arterial emboli, mostly with *S. viridans* type (Ann IM 1991;114:635); pulmonary emboli (60% in right-sided type); CNS including TIA, CVA, mycotic aneurysm, abscess, encephalopathy, and bacterial as well as aseptic meningitis (Curr Concepts Cerebro Dis 1991;26:19); renal failure

r/o acute rheumatic fever, collagen vascular disease, acute glomerulonephritis, marantic endocarditis. And atrial myxoma (Nejm 1995;333:1610): rare; occasionally familial; left:right = 4:1; pedunculated lesion causes sx when plugs or extends through A-V valve making it stenotic or insufficient; sudden CHF sx, cachexia, anemia, fever; murmur can be unusual, variable or mimic MS or MR; may have the clinical picture of SBE; cmplc: peripheral emboli, complete stenosis of A-V valve, FUO; find w echo (Nejm 1970;282: 1022), ESR markedly elevated; rx w surgical removal

Lab:

Bact: Blood cultures (Ann IM 1993;119:270), 10 cc × 3 adequate unless given antibiotics in past 2 weeks, then should do × 5 (Ann IM 1987;106:246); positive in 80%; if negative, r/o murantic (thrombotic type seen in cancer patients), *Brucella,* anaerobes, rickettsial Q fever, and fungi like histo and aspergilli; if *Strep. faecalis* (an enterococcus) reported by the lab, r/o *Strep. bovis* often so misidentified, associated with colon cancer (Nejm 1973;289: 1400), and very sensitive to penicillin

Hem: Crit <38% (50%); ESR up (80%)

Noninv: Echo (Nejm 2001;345:1318), 80% positive, 20% false negative; with transesophageal echos can get to 95% sens (Nejm 1991;324:795; 1990;323:165)

Serol: RA titer positive (50%) (Ann IM 1968;68:746); low C_3 complement

Urine: Rbc's (95%—K. Holmes, 1971; 29%—L. Weinstein, 1987)

Rx: Prophylaxis (p 451)

Therapeutic antibiotics (Jama 1995;274:1706): for *Strep. viridans* and *bovis,* penicillin or ceftriaxone or vancomycin iv × 4 wk or penicillin iv + aminoglycoside × 2 wk; for *Staph. aureus,* nafcillin or oxacillin or cefazolin or vancomycin + debatably 3–5 d gentamicin (Ann IM 1996;125:969 vs. 1982;97:496); for *Staph. albus,* gentamicin + rifampin + vancomycin (Ann IM 1983;98:447); for *Enterococcus faecalis,* penicillin or ampicillin/vancomycin + aminoglycoside × 4 wk unless sx >3 mo or on mitral valve in which case rx for 6 wk (Ann IM 1984;100:816)

Surgical interventions rarely needed except for valve ruptures and
infections of implanted valves (Ann IM 1982;96:650) but over time
(10 yr) 25% of mitral and 60% of aortic valves need surgery (Ann
IM 1992;117:567)

PERICARDITIS

Cause:
Acute: uremic, bacterial from a subdiaphragmatic abscess (Nejm
1967;276:1247), post-MI, viral especially Coxsackie,
postsepticemic (Ann IM 1973;79:194), mycoplasma (Ann IM
1977;86:544), malignancy invading pericardium
Chronic: tuberculosis, sarcoid

Epidem: Coxsackie viral type is probably the most common cause and
occurs in late summer and fall like other enteroviruses

Pathophys: Stiffening causes restriction of ventricular dias filling; incr
heart rate must compensate for decr stroke volume; can tolerate
1–3 L if slowly accumulates, only 300–400 cc if rapid accumulation
Paradoxical pulse if constrictive (exaggeration >10 mm Hg of normal
drop of systolic BP with inspiration) due to impaired venous return
and normal incr pulmonary vascular volume w inspiration (Mod
Concepts Cardiovasc Dis 1978;47:109,115)

Sx: Dyspnea; chest pain, often pleuritic and better when sits up

Si: Ascites, poor heart sounds, no PMI, tachycardia; pleural effusions on
left more often and larger than on right, unlike CHF (Nejm 1983;
308:696)
In constrictive pericarditis: incr CVP with Kussmaul's si, r/o RV
infarction; rapid Y descent and rebound, r/o infiltrating
myocardiopathy, eg, amyloid. Paradoxical pulse >10 mm Hg, r/o
asthma, RV myocardial infarction (Nejm 1983;309:551)

Crs:

Cmplc: Pericardial tamponade

Lab:
Noninv: EKG may show electrical alternans, ie, alternate QRSs have
higher and lower voltages; ST elevation, and/or PR elevations in
limb and precordial leads, which exclude early repolarization,
which usually has precordial lead (ST's) or limb (PR's) involvement
only (Nejm 1976;295:523); T's invert only after ST's back to normal
Echo shows pericardial fluid and and may show tamponade
hemodynamics

Xray: Chest shows large heart, "boot-shaped." CT may show calcifications in 27% of constrictive types, usually chronic, 2/3 w/o a dx, occasionally is tbc (Ann IM 2000;132:444)

Rx: (Mod Concepts Cardiovasc Dis 1979;48:1)

ASA or other NSAID rx avoiding indomethacin and/or steroids if ASHD and recent MI (Circ 1996;94:2341)

If constrictive, tap under echo or EKG guidance; pulmonary edema can develop if tap too much too fast leading to an overload of a deconditioned heart (Nejm 1983;309:595); if constrictive and chronic, surgical pericardectomy

MYOCARDITIS/DILATED CARDIOMYOPATHIES

Nejm 2000;343:1388; 1994;331:1564

Cause:

- Arrhythmias: ectopic atrial and permanent junctional reentrant tachycardias, reversible cardiomyopathy if ablate focus (R. Fletcher 1/00)
- Collagen vascular causes including SLE, polyarteritis nodosa, endocardial fibroelastosis (occasionally seen in children due to a treatable inherited carnitine deficiency—Nejm 1981;305:385), sarcoid, carcinoid (last two may be restrictive and/or congestive)
- Deficiencies like hypophosphatemia from antacid binding, reversible (Ann IM 1978;89:867); thiamine (beriberi), selenium, carnitine
- Endocrine: thyrotoxicosis (Nejm 1982;307:1165) and hypothyroidism; pheochromocytoma (Nejm 1987;316:793); homocystinuria (p 241), hypocalcemia
- Lymphocytic myocarditis (Nejm 1997;336:1860)
- Idiopathic (<50%)
- Infectious from any severe bacteremia, eg, meningococcal, diphtheria, mycoplasma (Ann IM 1977;86:544); viral (Mod Concepts Cardiovasc Dis 1975;44:11) including CMV, influenza, echo, Coxsackie B, yellow fever, mumps, polio, rubella, HIV (Nejm 1998;339:1093); parasites including toxoplasma, Chagas' disease
- Ischemic
- Genetic neurologic/myopathic causes (30%) including Friedreich's ataxia; dyskalemic myopathies; muscular dystrophies including

limb girdle, Emery-Dreifuss (Ann IM 1993;119:900), and myotonic; Refsum's disease; familial sarcomere protein gene mutations (Nejm 2000;343:1688) and other autosomal dominant genetic causes affecting cellular function (Nejm 1999;341:1715; 1996;335:1224)

- Peripartum (Nejm 2001;344;1567, 1629); onset 1 mo prior or up to 6 mo post partum w variable outcomes but usually some residual dysfunction
- Toxic agents like alcohol (Ann IM 1974;80:293; Nejm 1972;287:677), daunorubicin (Daunomycin) (p 330) and bleomycin, cobalt in beer (Ann IM 1969;70:277), arsenic (p 23); lead, cocaine, mercury, carbon monoxide, phenothiazines; most reversible except chemotherapy drugs.

Epidem: Idiopathic type prevalence = 36/100,000 (Circ 1989;80:564): blacks:whites = 2.5:1; males:females = 25:1.

Pathophys: Dilation of both ventricles; mural thrombi

Sx: CHF sx's; muscle weakness in alcoholic type since 83% have skeletal myopathy as well (Ann IM 1994;120:529)

Si: Afib and other supraventricular arrhythmias; S_3 gallop (Ann IM 1969;71:545); CHF si's

Crs: (Nejm 2000;342:1077) Often chronic and indolent; in alcoholic type, it can rapidly resolve with abstinence. Postpartum type has best prognosis (90% 5 yr survival); idiopathic, ischemic, daunorubicin, and infiltratives types = 50% 5 yr mortality; HIV type, 25% 3 yr mortality

Cmplc: Systemic emboli from mural thrombi and Afib

r/o hypertrophic (IHSS); "hibernating myocardium," ie, ischemic myocardopathy reversible w revascularization (Nejm 1998;339:173); and **restrictive myocardiopathies** (Nejm 1997;336:267): amyloid, hemachromatosis, familial, idiopathic, endomyocardial fibrosis, eosinophilic cardiomyopathy, sarcoid, Gaucher's, Fabry's, and Hurler's disease

Lab:

Chem: Phosphate level (Ann IM 1978;89:867)

Noninv: EKG may show Afib (20%), cloven T waves especially in alcoholic type (Ann IM 1969;71:545), arrhythmias, blocks, Q waves, or LVH. Echocardiogram most helpful, EF <45%

Path: Endocardial bx (Nejm 1982;307:732) in peripartum and all types to dx infiltrative disease; not helpful in dilated types, IHSS, Wilson's disease, etc. (complete list—Ann IM 1982;97:885; Nejm

1983;308:12); but does not correlate well with clinical findings or prognosis (Nejm 1985;312:885)

Rx: Anticoagulate acutely and chronically; prednisone rx even when inflammatory by bx is no help (Nejm 1989;321:1061) or even w additional immunosuppressive drugs (Nejm 1995;333:269); perhaps human growth hormone 4 IU sc qod (Nejm 1996;334:809, 856); transplantation, 75% 5-yr survival (Mod Concepts Cardiovasc Dis 1986;55:37)

of CHF using vasodilators

of PVCs; improve EF w digoxin, ACEIs, β blockers, amiodarone (Mayo Clin Proc 1998;73:430)

IDIOPATHIC MYOCARDIAL HYPERTROPHY AND SUBAORTIC STENOSIS
Nejm 1997;336:775

Cause: Genetic, over 10 different mutations can cause, one on chromosome #14 (Nejm 1992;326:1108; 1989;321:1372), autosomal dominant with nearly complete penetrance when measure thickness of interventricular septum (Ann IM 1986;105: 610; Nejm 1973;289:709)

Epidem: Prevalence = 1/500; male:female = 4:1 in sporadic type, but equal in genetic type (E. Braunwald, 1978); higher incidence in Fabry's disease (Nejm 1982;307:926)

Pathophys: 50% due to mutations in the myosin heavy chain gene (Nejm 1992;326:1108; 1991;325:1753). Abnormal intraventricular septum produces dynamic aortic root obstruction and subaortic stenosis; mitral regurgitation is due to anterior mitral leaflet being distorted by the septum; obstruction is worsened by diuresis and vasodilators, and increases in contractility, eg, by digoxin, PVCs, catechols, and exercise. Reentrant PVCs because of different refractory periods in different muscle groups (Nejm 1980;302:97). Incr calcium channels increase the muscle sensitivity and contraction strength (Nejm 1989;320:755). Myocardial bridging of epicardial coronary arteries also occurs and causes myocardial ischemia/infarcts (Nejm 1998;339:1201)

Sx: Onset age 15–46 yr, positive family hx in 1/3 (E. Braunwald, 1978); syncope (3/18), dyspnea (13/18), chest pain (7/18), angina that starts when exercise stopped, palpitations

Si: LVH by palpation and double PMI, with diphasic arterial systolic peak murmur

Aortic murmur without radiation into neck (Nejm 1988;318:1575), decreases with leg elevation and squatting, which increase venous return; worse with isoproterenol, exercise, standing, amyl nitrite inhalation, alcohol ingestion, and Valsalva maneuver

Crs: Two types: slowly progressive (Ann IM 1972;77:515) and generally benign (Jama 1999;281:650; Nejm 1989;320:749); and "malignant," with premature death in young adulthood w myosin heavy chain mutation (Nejm 1992;326:1108)

Cmplc: Sudden death by Vtach/fib (Nejm 1988;318:1255) correlates w LV wall thickness (Nejm 2000;342:1778); endocarditis; Afib often

r/o **"athlete's heart"** w LV wall thickness always <16 mm, rarely >13 mm (Nejm 1991;324:295) which overlaps w IHSS in men but not in women (Jama 1996;276:210)

r/o other causes of sudden death in athletes (Nejm 1998;339:364): cardiomyopathy (22%), ASCVD 15%), anomalous coronary artery (12%), IHSS (2%) (see screening cardiac exam p 682)

Lab:

Noninv: EKG shows LVH, big Qs in V_{1-2} (hypertrophied septum) Holter for malignant PVCs. Nonspecific EKG changes occur in affected children before echo changes (Nejm 1991;325:1753)

Echo shows hypertrophied septum and LV wall and systolic anterior motion of mitral valve; Doppler shows subvalvular gradient

Path: Endocardial bx shows chaotic muscular disorder (Nejm 1977; 296:135). Genetic PCR studies of peripheral lymphocytes can detect in presymptomatic stage (Nejm 1991;325:1753)

Xray: Chest shows LVH

Rx: β blockers or verapamil (Mod Concepts Cardiovasc Dis 1990;59:1; Ann IM 1982;96:670); disopyramide (Norpace—Nejm 1982; 307:997) 150–200 mg po qid. Avoid digoxin, diuretics, catechols, alcohol (Nejm 1996;335:938), nitrates and other vasodilators.

Surgical myotomies when resting obstruction >75 mm or class II sx despite medical rx; 80% success (Ann IM 1972;77:515)

of Afib: amiodarone and warfarin anticoag

of Vtach/sudden death: amiodarone, implantable defibrillator (Nejm 2000;342:365, 422)

CARDIOLOGY

2.6 VALVULAR HEART DISEASE

MITRAL VALVE PROLAPSE SYNDROME
(Barlow's Syndrome)

Nejm 1989;320:1234; Ann IM 1989;111:305; Mod Concepts
Cardiovasc Dis 1979;48:25

Cause: Genetic, autosomal dominant; decreased penetrance in males; less
frequent over age 50

Epidem: Associated with various inherited connective tissue diseases
including Ehler-Danlos syndrome, Marfan's, osteogenesis
imperfecta, pseudoxanthoma elasticum (Nejm 1982;307:369), and
von Willebrand's disease (Nejm 1981;305:131). Prevalence <2.5%
in adults (Framingham—Nejm 1999;341:1,8)

Pathophys: Abnormal cordae and valve, not papillary muscle. Atrial
muscle in valve may also produce electrical atrial and ventricular
bypass tracts and reentrant arrhythmias (Nejm 1982;307:369)

Sx: Palpitations (premature junctional beats, PACs, PVCs), anxiety often
leads to discovery although no more prevalent in anxious pts than
in normals

Si: Midsystolic click (92%), late systolic murmur (85%) which moves
toward S_1 with standing or other decrease in venous return.
Tricuspid prolapse may occur too (6/13—Nejm 1972;287:1218)

Crs: Same as matched controls at Mayo (Nejm 1985;313:1305); 90%
10-yr survival, <10% get major cmplc listed below

Cmplc: Sudden death rarely (2.5% at Mayo?—Nejm 1985;313:1305);
PVCs associated with sx, present in 16% of children with Barlow's
on ETT (J Peds 1984;105:885); endocarditis (1% at Mayo—Nejm
1985;313:1305; 3%—Nejm 1989;320:1031); CVA/TIAs (Nejm
1980;302:139) vs no incr rates (Nejm 1999;341:8); Graves' disease
(Nejm 1981;305:497); valvular insufficiency requiring surgery in
6% (Nejm 1989;320:1031)

r/o other causes of chronic mitral valve regurgitation (Mod Concepts
Cardiovasc Dis 1979;48:25), benign MVP w insignificant mitral
regurgitation = 2/3 of all w MVP (Nejm 1989;320:1031)

Lab:
Noninv: EKG normal in 76%; may show "inferior ischemia" or PVCs
Echocardiogram

Rx: SBE prophylaxis when mitral regurgitation present (ie, a murmur)
Propranolol or other β blocker rarely needed

Surgical valve replacement occasionally (<5%) necessary if severe
mitral regurgitation, esp in men >60 yr old

VALVULAR HEART DISEASE
Nejm 1997;336:32

Including AS (Nejm 1987;317:91; Ann IM 1987;106:292), AI, MS, MR
(Nejm 2001;345:740), TS, and TI

Cause: Many are rheumatic (p 795)

Epidem: AS most common in elderly now; MS/MR in females age 20–40;
TS/TI always accompanies mitral or aortic disease but occurs in
only 2–4% of patients with RHD

Pathophys: Rheumatic pancarditis causes chordae fibrosis and shortening,
and valvular vegetations at points of trauma. MS always present in
RHD to some degree; hemoptysis in MS is due to shunts from
pulmonary veins to bronchial veins. 70% of all patients with
chronic MR in the 1960s was due to RHD, while 30% was due to
chordae rupture from myocardial infarction, endocarditis, and
trauma. Severe AI alone rarely is due to RHD; usually from trauma,
syphilis, dissecting aneurysm, endocarditis, SLE (Ann IM 1969;
71:81), RA, ankylosing spondylitis. AS now rarely (10%) is due to
RHD, most is calcific aortic stenosis on bicuspid or previously
normal valves

Sx: MS: exertional dyspnea, orthopnea, hemoptysis

MR: exertional dyspnea, orthopnea

AS: angina, CHF, syncope

AI: gradual CHF sx

Si: MS: atrial fibrillation; mid-diastolic murmur with presystolic
accentuation even in atrial fibrillation (Nejm 1971;285:1284);
opening snap; loud S_1

MR: loud systolic murmur, radiates to axilla

AS: CHF, loud systolic murmur radiates into carotids; worsens with
amyl nitrite inhalation in contrast to MR and VSD

AI: early diastolic murmur; this typical murmur is present in 73%
(sens), and is heard only 8% of the time in patients w/o AI (92%
specif—Ann IM 1986;104:599). Austin-Flint murmur of functional
MS narrowed by AI regurgitant jet. Very soft S_1 as mitral valve
floats closed from the AI; indicates urgent need for surgery

Crs: MS: slow progression

CARDIOLOGY

AS: if heavily calcified, <0.07cm^2 but asx, 80% 4 yr mortality (Nejm 2000;343:611, 652); after angina 50% survive 5 yr; after syncope 50% survive 3 yr; after CHF 50% survive 2 yr

Cmplc: MS: CHF, SBE, emboli

AS: angina, sudden death, CHF, gi angiodysplasia with gi bleed, disappears after valve replacement (Ann IM 1986;105:54). After onset of any of the 3 sx, mortality is 75% at 3 yr unless valve replaced (Mayo Cl Proc 1987;62:986)

Lab:

Cardiac cath: MS significant valve diameter <1.2 cm^2, no sx if >2.5 (L. Cobb, 1971). AS significant if <0.07cm^2/m^2 (Nejm 1997;336:32)

Noninv: 2D echo and Doppler for valves, chamber sizes, and estimates of valve diameters or regurgitation amounts (Mod Concepts Cardiovasc Dis 1989;58:55, 61); in AI, 90$^+$% sens/specif (Ann IM 1986;104:599)

Xray: Chest, in MS shows large LA, PA, and RV, and may show valvular calcifications; in AS, may show 4-chamber enlargement, valvular calcifications usually only with significant disease

Rx: MR: repair before EF <60% or end diastolic ventricular dimension <45 mm; if due to full flail leaflet, repair sooner rather than later since prognosis w/o repair poor (Nejm 1996;335:1417)

MS: may do closed commissurotomy or percutaneous catheter commissurotomy via interatrial septum (Nejm 1994;331:961) which may diminish embolization if done early (Ann IM 1998; 128:885); valve replacement if calcifications/clot, porcine (Nejm 1981;304:258) or bovine pericardium w higher structural failure rates vs mechanical w higher bleeding cmplc (Nejm 1993;328:1289). Control Afib w digoxin or β blocker; anticoagulate w warfarin especially if Afib, concomitant AI, or clot by echo (Ann IM 1998;128:885)

AI: nifedipine po long-term reduces/delays LV dysfunction development and consequent valve replacement (Nejm 1994;331: 689, 736). Repair before EF <55% or end diastolic ventricular dimension <55 mm

AS: valve replacement if angina, CHF, or syncope; even in elderly if healthy (Nejm 1988;319:169; Ann IM 1989;110:421), and perhaps before sx develop

CHF: anticoagulate if platelet survival <3 d (Nejm 1974;290:537) or evidence of emboli; rheumatic fever penicillin prophylaxis; SBE prophylaxis

Surgical: valve choices (Nejm 1996;335:407); w mechanical valve replacement, ideal protime INR is 3–4 or 3–5 for maximal benefit/risk ratio (Nejm 1995;333:11); w bioprosthetic valves, warfarin to INR = 2–3 × 3 mo, then just ASA unless other embolic risk factors like Afib, dyskinetic segment, etc.; in pregnancy after valve replacement, warfarin is teratogenic in first trimester (25%) so heparin is used but is less than adequate anticoagulation (Nejm 1986;315:1390) and usually combined w ASA. (For normal and abnormal heart sounds w various valves see table in Nejm 1996;335:410)

2.7 CONGENITAL HEART DISEASE

ATRIAL SEPTAL DEFECTS (ASD): PRIMUM AND SECUNDUM TYPES

Nejm 2000;342:256

Cause: Congenital malformations

Epidem: Primum: 1–2% of all CHD; most common type of CHD in Down's syndrome (25%)

Secundum: 10–15% of all CHD; associated w anomalous pulmonary venous return

Pathophys: Primum: A-V canal defects including low ASD, high VSD, cleft mitral and/or tricuspid valves or even a common A-V valve

Secundum: mid or upper ASD allows left to right shunt

Sx: Primum: dyspnea, fatigue, pulmonary infections, and CHF in infancy in complete form, later in incomplete types

Secundum: rarely any in infancy or childhood; later dyspnea w CHF and pulmonary HT, palpitations if arrhythmias

Si: Primum: cyanosis mild or absent. Harsh systolic murmur, apical, pansystolic from MR (33%), TI or VSD (75%). P_2 incr; splitting present; CHF; RVH

Secundum: mild systolic murmur (pulmonic) at upper left sternal border; mid-diastolic rumble at lower left sternal border from high flow. S_2 wide and fixed; RVH

Crs: Primum: complete types cause CHF in infancy and death in 1–2 yr if not repaired; incomplete types get sx later, but survive less well than secundum types

Secundum: occasionally CHF sx in 2nd–3rd decade; or may be asx throughout adult life, but overall decr in life expectancy

Cmplc: Primum: CHF, pulmonary hypertension, supraventricular arrhythmias (Aflut or Afib) especially if surgically closed after age 40 (Nejm 1999;340:839), SBE rarely, incr incidence of rheumatic fever; r/o partial anomalous pulmonary venous return

Secundum: CHF and pulmonary HT late; strokes, multiple in patent foramen ovale pts, esp if divers (Ann IM 2001;134:21)

Lab:

Noninv:

Primum: EKG: left axis, pRBBB, R and LVH, counterclockwise rotation

Secundum: EKG axis normal or RAD, partial and full RBBB, RVH and strain; clockwise rotation.

Echo: diagnostically abnormal in 90% (Ann IM 1976;84:246) w doppler, in 100% w TEE

Xray: Primum: chest shows small aortic knob; RVH and incr pulmonary flow. If MR, then large left atrium and LV. Angiography shows "gooseneck deformity" of LV outflow tract; serrated mitral valve leaf; rest depends on particular variant

Secundum: chest shows small aortic knob; RHV + incr pulmonary flow; no LA enlargement, unlike patent ductus or VSD

Rx: Primum: surgical early if sx; can't if fixed pulmonary hypertension. Open repair or pulmonary artery banding in infants with severe sx. Operative mortality: 40% if complete, 15% if partial. Do it at age 5+ ideally; cmplc: complete heart block

Secundum: open repair with bypass at age 5+ if shunt >1.5 ratio, 95+% 10-yr survival even in adults >40-yr age (Nejm 1995;333:469); can't if significant right to left shunt. Operative mortality = 1–5%, 50% if right to left shunt, 15–20% if CHF or pulmonary HT; cmplc: return of shunt, and can never be sure it isn't anomalous pulmonary veins or sinus venosum

VENTRICULAR SEPTAL DEFECT

Nejm 2000;342:256; Ann IM 2001;135:812

Cause: Congenital malformation

Epidem: 20% of all CHD; associated with triad of 3rd degree heart block, ventricular septal defects, and corrected transposition

Pathophys: Causes an L-to-R shunt, which in end-stage disease reverses to an R-to-L shunt (Eisenmenger's syndrome) with clubbing and cyanosis

Size of defect is crucial to sx, location unimportant. At birth, high hematocrit keeps PA pressure up and thus low shunt flow and minimal murmur; with dropping crit postpartum these appear (Nejm 1982;306:502)

Sx: Asually asx; can develop dyspnea, fatigue, and pulmonary infections

Si: Loud harsh pansystolic murmur at lower left sternal border, widely transmitted over precordium. Apical diastolic rumble if large shunt; loud P_2 if pulmonary hypertension

Crs: Spontaneous closure in 1/3 in childhood; life expectancy >65 yr if shunt <2:1

Cmplc: SBE (5–30% lifetime risk), CHF, pulmonary hypertension; with Eisenmenger's, 2/3 die in pregnancy (Nejm 1981;304:1215)

Lab:

Noninv: EKG normal unless huge L-to-R shunt causing LVH; RVH suggests fixed pulmonary hypertension

Echo w Doppler

Xray: Chest usually normal; with larger defects causing LVH and prominent pulmonary vasculature and a large left atrium. Small aortic knob

Rx: SBE prophylaxis (p 451)

Surgical (Mod Concepts Cardiovasc Dis 1977;46:1); indications: L-to-R shunt >2:1 or CHF; PA banding in infants; optimal age for final repair is 5 yr; contraindicated if R-to-L shunt. Operative mortality: 1–5%, increases to 15% if pulmonary HT (>70% of systemic pressures); banding mortality 25%. Surgical cmplc: complete heart block (rare), AI (rare)

PATENT DUCTUS ARTERIOSUS (PDA)

Nejm 2000;342:256

Cause: Persistence of patent ductus postpartum

Epidem: 10% of all CHD; female:male = 3:1; incr incidence in RDS infants rx'd w fluids, furosemide (prostaglandin E effect—Nejm 1983;308:743)

Patent Ductus Arteriosus (PDA), continued

Pathophys: L-to-R shunt, which in end-stage disease reverses to an R-to-L shunt (Eisenmenger's syndrome) with clubbing and cyanosis
Persistence of normal fetal channel between left pulmonary artery and aorta just distal to left subclavian artery

Sx: Usually asx; can develop dyspnea, fatigue, and pulmonary infections

Si: "Machinery" murmur maximum at left base, r/o coronary AV fistula, ruptured sinus of Valsalva; bounding pulses indicate wide pulse pressure; pink fingers, blue toes with Eisenmenger's

Crs: Case report of pt who lived to age 90 (Nejm 1969;280:146), 2/3 die by age 60

Cmplc: SBE, CHF, pulmonary hypertension; with Eisenmenger's, 2/3 die in pregnancy (Nejm 1981;304:1215)
r/o coarctation of aorta

Lab:
Noninv: EKG normal; occasionally LVH; if has RVH, suggests fixed pulmonary hypertension

Xray: Chest normal with small PDA; or w larger one, LVH, enlarged aortic knob with dilatation of the proximal relative to the distal aorta, and a large LA with prominent pulmonary vasculature

Rx: Indomethacin iv in neonates (Nejm 1981;305:67,97; Med Let 1981;23:95); prophylactically if <1 kg (Nejm 1982;306:506) although 18 mo survival w/o neurologic impairment not improved (Nejm 2001;344:1966). Or ibuprofen iv q 24 h × 3 to premies <30 wk gestation successfully prevents as well w less renal failure but not available (Nejm 2000;343:674,728; Jama 1996;275:539)
SBE prophylaxis (p 451)
Surgical: indications, lesion persistence or CHF; procedure, division and closure; optimal age for final repair, age 2–12 yr; contraindications, bacterial infection of PDA; operative mortality, 0.5–10%; cmplc: recurrent laryngeal nerve injury (rare), reopening of ductus after ligation, or mycotic aneurysm (rare)

AORTIC STENOSIS
Nejm 2000;342:256

Cause: Congenital malformations
Epidem: 3% of all CHD; occasionally associated with a syndrome of retardation, hypercalcemia, facial distortions, and supravalvular AS

Pathophys: Anatomic obstruction at supravalvular, valvular, or infravalvular (p 94) areas; bicuspid valve is most common type present in 2–3%

Sx: Often asx; or occasionally only mild fatigue and exertional dyspnea; angina and/or syncope are ominous; CHF late; dysphagia (Nejm 1967;276:832)

Si: BP normal; narrow pulse pressure; loud ejection murmur maximum at base; no MR unlike in IHSS; ejection click (split first heart sound); CHF si's

Crs: Like acquired AS (p 97)

Cmplc: Ischemia, Vtach/fib, CHF, SBE, heart blocks (Ann IM 1977;87:275)

r/o bicuspid aortic valve (1–2% of US population has)

Lab:

Noninv: EKG is normal; or LVH and strain. 2D echo

Xray: Chest shows LVH, dilatation of ascending aorta

Rx: SBE prophylaxis (p 451)

Surgical (Mod Concepts Cardiovasc Dis 1977;46:1); if valve area <0.7 cm^2/m^2; open valve replacement with bypass; operative mortality = 1–5% for commissurotomy, 10% for subvalvular type; cmplc: aortic insufficiency, SBE, 13% incidence over 25 yr (Jama 1998;279:599)

PULMONIC STENOSIS

Nejm 2000;342:256

Cause: Congenital malformations

Epidem: 5% of all CHD

Pathophys: RV outflow (10%), valvular (90%), or infundibular (rare alone)

Sx: Often asx; or occasionally only mild fatigue and exertional dyspnea; cyanosis and CHF in severe cases

Si: P$_2$ diminished; loud ejection murmur at upper left sternal border neck and back; CHF including hepatomegaly in children; ejection click, decreases with inspiration

Crs: Very stable (Nejm 1972;287:1159, 1196)

Cmplc: SBE, CHF

Pulmonic Stenosis, continued

Lab:
   Noninv: EKG is normal, or LVH + strain; P pulmonale
   Echocardiogram
Xray: Chest shows PA dilatation, RVH, diminished pulmonary
   vasculature
Rx: SBE prophylaxis (p 451)
   Surgical if gradient >60 mm or area <0.7 cm^2/M^2; operation type
   either open commissurotomy with bypass, which has a high
   incidence of valve incompetence post op, or percutaneous balloon
   valvuloplasty in children and adults (Nejm 1996;335:21,
   1982;307:540); operative mortality is 1–5%; cmplc: pulmonic
   insufficiency (13%), which usually disappears w time

TETRALOGY OF FALLOT
   Nejm 2000;342:334

Cause: Congenital malformation
Epidem: 10% of all CHD; 50–70% of cyanotic CHD; 85% of adult
   cyanotics
Pathophys: VSD and pulmonic stenosis of varying positions and severities,
   and dextroaorta with right-sided aortic arch (25%)
Sx: Cyanosis onset after age 3 mo unless total pulmonary atresia present;
   dyspnea; squatting relieves sx
Si: Cyanosis, clubbing; P$_2$ decreased; loud systolic along left sternal
   border; absent in severe cases
Crs:
Cmplc: Hypoxic spells (paroxysmal dyspnea with marked cyanosis
   leading to unconsciousness); brain abscess; paradoxical embolism;
   relative anemia; SBE; CHF (rare); pneumonia; gout; hemoptysis;
   pulmonary artery dissection; sudden death from ventricular
   arrythmias even after repair
Lab:
   Noninv: EKG shows right axis, RVH + strain; in acyanotic form, LVH
   Echocardiogram
Xray: Chest shows small heart, "boot-shaped," diminished pulmonary
   vasculature; right-sided aortic arch (25%)

Rx: Preventive: SBE prophylaxis (p 451)

Surgical: "open" total correction, patch VSD, resect pulmonary infundibulum, incise pulmonary valve (for age 3–5 yr); mortality <3% in children and <10% in adults, good (86+%) 30-yr survival if survive the surgery (Mayo—Nejm 1993;329:593); cmplc: heart block (rare) and pulmonary insufficiency

COARCTATION OF THE AORTA

Nejm 2000;342:256

Cause: Congenital malformations

Epidem: 5% of all CHD; male:female = 4:1

Pathophys: Associated with PDA often, and bicuspid aortic valve (70–90%). Hypertension is renal via angiotensin (Nejm 1976; 295:145)

Sx: Rarely sx (CHF, leg pains, headache) in childhood; CHF in 3rd–4th decades

Si: Hypertension in arms, normal or low BP in legs; decreased/delayed femoral pulses; systolic murmur (75%) in left upper back or pulmonic areas

Crs:

Cmplc: SBE on bicuspid aortic valve; intracranial bleeding; hypertensive encephalopathy; ruptured/dissected aorta; hypertensive cardiovascular disease

Lab:

Noninv: EKG normal, or LVH; if RVH, suggests a PDA beyond the coarc ("fetal type")

Xray: Chest, normal heart, and pulmonary vasculature; coarctation visible on plain chest occasionally; rib notching in older patients

Rx: Surgical for both (Mod Concepts Cardiovasc Dis 1977;46:1) resection of coarcted segment and end-to-end aortic anastomosis ideally done at age 5–15 yr; operative mortalities >20% in infancy, <1% age 5–15 yr, 10% over age 30; cmplc: spinal cord ischemia (rare); acute necrotizing arteritis of mesenteric vessels (rare); hypertension postop in most

CONGENITAL HEART DISEASE: MISCELLANEOUS

SYNDROMES

Ebstein's anomaly (Nejm 2000;342:336): Low tricuspid valve ("atrialization of RV"); ASD with right-to-left shunt, cyanosis, and clubbing; PAT and other arrhythmias; exertional dyspnea; lucent lung fields; pRBBB, WPW type B (20%), P pulmonale, SBE diathesis, but no RVH unlike tetralogy

Eisenmenger's syndrome: (Nejm 2000;342:339; Ann IM 1998;128:745)
Pathophys: Left to right shunting from ASD, VSD, or PDA,
Sx: Dizziness
Si: Clubbing, cyanosis, RVH, pulmonary insufficiency murmur (Graham-Steell)
Crs: 45% 25 yr survival; worsened by higher altitudes
Cmplc: Thromboembolism (PE, CVA); high mortality w surgery or pregnancy; gout; gall stones; renal failure
Lab: Echo, Holter for arrythmias
Rx: Phlebotomy to keep crit <60%; heart-lung transplant if medical management failing

Holt-Oram syndrome: (Nejm 1994;330:885) Abnormal gene on chromosome #12, autosomal dominant; 1/100,000 births; ASD and/or VSD; radius, thumb, or shoulder girdle bony changes

Kartagener's syndrome: Autosomal recessive; ciliary microtubular defect, also immobilizes sperm (Ann IM 1980;92:520; Nejm 1979;300:53); bronchiectasis; sinusitis; MS, ASD, and situs inversus totalis in many

Pectus excavatum: Diminished cardiac output at maximal exercise even with moderate pectus; restrictive lung disease and pulmonary hypertension w severe disease; surgically correctible (Nejm 1972;287:207)

Transposition of the great vessels (Nejm 2000;342:337): Anomalous origins of aorta from RV and PA from LV, w VSD, ASD, and PDA allowing communication

Rx: Post-partum, stat prostaglandin E to keep PDA open + creation of ASD by balloon catheterization; eventually surgically switch aorta and PA

DIFFERENTIAL DX OF CONGENITAL HEART DISEASE

Preop catheterization only occasionally necessary (Mod Concepts Cardiovasc Dis 1986;55:20; Nejm 1981;305:1235). See Table 2.7.1

Table 2.7.1

	Xray	EKG	Differential Dx
Cyanotic	Decreased pulmonary vascularity	RVH	Severe PS w VSD (tetralogy or ASD) Severe pulmonary vascular obstruction ("Eisenmenger's physiology") w ASD, VSD, ductus, etc.
		LVH	Tricuspid atresia
		Concentric ventricular hypertrophy	Truncus w hypoplastic PA
	Decreased pulmonary vascularity w huge RA	RAH and pRBBB	Ebstein's
	Increased pulmonary vasculature	RVH	Postductal coarctation Complete transposition of pulmonary veins
		Combined ventricular hypertrophy	Transposition of great vessels, or Single ventricle, or Truncus
Acyanotic	Normal pulmonary vasculature	RVH LVH Normal	PS or MS MR, AS, AI, coarctation Mild of all above

Table 2.7.1 *(continued)*

	Xray	EKG	Differential Dx
Acyanotic (*cont.*)	Increased pulmonary vasculature	RVH	ASD, secundum type, or Incomplete transposition of pulmonary veins, or All L to R shunts w increased RV pressures
		LVH	VSD, small to moderate, or PDA, small to moderate, or ASD, primum type, or Common AV canal, or AV fistula including aorta/ pulmonary fenestration
		Normal	Mild forms of all above

2.8 PERIPHERAL VASCULAR DISEASE

ABDOMINAL AORTIC ANEURYSM

Cause: Unknown mix of genetic, mechanical, and other factors

Epidem: 15,000 deaths/yr in US, 6% prevalence at age 80 yr in men, 4.5% at age 90 in women; 18% incidence in brothers >60 yr of affected pts (Ann IM 1998;130:637)

Pathophys: Spontaneous rupture at 5–7 cm diameter

Sx: Age >55 yr; pain, usually in back, can be buttock or testicular; rarely can be colicky; may dissect down to give perianal hematoma (Nejm 1969;280:548)

Si: Pulsating abdominal mass; shock

Crs: If >5 cm diameter by ultrasound, 3–12% (Nejm 1993;328:1167) vs 25% (Nejm 1989; 321:1009, 1040) rupture in 5 yr; if <5 cm diameter only 5% rupture in 8 yr (Nejm 1989;321:1009). After rupture, 62% die before getting to hospital, 30% in hospital, and <8% survive

Cmplc: Rupture into bowel, peritoneal cavity, vena cava, retroperitoneum; disseminated intravascular coagulopathy (Nejm 1971;285:185). **Cholesterol emboli,** sometimes precipitated by warfarin in 3–12 wk, presents with livedo reticularis without hypotension (the usual cause), pain, worsening renal failure; no rx possible, dx w bx's of skin, kidney, etc (Nejm 1993;329:38). Incr morbidity and mortality from other ASCVD (Ann IM 2001;134:182)

Lab:

Urine: Microscopic hematuria sometimes

Xray: KUB shows calcification in aorta; with rupture, bilateral loss of psoas shadow; lateral abdomen may show aneurysm in calcified aorta >5 cm

Ultrasound, 100% sens and easy way to follow

Rx: Prevent by screening w abdominal exam (90% sens, 65–85% specif in thin pts >50—Arch Int Med 2000;160:833) and/or ultrasound in males age >65 (P. Frame—Ann IM 1993;119:411; Can Med Assoc J 1991;145:783); do surgery if ≥5.5 cm, no surgery if ≤4 cm; between 4 and 5.5 cm, follow q 3–6 mo (Lancet 1998;352:1649, 1656; Ann IM 1990;113:731)

Surgical excision and Dacron replacement; can only do if renal vessels spared; mortality <5% if done electively, 50% if done emergently; cmplc: spinal cord infarct and paraplegia (rare—Nejm 1969;281: 422). In fragile pts, endovascular stent possible (Nejm 1997;336:13, 1994;331:1751)

ACUTE AORTIC DISSECTION

Jama 2000;283:897; Nejm 1997;336:1876, 1987;317:1060

Cause: Atherosclerotic; traumatic usually at ligamentum arteriosum in chest (Nejm 1970;282:1186); Marfan's syndrome (medial cystic necrosis of aorta), or Ehler-Danlos syndrome

Epidem: 1.5× as common as ruptured abdominal aortic aneurysm. Incr incidence w hypertension, Marfan's syndrome (medial cystic necrosis of aorta), and Ehler-Danlos syndrome. No increase in syphilitic, rheumatoid, or atherosclerotic (?) aortitis

Pathophys: Medial rupture of vasovasorum causes a dissecting hematoma which ruptures back into lumen, usually, though not always, distally creating a double-barreled lumen. Lathyrism is an experimental duplication by feeding sweet peas to rats thereby creating defective collagen formation

Stanford classification: type A = ascending aorta involved; type B = no involvement of ascending aorta, descending only

Sx: Pain (95%), thoracic, abdominal or in back; often migrating

Si: BPs in legs and arms unequal; asymmetric pulses (15%), aortic
insufficiency murmur (32%)

Crs: Mortality 1%/hr, 50% overall in type A with ascending aorta
involvement; 5% overall for type B

Cmplc: Organ ischemia due to vessel occlusion
r/o aneurysm of thoracic aorta (Jama 1998;280:1926) especially in
elderly women; rx by aggressively rx'ing HT, or if partial rupture or
≥6cm w surgery or endovascular stent (Nejm 1994;331:1729)

Lab:
Chem: Smooth muscle myosin heavy chain protein elevation
>25 μgm/L within 3 yr of onset of sx, 90+% sens and specif for
proximal dissection (Ann IM 2000;133:537)
Noninv: Transesophageal echo (TEE) (97% sens, 77% specif); also
very accurate for traumatic aortic rupture (Nejm 1995;332:356); or,
less good, transthoracic echo (57% sens, 83% specif) (Nejm 1993;
328:1,35)

Xray: (Nejm 1993;328:1,35)
Plain chest xray may show aortic knob widening
CT of chest (Ann IM 1984;101:801) w contrast (94% sens, 87% specif)
MRI (98% sens, 98% specif)
Aortogram to define point of origin, aortic insufficiency, and any vessel
compromise but MRI + TEE may obviate need for this

Rx: 1st: Nitroprusside 25–50 μgm/min w β blockers (Med Let
1987;29:18) such as propranolol 0.05–0.15 mg/kg iv q 4–6 h
2nd: Trimethaphan (Arfonad) 1–2 mg/min iv
Surgical for all type A (ascending aorta involvement) and many type B;
20+% mortality
Stent grafts possible for both types A and B (Nejm 1999;340:1539,
1546,1585)

DEEP VENOUS THROMBOPHLEBITIS
Nejm 1996;335:1816

Cause: Venous stasis and intimal injury; coagulation abnormalities; iv's
are an occasional cause; 2/3 due to particulates in iv, 1/3 chemical
and/or needle irritation, <1% bacterial (Nejm 1985;312:78);
trauma pts have a 60% incidence, 18% is proximal DVT (Nejm

1994;331:1601). Usually lower extremities; upper extremity DVT has similar causes though less common (Ann IM 1997;126:707)

Inherited/acquired protein deficiencies (Nejm 2001;344:1222); one of these deficiencies is present in 31% of outpatients with lower and 9% of pts w upper extremity DVT (Ann IM 1997;126:707); a h/o DVT in the family or at a young age does not increase the likelihood (Nejm 1990;323:1512):

- Factor V (Leiden) mutation (Ann IM 1998;128:15; 1997;127:895, Nejm 1997;336:399) in 25–40% of pts w idiopathic DVT (Nejm 1999;340:901), a heterozygous single amino acid point mutation causing resistance to protein C. 3–5% prevalence in US white population (Jama 1997;277:1305); one study finds DVT risk incr only if assoc w 20210A mutation (Nejm 1999;341:801). Also associated w incr fetal loss, miscarriage, and stillbirth in both hetero- and homozygotes (Ann IM 1999;130:736), and perhaps w a slight increase in CVAs (Ann IM 1996;125:264 vs 1997;127:895). But screening of asx population is not worth anticoagulation risks since annual incidence of DVT is <1% (Ann IM 2001;135:322,367; 1997;127:895), nor is screening prior to joint replacement indicated since no incr risk (Ann IM 1998;128:270)
- Prothrombin gene position 20210 mutation of G to A; most common abnormality after factor V (Leiden) (Ann IM 1998;129:89; Blood 1996;88:3698), present in 5% w idiopathic DVT (Nejm 1999;340:901)
- Protein C deficiency or resistance: normally inactive protein C circulates in blood, is activated by clot on endothelium and that activated form breaks down activated factors V_a and VIII_a; deficiency is autosomal dominant, vitamin K-dependent (Nejm 1986;314:1298; 1983;309:340); but many with heterozygous protein C deficiency have no thrombosis, so there may be some other associated defect in some (Nejm 1987;317:991); homozygous protein C deficiency causes neonatal purpura fulminans (Nejm 1991;325:1565)
- Protein S deficiency (Ann IM 1998;128:8): a protein C cofactor, also autosomal dominant (Ann IM 1993;119:779) and vitamin K-dependent, associated with nephrotic syndrome (Ann IM 1987;106:677; 1987;107:42; Nejm 1984;311:1525); 1.5–7% prevalence in pts w DVT; homozygous state causes neonatal purpura fulminans; 50% of affected pts will have sx by age 30. Can also occur as an acquired autoimmune deficiency (Nejm 1993;328:1753)

CARDIOLOGY

- Antithrombin III deficiency: autosomal dominant (Ann IM 1992; 116:754; Nejm 1983;308:1549)

Lupus anticoagulant or anticardiolipin (phospholipid) antibodies in SLE or ITP or **primary antiphospholipid syndrome** (Ann IM 1996;125:747; 1992;117:303,997; 1992;116:293) w elevated PTT, present in 5% of pts w idiopathic DVT (Nejm 1999;340:901), manifest by arterial thrombi and DVTs, rx'd w warfarin to INR >3 (Nejm 1995;332:993, 1025), and thrombocytopenia rx'd w steroids and/or danazole (Ann IM 1994;121:767)

Idiopathic factor VIII levels >243 IU/100 cc (Nejm 2000;343:457)

Homocystinemia (p 241) (Nejm 1996;334:759; Ann IM 1995;123:746)

Epidem: Associated w occult cancers (15%), may be either superficial migratory or DVT type (Ann IM 1982;96:556); cancer present in 10% w one identifiable episode, >20% w more than one idiopathic episode (Nejm 1992;327:1128). Incr incid (Nejm 2001;344:1222) w pregnancy, BCP use (Nejm 2001;344:1527), ERT, elevated factor VIII levels

Pathophys: See above

Sx: None; or calf pain; unlateral edema

Si: None; or Homan's sign, or incr calf diameter

Crs: (Arch IM 2000;160:769; Ann IM 1996;125:1) 75% 5-yr survival, 25% recurrence over 5 yr

Cmplc: Pulmonary embolus (14%), but incidence is decr to <0.4% w and after rx (Jama 1998;279:458); in idiopathic upper extremity DVT, PE rate is 26% (Ann IM 1999;131:510)

Chronic postphlebitic syndrome (edema, pain, stasis dermatitis, and ulcers) in 30% after 5 yr, incidence can be decr by half w post episode use of compression stockings × 2–3 wk (Lancet 1997;349: 759); rx sx w herbal Venastat I po bid, avoid in pregnancy (Rx Let 1998;5:17)

Thrombotic skin necrosis, especially of penis with protein C deficiency and warfarin rx; rx with vitamin K, avoid by using heparin rx (Sci Am Text Med 1984)

r/o superficial phlebitis rx'd w local heat and NSAIDs

r/o occult cancer w H+P, chest xray, and standard labs, don't pursue further unless abnormalities found there (Nejm 1998;338:1169; Ann IM 1996;125:785) vs more extensive noninv studies (Nejm 1998;338:1221)

Lab: (Ann IM 1998;128:663).

Hem: D-dimer (fibrin split products) 86–93% sens, 77–82% specif for proximal DVT, but lower specif when prevalence higher, eg, w carrier (Ann IM 1999;131:417; Circ 1995;91:2184), and lower sens w newer latex agglutination 5 min bedside tests (SimpliRED, and others) (Ann Emerg Med 2000;35:121); if <1092 ng/cc, no DVT (Stroke 1996;27:1516)

Noninv: Beware that many noninv labs and xray depts call the femoral vein "the superficial femoral vein" when it really is a deep vein (Jama 1995;274:1296); all detect above knee DVT; below knee DVT not significant unless extends above, hence do at least one follow up test 5–7 d later if first neg.

Ultrasound (Ann IM 1998;129:1049), simple compressibility of groin and popliteal space (Ann IM 1998;128:1), or duplex: noncompressibility with probe (91% sens, 99% specif—Nejm 1989;320:342; or better—Arch IM 1991;151:2217; Ann Emerg Med 1991;20:494; vs 91–95% sens, 83% specif—Arch IM 1992;152:1901) all in pts w sx; 6–10% of positives will be missed with a single test (Ann IM 1998;128:1, Nejm 1993;329:1365); but in asx high-risk pts sens only 38% though specif 92% (Lancet 1994;343:1142; Ann IM 1992;117:735). If ultrasound negative, McMaster protocol (Jama 1998;279:1094): 1 point each for h/o cancer or pedisposing activity, local tenderness or cord over deep vein system, edema in ankle, >3 cm calf difference, and /or distended collateral veins (not varicosities); a score of ≥3 points indicates high probability and need for venogram; if 1–2 points, probability is moderate and f/u ultrasound in 1 week adequate.

Impedance plethysmography (IPG) (Ann IM 1993;118:25; Arch IM 1992;152:1901); not as good or frequently used as ultrasound. Valid in pregnancy if done in the decubitus position (Ann IM 1990;112:663)

Xray: Venogram, but 2% of the time it causes DVT itself

Rx:

Prevention:

- Avoid estrogen as BCPs or ERT; although in factor V Leiden, incid of thromboembolism <2% (Ann IM 2001;135:322)
- LMW heparin (Am J Med 1999;106:660; Nejm 1993;329:1370) like enoxaparin 30–40 mg qd and graduated compression stockings in neurosurg pts (Nejm 1998;339:80), (NNT from 3–5) in hip replacement pts (Jama 1994;271:1780), but regular heparin

and warfarin are also effective; use throughout pregnancy if h/o DVT, 3 miscarriages, or even one still birth (Nejm 2001;344:1222)

- Unfractionated heparin bid, indiscriminantly administered to general medical (Ann IM 1982;96:561) and in surgical patients (Nejm 1988;318:1162), increases survival; q 8 h, adjusting dose to keep PTT >31 sec works best in hip replacement patients (Nejm 1983;309:954); 500 U w or w/o dihydroergotamine 2 h before and q 12 h after hip surgery, decreases DVT incidence from 25% to 10% (Med Let 1985;27:45)
- Pneumatic calf compression postop probably as good as above (Med Let 1985;27:45)
- Elastic compression stockings for people over age 55 flying >8 hrs decreases incidence from 12% to 0% (NNT = 9) (Lancet 2001;357:1485)
- ASA qd helps some (Lancet 2000;355:1295)
- Experimental: prophylaxis w desirudin (Revasc) (recombinant hirudin) (Nejm 1997;337:1329,1383), or w polysaccharide (Nejm 2001;344:619), ? more effective than LMWH

Therapeutic:
- Heparin iv × 5 d , unfractionated iv, or low molecular weight heparins better than unfractionated heparin for acute DVT (Nejm 2001;344:626; Ann IM 2001;134:191) because faster thrombus regression and less frequent thrombocytopenia (Nejm 2001;344:673), and allow home rx: enoxaparin (Lovenox) 1mg/kg sc qd or bid (Nejm 1996;334:677; Ann IM 1996;124:619), or others (p 36)
- + warfarin (p 36) started on day 1 (Nejm 1992;327:1485); overlap heparin and warfarin w adequately prolonged INR (>2) at least 2 d before stopping to avoid hypercoag state (Nejm 1996;335:1822); continue warfarin × 6 mo (Nejm 1999;340:901,955; 1995;332:1661) vs 3 mo (Nejm 2001;345:165) if no specific cause, × 1–2 mo if transient specific cause, and lifelong if recurrent idiopathic type (Nejm 1995;332:1710) after 2nd episode does prevent recurrence but w a 10% bleeding risk (Nejm 1997;336:393). If due to antithrombin III deficiency, anticoagulate after first episode.
- Thrombolysis perhaps (no—Nejm 1994;330:1864)
- IVC filter to reduce pulmonary embolus rate from 4% to 1.5%, but subsequent recurrent DVT is 20+% vs 11%, and short and long term mortality the same (Nejm 1998;338:409)

PERIPHERAL VASCULAR OCCLUSION AND ISCHEMIA

Nejm 2001;344:1608; 1991;325:577

Cause: ASCVD causes thrombotic type; embolic from post-MI (10%), mural thrombus, atrial fibrillation (75%), and valvular heart disease (15%)

Epidem: 30% of patients with premature (age <50 yr) peripheral and CNS thromboembolic vascular disease are heterozygotes for homocystinuria variants (p 241) (Nejm 1985;313:709)

Pathophys:

Sx: Cold, pale extremity; decreased sensation and motor strength; pain usually but not always, worse with elevation; claudication, progresses to rest pain (r/o spinal stenosis in elderly)

Embolic incidence to: femoral (34%), brain (20%), popliteal (14%), iliac (13%), viscera (10%), aorta (9%), axillary (5%)

Si: Pale with elevation >1 min, then dependent rubor (reactive erythema) when first put down (Mod Concepts Cardiovasc Dis 1976;45:91); diminished or absent pulses; mottled skin; ischemic ulcers; gangrene

Crs: In embolic, without rx, extremity loss is: axillary 10%, popliteal 12%, femoral 40%, aorta 80%

Cmplc: Gangrene of extremities

r/o:

- Vnous occlusion
- Abdominal aortic aneurysm with **cholesterol emboli,** sometimes precipitated by warfarin in 3–12 wk (Circ 1967;35:946) angiography or surgical aortic manipulation, presents with blue toes and livedo reticularis without hypotension (the usual cause), pain, may see emboli in retinal vessels, elevated amylase/lipase, low complement, worsening renal failure, no rx possible, dx w bx's of skin, kidney, etc. (Nejm 1993;329:38)
- **Thromboangiitis obliterans (Buerger's disease)** (Nejm 2000; 343:864): Rare (in US) disease of young male smokers, due to endarteritis obliterans of vasa vasora, presents w claudication especially of instep and has a positive Allen's si (with posterior occlusion of radial and ulnar arteries and the rapid release of 1 leads to rapid filling on that side alone, and is delayed several seconds on other) and superficial thrombophlebitis (40%), treat by stopping smoking, vasodilators, and hyperbaric oxygen to rx ulcers (Nejm 1998;339:672)

Lab:
   Noninv: Doppler studies for segmental systolic BPs and Doppler wave forms (Nejm 1983;309:841)
Xray: Duplex ultrasonography (Brit J Surg 1996;83:404)
   Angiography only if plan to do surgery as you would if embolic
Rx: Stop cigarettes, weight loss; exercise program of walking to pain tolerance >30 min at least tiw for at least 6 mo helps (Jama 1995; 274:975; Ann IM 1990;113:135); β blockers may, but don't usually, worsen sx (Arch IM 1991;151:1769) unless coincident nifedipine use (BMJ 1991;303:1100); ASA 325 mg po qd (Lancet 1992;340: 143); anticoagulation with heparin then warfarin

Medications
   • ASA i po qd
   • Cilostazol (Pletal) (Med Let 1999;41:44; Rx Let 1999;6:8) 50–100 mg po bid; platelet inhibitor and vasodilator; half-life incr by erythromycin, ketoconazole, diltiazem, omeprazole, grapefruit. Adverse effects: headache, diarrhea, dizziness, worse CHF
   • Pentoxifylline (Trental) 400 mg po tid for claudication (Can Med Assoc J 1996;155:1053; Ann IM 1985;102:126)
   • Ticlopidine (Ticlid) 250 mg po bid decr claudication and need for bypass surgery, and increases graft patency post-op (Nejm 1997; 337:1726)
   • Heparin sc qd helps modestly (Am J Med 1999;107:234)
   • Ginko (Am J Med 2000;108:276) 120–160 mg po qd
Bypass surgery if ulcers or intolerable pain
of acute thrombotic or embolic occlusion: embolectomy within 6 h with Fogarty catheter; or thrombolysis iv × 2$^+$d w indwelling catheter using urokinase for acute (<2 wk) or chronic obstruction, w f/u angioplasty, helps 50–80% (Nejm 1998;338:1105 vs 1148; Ann IM 1994;120:40).

SUBCLAVIAN STEAL SYNDROME
   Jama 1972;222:1139; Nejm 1967;276:711

Cause: Atherosclerosis of subclavian artery
Epidem:

Pathophys: Steal syndrome due to retrograde vertebral arterial flow to arm which, with exercise, siphons ("steals") blood from cerebral circulation

Sx: Precipitated by arm exercise (20%), head turning to side, standing. Dizziness (11/13); transient blurred vision (6/13); syncope (4/13); aphasia (4/13); dysarthria (3/13); dementia (6/13)

Si: Diminished capillary filling with arm elevation; diminished pulse in arm (13/15); left arm to right arm BP differences of >20 mm Hg (11/13); bruit in 8/9 incomplete blocks, 1/6 complete blocks; lateralizing motor or sensory changes (4/13)

Crs:

Cmplc: CVA

Lab:

Noninv: Doppler analysis as good as angiography; 30-msec delay in pulse measurable

Xray: Angiography; MRA or duplex scanning of neck to detect retrograde vertebral flow

Rx: Surgical reconstruction; carotid vertebral bypass when on left; vertebral artery ligation especially when on left; on right can precipitate a carotid steal; a minor procedure. Contraindications: vertebral thrombosis, high technical risk, hemodynamically insignificant risk; morbidity/mortality: 1/13 postop mortality; 2/13 have residuum from preop stroke; cmplc: contralateral steal syndrome, especially if repair a total occlusion and a partial exists on other side (Nejm 1967;277:64)

2.9 MISCELLANEOUS

CARDIAC EXAM

Auscultatory BP gap: Loss of Korotkoff sounds between systolic and diastolic pressures; in HT pts correlates w ASHD (Ann IM 1996; 124:877)

Ejection clicks: Systolic click as blood enters a dilated pulmonary artery or aorta, seen with ASD, PDA, mild pulmonic stenosis or aortic stenosis

Gallops: (Nejm 1968;278:753)

S₃ (Nejm 1992;327:458), ventricular gallop: idiopathically normal in people under age 35 (Nejm 1983;308:498); any LV dilatation, not hypertrophy, due to early LV filling with high atrial filling pressure pushing forward flow, eg, in CHF (overly compliant ventricle), and MR (abnormally high, early A-V flow)

S₄, atrial gallop, due to any LV hypertrophy (diminished compliance) with slowed diastolic filling and significant atrial push, eg, in HT, AS, post-MI where there is an "indurated" noncompliant wall

Heart sounds, timing of: With JVP and EKG: c wave is not due to carotid artery (starts sooner in patients with LBBB—Nejm 1971;284:1309). See Fig. 2.9.1

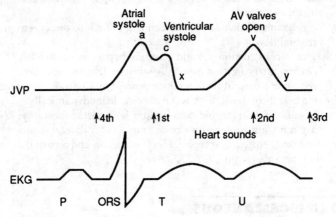

Figure 2.9.1

Hepatojugular reflux: 10–30 sec midabdom compression causes an incr JVP, which falls immediately with release; correlates with PCWP ≥15 mm Hg (Ann IM 1988;109:456), 10% false pos and neg, false pos from isolated right ventricular disease

JVP clinical estimate of cm above angle of Louis (manubrial-sternal junction), which is 5 cm above LA; upper limit of normal = 7–9 cm; at 45° angle, JVP only visible if >7 cm (Jama 1996;275:630)

LVH, by xray = >1.5 cm behind inferior vena cava on lateral, 2 cm up from diaphragm
By PE, apical pulse sustained throughout systole

LV enlargement without LVH by PE: apical impulse >3 cm^2 in L lateral decubitus position is reliable (>90% sens/specif—Ann IM 1983;99: 628; 100% sens, 30% specif—Jama 1993;270:1943) for LV dilatation, much better than position relative to sternum or midclavicular line supine; but dullness >10.5 cm from midsternum is 90% sens, 30% specif (Jama 1993;270:1943)

Maneuvers during cardiac exam to bring out and suppress various heart sounds (Nejm 1988;318:1572; for sens/specif—Ann IM 1983;99:346):
• Valsalva, squatting, inspiration, and leg raising increase venous return and thus R-sided murmurs
• Squatting to standing decreases venous return and hence diminishes R-sided murmurs
• Hand grip or, even more so, bilateral arm BP cuffs at 20 mm above systolic pressure for 20 sec (Ann IM 1986;105:368), increases peripheral vascular resistance and hence L-sided regurgitant murmurs like MR, AI, and VSD
• Amyl nitrite inhalation (reduces peripheral vascular resistance) decreases mitral regurge, AI, and VSD murmurs (Mod Concepts Cardiovasc Dis 1975;44:23) but reflex tachycardia may mask
• Carvallo's maneuver (deep inspiration) in 80%, and by hepatojugular reflux in 66% (Ann IM 1984;101:781) to emphasize tricuspid regurgitation
• Respiratory variations of heart sounds (Mod Concepts Cardiovasc Dis 1981;50:37)

Murmur mimics: Austin-Flint murmur is a "murmur of mitral stensosis" caused by aortic insufficiency; Graham-Steell murmur is a "murmur of AI" caused by MS-induced pulmonic insufficiency

Palpitations (Nejm 1998;338:1369)
Cause: SVT (Afib, AVNRT, AVRT), Vtach, PVCs, anxiety/panic disorder
W/u: H+P, EKG, Holter or event monitor, ?electrophysiologic testing
Rx: β blockers for nonspecific rx

Pediatric murmurs, benign: (p 686)

Pericardial rubs: 18% monophasic, 24% diphasic, 58% triphasic (atrial systole, ventricular systole, and protodiastolic components), 22% palpable (Nejm 1968;278:1204)

Pericardial tamponade: JVP incr, BP decreased, distant heart sounds, paradoxical pulse, Swan-Ganz numbers show equal pressures, ie, RAP = RVDP = PADP = PCWP, r/o acute RV infarct w functional pericardial tamponade from acute RV dilatation (J. Love 3/95; Nejm 1983;309:39,551)

Split heart sound: differential dx:
1st sound split: RBBB (r/o click)
2nd sound, wide or fixed split: RBBB, pulmonary stenosis, pulmonary hypertension, ASD; rarely VSD, PVCs, MR (Mod Concepts Cardiovasc Dis 1977;46:7)
2nd sound, paradoxical splitting: LBBB, aortic stenosis, WPW syndrome type B, PDA, IHSS (Mod Concepts Cardiovasc Dis 1977;46:13)

Swan-Ganz use: Associated w severity adjusted incr morbidity + mortality and use should be curtailed (Jama 2001;286:309; 1996;276:889,916); maybe use in hypotension to manage iv nitroprusside and/or pressors like dobutamine and dopamine (Ann IM 1983;98:53; Nejm 1976;295:1404) especially in R ventricular infarct patients with hypotension

Syncope differential dx: (Nejm 2000;343:1856; Ann IM 1997;126:989; 1997;127:76; Mod Concepts Cardiovasc Dis 1991;60:49)
• IHSS
• Arrhythmic, eg: long QT, SVT, Vtach, heart block
• Vasovagal (Ann IM 2000;133:714; including reflux and pharyngeal stimulation (Ann IM 1992;116:575)
• Orthostatic/postural hypotension: (Mod Concepts Cardiovasc Dis 1985;54:7; in elderly—Nejm 1989;321:952) (p 562) rx.
   Testing: supine BP after 2 min, then standing BP after 1 min; positive if P incr >30/min, and or sys BP decr >20 mm Hg (Jama 1999; 281:1022)
   Reflex vasodilatation: psychiatric, carotid sinus pressure, swallow and micturition syncope, inferior MI. Or neurally mediated hypotension

(Jama 1995;274:961); in the latter, strong ventricular contractions may cause via C-fiber-induced peripheral vasodilatation (Ann IM 1991;115:871); bring out with tilt table and isoproterenol infusion; but such maneuvers cause syncope in patients with no h/o blackouts almost as often (Ann IM 1992;116:358), although if bradycardia and hypotension occur quickly on tilt table alone, dx may be more secure (Nejm 1993;328:1117); associated w chronic fatigue syndrome: pacer rx no help (Nejm 1993;328:1085); rx by avoiding diuretics, vasodilators and tricyclics, increase salt intake, try fludrocortisone (Florinef), β blockers, and anticholinergics like disopyramide (Norpace) (Jama 1995;274:961), or SSRI like paroxetine 20 mg qd (J Am Coll Cardiol 1999;33:1227)

Decreased venous return: blood loss, third spacing, cough/exertion, syncope, venous pooling from varicosities; postprandial splanchnic blood pooling probably is most common cause of orthostatic hypotension in elderly (Ann IM 1995;122:286); caffeine no help

Decreased peripheral resistance: arteriovenous malformation, heat

Circulating vasodilator: carcinoid, mastocytosis

Renin excess and aldosterone deficiency states

Autonomic neuropathy (p 562 for w/u and rx)

Miscellaneous: deconditioning, starvation, pulmonary embolus, pheochromocytoma, CNS tumor, marijuana, sepsis, billowing mitral valve, Addison's disease

Wide pulse pressure: Differential dx: thyrotoxicosis, aortic insufficiency, calcific arteriosclerosis, arteriovenous shunt

PERIOPERATIVE RISK ASSESSMENT

Point systems and risks

Stable angina by itself not a risk. Post-MI cardiac cmplc of surgery are 5.8–30% at 0–3 mo, 2.3–15% at 3–6 mo, 1.5–5% at 6 mo and beyond (Anesthesiol 1983;59:499; Jama 1972;220:1451). W/u beyond chest xray and EKG (like ETT) only needed if functional status unclear or high risk as defined by points below (Nejm 1995;333:1750)

Point Systems; 4 extant systems all perform comparably and only ID 2/3 of the risk (Ann IM 2000;133;356,384; Nejm 1997;337:1132; Ann IM 1997;127:309,313; 1983;98:504; Nejm 1977;297:845). See Tables 2.9.1 and 2.9.2

Table 2.9.1 Goldman Criteria

Condition	Points
age >70 yr	5
MI w/i 6 mo	10
S_3 or JVD	11
Significant valvular AS	3
Rhythm other than NSR or PACs	7
>5 PVCs/min documented anytime in past	7
Generally poor health, eg, pO_2 <60, creatinine >3 mg %, pCO_2 >50, abnormal PFTs, K <3.0 mEq/L, HCO_3 <20, BUN >50	3
Intraperitoneal or thoracic, or aortic operation	3
Emergency operation	3

Table 2.9.2 Risks

Points	Class	Surgical Risk of Nonfatal Cardiac Cmplc (%)	Surgical Risk of Cardiac Death
0–5	I	0.7	0.2
6–12	II	5	2
13–25	III	11	2
26+	IV	22	56

Or use medical conditions risk index table (Ann IM 1997;127:311) which suggests if ≥20 points, periop cardiac risk = 10–15% and should consider more w/u.

Preop cardiac surg w/u for noncardiac surgery unnecessary unless medically unstable (Nejm 1999;341:1838; Ann IM 1996;124:767); plain echocardiographic assessment not helpful (Ann IM 1996;125:433), but dobutamine stress echo (Jama 2001;285:1865) may be helpful in high risk pts, esp those not on β blockers

Periop atenolol 10 mg iv pre and post op + 50 mg po bid until d/c, decreases cardiac morbidity/mortality × 11% over 2 yr (Nejm 1996;335:1713,1761), or other β blocker (Nejm 1999;341:1789)

Pulmonary evaluation (Nejm 1999;340:937): maximize COPD/asthma states w antibiotics if infected, steroids, and preop training for postop incentive spirometry; PFTs controversial. Also maximize postop pain control

Geriatric surgical cardiac risk (Ann IM 1985;103:832): those who pass above criteria as low risk can be given a 2-min ETT supine to raise pulse >99; those unable to do that suffer a 20% severe cardiac cmplc

rate, whereas those able to do it have only a 1.5% severe cardiac cmplc
rate

2.10 EKG READING

GENERAL

- Always use limb leads rather than V leads for measurements where possible
- Peri-infarction block not a clinically useful concept
- Qs <0.04 sec wide or <1/3 of R height are insignificant (eg, septal) except in the face of LBBB
- Pediatric differences: big R in V_1+ RAD in infants; former may persist to age 5, latter gone in 2–3 yr. Anterior T inversions out to V_4 may last into early teen years
- Interval calculation:
    PR = beginning of P to beginning of QRS
    QRS = beginning of QRS to J point where QRS joins ST segment
    QT = beginning of QRS to end of T; upper limit of normal (see Table 2.10.1 and Figure 2.10.1)
- Axis calculation:

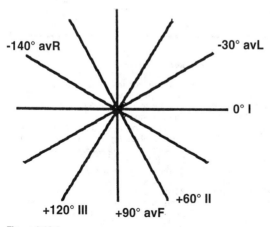

Figure 2.10.1

Table 2.10.1 Normal Q-T Intervals and Their Upper Limits of Normal

Heart Rate/min	Normal Q-T Intervals		Upper Limits of Normal Q-T Intervals	
	Men and Children (sec)	Women (sec)	Men and Children (sec)	Women (sec)
40.0	0.449	0.461	0.491	0.503
43.0	0.438	0.450	0.479	0.491
46.0	0.426	0.438	0.466	0.478
48.0	0.420	0.432	0.460	0.471
50.0	0.414	0.425	0.453	0.464
52.0	0.407	0.418	0.445	0.456
54.5	0.400	0.411	0.438	0.449
57.0	0.393	0.404	0.430	0.441
60.0	0.386	0.396	0.422	0.432
63.0	0.378	0.388	0.413	0.423
66.5	0.370	0.380	0.404	0.414
70.5	0.361	0.371	0.395	0.405
75.0	0.352	0.362	0.384	0.394
80.0	0.342	0.352	0.374	0.384
86.0	0.332	0.341	0.363	0.372
92.5	0.321	0.330	0.351	0.360
100.0	0.310	0.318	0.338	0.347
109.0	0.297	0.305	0.325	0.333
120.0	0.283	0.291	0.310	0.317
133.0	0.268	0.276	0.294	0.301
150.0	0.252	0.258	0.275	0.282
172.0	0.234	0.240	0.255	0.262

Reprinted by permission from Chung EK. Pocket guide to ECG diagnosis. Cambridge, MA: Blackwell Science, 1996:30–31.

Table 2.10.2

EKG Segment	Dx	Criteria/Abnormalites
P waves	RAE	P >2.5 mm high in II, III, avF, or V_1; or >1.5 mm in V_2
	LAE (+/or conduction delay)	P =.12 sec in II, III, or avF (volume only, eg, mitral stenosis), or P >1 mm^2 negative area in V_1 (33% false neg; mitral regurg. volume and/or pressure can cause—Circ 1969;39:339, Am J Cardiol 1977;39:967)
PR interval, Short	LGL	<.12 sec with no delta wave
	WPW	<.12 sec with delta wave present
Long	1st degree heart block	>.20, or >.22 sec if rate slow (<60)
Elevated	Pericarditis (p 91)	In both limb and precordial leads, usually associated w ST elevations there as well (Nejm 1976;295:523)

Table 2.10.2 *(continued)*

EKG Segment	Dx	Criteria/Abnormalites
QRS		
Axis deviation and hemiblocks	LAD + LAHB	Axis <−45° (? <−30°) and small Q_I and/or small R_{III}; but no LBBB
	RAD + LPHB	Axis >105°, >90° if age >50, and R_I +/or Q_{III} but don't call if RVH
	Bifasicular block	Either of above + RBBB
Bundle branch blocks	pRBBB	QRS <.10, S_I, S_{II}, S_{III}, + RSR' in V_1 or avR
	RBBB	QRS =.10 sec and (almost always), S_I, S_{II}, S_{III}, and RSR' in V_1 or other evidence of forces to R shoulder like terminal R in avR or terminal S in V_6
	IVCD	QRS >.10 but <.12 sec without above pattern and with an avL septal Q and/or a V_1 septal R
	pLBBB	Like IVCD but without avL septal Q or V_1 septal R
	LBBB	QRS >.12 sec, big slurred R_I and QS in V_1; rarely benign (Ann IM 1969; 70:269), if new, 50% 10-yr mortality (Ann IM 1979;90:303)
	Bilateral BBB	1st one then other over time (slowed not fully blocked)
Low voltage	Myxedema, COPD, amyloid, obesity, MI damage, pericardial effusion	Voltage <10 mm in all leads; or overall voltage of QRS in I + II + III <15 mV (Chung).
Ventricular hypertrophies	LVH; When prolonged ventricular activation time (first .04 sec) and LVS, increased ASHD; 60% 12 yr, 50% males >45 2 yr mortality (Ann IM 1970;72:813)	Single precordial S or R >25 mm (relatively nonspecific criterion); or SV_2+ RV_6 or SV_1+ RV_5 >35 mm (good); or R_{avL} =11 mm (better criterion), or R_{avL}+ SV_3 >28 (J Am Coll Cardiol 1985;6:572) (better); or R_I + S_{III} >23 mm (best). Can't read in LBBB
R > S in V_1	RVH	RV_1 > S + T inverted in V_1; or RV_1 + SV_5 >10.5 mm (Am Hrt J 1949; 38:273); or RV_1 >10 mm w RBBB
	RVH and strain	Above + inverted Ts and/or depressed STs in V_{1-3}
	RBBB	see above criteria
	WPW type A	Short PR and delta wave
	Direct posterior MI	Initial RV_1 >.04 sec wide + Ts upright in V_1
	Dextrocardia	Increasing R voltage right precordial leads V_1R to V_6R

CARDIOLOGY

Table 2.10.2 *(continued)*

EKG Segment	Dx	Criteria/Abnormalites
QRS *(cont.)*		
MI patterns	Anterior MI, r/o COPD and poor lead placement	Poor R wave progression, ie, R < S still in V_4
all w initial ST elevations, then T inversions + Qs if transmural, r/o LBBB, WPW, cardiomyopathy	Anterior septal MI	Qs in V_{2-3}
	Anterior MI	Loss of R force across precordium or Q waves in V_{3-4}
	Anterior lateral MI	Qs in V_{5-6}
	High lateral MI	Qs in I, avL, V_6
	Inferior wall MI	Qs in at least two of II, III, or avF
MIs w LBBB (Am Hrt J 1988;116:23); all w about 25% sens, >90% specif)	Septal MI	LBBB + new "septal" Q in avL or R in V_1; really is RV forces seen through infact "window" of septum; or LBBB + Q wave in =2 leads V_{3-5}; or LBBB + late notching of S in =2 leads V_{3-5}
	Any area MI	LBBB + evolving ST-T changes; or (Nejm 1996;334:481) on initial EKG, =1 mm ST elevations concordant w QRS, =1 mm ST depressions in V_1, V_2, or V_3, =5 mm ST elevations opposite direction from QRS in any lead; or upright T in V_5 or V_6
Pulm embolus patterns		$S_1Q_3T_3$, very specific but only w massive emboli (Am J Emerg Med 1997;15:310); anterior T wave inversions (68% sens) (Chest 1998;113:850); or =3 of the following (70% sens) (Am J Cardiol 1994;73:298): RBBB or pRBBB, S in I and aVL =15 mm, poor R progression, Q in III and F not II, RAD >90°, voltage <5 mm in limb leads, T inversions in II + F or V_1–V_4
ST segments		
Depressions	Significant (2+ vessels w >50% occlusions) ischemia	ETT induced >1 mm at $.08^+$ sec past J point and horizontal or downsloping; greater likelihood w increased depression, as move from upsloping to downsloping, and w pre-test likelihood (Nejm 1979;300:1354)
	LV strain; subendocardial ischemia/infarct, dig effect	Depressions w or w/o partial T inversions
	Reciprocal changes of MI	Elevations > depressions

Table 2.10.2 *(continued)*

EKG Segment	Dx	Criteria/Abnormalites
ST segments *(cont.)*		
Elevations	Acute injury	Reciprocal changes often also present
	Pericarditis	Reciprocal changes not present; always involve limb and precordial leads, axis $0°-+30°$ (Nejm 1976; 295:523), Ts don't invert until STs normal
	LV aneurysm	Persistent elevations after transmural MI
	Early repolarization	Young patient, upward coving, usually precordial leads, axis $0°-+30°$ (Nejm 1976; 295:523), no evolution; a normal variant
QT intervals		
Short (<.20 sec)	Hypercalcemia	ST segment really short, not the T wave portion
	Dig effect	
Long (see table 2.10.1)	Hypocalcemia	ST segment long w normally shaped Ts though may be inverted
	Hypokalemia, quinidine, phenothiazines, MI, CVA, myotonic dystrophy, myxedema	QT long w flat Ts; U waves; w or w/o ST depressions
T waves		
Peaked	Hyperkalemia	>10 mm high (evolve to wide QRS, and later sine wave pattern), narrow
	Hyperacute MI	>10 mm high, wider
Inversions	LV strain, subendocardial ischemia	Inverted asymmetrically
	LVI	Inversions w/o ST depressions
	RV strain	Isolated to V_{1-3}
	Old MI and/or IMMI or BBB	Inverted symmetrically and >5 mm
	Juvenile pattern	Under age 12 and inverted V_{1-4}
	Hyperventilation; GI disease like cholecystitis (Ann IM 1992;116:218), may elevate STs as well	Inverted asymmetrically and reversion to normal w atropine or isoproterenol
	Subarachnoid bleed	Symmetric, deep inversions across precordium

ASMI = anterior septal MI; ETT = exercise tolerance test; IMMI = intramural MI; IVCD = intraventricular conduction delay; IWMI = inferior wall MI; LAD = left axis deviation; LAE = left atrial enlargement; LAHB = left anterior hemiblock; LGL = Lown-Ganong-Levine syndrome; LPHB = left posterior hemiblock; LVH = left ventricular hypertrophy; LVI = left ventricular ischemia; LVS = left ventricular strain; pLBBB = partial left bundle branch block; pRBBB = partial right bundle branch block; RAD = right axis deviation; RAE = right atrial enlargement; RVH = right ventricular hypertrophy; SEI = subendocardial ischemia; WPW = Wolff-Parkinson-White.

2.10 EKG Reading **127**

Chapter 3
Dermatology

D. K. Onion and E. Sahn

3.1 MEDICATIONS

ANTIFUNGAL AGENTS
  (Rx Let 1999;6:21; Med Let 1997;39:63)

Topicals:
- Butenafine (Mentax) cream qd × 4 wks for tinea pedis, 80% cure
- Ciclopirox (Loprox) 1% lotion/cream bid for tinea, $27/15 gm
- Clotrimazole (Lotrimin) topical × 2–4 wk; used vs monilia and tinea; OTC, inexpensive
- Econazole (Spectazole) cream, for tinea, $12/15 gm
- Haloprogin (Halotex) (Med Let 1988;30:99) topical; used vs tinea, 5% absorbed; $12/15 gm
- Ketoconazole (Nizoral) cream, $15/15 gm; shampoo (Med Let 1994;36:68) $16/4 oz
- Miconazole (Monistat) topical × 2–4 wk; used vs tinea and monilia; $2/15 oz generic, OTC (Micatin)
- Naftifine (Naftin) topical; used vs non monilial dermatophytes; $17/15 gm gel
- Nystatin (Mycostatin) topical; used vs monilia
- Selenium sulfide (Med Let 1994;36:68) 1% OTC or prescription 2.5% shampoo; for t. versicolor and dandruff by decreasing spore spread; $2.70/4 oz generic
- Sulconazole (Exelderm) cream vs tinea; $10/15 gm
- Terbinafine (Lamisil) cream vs tinea bid × 1–2 wk; $28/15 gm, OTC

- Terconazole (Terazole) topical; similar to ketoconazole for vaginal candidiasis
- Tolnaftate (Tinactin) topical × 2–4 wk; used vs tinea, 70$^+$% effective; OTC, cheapest and most cost effective (Jama 1994; 272:1922)
- Undecylenic acid (Cruex, Desenex) creams

Oral/Systemic:

- Fluconazole (Diflucan) (J Am Acad Derm 1994;30:684; Ann IM 1990;113:183); 50–400 mg po qd, eg, 150 mg po × 1 for vaginal candidiasis (Med Let 1994;36:81); vs candida, dermatophytes, and t. versicolor; none of H_2 blocker interference or testosterone problems of ketoconazole
- Griseofulvin (Fulvicin) 250 mg po bid × 4 wk ($22) for skin, × 6–8 wk for foot skin, 500 mg po bid × 6$^+$ mo for fingernails and × 12 mo for toenails ($710); best absorption with a fatty meal, used vs monilia and tinea, prevents infection of newly formed skin; drug of choice in children w t. capitis. Adverse effects: gi intolerance, SLE, sleepiness and headache resolve with continued use
- Itraconazole (Sporonox) (J Am Acad Derm 1994;30:684; Med Let 1993;35:7) 100–200 mg po qd × 6–12 mo for onychomycosis (Med Let 1996;38:5); or pulsed doses of 200 mg po bid 1/4 wks × 3–4 mos; 100 mg po qd × 2–4 wk for t. corporis; vs *Candida,* dermatophytes, and t. versicolor but cmplcs don't justify use usually; also used vs histo, blasto, invasive aspergillosis; 80–90% effective, but amphotericin still better if life threatening; needs gastric acid to be absorbed, less toxic than ketoconazole but adverse reactions (Med Let 1996;38:72) include incr toxicity of cytochrome C-metabolized drugs like erythromycin, benzodiazepams, cisapride, non-sedating antihistamines, as well as hepatotoxicity and CHF (Rx Let 2001;8:33); $5/d for 100 mg qd
- Ketoconazole (Nizoral) topical $12/15 oz; 200–400 mg po qd ($2–4/d); more toxic than griseofulvin; vs candida, dermatophytes, and t. versicolor. Adverse effects: nausea and vomiting, hepatitis (can be fatal) so monitor LFTs q 2 wk, Antabuse-like effect, need gastric acid to absorb, antitestosterone synthesis causes impotence and gynecomastia (Nejm 1987;317:812); decr levels with rifampin (Nejm 1984;311:1681), INH, anticholinergics, and H_2 blockers;

increases effects/levels of warfarin, cyclosporin A, oral
hypoglycemics, and phenytoin
- Terbinafine (Lamisil) (Med Let 1996;38:72) 250 mg po qd × 6 wk
  for fingernails (90% cure), × 12 wk for toenails (40–80% cure),
  or pulsed rx w 500 mg qd 1/4 wks × 3 mos slightly less effective.
  Adverse reactions: headache, gi, taste changes; occasional rash and
  hepatitis (follow LFTs); rare pancytopenias, red eye and
  anaphylaxis; $5/d

ANTIVIRAL AGENTS

- Acyclovir for herpes simplex, zoster, and varicella especially in children
  (Peds 1993;91:674)
- Cimetidine 300 mg po tid × 8 wk for warts in children (Arch Derm
  1996;132:680; J Am Acad Derm 1994;28:794)
- Imiquimod (Aldara) (Rx Let 1997;4:35) topically tiw × 3–4 mo; for
  common and venereal warts and molluscum (Rx Let 2000;7:10); avoid
  in pregnancy; cost $100/mo
- Interferon α-2b used vs warts locally by injections (Med Let 1988;30:70)

TOPICAL STEROIDS
(Med Let 1986;28:57)

Most come in 15, 30, 45, 60, 120 and 240 gm tubes, or as solutions 20 or
60 cc

Adverse effects: local skin atrophy especially on face and with intralesion
injections, never occurs with simple hydrocortisone though;
hypopigmentation and telangiectases; adrenal suppression may occur
when over 2 wk rx especially with occlusive dressings

Topical Steroid Potency Rankings (Am J Med 1999;107:599)

3.2 DERMATOSES

ACNE VULGARIS
Nejm 1969;280:1161

Cause: Hormonal changes of puberty; bacterial (corynebacterium)?,
iodides and bromides, phenytoin (Nejm 1972;287:148)

Epidem: Teenagers; XYY genotype may correlate, especially with early age
of onset (Ann IM 1970;73:270); associated with seborrheic dermatitis

Pathophys: Hypertrophic sebaceous glands lead to incr sebum production and desquamation, especially with androgen stimulation, w comedone formation; sebum undergoes lipolysis by bacteria which, in turn, causes inflammation. Cystic acne is associated with incr androgen levels from partial adrenal 2I-OH deficiency or polycystic ovaries, hence low-dose dexamethasone and/or birth control pills help (Nejm 1983;308:981)

Sx: Acne; iodide and bromide types lack comedones and may be in unusual places

Si: Papules on erythematous base, pustules, comedones

Crs:

Cmplc: **hidradenitis** in axilla or groin, rx with topical and systemic antibiotics, and antibacterial soaps, intralesional steroids; birth control pills occasionally helpful. Avoid I+Ds; rx severe cases with excision of apocrine gland-bearing skin

r/o **acne rosacea** which is central facial; has telangiectases, papules, and pustules w/o comedones or scarring; rx with dietary vasodilator restriction, topical rx with metronidazole 0.75% cream bid (Med Let 1989;31:75), and po tetracycline as below

Lab:

Rx: (Nejm 1997;336:1156)

Mild:

- Avoid facial creams; wash face bid and hair qod
- Topical rx (Med Let 1996;38:53) (all cost $20/bottle) with:
    Benzoyl peroxide, resorcinol, salicylic acid (Pernox, Xerac, Fostex, Banoxyl, Syntex, Abiotin)
    Tretinoin (Retin A, Avita) 0.025, 0.05, or 0.1% cream or gel. Adverse effects: stings transiently first week, sun sensitivity and incr skin cancer risk, and rarely if hepatic dysfunction can get neuropsych toxicity (Ann IM 1996;124:227)
    Tazarotene gel (Tazorac)
    Adapalene gel (Differin) (a retinoid) q hs
    Erythromycin 2% soln gel or cream bid, or 2, 3, or 5% soln w benzoyl peroxide gel (Benzamycin)
    Clindamycin 1% gel, solution or lotion (Nejm 1980;302:503); combined w benzoyl peroxide (BenzaClin) not as good (Rx Let 2001;8:21)
    Azelaic acid (Azelex) 20% cream bid

DERMATOLOGY

Acne Vulgaris, continued

Moderate:
- Birth control pills w 50^+ μ gm of estradiol in women, avoid norethindrone-and norgestrel-containing ones since these have some androgen effect
- Tetracycline 250–500 mg po bid until better, then qd and taper; because of sunburn, use sunscreen or stop in summer, especially w doxycycline (Nejm 1976;294:43); beware of pregnancy in women, because it stains infants' teeth
- Clindamycin po as good or better
- Erythromycin also works
- Azithromycin 250 mg po biw-tiw or less, expensive (Rx Let 1999;6:62)

Severe/Cystic:
- Retinoids:
  Isotretinoin (Accutane) 1–4 mg/kg po qd × 4 mo after derm consult; 100^+/mo; 95% remissions (Med Let 1982;24:79; Nejm 1979;300:329). Adverse effects (FDA Bull 13:21): 33% teratogen in 1st trimester (Nejm 1985;313:837), now legally virtually prohibited for potentially pregnant women (Nejm 1989;320:1007); elevated uric acid; regional ileitis; corneal opacities; elevated lipids may cause atherosclerosis (Nejm 1985; 313:981); pseudotumor cerebri; hyperostosis, at least at higher doses which are used in ichthyosis (Nejm 1983;308:1012); arthritis and fatigue limit use in athletes (R. Kenney 12/85)
  Acitretin (Soriatane) (Rx Let 1997;4:64) po qd; less long acting metabolites than isotretinoin but alcohol counteracts this advantage by converting it to those toxic forms
- Low-dose dexamethasone, w or w/o birth control pills (Nejm 1983;308:981)
- Intralesional steroids
- Cryotherapy

ALOPECIA AREATA

Cause: Probably autoimmune
Epidem: Common; 17/100,000 population

Pathophys: Nonscarring alopecia

Sx: Sudden loss of hair in round or oval patches

Si: Nonscarring patchy hair loss; "exclamation mark" hairs; when regrows, may come in white ("hair turned white overnight")

Crs: Waxes and wanes

Cmplc: r/o other nonscarring alopecia: local active infection, drugs (chronic heparin, colchicine, methotrexate, bc pills, cyclophosphamide), xray rx, hypo- and hyperthyroidism, secondary syphilis (eyebrow and "moth-eaten" occipital hair), t. capitis, **trichotillomania** (nervous tic in which pt pulls own hair out). These contrast with scarring alopecia: trauma, lichen planus, tertiary syphilis, discoid lupus, postinfectious (deep mycosis, typical and atypical tuberculosis, pyoderma)

Lab:

Rx: (Nejm 1999;341:964)

Steroids: topical clobetasol (Temovate) bid or intralesional triamcinolone

Minoxidil topically as 2% ointment or lotion, or 5% solution, helps 85% within 6 wk (BMJ 1983;287:1015), may only prevent further loss and must be continued forever. Adverse effects: minimal systemic absorption and its effects; cost: $2/d for 1 cc bid, OTC less costly

Anthralin (Drithocreme) 0.1% × 2–4 h qd

If resistant, 5% minoxidil + 0.5% anthralin (Arch Derm 1990;126:756); or rarely topical immunotherapy like diphenylcyclopropenone (Derm Clinics 1996;14:739)

DERMATOLOGY

CAPILLARY HEMANGIOMAS, STURGE-WEBER SYNDROME, AND PORT WINE STAINS (PWS)

Nejm 1999;341:173; 1967;277:333

Cause: Congenital

Epidem: PWS: 3/1000 births

Pathophys: CNS, skin, and other organ (eg, liver) hemangiomas

Sx: Skin lesions usually flat, though may be rounded; seizures in Sturge-Weber

Si: Thrills and bruits, hemiparesis and/or other neurologic si's

Crs: Capillary ("strawberry") hemangiomas: 25–50% present at birth, rest appear within 2 mo; maximum growth by 6–12 mo; involution begins in 16% at 6 mo, 65% at 12 mo, gone in 98% by age 9 yr

Sturge-Weber and port wine stains gradually darken and thicken until middle age; no involution

Cmplc: CHF; thrombocytopenia (Kasabach-Merritt syndrome) due to platelet trapping; spinal cord mass lesion si's due to hemangioma there, often (20%) w overlying arteriovenous malformation in same dermatome (Nejm 1969;281:1440)

Glaucoma in 45% if both 1st and 2nd branches of Vth cranial (trigeminal) nerve involved in Sturge-Weber syndrome

Lab:

Xray: Skull in Sturge-Weber may show parallel lines of vessel ("tramline") calcification

MRI in Sturge-Weber to find leptomeningeal hemangiomas

Rx: of capillary hemangiomas: treat symptoms (bleeding, pain, ulceration, or infection). Will usually involute. If life-threatening cmplc or severe deformity of adjacent structures, use intralesional or systemic steroids; pulsed dye laser; or if that fails, interferon α-2a sc qd (Nejm 1992;326:1456)

of port wine stains: flashlamp pulsed tunable dye laser rx under age 5 up to early adulthood works in 95+% (Nejm 1998;338:102; 1989;320:416; Med Let 1997;39:10; 1991;33:104)

DERMATITIS HERPETIFORMIS

Nejm 1983;308:816; Ann IM 1980;93:857

Cause: Genetic association in 90% (HLA B8 and DR_w3—Ann IM 1982;97:105) but not clinically hereditary

Epidem: Associated with Hashimoto's thyroiditis, hypothyroidism, hyperthyroidism, and thyroid nodules in 50% (Ann IM 1985;102:194); pregnancy; hypoparathyroidism

Males > females

Pathophys: IgA deposition at dermal/epidermal junction, because is allergic in etiology (J Am Acad Derm 1992;27:209, Ann IM 1982;97:105)

Sx: Debilitating itch and rash; precipitated by UV, steroids, and infection (Ann IM 1984;100:677)

Si: Umbilicated, grouped vesicles, r/o other viral (h. simplex, h. zoster, variola, varicella)

Crs:

Cmplc: Lymphomas

r/o pustular psoriasis, often indistinguishable even histologically (Ann IM 1984;100:677)

Lab:

Path: Small bowel bx shows sprue-like pathology even though asymptomatic; skin bx shows IgA at dermal-epidermal junction

Rx: Gluten-free diet, rice and oats ok (Nejm 1997;337:1884) but takes two years to help

Sulfapyridine 4 gm po qd

Dapsone 100 mg po qd; inhibits polys chemotaxis. Adverse effects: G6PD deficiency anemia precipitation, severe peripheral neuropathies

ECZEMATOUS DERMATITIS

Cause:

- *Atopic:* Genetic, often autosomal dominant, co-inherited w bronchial hyperresponsiveness and asthma (Nejm 1995;333:894); sometimes associated w interleukin-4 receptor mutation, enhancing allergy (Nejm 1997;337:1720, 1766)
- *Contact:* Rhus (poison ivy and others), mango rind (Nejm 1998;339:235), and gypsy moth caterpillar hairs (find with scotch tape—Nejm 1982;306:1300); by direct contact
- *Neurodermatitis* (psychiatrically self-induced)
- Type IV DHS reaction to allergen, eg, latex allergy in gloves, 82% of latex allergies are this, rarely are anaphylactic type I (Ann IM 1995;122:43)

Epidem:

Pathophys:

Sx:

Acute: Characterized by weeping vesicles, chronic by pruritus and lichenification

Atopic: H/o stress, allergies, asthma

    Contact: H/o contact, especially when wet; burning more than itching; appears within 24 h of contact, hyperpigmentation may occur later

    Neurodermatitis: H/o stress, dependent personality, self-excoriation

Si:

    Atopic: Medial, infraorbital skin pleat (Morgan-Dennie fold)

    Contact: Linear lesions somewhere

    Neurodermatitis: Scratching

Crs: No spread

Cmplc: r/o **"id" reaction** (autosensitization) which may follow any rash, especially chronic ones of lower extremities like stasis dermatitis; and Wiskott-Aldrich syndrome (p 377)

Lab:

    Serol: In atopics, IgE elevated ≥95 IU and/or ≥3 pos RAST tests to common allergens (Nejm 1997;337:1720) often

Rx: Prevent w/Lactobacillus Peripartum halves eczema incidence at age 2 (Lancet 2001;357:1076)

- Avoid vaccinations and herpes infections in atopic dermatitis
- Wet soaks with Domeboro's soln, etc., 10–20 min qid
- Topical steroids immediately after soaks, then emollients like Crisco, mineral oil, Lubriderm, Eucerin, petrolatum
- Antihistamines po, especially hydroxyzine, which can be taken in high doses but may be sedating; and antipain meds, since itching is a form of pain
- Doxepin (tricyclic antidepressant) 5% topical cream helps though is absorbed (Med Let 1994;36:99)
- Steroids, topically with occlusion; avoid systemic because of rebound
- Tar preparations occasionally help
- Crushed plantain (Nejm 1980;303:583; Shakespeare's Romeo and Juliet 1.2.52–53) for poison ivy
- Tacrolimus (Protopic) 0.03% or 0.1% ointment bid helps (related to cyclosporine) (Med Let 2001;43:33; Nejm 1997;337:816); cmplc: burning sensation, photosensitivity, possible immunosuppression, skin malignancies and lymphomas, eczema herpeticum; 30 gm of 1% = $60

NEUROFIBROMATOSIS OF VON RECKLINGHAUSEN (Neurofibromatosis Type I)

Jama 1997;278:51; J Am Acad Derm 1993;29:376; Ann IM 1990; 113:39; Nejm 1991;324:1283

Cause: Genetic, autosomal dominant or sporadic mutations in germline cells (Nejm 1994;331:1403); mutation on long arm of chromosome #17

Epidem: Incidence: 1/3000–3500 births

Pathophys:

Sx: Onset by age 5, variable depending on site of lesions

Si: Café-au-lait spots (90%); 6 spots, >1.5 cm in adults, or >0.5 cm in prepubertal patients (Peds 1992;90:924; J Peds 1990;116:845) are diagnostic; axillary or inguinal "freckles" (Crowe sign) are the same thing; "coast of California" smooth edges unlike "coast of Maine" edges of Albright's syndrome (bone cysts and fibrous dysplasia, precocious puberty; rx'd with testolactone—Nejm 1986;315:1115)

Neurofibromas: soft skin nodules; plexiform neurofibromas are subcutaneous nodules along nerve course; also present internally, especially in bone and CNS

Lisch nodules, dome-shaped pigmented hamartomas on iris; present in 100% by age 20 yr (Nejm 1991;324:1264)

Crs: Variable

Cmplc:

- Pheochromocytomas (in <1%; 10% of pheos have neurofibromatosis)
- Renal artery stenosis and hypertension
- Bony, especially vertebral, and joint complaints
- Optic pathway gliomas
- CNS lesions, some cause retardation; mass effect, especially at foramen magnum; lesions of eighth cranial nerve often, also of fifth and eleventh. But acoustic neuromas are from central type II neurofibromatosis, a distinct and separate genetic abnormality (p 170)
- Sarcomatous degeneration into neurofibrosarcomas in 5–10% (Nejm 1967;277:1363)
- Spinal nerve compression at neural foramina especially in chest
- Pulmonary
- Chronic myelogenous leukemia in children (Nejm 1997;336:1713)

Lab:

Rx: Monitor for cmplc's

Surgical excision of individual neurofibromas

DERMATOLOGY

PSORIASIS

Am J Med;1999;107:595; Nejm 1995;332:581

Cause: Probably polygenetic; 91% of patients have positive family history; associated with HLA antigens W17 and HLA 13 (Nejm 1972;287:738,740; 1972;288:704), HIV infection (Bull Rheum Dis 1990;39:5)

Epidem: Worst in winter, probably from dryness and lack of sunlight; 1–2% of US population, rare in US blacks

Pathophys: Abnormal control of epidermal cell division or differentiation; 5x normal number of cells are synthesizing DNA. Cells migrate through epidermis too fast, hence is an epidermal hyperplastic condition that never becomes neoplastic. No other organ involvement, except possibly synovium. In exfoliative stage, can lose protein and go into negative nitrogen balance. Perhaps trauma causes initial elbow/knee changes

Sx: Onset usually under age 30 yr; doubt dx if onset over age 60 yr
Precipitated by stress (emotional, alcoholic binge, postinfection, drug reaction especially propranolol, chloroquine, NSAIDs, and lithium)
Arthritis (5%), asymmetric like ankylosing spondylitis (Bull Rheum Dis 1987;37:1)

Si: Papulosquamous rash; papule with scale which, when picked, leads to punctate bleeding (inter-rete ridge capillary); occasional pustular variant. Elbow, knee, scalp, gluteal cleft, flexor surfaces are initial distribution often; nail pitting; Koebner's phenomenon: rash appears at site of scratch or trauma 2–3 wk later

Crs:

Cmplc: Gout; exfoliative dermatitis (r/o mycosis fungoides if age >45 yr); pustular exacerbation with fever, inflammation, and pain, associated with hypoparathyroidism (r/o dermatitis herpetiformis—Ann IM 1984;100:677)

r/o **guttate psoriasis:** small droplet-sized lesions erupt over 1 wk poststrep infection, positive throat culture and ASO titer up (Arch Derm 1992;128:39), or with perianal strep in children (Ped Derm 1990;7:97) and spontaneously resolve over 2 mo

Lab:
Path: Skin bx shows acanthosis (incr epidermal thickness); retention of nuclei; rete ridges deeper, bigger, and some fused; interridge capillaries tortuous and close to surface and so bleed when scale picked. Feulgen stain shows mitochondria, ribosomes, and DNA in stratum corneum

Chem: Uric acid incr (due to incr cell turnover?)

Xray: Hands look like RA except no osteoporosis; whittled-down tufts like scleroderma, "pencil in cup" dip's

Rx: of scalp: steroids, salicylic acid solutions, tar shampoos, mineral oil of other areas:

- Sunlight or other broad band UVB source, short of burn, which will cause flare
- Steroids topically (avoid systemic po steroids which can precipitate pustular psoriasis) for small areas, with occlusive plastic dressings; or injections, eg, dilute (1:3) triamcinolone with lidocaine. Adverse effects: widespread use leads to systemic absorption and adrenal suppression; can precipitate exfoliative erythroderm; skin atrophy; rebound much more likely than with anthralin
- Anthralin paste, 0.1%, 0.2%, or 0.4%, to rash qd for 10 min to 1 h, then removal with mineral oil, bath, and extensive hydrophilic ointment; or Z-tar emulsion topically × 1 h, then shower, follow with UV; avoid groin; stains hair, skin
- Calcipotriene (Dovonex) (Med Let 1994;36:70) ointment 0.005% bid; a vit D analog, as good as topical steroids, although tachyphylaxis potential unknown; often used w potent or superpotent topical steroid (KOO regimen) initially then taper steroid. Adverse effects: hypercalcemia at high doses because it is a vit D analog; $120/10 gm; or similar
- Tazarotene gel (Tazorac) (topical retinoid) (Med Let 1997;39:105; Rx Let 1997;4:45) 0.05 or 0.1% qd to <20% of body surface (<40 gm/wk); for stable plaque type psoriasis; avoid in pregnancy; $2/gm

2nd line meds:

- Calcitriol (Calcijex) (J Am Acad Derm 1992;27:983,1001)
- Methotrexate 2.5–5 mg q 12 h × 3 doses q 1 week, but check current guidelines (Arch IM 1990;150:889); 10% get liver disease (Am J Med 1991;90:711)
- Psoralen or methoxsalen po with UVA (PUVA) highly effective, used tiw × 10 wk helps 85% then maintenance q 1–4 wk, but increases incidence of squamous cell cancer × 3 (Nejm 1984;310:1156) including male genitals unless protected (Nejm 1990;322:1093) and melanoma risk w 10 yr lag (Nejm 1997;336:1041)
- Acitretin (Soriatane) (Med Let 1997;39:106) 25–50 mg po qd w food. Adverse effects: teratogenic for 3 yr after stop, elevated LFTs

DERMATOLOGY

can revert on rx, various anterior eye changes, all worse w
alcohol, pseudotumor cerebri esp w tetracycline; $7/pill

- Etretinate (Tegison) (vit A-like retinoid) po. Adverse effects: toxic
and teratogenic up to 2 yr post rx; now replaced by acitretin
- Cyclosporine works, though nephrotoxic (J Am Acad Derm
1995;32:78; Nejm 1991;324:1277)
- Hydroxyurea (J Am Acad Derm 1991;25:522)

Experimental (Nejm 2001;345:248, 284): immune suppression w
monoclonal antibodikes vs CD4 and CD8 T cells w TNF agents like
infliximab, etanercept, alefacept, and hu 1124, all of which modify
of arthritis: (p 789) (Arch Rheum 1996;132:215)

TUBEROUS SCLEROSIS (Adenoma Sebaceum)
Arch Derm 1994;130:348

Cause: Genetic; autosomal dominant in 25%, sporadic in 75% (Arch
Derm 1995;131:1460)

Epidem: 1/10,000 population

Pathophys: Large hamartomas of brain, skin, et al. White spots due to
decr synthesis of melanin, but since there is a normal number of
melanocytes, they are not vitiligo

Sx: Epilepsy, mental retardation in some

Si: Peri/subungual fibromas especially of toenail; angiofibromas of face
(adenoma sebaceum), may look like acne w/o blackheads;
hypopigmented macular patches ("ash leaf" macules or "white
confetti") on the legs, best seen under Wood's light (Nejm
1998;338:1887), especially at birth, are first si; collagenoma of
lower back skin looks like pig skin; fibrous plaques on forehead;
mulberry tumors in fundus; pitted tooth enamel

Crs: Variable

Cmplc: Seizures (75%); renal failure due to angioleiomyoma and
angiomyolipomas on ultrasound and CT (Nejm 1998;338:1886);
honeycomb lung; rhabdomyosarcoma of heart (Nejm
1967;276:957); hamartomas throughout body

Lab:

Xray: MRI/CT of head shows calcified tumors or gliomas, subependymal tubers (Nejm 1998;338:1886)

Rx: Monitor for cmplc

URTICARIA/ERYTHEMA MULTIFORME

Nejm 1995;332:1767; 1994;331:1272 (drug induced)

Cause + Pathophys:

Idiopathic (80%)

Direct histamine release by opiates, NSAIDs, IVP dye (steroids protect), thiamine, curare, dextrans, some antibiotics

Immunologic:

- C' activation by cryoglobulins (IgG or cold agglutinins produced by tumors, multiple myeloma, SLE, arteritis, etc.), or by B_1C globulin damage (snake venom, DIC). Angioneurotic edema is C' mediated but is not urticaria.
- Antibodies vs mast cells; or, in chronic urticaria, their IgE receptors (Nejm 1993;328:1599)
- Mast cells as "innocent bystanders," eg, SLE, serum sickness, viral (especially coxsackie) infections or post h. simplex with antigens in all lesions (Ann IM 1984;101:48), leukemias and other malignancies, drugs (especially sulfas, seizure meds, allopurinol, NSAIDs), parasites, hepatitis B, perhaps mononucleosis plus ampicillin; nearly all recurrent erythema multiforme and most primary episodes are due to h. simplex, but a few of the latter are due to mycoplasma and drugs (E. Ringle 1990)
- Mast cell fixed antibody (IgE), eg, to fish, bee sting, penicillin
- Type IV (DHS) immune reaction leads to vasculitis

Physical/"neurogenic":

- Cold urticaria (test with ice cube), perhaps IgE attaches to a cold-dependent skin antigen and releases platelet-activating factor (Nejm 1985;313:405; 1985;305:1074)
- Local heat urticaria
- Systemic heat urticaria, cholinergic; seen when core body temperature is elevated, starts around hair follicles; seen in runners, tennis players, etc.
- Light/solar

- Stress
- Dermatographia

Associated diseases: urticaria pigmentosa occasionally (p 142) and anaphylaxis (p 17)

Epidem: 25% of adult population has had chronic urticaria × wks-mos.

Sx: Urticaria (hives), mucosal angioedema with all but physical types; abdominal pain (gi histamine release)

Si: Target skin lesions of erythema multiforme, raised urticarial lesions et al.; bilateral symmetry always suggests drug-induced first

Crs: Except in vasculitis, immunologic, and physical types, most lesions last <24 h

Cmplc: Epidermal detachment of mucous membranes, locally in Stevens-Johnson syndrome w 5% mortality, or extensively in toxic epidermal necrolysis (p 155) w 30% mortality (Nejm 1995;333:1660) (r/o systemic diseases like SLE, dermatomyositis, scarlet fever [p 327])

Lab:

Path: Skin bx at site of recent urticaria to r/o vasculitis

Rx: Avoid ACE inhibitors and NSAIDs; 2% ephedrine spray for angioedema; H_1 receptor antagonist antihistamines like loratidine 10 mg po qd (p 176); H_2 blockers like cimetidine sometimes also helpful

of acute, see anaphylaxis (p 17)

of cold urticaria: cyproheptadine (Periactin) best; doxepin (Sinequan) 10–25 mg po bid (Nejm 1985;313:405)

of heat (cholinergic) type: hydroxyzine (Atarax, Vistaril)

of vasculitis: steroids

of mast cell types: ketotifen 2 mg po bid, stabilizes mast cells (Ann IM 1986;104:507); acyclovir for, at least, recurrent erythema multiforme

URTICARIA PIGMENTOSA, MASTOCYSTOSIS

Nejm 1992;326:639; Mod Conc Cardiovasc Dis 1985;54:1

Cause:

Epidem: Fairly common

Pathophys: Abnormal mast cell proliferation, either neoplastic or reactive to soluble mast cell growth factor (Nejm 1993;328:1302), especially in skin and gi tract; intermittent chemical or mechanical irritation leads to release of histamine and prostaglandin D_2, et al. (Ped Derm 1986;3:265; J Am Acad Derm 1982;7:709; Nejm 1980;303:1400)

Sx: Episodic attacks of flushing, itching, palpitations, headaches, orthostatic sx, hyperventilation, abdominal cramping; attacks may be precipitated by alcohol, narcotics, and aspirin; freckles all over body, if rubbed cause urticaria (urticaria pigmentosa) (J Invest Derm 1991;96:325)

Si: Orthostatic BP changes

Crs: Usually benign in children; may be severe in adults (J Intern Med 1996;239:157)

Cmplc:

Lab:

Chem: 24-h urine especially after attack, for histamine metabolites (N-methylimidazole acetic acid, N-methylhistamine) and prostaglandin levels

Path: Skin bx shows 4+ mast cells in skin lesions

Rx: Acutely, adrenalin

Chronically, prevent with:

- Avoidance of narcotics, alcohol, and aspirin
- Chlorpheniramine 8 mg po qid or other antihistamine (Med Let 1989;31:43)
- Cimetidine 300 mg qid po or other H_2 blocker
- Na cromolyn 100 mg po (not inhalation) qid (Nejm 1979;301:465) for gi sx
- Ketotifen 2 mg po bid stabilizes mast cells (Ann IM 1986;104:507)
- PUVA rx (psoralens and UVA)

of mast cell tumor load: interferon α-2b causes dramatic regression (Nejm 1992;326:619)

3.3 INFECTIOUS DERMATITIS

CANDIDIASIS (MONILIASIS, LOCAL)

(Including vaginal)

Nejm 1997;337:1896 (vaginal), Ann IM 1984;101:390

Cause: *Candida albicans,* or rarely *tropicalis (*Ann IM 1979;91:539) or *glabrata*

Epidem: Associated with diabetes, cancer, blood dyscrasias, multiple antibiotic use, steroids, TPN, thymoma with myositis (Jama 1972;222:1619), various endocrine conditions, eg, bcp use, hypoparathyroidism, hypothyroidism, and hypoadrenalism. One form is due to an inherited defect in suppressor T cells (Nejm 1979;300:164)

Pathophys: Normal flora, opportunistic invasion

Sx: Vaginitis, dyspareunia, vulvar rash, oral mucous membranes as thrush, which scrapes off, conjunctivitis or uveitis, nails, perianal (diaper rash), rectum, other skin folds

Si: Inflammatory reactions; skin lesions have whitish central lesion with satellite pustules

Crs:

Cmplc: r/o associated conditions listed above; trichomonal (p 476) and bacterial vaginosis (p 407)

Lab:

Bact: Pseudohyphae (40%) on 10% KOH exam of skin scrapings or vaginal discharge; culture on rice/Tween agar shows distinctive pseudohyphae and condiospores; vaginal pH = 4–4.5

Rx: (for vaginal regimens and costs—Med Let 2001;43:3): All vaginal rx costs ~$10–30/course

Topical (all 80^+% effective):

1st:

- Miconazole (Monistat) 2% cream bid to skin; or vaginally bid, or 100 mg qd × 7 d, or DS × 3 d, or 1200 mg × 1
- Clotrimazole (Lotrimin) 10 mg troches sl work for oral thrush (Nejm 1978;299:1201); or 5 gm of 1% cream or 100–200 mg tab vaginally qd × 7, 2 tab qd × 3 d, or 500 mg once
- Butoconazole (Femstat, Mycelex) 2% cream 5 gm qd × 3–6 d (Med Let 1986;28:68), or as Gynazole 5 gm × 1 ($28)
- Terconazole (Terazol) 0.4% or 0.8% crm or 80 mg vag tab qd × 3–7 d
- Tioconazole (Vagistat) 6.5% cream, 4.6 gm hs × 1

2nd:

- Nystatin 100,000 U topically qd-qid × 14 d; 50% effective for vaginal candidiasis

Oral/Systemic (all 80+% effective):
- Fluconazole (Diflucan) 150 mg po × 1; 80+% effective; BEST for vaginitis, as good as or better than other regimens (Med Let 1994;36:81), $12; 150 mg po q 1 wk to prevent recurrent vaginitis (Nejm 1997;337:1896)
- Ketoconazole (Nizoral) 200 mg po qd vs mucocutaneous type (Ann IM 1980;93:791); for vaginitis 400 po qd × 5 d, or qd × 14 d, then 100 mg po qd prophylaxis works for frequent recurrences (Nejm 1986;315:1455)
- Itraconazole (Sporonox) 200 mg po × 3 d (Antimicrob Agents Chemother 1993;37:89)
- Nystatin 5 million U po tid × 1–2 wk to clear gi tract or biw for chronic prevention of especially recurrent vaginal candidiasis

TINEA CAPITIS, CORPORIS, PEDIS, AND CRURIS (Onychomycosis, Ringworm, Athlete's Foot)

Cause: Dermatophytes, *Trichophyton* spp. most commonly; also *Microsporum, Epidermophyton*

Epidem: Perhaps genetic susceptibility; worldwide; incr in Cushing's patients. Tinea corporis seen in children with puppy or kitten; t. capitis especially common in black children

Pathophys:

Sx: Annular, red, scaly, pruritic rash

Si: Scaling rash head, body, groin, between toes; annular, ringworm appearance often; distorted white flaking nails w onychomycosis. Wood's lamp illumination shows yellow-green fluorescence w *Microsporum* spp.

Crs:

Cmplc: Secondary bacterial infections; kerion of scalp, inflammation that can lead to severe scarring
  r/o granuloma annulare (p 161) and pityriasis rosea (p 156), which both have similar round lesions; pustular psoriasis when on soles and/or palms; in groin, **erythrasma,** a diphtheroid skin infection that fluoresces coral red in Wood's lamp light, rx w topical or oral erythromycin

Lab:
  Bact: KOH prep shows branching hyphae. Culture on Sabouraud's
    media
Rx: (Med Let 1993;35:77)
  Topical:
  • Ciclopirox (Penlac nail lacquer) (Med Let 2000;42:51) qd to nails,
    wash off weekly, 50% effective, $180/yr
  • Clotrimazole (Lotrimin) OTC, may be more effective than
    tolnaftate and covers candida (Med Let 1976;18:101) and
    inexpensive
  • Tolnaftate (Tinactin); doesn't work in scalp, hair, nails, palms, and
    soles
  • Haloprogen (Halotex); expensive, absorbed (5%) (Med Let
    1988;30:99), etc. (p 128)
  • Selenium sulfide shampoo 2.5% (Selsun) to decrease spore count
    and intrafamilial spread
  Oral (J Am Brd of Fam Pract 2000;13:268) (use only for nails, topical
    resistant skin infections, or in immunocompromised):
  1st:
  • Terbinefin (Lamisil) (p 128) for nails, 250 mg po qd × 12$^+$ wks,
    <70% effective; $650/3mo; pulsed rx w 500 mg qd 1/4 wks ×
    3 mos slightly less effective
  2nd:
  • Itraconazole 100 mg po qd × 2–4 wk for t. corporis; 200 mg po
    qd × 3–6 mo for nails, $1200/3 mos (Med Let 1996;38:5), or
    pulsed doses of 200 mg po bid 1/4 wks × 3–4 mos
  3rd:
  • Griseofulvin 250 mg po bid × 4 wk for skin, × 6–8 wk for t.
    pedis, 500 mg po bid × 6$^+$ mo for fingernails, × 12$^+$ mo for
    toenails, $750; in children w t. capitis, 15 mg/kg qd × 8 wk; best
    absorption with a fatty meal, eg, whole milk or ice cream

TINEA VERSICOLOR

Cause: *Pityrosporum ovale*
Epidem: Common, 20% adults have; often appears at puberty

Pathophys: A very superficial infection

Sx: Patchy areas of skin especially on shoulders, chest, and arms which are dark in winter, pale (don't tan) in summer

Si: Macular and punctate lesions often coalesce into confluent, scaly patches. Woods lamp fluorescence not clinically useful

Crs:

Cmplc:

Lab:

    Bact: Skin scraping with KOH shows "spaghetti and meatballs" (short hyphae and spores)

Rx:

- Selenium 2.5% (Selsun) shampoo qd, leave on 20 min, × 14 d; often recurs
- Ketoconazole 2% shampoo 5 min/day × 3d (J Am Acad Derm 1998;39:944)
- Fluconazole (Diflucan) 50 mg po qd × 2 wk ($61) or 400 mg po × 1 ($25); 75% cure at 6 wk (Acta Derm Venereol 1992;72:74)
- Itraconazole (Sporonox) 100 mg po qd × 15 d ($74) (Clin Experim Dermatol 1990;15:101), or 200 mg po × 5 d ($50) (J Am Acad Derm 1990;23(part 2):551)
- Ketaconazole (Nizoral) 200 mg po qd × 5 d ($11), or 400 mg po × 1 ($9), repeating in 1 wk or monthly at 200 mg po qd × 2 (DICP 1991;25:395)

VENEREAL (Genital) WARTS

Cause: Human papilloma virus

Epidem: Venereal spread and highly infective; incidence ~40% in college women w resolution and reinfection common (Nejm 1998;338:423); prevalence higher in HIV pos women (Nejm 1997;337:1343). Cause of laryngeal papillomas from aspiration at delivery (Nejm 1983;308:1261)

Pathophys: Virus present in normal as well as wart skin (Nejm 1985;313:784)

Sx: 1–6 mo incubation. Pain at site

Si: Warts on genitalia; in male partners, often flat and hard to see (Nejm 1987;317:916)

Crs:

Cmplc: Cervical carcinoma (p 588) (Lancet 2000;355:2189, 2194),
especially types 16 and 18, intraepithelial neoplasia often within
2 yr of contagion (Nejm 1992;327:1272) and eventual cervical
cancer in an unknown but significant number (Nejm 1999;341:
1633); also associated with vaginal, endometrial, vulvar (Nejm
1986;315:1052), anal (Nejm 1997;337:1350; 1987;317:973),
laryngeal, and conjunctival (Nejm 1989;320:1442) cancers
r/o molluscum contagiosum (p 162)

Lab:

Rx: (Med Let 1999;41:90) to patient and partner; stain area w acetic acid
1st to bring out latent warts for rx, especially in men; all work for
common warts rx too.

- Podophyllin soln, leave on 8 h 1st time, 24 h subsequently, or as gel
  (Condylox) (Rx Let 1997;4:35); avoid in pregnancy because of fetal
  damage and even death with only 1–2 cc; use cryotherapy instead
- Trichloroacetic acid topically, OK in pregnancy
- Electrodessication, OK in pregnancy
- Liquid N_2, OK in pregnancy
- Imiguimod (Aldara) (p 130) topically tiw × 3–4 mo; avoid in
  pregnancy
- Interferon injections tiw × 3 wk (Ann IM 1988;108:675; Nejm
  1986;315:1059); qd × 1 mo then tiw × 6 mo helps for respiratory
  papillomas (Nejm 1991;325:613), consider doing this if surgery
  required on papillomas q 3 mo

3.4 SKIN CANCERS

BASAL CELL CARCINOMAS

Nejm 1992;327:1649

Cause: Idiopathic; actinic

Epidem: Older patients; associated with sun UVB exposure and light
complexion; arsenical rx and arsenical keratoses of palm;
>>500,000/yr in US, increasing rapidly; 4^+x as common as
squamous cell Ca

Pathophys:

Sx:

Si: Exposed areas; telangiectasias, pearly raised borders, no incr keratin; may be a pit if marked stromal reaction; and central ulceration occasionally; occasionally pigmentation, often stippled

Crs:

Cmplc: Slight incr risk of other cancers (5–20%) (Ann IM 1996;125:815); in those dx'd under age 60, risk incr for testicular, breast, and non-Hodgkins lymphoma

  r/o **congenital basal cell nevus syndrome** (Nejm 1986;314:700); genetic, autosomal dominant; in young pts w pitted palms, large head with frontal bossing and wide eyes, who have multiple basal cell carcinomas; cmplc: jaw cysts, ovarian fibromas, medulloblastoma; rx w topical 5-FU and tretinoin (J Am Acad Derm 1992;27:842)

Lab:

  Path: Excisional biopsy

Rx:

- Excision
- Electrodesiccation and curettage, least traumatic but avoid around eyes, ears, nose, scalp, or if >2 cm or recurrent
- Radiation w 3000–6000 rad total dose at 300 qd, 89% successful, or w radium needles also possible, avoid in basal cell nevus syndrome since can be carcinogenic
- Cryotherapy
- 5-FU topically on penis or if multiple lesions, usually is only palliative

Refer for Mohs' microsurgery or for surgical excision if aggressive histopathology, recurrent, >2 cm, or involves ears, temples, midface triangle, or scalp

SQUAMOUS CELL CARCINOMA

Nejm 2001;344:975; 1992;327:1649

Cause: Neoplasia from sun exposure directly (eg, Canadian fishermen—Nejm 1975;293:411) or medical PUVA, eg, for psoriasis; or from actinic keratoses, or other chronic irritation, eg, sites of chronic osteomyelitis drainage which have an especially bad prognosis (Nejm 1980;303:367); or in renal transplant pts w HLA

Squamous Cell Carcinoma, continued

B mismatches, possibly from diminished surveillance (Nejm 1991;325:843)

Epidem: >>100,000/yr in US; 100–150/100,000/yr, over age 75 incid is 1000–1500/100,000/yr increasing rapidly

Associated with UVB sun exposure in whites; arsenical rx with arsenical keratoses of palm; lip lesions w renal transplant (Nejm 1995;332:1052); perhaps herpes simplex type II, causing vulvar carcinoma in situ though may not be full-blown squamous cell carcinoma (Nejm 1981;305:517, 483); **xeroderma pigmentosa** (autosomal recessive inability to repair UV-damaged DNA-Nejm 1986;314:1423), rx with po isotretinoin (Nejm 1988;318:1633)

Pathophys:

Sx: Skin sore that won't heal

Si: Skin ulceration with varying degrees of subcutaneous and intradermal invasion; scale and erythema; cutaneous horn sometimes, r/o seborrheic and actinic keratosis

Crs: Mortality <1/500, 1500 deaths/yr in US

Cmplc: 30% incr risk of non-dermal cancers like multiple myeloma, lymphoma, leukemias as well as incr risk of dermal basal cell carcinomas (Am J Epidem 1995;141:916) as well as worse prognosis when get other cancers (Ann IM 1999;131:655)

r/o wart recently treated with podophyllin; **actinic keratosis** (senile or solar), which may be multiple, may progress to squamous cell carcinoma and may be excised, frozen, or treated w topical 5-FU or masoprocol 10% cream bid × 28 d (Med Let 1993;35:97), prevent w sunscreen (Nejm 1993;329:1147); keratoacanthoma looks clinically and pathologically very similar, rx like squamous cell cancer

Lab:

Path: Biopsy, excisional or wedge if dx uncertain; in situ lesions called Bowen's Disease

Rx: Prevent w PABA sunscreens; 5-FU 5% cream bid × 4 wk to actinic keratoses, produces inflammation, vesiculation, and resolution. β carotene does not prevent new tumors (Lancet 1999;354:723; Nejm 1990;323:789) but low-fat diet does dramatically (Nejm 1994;330:1272)

Therapeutic (J Am Acad Derm 1993;28:628): surgical excision or referral for Mohs' micrographic surgery if high risk (>2 cm; into sc

tissue, histopathology > well-differentiated grade I, or involvement
of scalp, nose, ears, eyelids, or lips); irradiation; isotretinoin
0.5 mg/kg bid po × months if resistant (to surgery + radiation) or
recurrent extensive disease (Ann IM 1987;107:499)

MALIGNANT MELANOMA
Nejm 1991;325:171; Ann IM 1985;102:546; Jama 1984;251:1864

Cause: UV irradiation damage esp. in childhood, even in cases of ocular
melanoma (Nejm 1985;313:789); high intensity burns, which reach
melancocytes worse than chronic sun exposure (Nejm
1999;340:1341)

Congenital nevi: melanoma occurs w highest frequency in those
>20 cm diameter at birth; most feel risk to some degree even <2 cm
but some say no risk there (Jama 1997;277:1439).

Atypical mole syndrome (AMS) (NIH Consensus Statement
1992;10:1), or older term, dysplastic nevus syndrome (DNS) (Nejm
1985;312:91; Ann IM 1985;102:458—both with pictures); on short
arm of chromosome #1 (Nejm 1989;320:1367)

Epidem: 8th most common cancer in US (20th in 1985) (Ann IM
1996;125:369); 1/80 lifetime risk in US

Increased in Celts, especially those with red hair

Congenital nevi occur in ~1% of pop, though rarely >20 cm diameter

AMS can be autosomal dominant or sporadic; 2–5% prevalence; of
familial type, 100% will get in lifetime and account for 10% of all
melanomas; 18% of sporadics will get in lifetime and account for
30–50% of all melanomas; incr prevalence in Hodgkin's patients
(Ann IM 1985;102:37); but a few atypical nevi do not imply AMS,
although incidence of melanoma is still higher (Jama 1997;277:1439)

Pathophys:

Sx: Black, blue, or gray lesions increasing in size; pain; pruritus; bleeding;
notched borders; asymmetric

Si: Central black (or blue-gray "hurricane gray" = variable pigment)
papule or nodule in center of lentigo, dysplastic nevus, or normal
skin; disorderly color, surface, and edges; inflamed; occasional
satellites; does not dimple if squeezed unlike dermatofibromas
(Nejm 1976;294:1511). Amelanotic melanomas most often on soles

DERMATOLOGY

Malignant Melanoma, continued

Crs:
    Stage I: survival by thickness, <0.75 mm has a 96% 5-yr survival, >4 mm has a 47% 5-yr survival

    Stage II: nodal mets, 36% 5-yr survival

    Stage III: distant mets, 5% 5-yr survival

Cmplc: 2nd or 3rd primary melanoma, especially in AMS (DNS)

    r/o other melanotic lesions including **tinea nigra palmaris** (Nejm 1970;283:1112), junctional, compound, or dermal nevi which may have halos; **lentigo maligna** (only a few bizarre melanocytes), seen most often in elderly, in sun-exposed areas, good prognosis, a precursor, **nevus of ota,** benign melanosis of eye and surrounding skin in 1st and 2nd branches of trigeminal nerve, seen in 1/200 Asians, rx w laser (Nejm 1994;331:1745)

Lab:
    Path: Excisional (or incisional or punch if too large; never curette) biopsy; melanoma is staged by thickness of tumor. Reverse transcriptase PCR study of sentinel nodes find tumor in 1/2 of nodes neg by standard path techniques, and recurrence rates are higher in those pts (Jama 1998;280:1410)

Xray: CT and gallium scanning especially good for metastases (Ann IM 1982;97:694)

Rx: (NIH Consensus Statement 1992;10:1)

    Prevent by excision of congenital nevi, at least those >20 cm or those that are changing, and of changing atypical moles; photographs can help to follow both

    of lesions: excision with 1–2 cm margins (Jama 2001;285:1819) though 1–2 mm adequate for diagnostic excisions

    of metastatic disease: follow w hx, PE and chest xray to monitor for mets (Jama 1995;274:1703)

      • Interferon α-2 iv may help (Ann IM 1985;103:32)

      • Radiation helps palliate local lesions

      • Chemotherapy by isolated perfusion of extremities being tried

      • Adoptive immunotherapy with tumor-infiltrating lymphocytes (lymphocyte-activated killer cells) + interleukin 2 helps 5–10% to remission when widely metastatic disease (Nejm 1990;323:570; Med Let 1990;32:85)

- Dacarbazine + tamoxifen (Nejm 1992;327:516)

Nonspecific delayed hypersensitivity stimulators like BCG (Nejm 1982;307:913) and levamisole (Nejm 1980;303:1143) are no help

CUTANEOUS T-CELL LYMPHOMAS: Sézary Syndrome, Mycosis Fungoides, and Reticulum Cell Lymphoma

Ann IM 1988;109:372

Cause: Malignancies of T-cell lymphocytes (Ann IM 1974;80:685)

Epidem: Mostly in older (age >40 yr) patients; associated with industrial solvent exposure in older studies, also chronic contact dermatitis

Pathophys: "Helper" T_4 lymphocyte lymphomas

Sézary syndrome has erythrodermic variants plus circulating malignant T cells

Sx: Erythematous, scaly plaques, nodules, and tumors

Si:

Stage I: Polymorphic indurated papulosquamous rash; polycyclic red-brown scaly plaques (r/o sarcoid, Behçet's syndrome)

Stage II: Generalized erythroderm and cutaneous nodules

Stage III: Organ invasions lead to "-megalies"

Crs:

Stage I: 12^+ yr average survival (Arch Derm 1996;132:1309)

Stage II: 5 yr average survival; after ulcerates, 3–5 yr no matter what rx

Stage III: 2.5 yr average survival

Cmplc: Meningeal involvement occasionally occurs with CNS symptoms, even when skin changes are in remission (Ann IM 1975;82:499)

Lab:

Rx: Topical nitrogen mustard, when disease limited to skin

PUVA in early stages (Arch Derm 1996;76:475)

Systemic rx w chemotherapy drugs and interferon is effective palliation, not curative (Ann IM 1994;121:592)

Irradiation

Extracorporeal photochemotherapy with UVA (Med Let 1988;30:96) of Sézary syndrome: etretinate and electron beam rx (J Am Acad Derm 1992;26:960)

3.5 MISCELLANEOUS

PAPULAR/VESICULAR RASHES

rv of all bullous diseases—Nejm 1995;333:1475

Dermatitis herpetiformis (p 134)

Dystrophic epidermolysis bullosa (Nejm 1980;303:776)
Cause: Autosomal recessive and dominant forms
Si: Severe blistering with minor trauma causing contractures and protein
  loss; die by age 30 yr in recessive forms
Rx: Phenytoin, formerly thought helpful, but not proven so (Nejm 1992;
  327:163)

Eczema (p 135)

Gonococcemia (p 411)
Si: A few acral lesions, some hemorrhagic

Pemphigoid, bullous (Jama 2000;284:350)
Pathophys: Anti-basement membrane antibodies, usually IgG, occasionally
  IgE (Nejm 1978;298:417) and IgA in mucus membrane variant
Sx: Similar to pemphigus but in aged, and usually hemorrhagic; less severe
  than pemphigus; itchy; tense blisters because epidermis intact above
  split
Rx: Topical or systemic steroids; immunosuppressants like azathioprine
  (Arch Derm 1994;130:753), cyclophosphamide, etc; antibiotics like
  tetracycline and niacinamide (Arch Derm 1986;122:670)

Pemphigus vulgaris
Epidem: Associated with HLA-DR$_w$4 in 91% (Lancet 1979;2:441);
  paraneoplastic type with lymphoma (Nejm 1990;323:1729)
Pathophys: Antiepithelial ("prickle") cell IgG-4 antibody (Nejm 1989;
  320:1463; 1989;321:631)
Si: Can push blister fluid into new areas of skin (Nikolsky's sign); normal
  skin sloughs and forms bullae when rubbed; middle age onset; scalp,
  mucosal membranes, and flexor surfaces primarily involved; "baggy
  blisters" because overlying epidermis is very thin, rarely hemorrhagic

Rx: Steroids, and follow antibody titers; cyclophosphamide; azathioprine; or nicotinamide and tetracycline (J Am Acad Derm 1993;28:998)

Pityriasis lichenoides et varioliformis acuta (PLEVA)
Epidem: Rare, in children
Si: Lichenoid papules with a continuum between the acute vesicles and the chronic scarring (J Am Acad Derm 1990;23:473)
Crs: Self-limited
Lab:
    Path: Biopsy shows a vasculitis

Scalded skin syndrome (J Am Acad Derm 1994;30:319)
Cause: Staph toxin in children w 1st impetigo episode
Si: Denudation and epithelial slough
Lab:
    Bact: Skin culture neg, staph in nose or impetigo areas
    Path: Skin bx to r/o toxic epidermal necrolysis
Rx: Penicillinase-resistant penicillins; topical rx like a burn

Toxic epidermal necrolysis (Lyell's syndrome) (Nejm 1995;333:1600)
Cause: Drug-induced in adults, esp sulfas, seizure meds, oxicam NSAIDs, and steroids
Pathophys: Cleavage at dermal-epidermal junction, extreme variant of Stevens-Johnson syndrome
Crs: 15–20% mortality
Lab:
    Path: Skin bx to dx
Rx: Burn unit; steroids

DERMATOLOGY

PAPULOSQUAMOUS RASHES

Ichthyosis
Cause: Familial, some autosomal and some sex-linked recessives (Nejm 1972;286:821)
Sx: Childhood onset
Si: Fine scales; if recent onset r/o Hodgkin's
Rx: Hydrophilic ointment with wraps q 3 d; or propylene glycol and water q 1 wk

Leprosy (p 408)

Si: Psoriaform rash with marked decrease in sensation

Lichen planus

Si: "Polygonal, pruritic (often very), purple papules"; flexor surfaces
especially wrist and mucous membranes; linear configuration often;
reticular pattern beneath (use mineral oil); looks white in blacks;
"mother of pearl" in mouth; scarring alopecia; r/o leukoplakia and
monilia

Rx: Topical steroids with occlusion for skin, systemic steroids for
alopecia; PUVA; in mouth, cyclosporine rinse, but costs $70/day!
(Nejm 1990;323:290)

Mycosis fungoides (p 153)

Pityriasis rosea

Cause: Probably viral

Si: Oval, scaling lesions in lines of cleavage; vest distribution; white raised
papular lesions in blacks; r/o t. corporis and other pap-squam
etiologies, especially syphilis

Crs: Recurs occasionally

Lab:
Serol: VDRL or RPR to r/o syphilis

Psoriasis (p 138)

Seborrheic dermatitis/dandruff

Cause: *Pityrosporum ovale* is a commensal yeast which causes dandruff

Epidem: Common

Si: Red color to skin, looks like acne rosacea but concentrated in
nasolabial folds

Rx: (Med Let 1994;36:68): Sebulex/Selsun (selenium) shampoos biw 1%
OTC and 2.5%, cost: $2.76/4 oz; or similarly priced OTC
pyrithione zinc (Head and Shoulders). Alternate same with sebutone
(tar); topical steroids hs, foams (Olux, Luxiq) elegant but costly;
topical ketoconazole (Nizoral) cream or 2% by rx or 1% OTC
shampoo biw, cost: $16/4 oz

Secondary syphilis (p 440)

Si: Rash on soles and palms; lymphadenopathy; red papules with scale; not pruritic

Allergic vasculitis

Cause: Any vasculitis (Nejm 1997;337:1512) including giant cell, Takayasu's, polyarteritis, Wegener's, paraneoplastic, inflammatory bowel disease, and immune complex types (anaphylactoid Henoch-Schönlein purpura, cryoglobininemia, SLE, RA, Sjögren's, Goodpastures, Behçet's, scleroderma, and drug- or virally induced, a continuum from urticaria to erythema multiforme (p 141)

Si: Bilaterally symmetric, palpable (r/o DIC), hematuria- and guaiac-pos stools, hemorrhagic bullae

Bacteremia

Cause: Meningococcus, staph, pseudomonas, GC, SBE

Si: Rash often asymmetric, not palpable; or may present as vasculitis with symmetric palpable purpura

Idiopathic thrombocytopenic purpura (ITP) (p 357)

Si: Splenomegaly, decr platelets, never palpable

Rickettsial diseases: Spotted fever, typhus, etc. (p 446)

Si: Early lesions may blanche; palms and soles; palpable

Scurvy

Cause: Vitamin C deficiency, seen in elderly on poor diets

Si: Purpura never palpable, corkscrew hairs, perifollicular hemorrhage especially on knees; hyperkeratotic papules

Rx: Vitamin C

Other causes: Leukemias, TTP, thrombocytosis, myelofibrosis

DERMATOLOGY

Arch Derm 1994;130:734

Pruritic urticarial papules and plaques of pregnancy (PUPPP) (J Am Acad Derm 1984;10:473)

Sx: In primigravida, 3rd trimester; very pruritic
Si: Papules and plaques begin in the striae on abdomen

Papular dermatitis of pregnancy (existence debated)

Crs: Incr fetal mortality reported (12%) without rx (J Am Acad Derm 1982;6:977)
Lab:
   Chem: Incr HCG (r/o mole) in urine
   Path: Biopsy is nonspecific
Rx: Cortisone 40 mg po qd produces total remission

Pemphigoid gestationis (Jama 2000;284:350), previously dermatitis or herpes gestationis

Si: Vesicles and bullae with onset any time during pregnancy; may flare at delivery
Crs: Recurs in subsequent pregnancies
Cmplc: Premature delivery sometimes
Lab:
   Path: Biopsy shows specific subepidermal vesicles with polys early, then eosinophils; C_3 deposition on epidermal basement membrane from low titer pemphigoid type IgG auto-antibodies
Rx: Systemic steroids

Melasma

Si: Pigmented diffuse facial "tanning" common in pregnancy or with bcp use
Rx: Stop bcp's; daily sunscreen (SPF 15$^+$); hydrocortisone cream; Retin A cream; benzoyl peroxide cream, hydroquinone 2–4%

Amyloidosis

Si: Waxy papule, rubbed causes purpura (weak capillaries), "pinch purpura"

Baldness, male pattern (androgenic alopecia) (Med Let 1998;40:25; Rx Let 1998;5:6)

Rx: (Nejm 1999;341:964) Minoxidil (Rogaine extra strength) 2 or 5% OTC, must maintain rx to keep effect. Adverse effects: dizziness. $30/mo

Finasteride (Propecia) 1 mg po qd; takes 6–12 mo to work, must maintain dose to keep effect. Adverse effects: may reversibly decr libido, decr PSA levels. $50/mo

Burns: Thermal, (rv of rx—Nejm 1996:335:1581); iv fluids to keep urine output >1/2 cc/kg/hr, >1 cc/kg/hr in children

Survival (Nejm 1998;338:362) based on age, extent, and whether or not concomitant inhalation injury

Café-au-lait spots

Cause: Albright's disease "coast of Maine" irregular edges, or neurofibromatosis "coast of California" smooth edges

Rx: (Med Let 1997;39:10)

Clubbing (Ann IM 1994;120:238)

Causes: SBE, IBD, lung cancer, abscesses, bronchiectasis, benign familial

Si: (Jama 2001;286:341)
- Loss of angle (Lovibond's) between base of nail and dorsal finger surface, hence positive Schamroth sign (no space when dorsal distal phalanges juxtaposed)
- Thickness of distal phalanx at nail bed > thickness at dip joint
- Soft nail bed

Xray: Phalanges and distal arm and leg have periosteal elevations

Decubitus ulcers (pressure sores) (Jama 1995;273:865; Ann IM 1981;94:661)

Cause: Immobility

Epidem: 18% prevalence in bedridden

DERMATOLOGY

Table 3.5.1 Types of Dressings with Some Examples of Products Commonly Used to Treat Pressure Sores

Type	Examples
Protective dressings	
Permeable	OpCit™, Tegaderm™
Hydrocolloid	DuoDERM™, Comfeel™, Tegasorb™, Ultec™
Petroleum gauze	Vaseline™, Xeroform™
Antimicrobial dressings	
Disinfectant solutions (The use of these agents remains controversial.)	Acetic acid, hydrogen peroxide, sodium hypochlorite (Dakin's), povidone iodine (Betadine™), chloramine-T (Chlorazene™)
Topical antibiotics	Silver sulfadiazine (Silvadene™), mupirocin (Bactroban™), metronidazole (Flagyl™)
Hypertonic antimicrobials	Hypertonic saline, sucrose (granulated sugar), NaCl gauze (Mesalt™)
Debriding	
Gauze dressings	Normal saline/disinfectant wet-to-dry gauze
Enzymatic products	Elase™ (fibrinolysin & DNAase), Santyl™ (collagenase), Granulex™ (trypsin), Panafil™ (papain)
Cavity filling	
Gauze dressings	Normal saline gauze, hypertonic saline gauze (Mesalt™)
Hydrocolloids	DuoDERM Hydroactive Gel™
Alginates	AlgiDERM™, DermaSORB™, Sorbsan™

Rx: (Med Let 1990;32:17)

    Prevent w alternating pressure mattress, air mattress (Jama 1993;269:1139), egg crate foam mattress 6.5 in. thick (Lancet 1994;343:568), turning; vitamin C 50 mg bid po

    Debridement with Granulex (trypsin) or surgery; hydrocolloid dressings like Duoderm. See Table 3.5.1

Erythema nodosum

Epidem: Associated w drugs esp. BCPs, sarcoid, tuberculosis, ulcerative colitis, regional enteritis, lymphogranuloma venereum, chancroid, cat scratch fever, histoplasmosis, coccidioidomycosis, drug eruptions, diphtheria, strep infections, rheumatic fever, SLE

Si: Very tender nodules, usually on anterior shin, w/o scarring

Rx: Bed rest, elevation; NSAIDs; colchicine; and, if severe, oral steroids

Granuloma annulare
Cause: Idiopathic
Epidem: In children often
Sx: Acral (arms, legs)
Si: Raised edges
Crs: Go away in mos. to years
Cmplc: r/o t. corporis which has a scale; sarcoid
Rx: Intralesional steroids

Hirsutism/hypertrichosis (p 627)

Hyperpigmentation
Cause: Postinflammatory, especially in blacks
Rx: Tretinoin 0.1% cream (Retin A, retinoic acid) qd × 40 wk over entire
area, not just the spots (Nejm 1993;328:1438)

Impetigo
Cause: Staph or strep superficial stratum granulosum (epidermal)
infection
Si: Bullae, usually rupture
Cmplc: AGN
r/o ecthyma contagiosum or orf infection from sheep, where skin is
invaded a little more deeply and requires longer conservative rx
(Cleve Clin J Med 1991;58:531)
Rx: Antistaph penicillin or topical mupiricin (Bactroban); wet compresses
× 20 min bid

Keloid
Rx: Prevent w imiquimod (Aldara)? cream post op hs × 8 wk (Rx Let
2001;8:29)
Inject with triamcinolone q 1 mo, causes flattening; topical Retin A;
expensive Silastic gel sheeting

Laceration (Nejm 1997;337:1140)
Cause: Trauma
Cmplc: r/o nerve, tendon, joint involvement which may need OR
Rx: Clean, debride, suture (see Table 3.5.2), or use octylcyanoacrylates
when available

DERMATOLOGY

Table 3.5.2 Characteristics of Absorbable and Nonabsorbable Sutures

Type of Sutura (Trade Name)	Degree of Knot Security	Tensile Strength	Duration of Wound Security*	Tissue Reactivity
Absorbable				
Surgical gut	Poor	Fair	5–7 days	Most
Chromic gut	Fair	Fair	10–14 days	Most
Polyglactin (Vlcryl)	Good	Good	30 days	Minimal
Polyglycolic acid (Dexon)	Best	Good	30 days	Minimal
Polydixanone (PDS)	Fair	Best	45–60 days	Least
Polyglyconate (Maxon)	Fair	Best	45–60 days	Least
Nonabsorbable				
Nylon (Ethilon)	Good	Good	NA	Minimal
Polypropylene (Prolene)	Least	Best	NA	Least
Silk	Best	Least	NA	Most

*This column indicates the period during which at least 50% tensile strength is retained NA denotes not applicable.

Reproduced with permission from Singer AJ, Hollander JE, Quinn JV. Evaluation and management of traumatic lacerations. Nejm 1997; 337:1142–1148.

Leukoplakia

Si: On mucosal surfaces

Lab:

  Path: Biopsy shows nuclei and plasma cells in stratum corneum

Rx: 13-cis-retinoic acid 1–2 mg/kg qd (Nejm 1986;315:1501)

Lichen sclerosis of vulva

Cause: Perhaps due to decr testosterone levels

Rx: Strong topical steroids (J Reprod Med 1993;38:25; Brit J Derm 1991; 124:461)

  Testosterone 2% topically bid (Nejm 1984;310:488), but causes masculinizing side effects (Obgyn 1997;89:297)

"Liver spots," actinic lentigines

Rx: Prevent w sunscreen SPF 15$^+$

  Tretinoin (retinoic acid) 0.1% cream qd (Nejm 1992;326:368), gentle cryotherapy, or laser (Med Let 1997;39:10)

Molluscum contagiosum

Cause: Molluscum contagiosum virus
Epidem: Can be venereally spread
Sx: Inguinal papules, anywhere in children
Si: Umbilicated inguinal, 1–4 mm, round, raised lesions
Rx: Excise, freeze, burn; or, in children, less traumatically w cantharidin 0.7% applied w toothpick, cover w tape, wash off in 4 hr; imiquimod (Aldara) (p 130) qd under band-aid

Orf ulcers (Nejm 1997;337:1131)

Cause: Parapox virus
Epidem: Contact w sheep in which is a common cause of skin lesions

Palm and/or sole rashes

Cause: Coxsackie A, hand-foot-mouth disease; dyshydrotic eczema (almost never contact) (p 657); endocarditis; erythema multiforme; Kawasaki's disease; atypical measles in patients previously vaccinated (Ann IM 1979;90:873–887); neisserial gonorrhea and meningococcus; psoriasis, especially pustular; rat bite fever; Reiter's; Rocky Mountain spotted fever; secondary syphilis; t. pedis

Pruritus differential dx

- Metabolic: gall bladder/pancreatic disease, uremia, hypo- or hyperthyroidism, polycythemia vera, lymphoma/leukemia, abdominal cancer, iron deficiency, diabetes
- Skin lesions
- Psychiatric delusions of parasites
- Real parasites, eg, hookworm, scabies, lice
- Dry skin (xerodermatitis)

Sarcoid

Si: Violet indurated plaque that blanches (p 821)

Spider bites, brown recluse

Crs: (Nejm 1998;339:379): Minimal inflammation in first 24 hr then severe inflammation and necrosis over 1 week which may need surgical debridement
Rx: High dose oral steroids, perhaps w Dapsone started in first 24 hr may prevent necrosis

DERMATOLOGY

Stasis ulcers

Rx: Prevent w Ace wraps, elastic stockings, elevation

Treat w stoma adhesive qd; Banoxyl, Zn oxide (Unna) boot, perhaps pentoxifylline (ACP J Club 2001;134:14); if <6 mo old and <5 cm^2 area, healing w q 1 wk Zn oxide boot likely w/i 6 mos (Am J Med 2000;109:15)

Sunburn (Med Let 1999;41:43)

Cause: UV or sun at 290–320 nm (UVB), or 320–340 nm (UVA II) wavelength; over 100 drugs can increase sensitivity (Med Let 1995;37:35)

Cmplc: Photoaging, actinec damage including keratoses, squamous cell Ca, basal cell Ca, melanomas

Rx: (Rx Let 1999;6:40)

Prevent w sun block SPF 15–30, eg, Uval, Solbar, benzones (Med Let 1993;35:54)

Telangiectasias

Cause: Idiopathic; alcoholic spider angiomata; aluminum workers in vest pattern (Nejm 1980;303:1278); **Osler-Weber-Rendu Syndrome** w autosomal dominant telangiectasias of brain, skin, gi tract, liver (Nejm 2000;343:931), etc.

Rx: SBE prophylaxis if possible pulmonary AVMs; support group (800-448-6389); various laser rx's possible (Med Let 1991;33:104); ε-aminocaproic acid rx may decrease bleeding in Osler-Weber-Rendu (Nejm 1994;330:1789)

Vitiligo

Cause: Genetic; chemical leukoderma, Addison's, Graves', pernicious anemia, t. versicolor, tuberous sclerosis (present at birth), autoimmune, nonspecific (Nejm 1977;297:634), albinism (genetic, associated with actinic keratoses, cancers, nystagmus)

Rx: Trimethylpsoralens 40 mg po qd + sunlight 2$^+$ h after taking; topical also possible but blisters easily; irreversible depigmentation with monobenzyl ether of hydroquinone (20%) as last resort

Wrinkles

Cause: Smoking and sun exposure both cause independently (Ann IM 1991;114:840) by decreasing skin collagen

Rx: Laser (Med Let 1997;37:10); topical tretinoins (Nejm 1997;337:1419)

Chapter 4
ENT

D. K. Onion

4.1 EAR

OTITIS EXTERNA (Bacterial, Allergic, Seborrheic, Fungal [Otomycosis], Viral [rarely])

Cause:

Bacterial: Staph, *Pseudomonas*

Fungal: Aspergillus niger

Viral: Herpes simplex and zoster

Epidem:

Bacterial: Most common type of otitis externa

Pathophys:

Bacterial: Local furunculosis that becomes more diffuse

Sx:

Allergic: 1^+ pain; 3^+ itching

Seborrheic: 1^+ pain; 1^+ itching

Bacterial: 3^+ pain, especially w movement of pinna

Fungal: 1^+ pain; 3^+ itching

Viral: 1^+ pain w herpes simplex; 3^+ pain w herpes zoster

Si:

Bacterial: Pain w tragal pressure and pinna traction; erythema and edema of external ear canal

Allergic: Acute: weeping small vesicles; chronic: fissures and scales

Seborrheic: Greasy scales, dandruff

Fungal: Looks like wet newspaper; black discharge is diagnositic

Viral: Vessels in ear may rupture, or form hemorrhagic bullae

Crs:
Cmplc:
Bacterial: Malignant otitis externa, a severe perichondritis, now only a problem in pts w resistant organisms or diminished resistance, eg, diabetes, cancer, or AIDS

r/o: Acute mastoiditis
Lab:
Bact: Culture if drainage
Rx: Avoid water in all types
Allergic: antihistamines; topical steroids
Seborrheic: keep hair away from ears; topical steroids
Bacterial/fungal: clean out well

Domeboro's soln, or 9:1 alcohol/vinegar soln gtts to acidify area, which prevents pseudomonas growth, w wick (eg, "Pope's otowick," a commercial sponge material) if necessary to get into canal

Topical antibiotics and steroids (Cortisporin or Cipro HC) gtts t-qid, or ofloxacin (Floxin) gtts bid (Rx Let 1998;5:8)

Glycerin to decrease swelling by hydroscopic action (VoSol)

Systemic antibiotics, eg, penicillin, dicloxacillin, cephalothin, or ciprofloxacin especially if *P. aeruginosa* (Nejm 1991;324:392) and if sensitive; malignant external OM, rx w ceftazidime (Rv Inf Dis 1990;12:173)

Viral: sedation; occasionally local antibiotics; ? acyclovir

OTITIS MEDIA

Nejm 1995;332:1560; Am J Pub Hlth 1977;67:472

Cause: Acute: most are bacterial (Jama 1994;273:1598): H. flu (25%), 40% are β-lactamase pos, if associated w conjunctivitis then 70% are H. flu non-β-lactamase types; pneumococcus (35%); *Moraxella (Branhamella) catarrhalis* (25%); other strep; viral (30%—Clin Ped 1972;11:204), although more (40%) may be virally induced (Nejm 1999;340:260), RSV, parainfluenza, and influenza

Chronic: above plus staph, *Proteus, Pseudomonas*

Serous type (chronic OM w effusion): fluid secretion w/o culturable organisms usually, although 1/3 may have organisms (Jama 1998; 279:296)

Significant genetic predisposition by twin studies (Jama 1999;282: 2125,2167)

Epidem: Some viral infections predispose, eg, RSV, influenza, and adeno (Nejm 1982;306:1377). Serous OM often follows infectious resolution

Pathophys: Rhinitis and sinusitis spread along eustachian tube. Cmplc from juxtaposition of several structures, eg, meninges, facial nerve, oval and round windows, semicircular canals, and lateral sinus. Allergic/atopic individuals have much higher persistent rates (D. Hurst, Otolaryngol-Head Neck Surg 2000;123:533; Laryngoscope 1999;109:471)

Sx: Pain, severe and deep, unbothered by external ear manipulation, may improve suddenly w spontaneous drainage; sense of fullness; diminished hearing acuity

Si: Decreased hearing; inflamed drum, often bulging; loss of light reflex, poor air movement and pain w pneumatic otoscopy

Crs: Acute usually improves within 48 h of starting antibiotics, and clears in <2 wk. Serous OM is persistent OM w effusion that lasts >3 mo w hearing loss

Cmplc:
- Ossicle necrosis especially of incus
- Chronic otitis w granulomas and polyps
- Mastoiditis leading to "erect ear" si, loss of post-auricular crease
- Meningitis and encephalitis
- Lateral sinus thrombosis w undulating fever and rigors, rx by tying jugular vein to stop spread
- Facial nerve paralysis, in chronic OM rx w surgical decompression
- Labyrinthitis, extension of infection through windows leading to vertigo, rx by destroying labyrinth
- Lateral semicircular canal involvement causes vertigo
- Chronic serous otitis
- Hearing acuity decrease w chronic involvement, but no diminished intellectual/verbal abilities if delay tubes (Nejm 1985;312:1529)

Lab: Tympanometry to evaluate middle ear effusions (Nejm 1982;307: 1074); not helpful <age 6 mo

Xray: CT of mastoids show haziness early, sclerosis and erosion later

Rx:
Prevent w
- Pneumococcal vaccine conjugated @ 2, 4, 6, and 12 mo age, decr overall incid by 6%, vaccine type pneumococcal episodes by 20% (NNT-2 = 5) (Nejm 2001;344:403)
- Influenza vaccines? (Nejm 1999;340:312)
- Prophylactic antibiotics, rarely used now: sulfisoxazole, or amoxicillin, or Tm/S all at half rx doses as single hs dose × 3 mo or w URIs (Med Let 1983;25:102); as good as tubes

of acute OM (see management flow chart—Nejm 1995;332:1560): antibiotics: 1st, amoxicillin 40 mg/kg/d, or 60–90 mg/kg/d if pcn-resistant pneumococcus possible (Rx Let 1998;5:61); 2nd, amoxicillin/clavulinic acid (Augmentin); 3rd, Tm/S (8/40 kg/24 h) in 2 doses; 4th, erythromycin + sulfa (Pediazole); 5th, cefaclor, et al. Or, if won't take po, ceftriaxone 50 mg/kg up to 1 gm × 1, may dilute w lidocaine to decr pain (Rx Let 1998;5:10). 5 d rx may be enough over age 2 (Rx Let 1998;5:42). Could give rx and tell to fill if not better on Tylenol in 48 hr since only ~1/7 cases over age 2 and otherwise low risk will need antibiotics, and benefit at 2 wk no different than placebo (Bmj 2000;320:350)

of serous OM: antibiotics may help clear (~1/3 over 1 mo after 2 wk rx) but many will clear spontaneously (Nejm 1987;316:432); steroids × 7–14 d w antibiotics (Arch Otolaryngol Head Neck Surg 1991;117:984)

Decongestants and antihistamines no help in acute or serous (BMJ 1983;287:654; Nejm 1983;308:297) though many practitioners still feel they help

Surgical: tubes help hearing acuity, but not verbal/intellectual losses (Nejm 2001;344:1179; 1985;312:1529); polyp and granulation tissue removal; prosthetic replacement for ossicle necrosis. Mastoiditis can be rx'd w simple mastoidectomy, mastoid tympanoplasty, or radical mastoidectomy if advanced. Adenoidectomy may help serous OM esp w tubes (Nejm 2001;344: 1188; 1987;317:1444; Jama 1999;282:945 vs 987)

CHOLESTEATOMA

Cause: Epidermal proliferation, though not a true neoplasia
Epidem:
Pathophys: Keratin layering arising in external canal or TM results in TM perforation (usually high on drum unlike OM), middle ear invasion
Sx: Conductive hearing loss; foul otorrhea several times a month; ear pain
Si: Pearl white growth seen through the drum, or, more often, within marginal perforations often in attic, posterior/superior area (pars flaccida) or filling whole canal; foul otorrhea
Crs: Progressive
Cmplc: Brain abscess; facial paralysis; labyrinthine fistula
Lab:
Xray: CT shows erosion of adjacent bone
Rx: Surgery

MENIERE'S DISEASE

Cause: Idiopathic
Epidem: Onset usually in 5th decade
Pathophys: Endolymphatic hydrops in scala media causes increased pressure. Probably due to diminished resorption causing organ of corti damage and semicirc canal involvement

Attack probably represents an endolymphatic rupture w mixing of endo- and perilymph; endolymph has an intracellular ionic content
Sx:

- Sensorineural hearing loss first; fluctuating ascending low-frequency loss early, then permanent high-frequency loss later
- Episodic tinnitus
- Episodic vertigo, violent, last an average 1/2–2 h only (10 min– 24 h min/max); 1–4 attacks/mo; unilateral in 85%

Si: Decreased auditory discrimination, in contrast to conductive losses; recruitment

Crs:

Cmplc: Complete hearing loss in affected ear

Lab: Audiometry shows sensorineural loss w/o air-bone gap. Recruitment of sound so that loudness increases abruptly w slight increase indecibel level, ie, abnormally loud above their abnormally high

ENT

threshold; this is the distinguishing feature between cochlear
(Meniere's, presbycusis) and retrocochlear disease

Rx: Salt, caffeine, and alcohol restriction

Medications:

- Benzodiazepams in low dose, tapered to minimally effective dose,
  like diazepam (Valium) 2 mg po tid (never more) initially then
  tapered over 1–2 wk to 2 mg qd; or lorazepam (Ativan) 1 mg sl/po
- Antihistamines (Benadryl)
- Antivertigo drugs (scopolamine, meclizine [Antivert],
  dimenhydrinate [Dramamine], phenothiazines)
- Diuretics prophylactically, eg, thiazides
- Streptomycin, perhaps, 2–3 gm im qd to produce bilateral nerve
  damage in 10–20 d (Arch Otolaryng 1967;85:156); an older
  method of rx

Surgical: rarely need; labyrinthectomy through middle ear if hearing
already gone there; endolymphatic saccule to subarachnoid space
shunt; sacculotomy; 8th nerve section

CEREBELLAR-PONTINE ANGLE TUMORS
Nejm 1991;324:1555; 1972;287:895

Cause: Acoustic neuroma (AN); rarely neurofibromatosis type 2, bilateral
acoustic neuromas (Jama 1997;278:51; Nejm 1988;318:684),
autosomal dominant on chromosome #22; meningioma; metastatic
cancer from lung, breast, prostate, kidney

Epidem: AN is most common; meningioma second most common, and
metastatic disease third most common

Pathophys: ANs arise in vestibular portion of eighth nerve and gradually
compress cranial nerves VIII and VII, then cerebellum, then IX, X,
and XI

Sx:

- Hearing loss unilaterally, sensorineural, first sx usually
- Vertigo, mild, slowly progressive, unilateral
- Tinnitus, unilateral often
- Facial palsies

- Dysphagia
- Facial numbness

Si: Sensorineural hearing loss; ataxia, peripheral (eg, fingers), uncrossed; sensory deficits in cranial nerves, eg, distal VII (taste), and V (pin and touch); caloric testing shows no response on affected side (95%)

Crs: Neurofibromatosis type 2 onset in teens and 20s

Cmplc: Neurofibromatosis type 2 is associated with meningiomas and gliomas

Lab:

CSF: Shows elevated protein (67% of those w sx); present earlier in perilymph tap, if done

Noninv: Brainstem auditory evoked responses 100% positive (Nejm 1984;310:1740)

Xray: MRI with contrast; CT with contrast

Rx: Surgical, stereotatic radiosurgery vs microsurgery (Nejm 1998;339: 1426); in elderly, first follow with q 6 mo CT or MRI to be sure progressing

SENSORINEURAL HEARING LOSS (DEAFNESS)

Nejm 1993;329:1092

Cause:

- Cochlear types include presbycusis in old age, high-frequency losses worst; Meniere's disease, unilateral in 85%; ototoxic drugs, eg, streptomycin, gentamicin, which can be unilateral; and exposure to loud noise, eg, rock and roll (Nejm 1970;282:467); idiopathic sudden (days) unilateral or bilateral loss due to anticochlear antibodies (Jama 1994;272:611)
- Neural (retrocochlear), often unilateral (Nejm 1967;276:1406); include most commonly viral, like measles, mumps, and adenovirus infections; neuroma, vascular occlusion, hypercoagulopathy, meningitis, syphilis, multiple sclerosis, collagen vascular diseases, trauma (often w vertigo) (Nejm 1982;306:1029), and cerebellar-pontine angle tumors
- Congenital genetic syndromes: maternally inherited diabetes and deafness (Ann IM 2001;134:721), and others

Epidem: Prevalence incr by smoking (Jama 1998;279:1715)

ENT

Pathophys:

Si + Sx: Diminished discrimination, poor verbal skills in children, Weber test goes to unaffected side, positive Rinne's test, no recruitment (except in Meniere's and presbycusis); if loss >40 db at 2000 cps in best ear in elderly, it causes significant dysfunction and is markedly improved by hearing aid (Ann IM 1990;113:188)

Crs:

Cmplc:

Lab: Audiometry shows no air-bone gap and diminished discrimination

Rx: Hearing aid amplification (Med Let 1998;40:62) w conventional analog aid (Chrystal Ear mail order cheap version = $300, up to $1000); 3 types: linear peak clipper not as good as compression limiter or wide dynamic range compressor by DBCT (Jama 2000; 284:1806). Programmable hearing aids; or digital hearing aids ($2900)

Rarely in the profoundly deaf, cochlear implant hearing aids, $20,000 (Jama 1995;274:1955, Nejm 1993;328:233, 281; Med Let 1985;27:51)

4.2 NOSE/THROAT

HEREDITARY ANGIONEUROTIC EDEMA
Ann IM 1976;84:580

Cause: Genetic, autosomal dominant, or rarely acquired, C'1a esterase inhibitor deficiency (Ann IM 2000;132:144)

Epidem: Most Western races

Pathophys: C'1a esterase inhibitor inactivates clotting factors XII and XI, the latter build up and release kallikreins/kinins causing pain, shock, etc. (Nejm 1983;308:1050)

Sx: Onset not until age 20–50 yr; frequently precipitated by trauma, psychologic stress, or pharyngitis; abdominal pain often leads to surgery

Si: Edema of skin, upper gi and respiratory tracts, recurrent, acute, nonpitting, nonpruritic, circumscribed, transient, involves localized areas

Crs:

Cmplc: Laryngeal edema causing asphyxia (26% patients die this way)

r/o:

- Much more common, benign **acquired angioedema** = 90% of patients w above sx; rx w prednisone 60 mg qd × 1 wk, then qod and decrease to 5–10 mg qod; plus hydroxyzine 25 mg tid helps decrease frequency and severity (Ann IM 1991;114:133); or if no response, then tranexamic acid (ϵ-aminocaproic acid-like drug) up to 1 gm po tid (Am J Med 1999;106:650)
- "Pseudo-angioedema" associated w lymphoma and colon Ca
- Uvular edema of Franklin's disease
- ACE inhibitor drug reaction angioedema (Jama 1997;278:232; Ann IM 1992;117:234)

Lab:

Immunol: Screen for C_4, if decr look for serum α_2-globulin inhibitor of C'1a (present in 90%, 10% have inactive, nonfunctioning C'1a esterase inhibitor)

Rx: Preventively screen family

for prophylaxis:

- Tranexamic acid 1 gm po tid (Am J Med 1998;106:650)
- Androgens, like danazol 200 mg tid, prevents attacks, little virilization (Ann IM 1980;93:809; Nejm 1976;295:1444; $1/pill); stanozol 0.5 mg b-qid good too, cheaper; oxymethalone 5–10 mg qd, can use 4 days preop too
- Steroids, like prednisone 60 mg qd × 1 wk, then qod and decrease to 5–10 mg qod; plus
- Hydroxyzine 25 mg tid helps decrease frequency and severity (Ann IM 1991;114:133)

for acute life-threatening attack or its prophylaxis: C'1a inhibitor from vapor heated pooled plasma concentrate (Nejm 1996;334:1630); + supportive care

ACUTE EPIGLOTTITIS (Bacterial Supraglottitis)

Jama 1994;272:1358 (adults); Nejm 1986;314:1133 (adults); Ann IM 1969;70:289

Cause: H. flu, type B, is predominant organism in children and adults; staph, *S. pneumoniae,* rarely other strep

Epidem: Primarily in children age 1–5 yr, but now more commonly in adults, eg, President George Washington; >10/million adults/yr Incidence 1.8 cases/100,000/yr in adults, 0.6/100,000 in children; M:F = 1.8:1 in adults

Pathophys: Obstruction of upper airway by edematous epiglottis

Sx: Extremely sore throat (95%), more than the dysphagia (94%), plus respiratory distress often over 6–24 hr

Si: Epiglottis and/or other supraglottic structures inflamed and edematous by direct or indirect laryngoscopy (safe to do in adults, not in children), need to sit erect (21%), muffled voice (54%), fever (50%), drooling (40%), stridor (15%); pharynx often (50%) normal

Airway intervention needed in 42% w stridor, 47% w need to sit erect

Crs: Sore throat × 2–4 d, dysphagia and respiratory distress 6–24 h

Cmplc: Sudden, unpredictable airway obstruction, 7% mortality without prophylactic airway; decreases to 1% with airway prophylactically placed

r/o angioneurotic edema, foreign body

Lab:

Bact: Blood culture

Xray: Lateral soft tissue film of neck shows narrowed glottis, 20% false neg, not as good as indirect laryngoscopy

Rx: Prevent w H. flu vaccination

Appropriate antibiotic, usually 2nd or 3rd generation cephalosporin like cefuroxime, or ampicillin plus chloramphenicol; no evidence that steroids help but most clinicians believe they do

Early prophylactic nasotracheal intubation in OR under anesthesia, especially in children where should not wait for stridor to intubate

ALLERGIC RHINITIS

Jama 1997;278:1849; Nejm 1991;325:860

Cause: Allergens including grass, tree, and ragweed pollens; dust; animal dander; fungal allergens like thermophilic actinomycetes in car air conditioners (Nejm 1984;311:1119)

Epidem: Airborne; prevalence = 5–20%, increased to 30% if atopic; peak incidence in childhood and adolescence

Pathophys: IgE produced, attaches to mast cells and releases mediators when antigen presents; basophils probably responsible for "late" (hours later) exacerbations (Nejm 1985;313:65); but not all w measurable IgE have the clinical syndrome; precipitating antigens most commonly are pollens, animal dander, house mites, insects, mold spores, and food

Sx: Nasal congestion, sneezing, rhinorrhea, pruritus of nose and eyes, sometimes cough, diminished olfaction

Si: Nasal polyps

Crs: Usually seasonal; recurrence rate of polyps high

Cmplc: Asthma in 20%

r/o **atrophic rhinitis** caused by *Treponema pallidum,* which somehow impairs cilial action; has a bad smell, crusted discharge, and positive STS

Lab:

Bact: Nasal smear shows eosinophils

Hem: Eosinophil count increase (66%)

Immunol: RAST tests, ~$7/antigen, qualitative not quantitative; done by putting antigen on filter paper, adding pt serum, washing, then adding hot anti-IgE, washed again, then counts made

Rx: Avoid antigens by using electrostatic precipitators, and covering and washing bedding

Humidified heat 30 min q 2 h to raise nose temperature >109°F (>43°C) cures coryza (Proc Natl Acad Sci 1982;79:4766); no, new studies disprove (Jama 1994;271:1109, 1112)

1st choice medications:

- Decongestant like pseudoephedrine; topical decongestants are better than systemic, but can lead to **rhinitis medicamentosa** if used >7 d; rx w steroid nose spray to get off, and systemic absorption increases CVA risk (Med Let 2000;42:113)
- Antihistamines (H$_1$ blockers) (Med Let 1994;36:78; Nejm 1994; 330:1663) like diphenhydramine (Benadryl), triprolidine (w pseudoephed = Actifed) or chlorpheniramine (w pseudoephed = Sudafed) 4 mg qid (cheap); but more driving impairment than a blood alcohol level of 0.1% (Ann IM 2000;132:354); possibly azelastine (Astelin) (Med Let 1997;39:45) ii sprays bilat bid, an H$_1$ blocker w systemic absorption, $50/mo

ENT

2nd choice meds:
- Non-sedating type antihistamines; metabolism is inhibited by grapefruit juice (Med Let 2001;43:35); all are nonsedating and have no anticholinergic side effects; $2/d
  - Fexofenadine (Allegra) 60 mg po q 12 hr; absorption decr 70% w any fruit juice (Rx Let 2001;8:32)
  - Cetirizine (Zyrtec) (Med Let 1996;38:21, 95) 5–10 mg po qd
  - Loratadine (Claritin) 10 mg po qd; cmplc: fulminant hepatic necrosis being reported (Ann IM 1996;125:738)
- LRAs like montelukast (Singulair) (Rx Let 2000;7:51)
- Na cromolyn 4% intranasal spray q 3–4 h (Med Let 1991;33: 115). Ophthalmic cromolyn helps if eye sx prominent

3rd choice: Topical steroids (Med Let 1999;40:16) like beclomethasone (Vancenase AQ2, Beconase AQ3) nasal spray ii bid ($25/mo); flunisolide (Nasalide) spray ii bid ($43/mo); budesonide (Rhinocort) ii bid ($43/mo) (Med Let 1994;36:63); fluticasone (Flonase) ii bid (Med Let 1995;37:5), $46/mo; triamcinolone, mometasone, all ~$45/mo

4th choice: Steroids po × 3 wk, then continue at 5 mg qd × 2–3 mo

5th choice: Skin test and desensitize next year; efficacy clear, at least for grass pollens (Nejm 1999; 341:468, 522), give × 3 yr, benefits last >3 yr after cessation

SINUSITIS

ACP position ppr—Ann IM 2001;134:495; Jama 1997;278:1850; Nejm 1992;326:319; Ann IM 1992;117:705; Nejm 1983;309:1149

Cause: Pneumococcus, H. flu, *M. catarrhalis,* strep, staph, occasionally anaerobes (Nejm 1974;290:735, 1351). Cystic fibrosis or heterozygous gene carrier (Jama 2000;284:1814)

Epidem: Associated w rhinitis (90%), dental caries (10%); occurs at any age >2 yr

Pathophys: Edema around sinus ostia blocks drainage; all sinuses drain to medial meatus, except ethmoidals to superior meatus, sphenoid occasionally to sphenoethmoid area, and lacrimal duct to inferior meatus

Sx: Dull headache; local pain off and on, a maxillary "toothache"; worse when leaning over; purulent nasal discharge; sx are unresponsive to decongestants; loss of smell and taste

Si: Rhinitis, postnasal discharge, pus on middle turbinate, loss of sinus transillumination (for frontals, light below medial supraorbital ridge; for maxillaries, light downward on midinferior orbital rim and look inside mouth—Nejm 1992;326:319)

Crs: Either acute ethmoidal or frontal sinusitis is an acute emergency requiring hospitalization, iv antibiotics, and consideration of surgical drainage

Cmplc: Orbital cellulitis, epi/subdural abscess, cavernous sinus thrombosis, osteomyelitis, asthma exacerbation

Lab:

Bact: Culture of nasopharynx correlates w sinus aspiration culture very poorly (30%—Nejm 1981;304:751)

Xray: Not routine, may get if chronic or recurrent: plain films show opacity (85% specif), air fluid levels (80% specif), or >6 mm mucosal thickening (Jama 1995;273:1015), and if normal then the dx is untenable; CT scans, 4 slice, especially for sphenoidal and ethmoids

Rx: Nasal local decongestants like epinephrine gtts 0.5–2%, or phenylephrine 0.25% in saline nasally qid for <7 d, and nasal steroids bid alone or with antibiotics (Jama 2001;286:3097)

Antibiotics (Jama 2001;286:1849; Rx Let 2000;7:49): amoxicillin × 10 d first in children (Nejm 1992;326:319) and adults (BMJ 1996; 313:325, Nejm 1981;304:750), or erythromycin, or erythro/sulfa (Pediazole), or Tm/S × 3 d bid as good as 10 d (Jama 1995;273: 1015); 2nd line drugs: cefpodoxime, cefaclor tid, cefuroxime bid, azithromycin, clarithromycin; except for ethmoidal and sphenoidal when should start w a penicillinase-resistant penicillin like amox/ clavulanic acid (Augmentin) high dose SR or ES, or 2nd generation fluoroquinolone

Surgical functional endoscopic sinus surgery for drainage if worsening despite medical rx; rarely enteronasal anterostomy (Caldwell-Luc procedure)

ENT

4.3 ENT CANCERS

LARYNGEAL CARCINOMA
Nejm 1982;306:910,1151

Cause: Chronic irritation causing neoplasia, esp. from smoking (90%) and drinking alcohol

Epidem: 10,000 new patients/yr in US; male:female ratio = 10–20:1; peak incidence age 45–65 yr

Pathophys: 75% involve true cords (glottic); important since true cord itself has poor lymphatic drainage, hence few mets; subglottic and supraglottic areas are "silent," ie, sx appear late

Cigarette and alcohol-induced mutations in p 53 gene, inactivation of which often induces cancer (Nejm 1995;332:712)

Sx: Glottic type: hoarseness

Supraglottic type: ear pain, throat lump, dysphagia, aspiration, muffled "hot potato" voice

Si: Tumor on laryngoscopy in all (supraglottic, glottic, and subglottic)

Crs: Supraglottic and subglottic have very poor prognosis even w all forms of rx. Glottic "a good cancer to have" since early sx and few mets

Cmplc: Aspiration, pneumonia, weight loss from dysphagia, airway obstruction

Lab:
Path: Bx shows squamous cell carcinoma; occult tumor cells invisible at margins and/or nodes, detectable by PCR assay (Nejm 1995; 332:429)

Rx: Prevent by stopping smoking. Even after dx, stopping will double cure rates and survivals for all head and neck cancers (Nejm 1993; 328:159); isotretinoin prevents the frequent occurrence (30%) of 2nd primary cancers (Nejm 1993;328:15; 1990;323:795)

Radiation, as long as isolated to one cord and not spread to other or ventricle, 90% cure of glottics; possibly hyperfractionated type (Nejm 1998;338:1798)

Surgery w laser, or transoral rx of in situ/early lesions; chordectomy; conservative laryngectomy procedures; conservative neck dissections when in piriform area or when neck nodes present

NASOPHARYNGEAL AND MAXILLARY SINUS CANCER

Nejm 1982;306:1151

Cause: Neoplasia

Epidem: Nasopharyngeal: most common cancer in Asians; chemical and fume exposures and associated w HLA-A2 locus (Nejm 1976;295:1101), w human papilloma virus #16 (Nejm 2001;344:1125), and w EBV (Nejm 1995;333:693; Ann IM 1986;104:331)

Pathophys: Cigarette and alcohol-induced mutations in p 53 gene, inactivation of which often induces cancer (Nejm 1995;332:712)

Early mets

Sx: Bloody nasal discharge

Nasopharyngeal: nontender neck mass (1st sx in 30%), unilaterally blocked ear

Maxillary sinus: loosening of teeth or dentures, malocclusion, and recurrent idiopathic epistaxis

Si: Serosanguineous: unilateral nasal discharge

Nasopharyngeal: nontender neck mass usually in posterior triangle, unilateral serous otitis ("any adult w a persistent serous otitis has a nasopharyngeal cancer until proven otherwise")

Maxillary sinus: gingivolabial fold loss

Crs:

Maxillary sinus: pain, proptosis, neural involvement

Cmplc:

Lab:

Path: Bx shows squamous cell carcinoma. In nasopharyngeal, fine needle aspiration of primary or metastasis shows EBV genome by PCR 25% of the time (Nejm 1992;326:17)

Xray: CT of maxillary sinus shows increased density or bony destruction w expansion of the maxillary sinus

Rx: Prevent by stopping smoking; stopping will double cure rates and survival for all head and neck cancers (Nejm 1993;328:159). Isotretinoin prevents the frequent occurrence (30%) of 2nd primary cancers (Nejm 1993;328:15; 1990;323:795)

Nasopharyngeal:

1st, radiation of primary and mets; possibly hyperfractionated type (Nejm 1998;338:1798)

2nd, surgery of primary and mets

3rd, chemotherapy w cis-platinum + 5-FU (Nejm 1992;327:1115)

Maxillary sinus:
   1st, surgery and/or radiation; possibly hyperfractionated type
      (Nejm 1998;338:1798)
   2nd, chemo w cis-platinum + 5-FU (Nejm 1992;327:1115)

SQUAMOUS CELL CANCER OF TONGUE AND TONSIL

Nejm 1982;306:1151

Cause: Neoplasia; ? from chronic irritation

Epidem: Always associated with:
- Smoking (increases relative risk × 27—Nejm 1995;332:712)
- Alcohol use (the two together increase the risk × 20—Arch Otolaryng 1983;109:746)
- Poor oral hygiene
- Snuff dipping in southern women (Nejm 1981;304:745)
- Betel nut chewing

Pathophys: Cigarette and alcohol-induced mutations in p 53 gene, inactivation of which often induces cancer (Nejm 1995;332:712)

Sx: Oral-pharyngeal lesion, bleeding or mass; neck mass; pain, local or referred to ear (otalgia)

Si: Hard, nontender mass, may ulcerate

Crs: Treatments cure ~30%

Cmplc: Local and/or rarely distant metastases

Lab:
   Path: Bx any lesion >14 d old w/o known cause (Nejm 1976;294:109); occult tumor cells invisible at margins and/or nodes detectable by PCR assay (Nejm 1995;332:429)

Rx: Prevent by stopping smoking; stopping will double cure rates and survivals for all head and neck cancers (Nejm 1993;328:159); and/or w isotretinoin (13 cis-retinoic acid) po at high dose × 3 mo, then low-dose maintenance to pts w leukoplakia; works but may not be worth it (Nejm 1993;328:15), but may be able to predict malignant conversion by DNA content analysis (Nejm 2001;344: 1270, 1323)

Surgical excision combined w radiation (hyperfractionated type—Nejm 1998;339:1798), and chemotherapy w cis-platinum + 5-FU (Nejm 1992;327:115), modestly improves survival

4.4 MISCELLANEOUS

Aphthous stomatitis

Cause: Unknown, viral vs immunologic, possibly stress related

Sx: Painful ulcers, r/o Behçets' syndrome, herpes simplex, coxackie infections (eg, herpangina, hand-foot-mouth disease) (p 505)

Rx:

- Amlexanox (Aphthasol) (Rx Let 1998;5:3) cream qid, decreases inflammation and speeds healing × 1 d $20/5 gm
- Phenelzine (MAOI) b-qid (Letter—Nejm 1984;311:1442)
- Na cromolyn decreases pain (Ann IM 1978;89:228)
- Tetracycline mouth washes, 125 mg/5 cc tid rinse and swallow
- Thalidomide (Nejm 1997;336:1487; Med Let 1998;40:103) 50–200 mg po qd × 2–4[+] wk; esp in AIDS pts; cmplc: teratogenicity, rash, somnolence, HIV proliferation, $0.75/50 mg

Cerumen (ear wax): Loosen w Ceruminex or Colace liquid (not syrup) (Rx Let 2000;7:63)

Cough (Nejm 2000;343:1715): Stop smoking is first rx for all

Acute and subacute:

- URI; rx w Actifed bid × 1 wk, or naproxen 500 mg po tid × 5 d, or iprotropium nasal ii t-qid × 4d
- Allergic rhinitis; rx w non-sedating antihistamines
- Bacterial sinusitis if tooth pain, poor transillumination, purulent nasal d/c; rx w Actifed, oxymetazoline spray bid × 5 d, and/or antibiotics vs H. flu and strep pneumo × 3 wk if sx < 4 wk
- COPD, rx as usual
- Whooping cough, no dx tests; if in community rx w erythromycin 500 mg qid × 14 d

Chronic: r/o GERD, ACEI use, allergic bronchitis rx w inhaled steroids, asthma, allergic rhinitis, COPD, chronic sinusitis

ENT

Epistaxis (nosebleed) (Wm Maxwell 1/98)

Rx: Prevent w short-term topical premarin cream bid (Rx Let 1999;6:66)

  1st, pack nose w cotton strips soaked w topical anesthesia +
  vasoconstrictor (4% cocaine does both)

  2nd, cauterize w silver nitrate or electric cautery

  3rd, pack, leave anterior packs in place 3d, posteriors 5 d, w

  • Vaseline strip gauze anteriorly, or Merocel pack, or Gelfoam

  • Balloon pack (Nozstop, etc), in anterior nose and in nasopharynx

  • Posterior pack or Foley catheters

  Refer to ENT if bleeding persists for internal maxillary artery ligation

Periodontal disease (rv—Nejm 1990;322:373); acute periodontitis and
necrotizing gingivitis are caused by a spirochete very similar to *T.
pallidum* (Nejm 1991;325:539)

Phonation, abnormal causes:

• Hollow voice from recurrent laryngeal nerve paralysis: air escape,
requires multiple breaths to say what should be able to say in one breath

- Left recurrent nerve causes: Cancer of lung (70%), aortic aneurysm,
mitral stenosis (rare)

- Right recurrent causes: Thyroid and other neck pathology

• Hoarseness from laryngeal cancer, benign polyps and nodules, or
laryngitis (whispers)

Temporomandibular joint syndrome: Many are psychiatric in origin
via anxiety (Nejm 1978;299:123) and bruxism; others feel dental
malocclusion is primary etiology. Orthodontic evaluation, surgery only
as a last resort

Tinnitus causes:

• Presbycusis most commonly in the elderly; audiogram will show
significant loss at 4000 cps

• Idiopathic type common

• Acoustic trauma

• Medications: aspirin, digitalis, streptomycin, gentamicin and other
aminoglycosides, quinidine, quinine

• Diseases: Meniere's

Xerostomia, postirradiation; rx w pilocarpine 5–10 mg po tid (Med Let
1994;36:76)

Chapter 5
Endocrinology/Metabolism

D. K. Onion

5.1 ADRENAL DISORDERS

CUSHING'S SYNDROME
Nejm 1995;332:791; 1994;331:629 (NIH—children)

Cause: (Nejm 1991;325:899)
- Cushing's disease from chromophobe or basophilic micro- or macroadenoma of pituitary
- Ectopic ACTH production by oat cell or other (ovary, pancreas, carcinoid) cancer, at least some of this type may be corticotropin hormone-releasing factor producers causing ACTH release indirectly through the pituitary (Nejm 1971;285:419); occasionally ACTH-producing carcinoid tumors, especially of lung (Ann IM 1992;117:209)
- Adrenal: Bilateral nodular hyperplasia or unilateral adrenal adenoma (15%) (ACTH receptor genetic defects—Nejm 1998; 339:27); rare primary pigmented nodular hyperplasia (Ann IM 1999;131:585) assoc w MEA and cardiac myomas; or carcinoma (<1% adults, 4% of children w Cushing's—NIH)

Epidem:

Pathophys: Glucocorticoids cause connective tissue dissolution, have an anti-vitamin D effect, cause proteolysis of muscle, lymphocyte/ monocyte inhibition (Nejm 1975;292:236), incr acid/pepsin secretion, incr gluconeogenesis, and decr glucose uptake. Aldosterone and androgens elevated too when ACTH is the mechanism

Sx: Muscle weakness, obesity/weight gain; growth retardation in children; easy bruising

Si: Muscle weakness; ecchymoses; moon face, buffalo hump; abdominal striae; truncal fat; osteoporosis and fractures; incr number and severity of infections; peptic ulcers; diabetes, nonketotic, insulin-resistant; psychoses; virilization; hypertension (47% in children); and edema

Crs: Excellent prognosis unless cancer or ectopic ACTH (usually cancer) (Nejm 1971;285:243)

Cmplc: See si above

Lab:

Chem: Serum cortisols, normal level is 10–25 μgm % (= 280–700 nM/L) in am, dropping to <7 μgm % in pm; after 1 mg dexamethasone at 11 pm, 8 am cortisol is <5 in normal; if >10, r/o Cushing's (100% sens, 90% specif—Ann IM 1990;112:738); false positives with phenytoin (Dilantin). If indeterminant then give 0.5 mg dexamethasone q 6 h × 48 h and measure cortisols; or get 24-h urinary free cortisol (6% false neg, fewer false pos) and/or 24-h urine cortisols × 3 ≥100 μgm/24 h

If above tests abnormal, then high-dose tests are done to differentiate cause, eg, baseline 8 am cortisol, 8 mg dexamethasone that night at 11 pm, then 8 am cortisol. Pituitary Cushing's patients, unlike adrenal tumors or ectopic ACTH production types, suppress value to <50% of baseline value (92% sens, 100% specif—Ann IM 1986;104:180, 68% sens in children; also see Nejm 1994;330:1295 for various test sens/specif)

CRH test: ACTH and cortisol incr after CRH given if pituitary tumor, not if ectopic ACTH or adrenal tumor (Ann IM 1985;102:344); 80% sens in children

Petrosal venous sampling for ACTH levels, simultaneous bilaterally reliably lateralize pituitary tumor (Nejm 1985;312:100)

Xray: (Ann IM 1988;109:547, 613)

CT, 60% false-negative rate due to small size of adenomas

MRI w gadolinium enhancement, 71% sens (52% sens in children), 87% specif; but 10% of the normal adult population have a lesion (Ann IM 1994;120:817)

Rx:
1st: Surgical transsphenoidal microadenomectomy, 90% successful (Nejm 1984;310:889 vs 76%—Ann IM 1988;109:487); bilateral adrenalectomy
2nd: Irradiation of pituitary, 83% successful in pts who fail surgery (Nejm 1997;336:172)
3rd: Aminoglutethimide, mitotane, metyrapone, and trilostane (Med Let 1985;27:87); bromocriptine; ketoconazole for its antisteroid synthesis effect (Nejm 1987;317:812)

CONN'S SYNDROME
Nejm 1998;339:1828; 1994;331:250

Cause: Bilateral adrenal hyperplasia; or unilateral adrenal adenoma secreting aldosterone

Epidem: 1–2% of all hypertensive patients

Pathophys: Increased aldosterone production causes Na^+ retention and K^+ loss leading to hypervolemia of 2–3 L, hypertension; H^+ loss causing metabolic alkalosis. Is there an anterior pituitary "aldosterone-stimulating factor"? (Nejm 1984;311:120)

Sx: Fatigue, weakness, tetany

Si: Hypertension; Trousseau's si, due to alkalosis; little edema, unlike secondary causes of incr aldosterone; proximal myopathy

Crs:

Cmplc: r/o **Liddle's syndrome,** an aldosterone-like effect is caused by an autosomal dominantly inherited renal tubular defect (Nejm 1999; 340:1177; 1994;330:178). **Bartter's syndrome** (Nejm 1999;340: 1180) and **licorice ingestion** (Nejm 1991;325:1223), both of which cause a normotensive hyperaldosteronism by peripheral angiotensin resistance and/or prostaglandin induction (Ann IM 1977;87:281,369; Nejm 1973;289:1022), rx'd w NSAIDs especially indomethacin (Ann IM 1977;87:281). Secondary causes of hyperaldosteronism. Rare unilateral adenoma or cancer of adrenal (Ann IM 1984;101:316)

Lab:
Chem: Aldosterone levels elevated; K^+ <3.7 mEq/L (80% sens) esp suspicious if Na^+ high or high normal; urine K^+ >30 mEq/24 hr; metabolic alkalosis w elevated HCO_3

Renin levels low, but elevated in secondary types of hyperaldosteronism

Adrenal vein sampling for lateralized aldosterone and cortisol levels

Saline infusion test: 2 L NS iv over 4 h decreases serum aldosterone to <10 ng% in normals (Ann IM 1984;100:300)

Captopril test: 25 mg po × 1 decreases serum aldosterone levels to <50% at 2 h in normals (Ann IM 1984;100:300) but not if Conn's present

Xray: CT very good to dx operable adenoma vs inoperable bilateral hyperplasia (Nejm 1980;303:1503)

Rx: Spironolactone 100 mg qid + antihypertensives (Ann IM 1999;1341:105)

Surgical adrenalectomy when unilateral lesion, though HT cured by this is only 35% (Ann IM 1995;122:877)

ADDISON'S DISEASE (Primary Adrenal Insufficiency)
Nejm 1996;335:1206

Cause: Idiopathic; autoimmune suppressor T-cell defect (Nejm 1979;300: 164); metastatic cancer; infection, especially tuberculosis, and meningococcemia w Friderichsen-Waterhouse syndrome; stress in pts chronically suppressed w steroids, possibly even inhaled beclomethasone (Nejm 1978;299:1387); HIV in AIDS pts (Ann IM 1997;127:1103)

Epidem: Peak incidence age 20–40 yr. Associated w HLA-B8 and DR 3/4, and thereby w pernicious anemia, myasthenia gravis, islet cell antibody IDDM, myxedema, vitiligo, alopecia, and primary gonadal failure

Pathophys: 80% of gland must be destroyed to get sx. ACTH and MSH similar, hence incr pigmentation; both mineralocorticoid and glucocorticoid deficiencies create the si and sx

Sx: Loss of "sense of well-being"; incr pigmentation, especially of scars, creases, and buccal mucosa; nausea, vomiting, and diarrhea; salt craving and weight loss; galactorrhea, rarely (Nejm 1972;287:1326)

Si: Hypotension, postural first and later even supine; cachexia; hyperpigmentation, vitiligo, longitudinal nail pigment streaks (Nejm 1969;281:1056); diminished axillary and pubic hair

Crs: 40% eventually develop other glandular failure as well (especially thyroid, gonadal)

Cmplc: r/o **hyporeninemic hypoaldosteronism** w hyperkalemia and metabolic acidosis due to depressed prostaglandin synthesis (Nejm 1986;314:1015,1041) seen in AODM and primary renal disease. **Adrenoleukodystrophy** in boys, a sex-linked abnormality of fatty acid metabolism (Nejm 1990;322:13). **Autoimmune polyendocrinopathy candidiasis/ectodermal dystrophy** (Nejm 1990;322:1829); 80% are hypoparathyroid, 70% are hypoadrenal, 60% of women with it are hypogonadal compared to 15% of men; by age 20, 100% have had significant candidal infections

Lab:

Chem: Na low, HCO_3 low; K elevated; ACTH elevated; 8 am cortisol <3 µgm is diagnostic, <15 µgm% when under stress, if >20 µgm% then dx is unlikely (D. Spratt 1/94)

Cosyntropin screening test of adrenal reserve: Get fasting blood cortisol, then give 250 µgm cosyntropin (ACTH analog) iv and draw repeat cortisol 30 min later (or im and 60 min later); a normal increases >6 µgm % to over 20 µgm % if adequate adrenal reserve (Nejm 1976;295:30)

Hem: CBC may show eosinophilia

Rx: Glucocorticoids like cortisol 25–30 mg po qd in am to mimic early am peaks; steroid equivalents in order of diminishing mineralocorticoid component: hydrocortisone 20 mg, prednisone 5 mg, methylprednisolone 4 mg, dexamethasone 0.75 mg

Mineralocorticoid, eg, fludrocortisone (Fluorinef) 100–300 µgm qd; adjust dose by renin level, which should be normal if adequate replacement; can cause significant supine hypertension over years (Nejm 1979;301:68)

Androgens can help reestablish sense of well-being and sexuality, especially in females, eg, dihydroepiandrosterone 50 mg po qd (Nejm 1999;341:1013)

In steroid-induced adrenal suppression (Nejm 1997;337:1285), slow tapering of steroids (Nejm 1976;295:30) should be done to allow recovery of pituitary/adrenal axis, decrease to a physiologic level of 20 mg hydrocortisone or other steroid equivalent q am, then taper q 4 wk to 10 mg qd by 2.5-mg increments; when 8 am plasma cortisol before pills is >10 μgm%, can stop and expect baseline adrenal function to be ok; still must supplement w 50 mg hydrocortisone or equivalent bid for minor and 100 mg tid for major illnesses (Jama 2002;287:236). When cosyntropin test (see above) is normal, no longer need such supplementation (Nejm 1976;295:30)

ADRENAL GENITAL SYNDROMES

Nejm 1994;331:250; 1990;323:1806; 1987;316:1519,1580

Cause: Genetic enzyme deficiencies; all autosomal recessive. In 21-OH, defect is in CYP21 gene for a microsomal cytochrome P450 enzyme (Nejm 1991;324:145)

Epidem: 21β-OH deficiency occurs in 1/14,000

Pathophys: See Fig. 5.1.1

Sx: Usually appears in children; although mild "adult adrenal hyperplasia" may not manifest until adulthood, mainly 21β-OH deficiency, rarely 11β- or 17-OH deficiency, which present w amenorrhea and hypertension

Si:

17-OHase: hyperaldosteronism, hypogonadism

3βde-OHase: virilization (female pseudohermaphroditism), salt loss, many die at birth

11-OHase: virilization (female pseudohermaphroditism), hypertension, hypokalemia

21-OHase: virilization (female pseudohermaphroditism), salt loss may manifest as SIDS in male infants where detected later because ambiguous genitalia not a clue

Crs: With rx, children grow up short but w normal sexual maturation (Nejm 1978;299:1392)

Cmplc: Iatrogenic Cushing's syndrome; Addisonian crisis; ovarian dermoids; precocious puberty, r/o **Albright's syndrome:** precocious puberty and other endocrine hyperfunctioning including thyroid, adrenal, and pituitary growth hormone, plus fibrous dysplasia of the bones and café-au-lait spots (Nejm 1991;325:688)

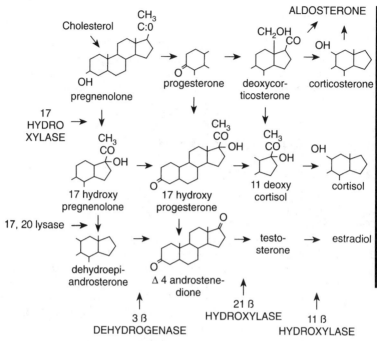

Figure 5.1.1

Lab:

> *Chem:* Plasma aldosterone incr in 11β-OH deficiency. In 21-OH deficiency, 17-OH progesterone, androstenedione, and testosterone all elevated
>
> *Urine:* 17-Ketosteroid steroids elevated in 11β-OH, 21β-OH 3βde-OH, and perhaps 17-OH deficiencies. 17-OH steroids elevated in 11β-OH deficiency

Rx: (Jama 1997;227:1077) Prevent w newborn screening?
of disease: use all 4 (Jama 1997;227:1073)

- Glucocorticoids, like hydrocortisone 25–30 mg/M²/d
- Mineralocorticoids as fludrocortisone (Florinef) 100–300 μgm qd for all ages, or more until reach normal renin levels; may also work prenatally if started within a month of conception to prevent

virilization of female infants (Nejm 1990;322:111); these
imperfectly decrease feedback production of more precursors
- Flutamide, an antiandrogen, also used to supplement this regimen
- Testolactone, inhibits androgen-to-estrogen conversion

5.2 DIABETES AND OBESITY

DIABETES MELLITUS

- Type 1, juvenile onset (JODM), usually IDDM
- Type 2, adult onset (AODM), usually NIDDM at least initially

Cause: (Nejm 1981;304:1454)

Type 1: hypoinsulinemia; has an autosomal genetic component;
HLA-linked to DQ antigens (Nejm 1990;322:1836); 90% are
autoimmune w measurable antibodies to islet cell antigens, insulin,
glutamic acid decarboxylase, et al. (Nejm 2000;342:301; 1994;331:
1428); perhaps associated w childhood exposure to cow's milk?
(Nejm 1992;327:302,348 vs Jama 1996;276:607; Nejm 1993;329:
1853). Viral infections like mumps and coxsackie (Nejm 1979;300:
1175) induce, probably through T cells (Jama 1997;277:1101) vs.
islet antigens

Type 2: insulin resistant (Nejm 1993;329:1988) adult type,
occasionally from hypophosphatemia (Nejm 1980;303:1259);
substantial genetic/familial component since 90% concordance in
identical twins; also associated w glycogen synthetase deficiency
(Nejm 1993;328:10), and chromosome #20 gene for glucokinase
deficiency (Nejm 1993;328:697)

Epidem: Prevalence of overt disease = 1.5%; 10% are chemically diabetic
at age 60 (P. Fialkow 1971); 0.3% of all obstetric patients. HLA
genes offer in utero selective advantage, hence persistence in gene
pool (Nejm 1986;315:1314)

Type 1: = 10–20% of all diabetics; anti-islet cell antibodies predict
onset (Nejm 1990;323:1167). Higher incidence/prevalence in
northern European populations (Nejm 1994;331:1428)

Type 2: = 80% of all diabetics; increases with parity with a 10–20 yr
delay (Nejm 1989;321:1214), and (Jama 2001;286:1945) with:

hypokalemia, β blockers, protease inhibitors, atypical
antipsychotics decr incid w ACEI use (Jama 2001;286:1882)

Pathophys:

Neuropathy (Ann IM 1987;107:546), retinopathy, and cataracts a
result of sorbitol accumulation from glucose via AR? (Ann IM 1992;
117:226; Nejm 1988;319:542); or perhaps due to "glycation" of
many body proteins like Hgb A_1C (Ann IM 1996;124, suppl #1:81)

Microvascular cmplc correlate w renin levels, which decrease w
intensive chronic rx (Nejm 1985;312:1412); nephropathy and
retinopathy are preceded in IDDM by elevated prorenin levels
(Nejm 1990;323:1101)

Infectious cmplc due to impaired PMNL phagocytosis from high blood
sugar levels (Ann IM 1995;123:919)

Insulin increases amino acid uptake, protein synthesis, glucose uptake,
FFA uptake, glycogen synthetase; decreases lipolysis, glycogenolysis

Muscle and fat tissues metabolize FFA when glucose <120 mg%. FFAs
inhibit glycolysis and hexose monophosphate shunt, hence TPNH
and all synthesis and repair; FFAs are metabolized to ketone bodies
causing acidosis, and are converted to triglycerides by the liver and
hence may contribute to atherosclerosis

Glucagon excess may be equally important in pathogenesis

In Type 2, genetic peripheral insulin resistance in the obese and incr
insulin levels cause eventual β-cell exhaustion (Ann IM 1990;113:
905,909) when genetically predisposed (Nejm 1996;334:777);
impaired/delayed insulin release to glucose load also allows hepatic
gluconeogenesis to persist 1–2 h, then insulin overshoot occurs
(Nejm 1992;326:22). But islet amyloid deposition may also
contribute (Nejm 2000;343:411)

In pregnancy, macrosomia due to incr substrate availability and some
maternal insulin/antibody complex absorbed by the fetus (Nejm
1990;323:309)

Sx: Polyuria, polydypsia, polyphagia, weight loss

Si: Necrobiosis lipoidica (95%) = pigmented skin plaques w white lipid
center, irregular, atrophic; fatty hepatomegaly; retinopathy w hard
exudates, microaneurysms and hemorrhages (Nejm 1983;309:527;
photos in 1993;329:320)

Crs: No worsening w acute stress (Nejm 1986;314:1078). Neuropathies
worsen over 5–10 yr when present, in ~50% (Nejm 1995;333:89)

Cmplc: (Nejm 1993;328:1676)

Acidosis/coma (p 200), and nonketotic, hyperosmolar coma (Nejm 1977;297:1452)

ASCVD rate doubled (Framingham heart study) from elevated lipids when Hgb A_1C levels >8% (Ann IM 1992;117:42), and perhaps from hypercoagulability induced by high glucose and insulin levels (Jama 2000;283:221); correlates w 5th finger first IP joint hypermobility ("prayer si"—Nejm 1981;305:191); large vessel not small vessel disease causes ischemic leg ulcers (Nejm 1984;311:1615)

Eating disorders in 30% of young type 1 women assoc w markedly incr microvascular cmplc

Eye: retinopathy (Nejm 1990;322:978) correlates w poor control (Nejm 1985;313:1433), but even with a return to normoglycemia w pancreatic transplant, retinopathy progresses (Nejm 1988;318:208); cataracts, assoc w doubled mortality rates (Nejm 1985;313:1438)

GI: nausea and vomiting; diarrhea often from bacterial overgrowth; fecal incontinence

Hypoglycemia at higher, "normal" blood levels in pts who usually run high (Nejm 1988;318:1487); patients report sx w only 15% of episodes (J Intern Med 1990;228:641) and awareness improves as severity and frequency improve though not neuropathic in etiology (Nejm 1993;329:834); driving significantly impaired between 47–65 mg% but pts fail to perceive it 50% of time (Jama 1999;282:750). Somogyi effect (Nejm 1988;319:1233; Ann IM 1983;98:219) due to decr epinephrine response to hypoglycemia during sleep (Nejm 1998;338:1657), r/o "Dawn phenomenon" from growth hormone surge (Nejm 1985;312:1473)

Infectious (Nejm 1999;341:1906) including emphysematous pyelonephritis and cholecystitis, necrotizing fasciitis, malignant otitis externa, and mucor infections

Nephropathy (1/3) and end stage renal disease 2.5% in 15 yr (Jama 1997;278:2069); genetic predisposition (Nejm 1989;320:1161); correlates w proteinuria (Nejm 1984;310:357; 1984;311:89), w inherited tendencies to hypertension (Nejm 1988;318:140,146) and ASHD (Nejm 1992;326:673), and w higher infection rates. GFR above normal until macroalbuminuria develops (Nejm 1996;335:1636)

Neuropathies including mononeuritis, eg, of 3rd nerve w pupil sparing unlike internal carotid aneurysm; impotence (60%—Ann IM 1971; 75:213); peripheral: sx of numbness daily (25% sens, 95% specif—Diabet Med 2000;17:105), stocking/glove, and diminished foot pain and flare contributing to ulcers (Nejm 1988;318:1306); radiculopathy (Ann IM 1977;86:166); decr visceral pain perception, eg, silent angina and MIs (Ann IM 1988;108:170) and decr COPD dyspnea (Nejm 1988;319:1369); autonomic, measure w expiratory-inspiratory respiratory variation in sinus rates, if <10, suspect it (Bmj 1982;285:559)

Obstetric: infant respiratory distress syndrome (Nejm 1976;294:357); congenital malformations (Nejm 1981;304:1331 vs 1988;318:671); definite increase in spontaneous abortions if blood sugar elevated (Nejm 1988;319:1617)

Skin ulcers of foot/ankle due to neuropathy w complicating osteomyelitis demonstrable by bone at base w blunt probing (66% sens, 85% specif—Jama 1995;273:721)

Syndrome X (diabetic) (Nejm 1999;340:1314): insulin resistance, type 2 diabetes, incr lipids, HT, ASCVD, and sometimes polycystic ovary disease

Lab:

Chem: Fasting blood glucose elevated >126 mg% (ADA) vs >140 mg% (Jama 1999;281:1203 vs 1222), or >200 mg% on 2 hr pc or random BS; FBS >110 but <126 mg%, or 2 hr 140–200 mg% = "impaired glucose tolerance." Home monitoring equipment and costs (Med Let 1992;34:115), or watch-like monitoring wrist band (Glucowatch) (Med Let 2001;43:42; Jama 1999;282:1839). Ob screen for gestational diabetes w 50 gm glucose po at 24–28 wk, get full GTT if 1 h sugar >140 mg% (MMWR 1986;35:201).

Hgb A_1C (glycosylated hemoglobin) >7.0% (90% specif, 99% sens), usually requires drug rx (Jama 1996;276:1247), increases fast but reflects glucose over past 2 mo (Nejm 1984;310:341); incr by Fe deficiency, decr by sickle cell disease, not a reliable screen to make dx; get q 3 mo and keep at least under 8% to prevent microvascular cmplc, under 7% dramatically reduces cmplc over 7 yr (Nejm 1993; 329:304, 977). Avg glucose over past 3 mo = 33 × Hgb A_1C - 86

Fructosamine office or home testing (In Charge, Duet) (Rx Let 1999;6: 56) reflects past 2–3 wk blood sugar rather than past 2–3 mo of Hgb A_1C; strips $4 each

Na^+ decr by incr glucose if not dehydrated; osmoles $= 2 \times Na +$ glucose/18; hence blood sugar/40 $\approx$ Na equivalents

Insulin and/or C-peptide levels abnormally low in type 1, unlike type 2 (Rx Let 2000;7:19)

Lipid profile, get LDL <100, or screen non-fasting w total and HDL and pursue further those w non-HDL >160 (J. Devlin 11/99)

NIL: EKG

Path: Liver bx if done shows incr nuclear, decr cytoplasmic glycogen; vessels show ASCVD; renal bx shows Kimmelstiel-Wilson lesion, glycogen in tubules, thickened basement membrane, which correlates w eye disease (Nejm 1985;312:1282)

Urine: Glucosuria r/o autosomal dominant nephrogenic diabetes (1/500 glycosurics); home monitoring as good as home blood glucose monitoring? (Diab Care 1990;13:1044)

Proteinuria: microalbuminuria >30 mg/24 h or >20 μgm/min requires rx; μgm albumin/mg creatinine ratio of >20–300) on spot urine indicates early disease (Nejm 1995;332:1251) vs >15 (Diab Care 1997;20:516)

Rx: Stepped care (Ann IM 1998;128:165; ADA in RxLet 1997;4:37):
- 1st: Lifestyle changes like diet, exercise and wgt loss
- 2nd: Po mono rx w sulfonylurea for lean pts, metformin for obese
- 3rd: Combo rx of #2 + acarbose
- 4th: Combo rx of #2 w insulin
- 5th: Insulin alone
- 6th: Insulin + troglitazone

Tight control in both types 1 and 2 (Lancet 1999;353:617; 1998;352: 837, 854) w avg Hgb A_1C ~7%, at least <8.1%, to prevent renal failure (Nejm 1995;332:1251) w tid insulin (Diab Care 1996;19: 195), improves (Nejm 1993;329:977):
- motor nerve conduction velocities (Ann IM 1981;94:307) as well as sensory and autonomic neuropathy (Nejm 1990;322:1031) and prevents development of all (NNT-5 = 4 for NCVs, and NNT-5 = 16 for clinical neuropathy—Ann IM 1995;122:561);
- proteinuria (Nejm 2000;342:381; 1994;330:15) and
- renal failure (Nejm 1991;324:1626);
- fetal anomalies and death (Nejm 1981;304:1331);
- retinopathy (Nejm 2000;342:381; 1993;329:304, 977);
- survival post-MI (NNT-2 = 13) (J Am Coll Cardiol 1995;26:57);

- endogenous insulin secretion if started early in type 1s (Ann IM 1998;128:517);
- quality of life and cost:benefit ratio (Jama 1998;280:1490)

ASA 650 mg po qd prevents ASHD cmplc (NNT-5 = 29—Jama 1992; 268:1292)

Stop hyperglycemia-producing meds (list—Ann IM 1993;118:536)

Experimental?: prevent cmplc w AR inhibitors? (Nejm 1988;319:548). ChemoRx w cyclosporine in new juvenile onset types can produce 1^+ yr remissions (Nejm 1988;318:663), or prednisone + azathioprine (Nejm 1988;319:599), but how different from usual "honeymoon"?; or pancreatic islet cell transplants, 100% 12 mo success! (Nejm 2000;343:230); possibly chromium 200^+ mg po qd (Rx Let 1998;5:10)

Diet: much unproven, go slow pushing (Nejm 1986;315:1224); total calories more important than ratios. High fiber, 25–50 gm qd, >50% soluble type, improves glycemic control and lipids (Nejm 2000;342:1392); fenugreek dietary legume supplement (Rx Let 1999;6:10); sugars no worse than starches (Nejm 1983;309:7); weight loss if overweight as most type 2s are

Exercise increases receptor sensitivity (Jama 1998;279:669) and glucose uptake, and glycogen synthesis in exercised muscles even in insulin-resistant pts (Nejm 1996;335:1357)

Oral hypoglycemics (Table 5.2.1)

Insulin U-100 sc, human (see Table 5.2.2). Best regimens (Nejm 1993; 329:977; Med Let 1989;31:363): hs N, am regular + NPH; or hs NPH, regular before each meal. In type 2s, can give 1 dose hs titrated up to get FBS <110 along w metformin 1000 mg po bid, resulted in best control w least weight gain (Ann IM 1999; 130:389)

Avoid leg injection w exercise since increases absorption (Nejm 1978; 298:79); can even inject through clothing?! (Diab Care 1997;20: 244). Pumps, external sc, or maybe implanted sc or intraperitoneal (Jama 1996;276:1322): dangerous in patients w autonomic neuropathy, β blockers, and/or hypoadrenal (Ann IM 1983;99:268) because of impaired glucose and epinephrine production response to hypoglycemia (Nejm 1983;308:485)

Rx of cmplc's:

Diarrhea: cholestyramine, metaclopramide (Reglan), opiates, antibiotics, clonidine (Ann IM 1985;102:197)

Foot ulcers/infections (Nejm 1994;331:854) w anaerobes and pseudomonas: avoid barefoot walking, get good shoes, rx calluses;

Table 5.2.1 Oral Hypoglycemics (Ann IM 1999;131:281)

Drug	Dose	Comment
Sulfonylureas:		
As good as insulin if get glucose control but HDL cholesterol not as good (Ann IM 1988;108:334), no value using w insulin (Nejm 1992;327:1453)		60–70% successful as single agent at 1st, but 6+% failure rate/yr thereafter; teratogenesis and hypoglycemia of newborn if use in pregnancy
1st generation:		Potentiated by warfarin, can cause hypo Na
Chlorpropramide (Diabinase)	250–500 mg qd	Renal excretion, multiday half life; cheap; antabuse-like effect
Tolbutamide (Orinase)	500–1000 mg bid	Hepatic metab; 5h half life; $5/mo
2nd generation		
Glipizide (Glucotrol)	2.5–20 mg bid	Hepatic metab; 2–4h half life; $15+/mo
Glyburide (Micronase)	2.5–10 mg qd	Hepatic metab; 10 h half life; $15+/mo
Glimepiride (Amaryl) (Med let 1996 38:47)	4–8 mg qd	Hepatic metab; 9 h half life; $20/mo
Biguanides		Won't cause hypoglycemia; decr hepatic gluconeogenesis, induce wgt loss, incr end organ insulin sens
Metformin (Glucophage) (Nejm 1996; 334:574; 1995;333:541; Med Let 1995;37:41); or w glyburide (Glucovance) (Med Let 2000;42:105) 1.25/250mg, 25/500, or 5/500	500–1000 mg hs, bid, or tid up to 2500 mg qd	Alone or w sulfonylurea or insulin (Ann IM 1999;131:182), esp if obese or high triglycerides; cmplc: gi sx, lactic acidosis (1/30,000 person-yrs) esp if creat >1.4 mg%, CHF (Rx Let 1998;5:18), and/or given angiographic dyes (hold pericath) or abnl LFTs; $47/mo, generic in 2001
Disaccharidase inhibitors		Inhibit pancreatic and brush border enzymes
Acarbose (Precose) (Med Let 1996;38:9; Diab Care 1997;20:248; Ann IM 1994;121:928)	50–200 mg po ac tid	Non-absorbable oligosaccharide; do not use w metformin; cmplc: hypoglycemia (rx w glucose not sucrose), flatulence, diarrhea, incr LFTs (monitor q 3 mos). $42/mo for 100 mg tid

Table 5.2.1 *(continued)*

Drug	Dose	Comment
Disaccharidase inhibitors (*cont.*)		
Miglitol (Glyset)(Rx Let 1999;6:9; Med Let 1999;41:49)	25–100 mg po tid	Similar to acarbose w/o LFT increases; use in type 2 w sulfonlylureas; multiple drug interactions including w sulfonylureas; $50/mo for 50 mg tid
Thiazolidinediones (glitazones)		Incr insulin sensitivity; use w insulin or sulfonylureas
Rosiglitazone (Avandia) (Med Let 1999;41:71); can use w sulfonylureas (Diabet Med 2000;17:40)	2–4 mg qd-bid	@ max dose w max metformin only 28% had HgbA$_1$C <7% (Jama 2000;283:1695); cmplc: fluid retention, hepatotoxicity including liver failure (Ann IM 2000;132: 118,121), get LFTs q2mo × 1yr, keep <3× nl; $75–100/mo
Pioglitazone (Actos) (Med Let 1999;41:112)	15–45 mg po qd	incr HDL w/o LDL incr; cmplc: fluid retention, no hepatitis yet but get LFTs q 2 mos; $75–100/mo
Troglitazone (Rezulin) (Nejm 1998;338:867,908)	200–600 mg po qd	Hepatitis (Ann IM 1998;129:36,38), pulled from US market in 2000
Meglitinides		Fast acting so can skip if miss a meal or take if eating irregularly;
Nateglinide (Starlix) (Med Let 2001;43:29)	60–120 mg tid ac	similar to sulfonylureas, can cause hypoglycemia; can use w metformin; hepatic metab; $80/mo
Repaglinide (Prandin) (Rx Let 1998;5:10,27; Med Let 1998;4:55,66)	0.5–4 mg po ac (0.5, 1, 2 mg tabs)	$67/mo for 1 mg tid

ENDOCRINOLOGY/METABOLISM

Table 5.2.2 Insulins

Insulin Type	Onset	Peak	Duration	Comment	Cost/ 1000 U
Lispro (Humalog) or Aspart (Novolog)	Minutes	30–60 min	3–4 h	(Med Let 2001;43:89; Nejm 1997;337:176) Helpful in pts w recurrent hypoglycemia; can give ac based on serving size. OK to mix w Humulins as long as draw up 1st (Rx Let 1999;6:9)	$50
Regular (Humulin-R)	15 min	2 h	6–8 h		$25
NPL (neutral protamine lispro)	15 min	2 h		plain or as 75/25% Humalog mix (Rx Let 2000;7:9)	
NPH (Humulin-N)	1 h	8–12 h	13 h		$25
Ultra-Lente (Humulin-U) qd hs	1 h	minimal	19 h		$25
Glargine (Lantus) qd hs	1.5 h	none	20 h	(Med Let 2001;43:65) 3 aa's altered from human insulin slows release; don't mix w others	$43
Inhaled				Experimental (Ann IM 2001; 134:203, 242)	

rx w parenteral imipenem, or ticarcillin + clavulanic acid (Timentin) (S. Sears 1991), or oral fluoroquinolone + clindamycin po × 10–14 d better than longer rx or more diagnostic testing to r/o osteomyelitis (Jama 1995;273:712); becaplermin (Regranex) gel qd (Med Let 1998;40:73; Rx Let 1998;5:11) helps ulcers heal moderately faster, $380/15 gm; surgical grafting w human skin (Dermagraft) (Diab Care 1996;19:350); perhaps granulocyte-colony stimulating factor 5 μgm sc qd × 7d (Lancet 1997;350:855). Automatic mechanical compression device at least 8 h/d helps heal faster (Arch Surg 2000;135:1405)

Gastroparesis: vomiting, poor emptying; rx w small volume, frequent feedings, metoclopramide (Reglan) 10 mg 30 min ac? (Ann IM 1983;98:86; 1982;96:444; Med Let 1982;24:67), or cisapride

(Propulsid) 10–20 mg po qid (Med Let 1994;36:1), which causes diarrhea in 30%, or erythromycin 250 mg tid (Nejm 1990; 322:1028)

Hyperlipidemia: agressive monitoring and rx since ASHD is incr 2–3x at least in type 2 pts (J.Devlin 3/96)

Hypertension: ACE inhibitors (Jama 1997;278:40); tight control decr morb and mortality (Arch IM 2000;160:2447); ok to use thiazides, β blockers and probably calcium channel blockers

Hypoglycemia: glucose tabs or gel if on disaccaridase inhibitors, otherwise candy; glucagon im

Impotence: (p 778)

Insulin resistance (Syndrome X): (Nejm 1991;325:938) type A (receptor unresponsive) assoc w acanthosis nigrans, polycystic ovary, and obesity (Nejm 1980;303:970); rare autoimmune type B assoc w other autoimmune syndromes especially lupus (Ann IM 1985;102:176); rx w U-500 regular insulin (Ann IM 1981;94:653), or insulin-like growth factor in extreme cases (Nejm 1992;327:853)

Ischemic heart disease: rx risk factors as aggressively as post-MI pts since 7 yr incid = 20^+% (Nejm 1998;339:229); prophylact w ASA qd (Am J Med 1998;105:494), and/or 1–2 alcoholic drinks qd (Jama 1999;282:239). CABG results in better survival long term than angioplasty (Nejm 2000;342:989)

Nephropathy/renal failure (Njem 1999;341:1127): prevent w ACE inhibitor rx (Ann IM 1998;128:982), and tight control; BP control; protein and PO_4 restriction (Nejm 1991;324:78); prevents progression of proteinuria to nephropathy (Jama 1994;271:275; Ann IM 1993;118:129; BMJ 1991;303:81) when microalbuminuria >20–200 mg/24 h (Ann IM 1993;118:577; BMJ 1992;304:339) and improves lipids (Ann IM 1993;118:246); ARAs equally good (Nejm 2001;345:851,861,870,910)

Neuropathy:
- TCA like amitriptyline or desipramine 75–150 mg po qd, both effective (Nejm 1992;326:1250) and slow progression in pts w established disease but creatinine <2.5 mg % (Nejm 1993;329: 1456, 1496);
- mexiletine (Diab Care 1997;20:1594);
- gabapentin (Neurontin) (Jama 1998;280:1831) 300–1200 mg po tid, adv effects: dizziness, somnolence, confusion;
- sorbinil 250 mg po qd? (Nejm 1988;319:548); adverse effects: rash, fever, myalgia may be severe (Ann IM 1991;114:720);

- capsaicin topical cream for painful neuropathy (Arch IM 1991; 151:2225), but questionable benefit and 0.075% OTC costs $27/oz (Med Let 1992;34:61);

Peri-operative management (Nejm 1970;282:1472)

Pregnancy: (Nejm 1999;341:1749) get Hgb A_1C level <9% before conception (Nejm 1981;304:1331); IQ of child inversely correlates w 3rd trimester maternal OH-butyrate levels (Nejm 1991;325:911); keep pc (not ac) blood sugars <140 mg % using diet and split dose am and pm NPH/regular insulin, roughly 2/3 dose in am and 1/3 in pm, am dose 2/3 NPH and 1/3 reg, pm dose 1/2 and 1/2 (Nejm 1995;333:1237). DO NOT USE ORAL AGENTS, although glyburide started in 2nd trimester reported to be safe and effective (Nejm 2000;343:1134, 1178)

Retinopathy (Nejm 1999;341:667): tight control, regular eye consults for laser rx (Ann IM 1992;117:226; 1992;116:660)

DIABETIC KETOACIDOSIS

Cause: Insulin-dependent diabetes mellitus

Epidem:

Pathophys: See Fig. 5.2.1

Coma from CSF acidosis, hence rarer in metabolic than respiratory acidosis because CO_2 crosses blood-brain barrier easily; HCO_3 rx may paradoxically induce/worsen coma (F. Plum, Nejm 1967; 277:605)

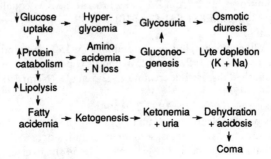

Figure 5.2.1

Sx: Malaise, confusion, nausea/vomiting, abdominal pain

Si: Kussmaul's (deep) respirations; stupor/coma; hypotension; dehydration

Crs: Onset over 2–3 d

Cmplc: Cerebral edema leading to coma w 90% mortality 6–10 h after starting rx especially in children (Nejm 1985;312:1147) w low pCO_2's, high BUNs, and who get bicarb rx (Nejm 2001;344:264, 302)

   r/o hypoglycemia; infection; appendicitis; nonketotic, nonacidotic hyperosmolar coma (Nejm 1977;297:1452) seen in the elderly w NIDDM; causes volume depletion, stupor, and coma

Lab:

   Chem: Glucose elevated

   Lytes: HCO_3 decr commensurate w anion gap, but hyperchloremic when not volume-depleted (Nejm 1982;307:1603); K low, though may be falsely high in DKA from pH shift of intracellular K to extracellular space for calculation (p 741). Osmoles, measured or calculated, may be incr if water-depleted; calculated osmoles = glucose/18 + 2 × Na + BUN/2.8 (Ann IM 1989;110:854)

   Ketones positive undiluted and out to as much as 1/8 diluted; may be negative if most ketone bodies are metabolized to hydroxybutyrate (measurable too)

   Amylase elevated (80%), 65% pancreatic, 35% salivary (Ann IM 1979;91:200)

Rx: (Nejm 1983;309:159)

   Follow q 1–2 h glucose, Na, K, HCO_3, ketones, urine output

   Insulin, regular, 0.33–0.44 U/kg iv push; then 7 U/h iv continuous until glucose <250 mg%; repeat push bolus in 1 h if glucose not decr >10%; then 2–6 U/h iv continuous (or im, or sc) until glucose <150 mg%; then routine maintenance. In children, regular insulin 0.1–0.2 U/kg iv push, then 0.1–0.2 U/h. Fluids: saline, or half-normal saline after 1st liter if osmoles elevated (ie, water-depleted), w 40 mEq KCl at 1 L/h until glucose <250 mg % then change to D5W or D5S

   NG tube since many die of emesis and aspiration from gastric atony

   HCO_3 iv rx only if HCO_3 <5 mEq/L or pH <7.1; gives paradoxical CNS acidosis (Nejm 1971;284:283), and right shift of hemoglobin dissociation curve

   PO_4 rx rarely needed? (Nejm 1985;313:447); maybe as K_2PO_4 if low (PO_4<0.1–0.5 mg %) to prevent insulin resistance (Nejm 1980; 303:1259)

OBESITY
Nejm 1997;337:396

Cause: 70% genetic, little environmental (twin studies—Nejm 1990;322: 1477, 1483)

Epidem: Prevalence incr in US, ~18% in 1998 (Jama 1999;282:1519), and varies inversely w breast feeding duration as infant (Jama 2001; 285:2453,2461,2506)

Pathophys: Many theories:
- Brain appetite/satiety center imbalance, "adipostat" set higher (eg, by sedentary lifestyle) or lower (eg, by regular exercise) (Nejm 1995;332:621,673,679)
- Fat tissue regulatory failure, incr numbers of fat cells in utero leads to fat adults (Nejm 1976;295:349)
- Psychiatric
- Cellular sodium pump thermogenesis decr (in rbc anyway—Nejm 1980;303:1017)
- Lower activity index (Nejm 1988;318:461,467,509)
- Insensitivity of brain to leptin, satiety regulator protein secreted by adipose cells? (Nejm 1996;334:292)

Sx: Frequently pts falsely report more activity and less intake than true, and falsely ascribe inability to lose weight to genetic resistance (Nejm 1992;327:1893)

Si: Triceps skin fold >23 mm; BP elevated (incr renin and aldosterone—Nejm 1981;304:930); ≥ 30 kg/M^2, or 20^+% over ideal body wgt (formula for IDBW: men = 106 lb + 6 lb/in over 5 ft; for women = 100 lb + 5 lbs/in over 5 ft)

Crs: Obesity in adolescence is associated w decr lifetime survival in men only (Nejm 1992;327:1350); also w lower education, income, and marriage rate, unlike other chronic disease states; is it genetics, discrimination, or both? (Nejm 1993;329:1008, 1076)

Cmplc: Sleep apnea (p 546); osteoarthritis of knees (Ann IM 1988;109:18); gallstones w weight loss (Nejm 1988;319:1567); fatty liver (75%) (Ann IM 2000;132:112); ASHD, diabetes, hypertension, premature death (Jama 1999;282:1523, 1530; Ann IM 1985;103:977); incr cervical and breast cancers and less frequent screening for them (Ann IM 2000;132:697)

r/o night eating syndrome (Jama 1999;282:657,689)

Lab:

Rx: (25 article rv supplement—Ann IM 1993;119(7 part 2):641–764)

Prevent gallstone formation w ursodeoxycholic acid 300 mg po bid or 600 mg qd, NNT = 4 (Ann IM 1995;122:899), cost $140/mo. ASA ii po bid probably decreases gallstone formation (Nejm 1988; 319:1567)

Diet, 600–800 qd mixed calories best; spares muscle and has fewest cmplc of starvation and/or high-protein regimens, like arrhythmias, especially ventricular, w prolonged QT (Ann IM 1985;102:121; Nejm 1980;303:735; 1980;302:477). New liquid diets now safe, cost ~$25/wk, but are successful long term in only 10–20% (Med Let 1989;31:22)

Exercise program, 45 min at 60–80% maximal pulse 3×/wk helps weight and HDL (Nejm 1991;326:461) no matter the genetic predisposition (Ann IM 1999;130:873)

Appetite suppressants (Jama 1996;276:1907) like:
- Fluoxetine (Prozac) 60 mg po qd;
- Sibutramine (Meridia) (Jama 2001;286:1331; Med Let 1998;40: 32; Rx Let 1998;5:14) 10–15 mg po qd × 1 mo, then cont'd × 1 yr if lose ≥2 kg in that first month for eventual 8 ±1 kg avg loss; many drug interactions; $112/30d
- Ephedra (mahuang)-containing supplements, but many health risks (Nejm 2000;343:1833)
- Herbal *Garcinia* sp. (hydroxycitric acid) no help (Jama 1998; 280:1596).
- NOT Phentermine (Ionamin) + fenfluramine (Pondimin) or dexfenfluramine (Redux), withdrawn from market because of fatal primary pulmonary HT and cardiac valve abnormalities (Nejm 1998;339:713,719; 1997;337:602; 1996;335:609), which stabilize after stop (Ann IM 2001;134:261, 267, 335)

Pancreatic lipase inhibitor, orlistat (Xenical) (J Intern Med 2000;248: 245; Med Let 1999;41:55; Rx Let 1999;6:25; 1997;4:33; Jama 1999;281:243,278) 120 mg po tid w meals. Adverse effects: fat soluble vitamin depletion, steatorrhea, possible incr breast Ca. $120/mo

Gastric bypass (gastric balloon rx ineffective—Med Let 1986;28:77), stapling or plication; or jejunum to distal ileum (colon originally) (Ann IM 1976;85:97); weight loss so produced creates great psychic effects (Nejm 1974;290:300); at 5 yr, 20% failure, 50% benefiting; similar to diet alone (Denmark—Nejm 1984;310:353; 1983;308:

995). Adverse effects (primarily w bypass procedures): most from
bypass blind loop bacterial overgrowth causing diarrhea and
immune complex diseases (Ann IM 1980;93:557; 1978;89:594);
fatty liver, cirrhosis, gallstones (Nejm 1974;290:921); immune
complex arthritis, rash (Ann IM 1980;93:557; Nejm 1976;294:
121), and nephritis (Ann IM 1976;84:594); diarrhea and
malabsorption; uric acid renal stones (20%) and hyperoxaluria
(MKSAP 1980); polyneuropathy, especially position sense, even in
stapled patients (Ann IM 1982;96:453); B_{12} and iron malabsorption
commonly (Ann IM 1996;124:469); metronidazole (Flagyl)
0.75–2 gm qd po helps all cmplc of blind loop (Ann IM 1980;
93:557)

Surgical liposuction, "tumescent" method w sc lidocaine + epinephrine
has cmplc of sudden death (5 cases—Nejm 1999;340:1471)

5.3 GONADAL DISORDERS

TURNER'S SYNDROME
Nejm 1996;335:1749

Cause: Genetic mutation or transmitted as ? "X-linked or autosomal
dominant expressed only in male." No incr w advanced maternal
age.

Epidem: Rare, incid = 1/1500–2500 females, prevalence = 50–75,000 in
US; more common in miscarriage fetuses

Pathophys: Part of mixed gonadal dysgenesis (see above); XO, X with
partial X or Y deletion, isochromosome of X or Y, ring chromosome
w deletion of X or Y. Lymphatic hypoplasia causes edema

Sx: Dwarfism (90% are <5 ft); primary amenorrhea; multiple moles
appear between age 4 and 15 yr

Si: Normal female genitalia; ankle edema; low hairline at base of neck;
neck webbing (20%); multiple nevi and nail anomalies; incr
carrying angle of elbow, short 4th metacarpal

Crs:

Cmplc: Diabetes mellitus; Hashimoto's thyroiditis in up to 50%;
congenital cardiovascular abnormalities, especially coarctation of

the aorta (15%); renal and gi congenital abnormalities occasionally; tumors in streak gonads if present; renal HT; scoliosis (10%); OM from malformations of mouth/nose

Lab:

Path: Streak gonads

Chromosome preps are Barr body-negative; get full karyotype to r/o XO-XY mosaicism w incr gonadal cancer incidence

Chem: FSH and LH incr (unlike hypogonadotrophic hypogonadism)

Xray: Prenatal ultrasound may show thickened nuchal fold, cystic hygroma, horseshoe kidney

Knee films show overgrowth of medial tibial condyle

Rx: Growth hormone rx in late childhood (Nejm 1999;340:502,557); ERT and cycled progresterone in adults; pregnancy possible esp w donated ova

Surgical removal of any streak gonad in all mosaics

KLINEFELTER'S SYNDROME

Cause: Genetic; mutation, in case of mosaics, in postconception fetus

Epidem: 1/250 male births (Nejm 1969;280:851); 1/20 aspermic males (Nejm 1969;281:969)

Pathophys: XXY, XXXY in at least some body cells (mosaicism)

Sx: Sexual immaturity, sterility

Si: Aspermic/hypospermic, male phenotype; small testes (<2.5 cm diameter); gynecomastia; diminished intelligence (IQ); vertical creases on upper lip as age (present in all females w/o ovaries)

Crs:

Cmplc: Breast cancer incidence is the same as for women (Nejm 1980; 303:795)

r/o "**supermale**" = XXYY, XYY; tall, aggressive; have varicose veins; may present looking like a Klinefelter's

Lab:

Chem: FSH and LH elevated (unlike hypogonadotropic hypogonadism)

Path: Testicular bx shows hyalinized tubules w clumped Leydig cells, r/o mumps orchitis

Chromosome preps show buccal Barr body-positive (85%); XXY or XXYY by full karyotype, unless miss in a mosaic

Klinefelter's Syndrome, continued

Rx: Testosterone 200 mg im in oil q 2–4 wk or pulse
Paternity possible w testicular sperm aspiration and in vitro
fertilization (Nejm 1998;338:588)

5.4 HYPERLIPIDEMIAS

r/o secondary causes (diabetes, hypothyroidism, hepatic and renal
disease and) first w FBS or Hgb A_1C, TSH, AST (SGOT).
See Table 5.4.1

HYPERCHOLESTEROLEMIA
Ann IM 1990;112:780; Arch IM 1988;148:36

Cause: Polygenic and dietary
Epidem: High prevalence in US decreasing by 10 mg%/10 yr now (Nejm
1991;324:941)
Pathophys: Elevated low-density lipoprotein (LDL) cholesterol increases
risk of atherosclerotic disease, while incr high-density lipoprotein
(HDL) cholesterol reflects lowered risk because is contained in a
transport protein that transports lipids from the periphery to the
liver for excretion. Apolipoprotein E4 allele associated w highest
LDL and CAD risks (Jama 1994;272:1666)
Sx and Si: Often none; arcus senilis, xanthomata in 85% of those w LDL
receptor defects
Crs: Levels >210 mg% at age 22 yr associated w higher ASHD rates at
age 20 yr (5%), age 25 (10%), age 30 (15%), and years later (Nejm
1993;328:313)
Cmplc: Principally ASHD, eg, angina and MIs; peripheral disease as well
r/o familial type II hypercholesterolemia (p 213); and secondary causes
of hypercholesterolemia: myxedema, obstructive liver disease,
porphyria, nephrosis (Nejm 1985;312:1544), dysproteinemias
Lab:
Chem: Lipid profile now usual initial test, rather than just total
cholesterol, for:

Table 5.4.1 Primary Lipoprotein Disorders Amenable to Treatment with Diet and Drug Therapy*

Alternative Novelative Classifications	Disorder	Mechanisms	Complications	Treatment[†]
Type I + V	Familial hypertriglyceridemia[‡]	Decreased serum triglyceride removal resulting from decreased LPL activity Increased hepatic secretion of triglyceride-rich VLDL	Pancreatitis at triglyceride concentrations >2000 mg per deciliter(22.6 mmol/ liter); low risk of CAD	Diet and weight loss Fibrate Nicotinic acid n-3 fatty acids Oxandrolone
Type II + V	Familial combined hyperlipidemia[‡]	Increased hepatic secretion of apolipoprotein B-containing VLDL and conversion to LDL Accumulation of VLDL, LDL, or both, depending on efficiency of their removal	CAD, PVD, stroke	Diet and weight loss Statin Nicotinic acid Fibrate[§]
Type III	Remnant removal disease familial dysbetalipoproteinemia	Increased secretion of VLDL Impaired removal of remnant lipoproteins resulting from homozygosity (ϵ_2/ϵ_3) or heterozygosity (ϵ_2/ϵ_3 or ϵ_2/ϵ_4) for apolipoprotein E ϵ_2	PVD, CAD, stroke	Diet, weight loss Fibrate[§] Nicotinic acid Statin

Table 5.4.1 (continued)

Alternative Nonelative Classifications	Disorder	Mechanisms	Complications	Treatment[†]
Type II	Familial or polygenic hypercholesterolemia	Diminished LDL-receptor activity Defective apalipoprotein B that is poorly recognized by LDL receptor	CAD, occasionally PVD, stroke	Diet Statin Bile-acid–binding resin Nicotinic acid
	Familial hypoalphalioproteinemia (low HDL syndrome)[¶]	Diminished apolipoprotein AI formation, increased removal, increased CETP or hepatic lipase activity	CAD, PVD, (may be associated with hypertriglyceridemia)	Exercise and weight loss Nicotinic acid Fibrate[§] Statin

*LPL denotes lipoprotein lipase, VLDL very-low-density lipoprotein, CAD coronary artery disease, PVD peripheral vascular disease, HDL high-density lipoprotein, and CETP cholesterol-ester transfer protein.

[†]The treatment may be given alone or in combination; the primary treatment is listed first, followed by other treatments in decreasing order of importance.

[‡]Diabetes mellitus can greatly exacerbate the condition. The hyperlipidemia of diabetes is closest mechanistically to familial combined hyperlipidemia.

[§]Combined treatment with a fibrate and a statin can increase the risk of myopathy.

[¶]This disorder is characterized by low concentrations of HDL cholesterol.

Reproduced with permission from Knopp RM. Drug therapy for liquid disorders. Nejm 1999;341:500. Copyright 1999, Mass. Medical Society. All rights reserved.

Total cholesterol (mM/L = mg%/40); fasting unnecessary; falsely decr by acute MI/inflammation

LDL, fasting, = total - HDL - TG/5 if TG <400

HDL, fasting <40 mg% is itself high risk; incr by chromium in brewer's yeast, alcohol ingestion (Ann IM 1992;116:881), weight loss (Jama 1995;247:1915) alone or induced w exercise; decr by uremia, type 2 diabetes, smoking, high carbohydrate diet (>60% of calories), and many drugs like β blockers, anabolic steroids, and progresterones

Rx: PREVENTION SCREENING AND RX (Natl Choles Educ Program [NCEP]—Jama 2001;285:2486). Use diet and exercise first, meds after 3+ mo.

1st, LDL rx of all pts ≥160 mg% (4.1 mM/l)

if >130 mg% (3.4 mM/L), rx pts w 2+ risk factors (smoking, HT, low HDL, Fm h/o ASCVD before age 55 in men or 65 in women, age >45 men or 55 women);

if >100 mg%, rx pts w h/o ASHD, periph artery disease, carotid disease, or AAA, hence secondary prevention; or if 10 yr ASHD risk >20% by Framingham tables (see NCEP charts— Jama 2001;285:2486)

2nd, after above accomplished, rx triglycerides >200 mg% and/or low HDL w nicotinic acid or fibrate

Screening and primary prevention drug rx w pravastatin 40 mg po hs in asx men over age 40 w LDL ≥150 mg % had improved survival, NNT-5 = 40 (Nejm 1995;333:1301); while lovistatin 20–40 mg po qd in pts w avg LDL and total cholesterols but low HDL, men and women up to age 75 decr ASHD events, NNT-5 = 50 (Jama 1998; 279:1615, 1679) but significant limitations (ACP J Club 1998; 129(3):58). Previous increases in violent deaths among men w cholesterol reductions not seen in recent statin primary prophylaxis studies, but decrements in attention and psychomotor speed are induced by dietary or statin cholesterol lowering (Am J Med 2000; 108:538:547)

But appropriateness in women, young and old, has been disputed unless h/o ASCVD (AnnIM 2000;132:769,780,833; 1996;124:518 vs 505; Jama 1995;274:1152); in children who may be harmed by rx (Jama 1995;273:1429,1461 vs Peds 1991;87:943) although statins experimentally used in adolescent boys w heterozygous familial hypercholesterolemia (Jama 1999;282:137); and in elderly, especially women, and in men and women over 70 (Jama 1994;272: 1335,1372; Ann IM 1989;110:622 vs yes for elderly men—Ann IM

1990;113:916); statins and gemfibrozil cause cancer in animals at levels similar to human blood levels (Jama 1996;275:55)

Secondary prevention, is data supported (Nejm 1997;336:332; Ann IM 1996;124:518 vs 505; Jama 1995;274:1152), by decreasing cholesterol in patients w known CAD, eg, Scandinavian simvastatin study of CAD pts showed a 9% absolute risk reduction = NNT-5 = 11 (Lancet 1994;344:1383)

Exercise, at least walk 2 mi qd or run up to 40 mi q wk helps HDL and ASHD risk in men and women (Nejm 1996;334:1298)

Diet: helps decr LDL only if combined w exercise (Nejm 1998;339:12)

Lose weight

Low cholesterol <300 mg qd (Nejm 1993;328:1213)

Polyunsaturated and monounsaturated fats like olive oil (Nejm 1986; 314:745) or canola or soy oil, any of which reduce death in post-MI pts from 5% to 1%/yr (Lancet 1994;343:1454); phyto-estrogens like sitosterol or sitostanol-ester margarine reduce LDL by 10–15% and may improve ASHD (Med Let 1999;41:56; Nejm 1995;333: 1308); stearic and oleic, but not palmitic saturated fats are ok (Nejm 1988;318:1244); but transoleic fatty acids just as bad, so margarine no good (Nejm 1990;323:439); partially hydrogenated (trans) fatty acid worsen LDL (Nejm 1999;340:1933,1994), so liquid oils better than semi liquid, better than soft, better than stick margerines, and because of better total/HDL ratios, butter not as bad as stick margerine

Fish or fish oil pills decrease triglycerides, but elevate LDL (Ann IM 1989;111:900); slows or reverses ASHD progression (Ann IM 1999;130:554), and also help BP (Nejm 1990;322:795)

Oleic and α-linolenic acid in walnuts (Ann IM 2000;132:538; Nejm 1993;328:603)

Soy protein 20–40 gm qd (Nejm 1995;333:276)

Alcoholic drinks 2–4 qd (Nejm 2001;344:549; BMJ 1996;312:731, 736)

Garlic 1/2–1 clove qd (decreases cholesterol by 9%—Ann IM 1993; 119:545) vs no help by double blind RCT (Arch IM 1998;158: 1189; Jama 1998;279:1900)

Soluble fiber (Nejm 1993;329:21) like psyllium (Metamucil) 4.3 gm pkt in water b-tid (5% cholesterol reduction—Ann IM 1993;119:545;

Arch IM 1989;151:1597; 1988;148:292) or oat bran 56 gm qd (Jama 1991;265:1833) or beans 100 gm/d (Med Let 1988;30:111)

Medications (Nejm 1999;341:498; Med Let 2001;43:43): All have a nearly 50% 1-yr cessation rate by pts in practice except HMG CoA reductase drugs (25%) (Nejm 1995;332:1125)

HMG-CoA reductase inhibitors (statins) (Med Let 1998;40:13,117; Rx Let 1998;5:2); po hs (because cholesterol synthesis occurs mostly at night, all may also stabilize plaques, retard thrombosis (Jama 1998;279:1643), and decr vascular inflammation (CRP levels—Jama 2001;286:64); no benefit to prevent restenosis after angioplasty (Nejm 1994;331:1331); and all may slow osteoporosis and fracture rates (Jama 2000;283:3205,3211,3255 vs Jama 2001;285:1850); cmplc: mild asx hepatitis (1–2%), check LFTs q 6–12 mos (Rx Let 1998;5:44); severe myopathy heralded by myalgias and incr CPK, more frequently seen w concomitant grapefruit juice (Rx Let 1999;6:55), verapamil (Rx Let 1998;5:62), erythromycin, ketoconazole, itraconazole, niacin or gemfibrozil use w CYP3A4 metabolized statins (lovistatin, simvastatin, and to a lesser extent, atorvastatin and cerivastatin); all cost $40–60/mo for standard dose

- Atorvastatin (Lipitor) (Med Let 1997;39:29; Jama 1995;275:128) 10–80 mg po qd; lowers choles more than others, also decr TGs by 40%, long half-life, no CNS effect
- Cerivastatin (Baycol) (Med Let 1998;40:13) pulled from market 2001
- Fluvastatin (Lescol) qd (Arch IM 1991;151:43; Nejm 1988;319: 24) 20 (10–40) mg po qd, no CNS effect; $36/mo at 20 mg
- Lovastatin (Mevacor) (primary prevention—Jama 1997;278:313) 20–40 mg po hs
- Pravastatin (Pravachol) 40 mg po hs, worked as primary prevention in Scottish trials (Nejm 1995;333:1301) but cost was $35,000/yr life saved (BMJ 1997;315:1577); no CNS effect
- Simvastatin (Zocor) (primary prevention—Jama 1998;279:1615; 1997;278:313) 10–40, occasionally 80 mg po hs; raises HDL (Rx Let 1999;6:51) and lowers triglycerides as well as atorvastatin (Rx Let 1998;5:44)

Cholesterol binders; all can incr TGs (L. Keilson)

- Cholestyramine 24 gm qd divided (Ann IM 1990;150:1822)

- Coleserelam (Welcho) (Med Let 2000;42:102) 625 mg tabs, 3–6
  po qd or divided; fewer gi side effects and drug interactions, can
  take w statins; $150/mo
- Cholestipol 5–10 gm b-tid (Nejm 1990;323:1290), alone or w
- Psyllium 2.5 gm po tid decr lipids more than cholestipol alone, is
  better tolerated, and costs 1/2 as much (<$500/yr) (Ann IM 1995;
  123:493); or

Nicotinic acid (niacin) 100 mg po hs, or 125 mg bid incr gradually
over 2 mo to 1 gm qid; or slow-release forms like Niaspan up to
2 gm po hs. Raises HDL the most of all the drugs, helps triglycerides
too. Adverse effects: flushing, which is helped by 300 mg ASA half
hour before each dose; aggravation of glucose intolerance;
hepatotoxicity; rhabdomyolysis sometimes when give w statins

Fibrates: gemfibrozil (Lopid) 600 mg bid, similar to clofibrate
(Atromid); decreases triglycerides and raises HDL, can decr
recurrent MIs in pts w LDL <130 but HDL <40 (Jama 2001;285:
1585; Nejm 1999;341:410). Adverse effects: gallstones (Am J Med
2000;108:418), rhabdomyolysis when give w statins

Fenofibrate (Tricor) (Med Let 1998;40:68; Rx Let 1998;5:28)
67–220 mg po qd, similar to gemfibrozil, used especially for
triglyceride elevations; can also cause rhabdomyolysis w statins

Estrogen/progestin replacement rx in post menopausal women, nearly
as effective as statin rx in lowering lipid levels (Nejm 1997;337:595)
though controversial (p 624)

TYPE I HYPERLIPIDEMIA

Nejm 1985;312:1300

Cause: Genetic or diabetics, autosomal recessive (Nejm 1991;324:1761)

Epidem: Rare except in Quebec French Canadians 1/40 of whom have the
gene; overall the gene prevalence is 1/500 (Nejm 1991;324:1761)

Pathophys: Lipoprotein lipase deficiency causes an increase in chylomicrons, not lysed by heparin (PHLA)

Sx: Recurrent abdominal pain (old surgical scars); early life onset (months
old to age 10 yr)

Si: Lipemia retinalis (picture—Nejm 1999;340:1969); hepatospleno-megaly; eruptive xanthomata (pimple-like correlate w chylomicrons)

Crs: Complete reversal w rx

Cmplc: Pancreatitis; possibly ASHD (Nejm 1996;335:848)

Lab:

> *Chem:* Cholesterol may be incr; total cholesterol/HDL ratio <4.5. TG >1000 mg%, often >1500 mg%; supranate milky; infranate clear; post heparin lipolytic activity low

Rx: Diet, low fat (<20% of calories); stop alcohol; avoid estrogens and cholesterol binders, which worsen (L. Keilson 5/97)

> Gemfibrozil or clofibrate, or niacin if sx

TYPE II HYPERLIPIDEMIA (Familial Hypercholesterolemia)

Nejm 1985;312:1300

Cause: Genetic, autosomal dominant

Epidem: Common, 1/200 prevalence

Pathophys: Decreased LDL receptors cause incr LDL and sometimes VLDL (Nejm 1986;314:879; 1984;311:1658); or, more rarely due to mutations in apolipoprotein B gene, which impairs receptor binding (Nejm 1998;338:1577). Apolipoproteins of LDL and HDL correlate better w familial risk than the cholesterol levels in each component (Nejm 1990;322:1494; 1986;315:721). Uremia and β blockers decrease HDL

Sx:

Si: Arcus senilis, tendinous xanthomata (80% over age 20 yr have them), tuberous xanthomata in homozygotes, xanthelasmas (only 50% in a general population are associated w type II disease, ie, 50% specif)

Crs: Malignant; MIs in pts age 30–40 yr, even in teens in homozygotes

Cmplc: Increased ASHD with MIs

> r/o secondary causes of hypercholesterolemia (p 206)

Lab: *Chem:* Cholesterol very high, w high LDL; TG normal in IIa, slightly elevated in IIb; supranate and infranate clear in both, PHLA normal in both.

Rx: Standard rx of hypercholesterolemia (p 209), statins + resins more effective than either alone

> Liver transplant in severe familial (Ann IM 1988;108:204)

TYPE III HYPERLIPIDEMIA
Nejm 1985;312:1300; Ann IM 1983;98:622

Cause: Genetic, autosomal dominant (Ann IM 1975;82:141)

Epidem: 1/500 (Castelli, 1983); adults only; males > females (estrogen protects—Ann IM 1977;87:517); associated w obesity, diabetes, gout

Pathophys: Abnormal apolipoprotein E 2/2 homozygote, dysfunctional β-lipoprotein causes an increase in VLDL remnants and chylomicrons plus other undefined factors, possibly obesity and diabetes

Sx: Xanthomas and xantholasmata

Si: Tuberoeruptive and palmar xanthomata (75%); xanthelasmas (25%) (r/o diabetes, type II hyperlipidemia, and normal variant)

Crs: Poor, questionably helped by rx

Cmplc: ASHD with MIs

Lab:

Chem: Cholesterol may be incr or normal; total cholesterol/HDL ratio <4.5; TG 400–1000 mg%; supranate milky; infranate cloudy; lipoprotein electrophoresis shows broad β slur; apolipoprotein E 2/2; PHLA normal

Uric acid elevated (40%)

GTT abnormal (55%)

Rx: Diet to lose weight, stop alcohol, decrease intake to <300 mg cholesterol qd and fat <30% of calories

Nicotinic acid 2–3 gm qd works but more side effects than diet alone; or as 2nd choices, clofibrate 2 gm qd (works by increasing cholesterol in bile, hence can cause gallstones) or gemfibrozil (Med Let 1982;24:59)

TYPE IV HYPERLIPIDEMIA
Nejm 1985;312:1300

Cause: Genetic, autosomal dominant; or alcohol

Epidem: Associated w diabetes (70%), obesity, hyperuricemia; very common, 50% of patients age <45 yr w ASHD at UCLA had it (Ann IM 1968;69:21)

Pathophys: Elevated VLDL; carbohydrate-induced, causes liver to overproduce TG

Sx: None until MI

Si: None until MI

Crs:

Cmplc: MIs

> r/o other causes of increased TG, including drugs (thiazides, BCPs, estrogens, β blockers, isotretinoin), burns and trauma, sepsis, SLE, MIs, glycogen storage diseases, obesity, alcohol

Lab:

> *Chem:* Cholesterol incr or normal; total cholesterol/HDL ratio incr; TG 150–1000 mg%; supranate clear; infranate cloudy; PHLA normal; lipoPEP shows incr pre-β-lipoprotein
> Uric acid increased
> GTT abnormal (70%)

Rx: Lose weight; rx diabetes; avoid alcohol, estrogens; diet of cholesterol <300 mg qd; exercise

> Nicotinic acid (niacin) (p 209)

TYPE V HYPERLIPIDEMIA

Nejm 1985;312:1300

Cause: Genetic, autosomal dominant

Epidem: Associated w diabetes, hyperuricemia, alcohol use; rare

Pathophys: Elevated chylomicrons and VLDL; a combination of types I and IV characteristics; fat- and carbohydrate-induced, ie, a type IV w a relative lipoprotein lipase deficiency from incr VLDL synthesis by the liver so that dietary TG more easily overwhelms it

Sx: "Pimples," recurrent abdominal pain

Si: Hepatosplenomegaly, lipemia retinalis (picture—Nejm 1999;340: 1969), eruptive xanthomata

Crs:

Cmplc: Pancreatitis, no MIs (debatably—Nejm 1996;335:848)

> r/o other causes of elevated triglyceride including drugs (poor diabetic control, thiazides, BCPs, estrogens, β blockers, isotretinoin), burns and trauma, sepsis, SLE, MIs, glycogen storage diseases, obesity, alcohol

Lab:

> *Chem:* Cholesterol elevated; total cholesterol/HDL ratio incr; TGs 1000+ mg%; supranate milky; infranate cloudy; PHLA low

Uric acid increased
GTT abnormal (70%)

Rx: Avoid estrogens and cholesterol binders, which increase TGs
(L. Keilson 5/97)

Decrease dietary fat to <20% of calories; no alcohol, lose weight

Gemfibrozil, niacin, or clofibrate if pancreatitis or xanthomata

5.5 PARATHYROID/CALCIUM/MAGNESIUM DISORDERS

HYPERPARATHYROIDISM

Nejm 2000;343:1863; 1999;341:1249; 1980;302:189; Ann IM 1973;79:566

Cause:

- Parathyroid adenoma (90%); vast majority are single, 4% double
- Carcinoma (4%) of parathyroids (Nejm 1983;309:325)
- Secondary: renal failure w autonomous PTH from hypertrophied gland

Epidem: Most commonly sporadic nonfamilial; prevalence now dropping, unclear why (Ann IM 1997;126:433)

Sometimes associated w multiple endocrine neoplasia (MEN) syndrome (Nejm 1990;322:723)

MEN type I: (95% have elevated PTH—Nejm 1986;314:1287) Hyperparathyroidism; adenomas of pituitary (30%), often prolactin-producing; pancreatic adenomas, especially gastrinomas (causing ZE syndrome) or insulin-producing ones (37%). Autosomal dominant from loss of suppressor gene on chromosome #11 (Nejm 1989;321:218)

MEN type II: Hyperparathyroidism, pheochromocytomas, and medullary carcinoma of thyroid

Pathophys: PTH is stimulated by low calcium; increases renal calcitrol (activated, 1,25-OH vit D) production (Ann IM 1994;121:633), which in turn increases gi calcium absorption, osteoclastic activity, and renal tubule calcium resorption and PO_4 loss. Relative imbalance of latter can cause stones (Nejm 1980;302:421)

Sx: Of hypercalcemia (p 219)

Si: Of hypercalcemia, esp fatigue and muscular weakness (Ann IM 1975; 82:474); palpable neck tumor occasionally

Crs: Carcinoma is invariably fatal

Cmplc: Renal stones in 20% of patients w elevated PTH, 5% of patients w stones have elevated PTH; and eventually some renal failure

Osteoporosis, esp of distal cortical bone (Colles fx's), or even von Recklinghausen's syndrome w generalized decalcification and fractures, brown tumors and bone cysts, and renal stones

r/o hypocalciuric hypercalcemia (p 219), which is not helped by parathyroidectomy

Lab:

Chem: Serum Ca^{2+} >10.5 mg%, 30% false neg. PTH/Ca ratios (Ann IM 1979;91:782). Urinary Ca^{2+} >250 mg/24h (females), >300 mg/24 h (males); 10% false pos, 30% false neg

Xray: Hands occasionally show punched-out lesions in phalanges, subperiosteal bone resorption distally w unique lacy appearance; dental films may show erosion of lamina dura, but many false pos and neg; clavicle may have distal end resorption

Scan w technetium/sestamibi can distinguish adenoma from hyperplasia (J Nuc Med 1992;33:1801; Arch Surg 1996;131:1074)

Rx: Surgical excision, even if asx (Nejm 1999;341:1249,1301), esp if young, osteoporosis, high serum calcium levels >12 mg%), and/or renal stones; less urgent if asx since no increase in vertebral fractures (Ann IM 1991;114:593; 1988;109:959); 5% of population have mediastinal and/or paraesophageal parathyroids

Estrogen replacement in postmenopausal female w mild disease (Ann IM 1996;125:360; Nejm 1986;314:508,1481) (p 624)

Calcium receptor agonist (R-568) in the future?

of hyperCa (p 219)

HYPOPARATHYROIDISM

Nejm 2000;343:1863

Cause: (D. Spratt 3/92)
- Postthyroidectomy
- Acquired: renal failure, hypomagnesemia, alcoholism (by hypo-magnesemia or direct suppression of PTH—Nejm 1991;324:721)

Hypoparathyroidism, continued

- Familial types from genetic hormone defects
- **Autoimmune polyendocrinopathy candidiasis/ectodermal dystrophy** (Nejm 1990;322:1829); 80% are hypoparathyroid, 70% are hypoadrenal, 60% of women and 15% of men with it are hypogonadal; by age 20, 100% have had significant candidal infections

Epidem: Associated w Addison's, PA, Hashimoto's, diGeorge syndrome (3rd and 4th pharyngeal pouches)

Pathophys: PTH necessary for osteoclastic response to low calcium, renal tubular calcium resorption and PO_4 excretion, and vit D activation
Alkalosis due to blocked PTH stimulation of organic acid production in bones (Ann IM 1972;76:825); monilia infections due to suppressor T-cell defects (Nejm 1979;300:164)

Sx: Of hypocalcemia: circumoral paresthesias, carpal-pedal spasms, stridor, seizures (brief, mild), bronchospasm, gi cramps, anxiety, cataracts

Si: Of hypocalcemia: tetany (carpal-pedal spasm, Chvostek's si and Trousseau's si); cataracts, vascular corneal opacities (band keratopathy), psychiatric changes, dystonias, and dyskinesias (Nejm 1972;286:762)

Crs:

Cmplc: Pustular psoriasis and dermatitis herpetiformis (Ann IM 1984; 100:677)

r/o: **Pseudohypoparathyroidism** which is genetic, sex-linked vs dominant; associated w hypopituitarism, especially types w low TSH and gi lactase deficiency; end-organ (bone and kidney) defect in cyclic AMP protein receptor for PTH as well as other hormones, eg, TSH (Ann IM 1986;105:197); si of hypercalcemia and mental retardation, short stature and phalanges; hypoplastic carious teeth; dx w Ellsworth-Howard test: iv PTH causes no increase in phosphate excretion (<25 mg/h) and/or no increase in cAMP excretion (Ann IM 1988;109:800)

Familial hypercalciuric hypocalcemia from defective calcium sensing receptor (Nejm 1996;335:1115)

Lab:

Chem: Hypocalcemia, r/o hypoalbuminemia (p 829 for correction formulas), lung cancer or its rx, leukemia, ricketts/osteomalacia, thyrocalcitonin-producing medullary carcinoma of the thyroid?, pancreatitis

Serum PO_4 elevated; metabolic alkalosis

Urine: Hypocalciuria

Xray: Skull films may show basal ganglia calcification (Nejm 1971; 285:72)

Rx: (D. Spratt 3/92)

1st: Vitamin D_3 50,000–100,000$^+$ U qd; or 1,25-$(OH)_2$ vitamin D (Rocaltrol), expensive; narrow margins of safety for hypercalcemia

2nd: Calcium po

3rd: Chlorthalidone 50 mg po qd or other thiazide, w low-salt diet, avoids renal stones of vit D rx (Nejm 1978;298:577)

Experimental: synthetic PTH, cmplc may be substantial (Jama 1996; 276:631)

HYPERCALCEMIA
Nejm 1992;326:1196

Cause/Epidem/Pathophys:

- Hyperparathyroidism (p 216) via renal calcitriol (activated vit D) production (Ann IM 1994;121:633,709)
- Cancers, especially lung, breast, and hepatoma (Nejm 1992;327: 1663), by:
  - PTH-like protein secretions, w T-cell leukemias/lymphomas (Nejm 1990;322:1106; Ann IM 1989;111:484)
  - Secretion of other bone-resorbing substances
  - Tumor conversion of 25-OH vitamin D to 1,25-OH vitamin D (calcitriol)
  - Local osteolytic mets
- Sarcoid, Hodgkin's lymphoma, non-Hodgkin's lymphoma, cat scratch disease (Jama 1998;279:532), and tbc, via extrarenal calcitriol (activated vit D) production in granulomas (Ann IM 1994;121:633,709)
- Vitamin D intoxication (Nejm 1992;326:1173) including the milk-alkali syndrome (Ann IM 1982;97:242)
- Immobilization
- Thyrotoxicosis
- Thiazides rarely (Nejm 1971;284:828)

- Vitamin A intoxication (Ann IM 1974;80:44)
- Disseminated coccidioidomycosis (Nejm 1977;297:431)
- Benign familial hypocalciuric hypercalcemia (autosomal dominant) (Ann IM 1985;102:511; Nejm 1980;303:810)
- Adrenal insufficiency

Sx: Fatigue, weakness, sleepiness, nausea/anorexia, constipation, polyuria/dypsia, and volume depletion

Si: Confusion, delirium, drowsiness, coma

Crs:

Cmplc: Pancreatitis, incr risk of digoxin toxicity

Lab:

Chem: Calcium elevated (p 829 for corrections for low proteins) ≥10.5 mg%; sx usually between 11–12 mg%, really toxic over 14 mg%

Noninv: EKG, Short QT interval w normal T wave, segment from QRS to beginning of T shortened

Xray:

Rx: Acute rx for Ca^{2+} >13 mg%, to decrease within hours:

- Normal saline 2.5–4 L/24 h iv to assure intravascular volume adequately replaced (CVP or Swann monitoring), avoid furosemide (Nejm 1984;310:1718) initially, but often needed after volume replaced to prevent volume overload and accelerate renal calcium clearance
- Pamidronate (Aredia) 60–90 mg iv over 24 h (Med Let 1992; 34:1), or 4–8 mg/hr

Chronic rx, work over 1–5 d, worth doing even w metastatic cancer since diminishes sx and allows hospital discharge (Ann IM 1990; 112:499):

- Bisphosphonates, eg, pamidronate (Aredia) 60–90 mg iv infusion over 8–24 h (Med Let 1992;34:1) or 1200 mg po qd × 5 d
- Steroids (Ann IM 1980;93:449) primarily for sarcoid pts, eg, prednisone 20 mg po tid (Ann IM 1980;93:269) or iv × 3–4 d
- Calcitonin 4 U/kg q 6 h sc or im, relatively weak agent alone
- Indomethacin (rarely helpful if due to cancer)
- Gallium nitrate iv infusion, experimental (Med Let 1991;33:41; Ann IM 1988;108:669) 200 mg/M^2 in 1 L continuous infusion qd × 5 d

HYPOMAGNESEMIA

Nejm 1968;278:772

Cause: GI fluid and electrolyte loss rx'd w Mg-free fluids; malnutrition; fistulae; burns; diuretics; cisplatinum-induced renal disease (Ann IM 1981;95:628)

Epidem: Associated w large gi fluid losses and malnutrition, eg, w ulcerative colitis, regional enteritis, chronic alcoholism, toxemia of pregnancy, primary hypo-/hyperparathyroidism, primary hyperaldosteronism, thyrotoxicosis, RTA, diuretic phase of ATN

Pathophys: Low Mg inhibits PTH secretion, which in turn causes hypocalcemic si and sx (Nejm 1970;282:61). Alcohol inhibits PTH secretion, thus also contributing (Nejm 1991;324:721)

Sx: Cramps

Si: Carpopedal spasm, Chvostek's si, Trousseau's si, delirium, muscle tremor and bizarre movements, convulsions, hypotension

Crs: Ataxias take months to clear

Cmplc: Hypocalcemia; hypo K^+ in cisplatinum type (Ann IM 1981; 95:328)

Lab:

Chem: Mg^{2+} <1.6 mEq/L. Alkaline phosphatase low

Noninv: EKG shows low-voltage and T-wave abnormalities

Rx: 40–80 mEq $MgSO_4$ (10 cc of a 50% hydrated soln) iv in 1 L D5S or D5W over 3 h

HYPERMAGNESEMIA

Nejm 1968;278:772

Cause: Renal failure, often parallels K^+ (Nejm 1969;280:981). Chronic Mg containing antacid and laxative use. Enemas, especially in megacolon, w Mg-containing soaps

Epidem: Less common than hypomagnesemia

Pathophys: Avg qd intake = 20–40 mEq; total body stores = 2000 mEq, half in bones, rest intracellular

Sx: Difficult defecation, urination; nausea; drowsiness at pharmacologic doses only

Si: Depressed DTRs, hypotension (Ann IM 1975;83:657)

Crs:

Cmplc: Heart block, respiratory paralysis

Lab:
  Chem: Mg^{2+} >2.2 mEq/L
  Noninv: EKG shows heart block
Rx: Calcium gluconate 5–10 mEq (10–20 cc of 10% soln iv)

5.6 PITUITARY DISORDERS

GALACTORRHEA/AMENORRHEA SYNDROME
  Nejm 1991;324:1555; 1985;312:1364; Ann IM 1986;105:238

Cause: Abnormal prolongation or initiation of prolactin production
  1/3 are true primary hyperprolactinemia, over half of these are due to
    micro-/macroadenomas and empty sella syndrome (Ann IM 1986;
    105:238); the rest are idiopathic, including Argonz-Del Castillo
    syndrome (spontaneous), and postpregnancy (Chiari-Frommel
    syndrome)
  2/3 are secondary types, from hypothyroidism; renal failure; cirrhosis;
    hypothalamic disease; and medications like reserpine, pheno-
    thiazines, verapamil (Ann IM 1981;95:66), metoclopramide (Ann
    IM 1983;98:86), and cimetidine (Nejm 1982;306:26)
Epidem:
Pathophys: Hypothyroidism causes the syndrome because TRH itself
    causes prolactin release. Prolactin inhibits LH secretion and peak
    thereby inhibiting menses
Sx: Amenorrhea (90%); may be masked by bcp use, and therefore present
    only as galactorrhea
  Galactorrhea or elicitable lactation
  In males, complaints of impotence and decr libido (Nejm 1978;299:
    847); presentation is later, so have higher incidence of
    hypopituitarism and visual field losses (Ann IM 1986;105:238)
Si: Galactorrhea, ie, any amount of milky substance expressible, no
    correlation of amount w prolactin level or tumor size
Crs: Usually benign, especially the idiopathic or microadenoma types
    (Ann IM 1984;100:115), although skeletal and cardiovascular
    consequences of hypogonadism, if present, must be considered

Cmplc: Panhypopituitarism

Visual field cuts w macroadenoma (>1 cm) especially during pregnancy, rare w microadenomas (Ann IM 1994;121:473)

Osteoporosis due to low estrogen levels (Nejm 1980;303:1511), reversible w rx (Nejm 1986;315:542)

ASHD from hypogonadism (estrogen lack)

Lab:

Chem: Prolactin >100 ngm/cc is likely adenoma, returns to normal w rx

Path: Prolactin-staining microadenoma, but 27% of normals in autopsy series also have? (Nejm 1981;304:156)

Xray: MRI (Nejm 1991;324:1555), but 10% false pos in general population (Ann IM 1994;120:817); CT, 15–20% false pos (D. Federman 3/85)

Rx: Pregnancy and nursing risks are small w idiopathic or microadenomas

Medical rx w dopamine agonists like:

Bromocriptine (Parlodel) 1.25–20 mg po qd divided, eg, 1.25–2.5 mg po hs with snack × 3–7 d, then 2.5 bid incr to tid gradually; try for higher doses until prolactin level is suppressed to decrease tumor size (Nejm 1985;313:656) in about 1/2. Adverse effects: hypotension, cost, nausea, peptic ulcer disease, headache, dizziness, Raynaud's at high doses

Cabergoline (Dostinex) 0.25–1 mg po biw, better tolerated and twice as effective, 83% become normoprolactinemic vs 59% w bromocriptine (Nejm 1994;331:904)

Surgical transsphenoidal resection if fail medical rx; 60–80% success at 1 yr if <10 mm diameter, 25–40% success if >10 mm; >50% recur over 2–5 yr (Nejm 1983;309:280)

GROWTH HORMONE DEFICIENCY

Cause: Idiopathic or associated w other pituitary lesions; genetic, autosomal recessive

Epidem: Dwarfism is associated w other pituitary defects 50% of the time

Pathophys: Growth hormone is responsible for growth stimulation and lipid mobilization/protein sparing. In pygmies and some genetic dwarfs (Nejm 1971;284:809), defect is in end-organ responsiveness from growth hormone receptor deficiency (Nejm 1990;323:1367)

Insulin-like growth factor mediates these effects and alone is responsible for most prenatal growth (Nejm 1996;335:1363)

Sx: Dwarfism in children: height impairment is often greater than weight impairment, ie, "pudgy" kids; 50% are <3d percentile at 1 yr

Si: In children, short stature, decr growth velocity, delayed bone age in adults, osteoporosis, hyperlipidemia, diminished muscle strength and vitality

Crs:

Cmplc: Hypoglycemia often, especially if ACTH deficiency too r/o growth hormone receptor insensitivity due to mutation, partial or complete (Laron dwarfism) (Nejm 1995;333:1093)

Lab:

Chem: Hypoglycemia, especially if there are combined HGH and ACTH deficiencies present (Nejm 1968;278:57)

HGH (IGF-1) levels low for age, or fails to elevate w stimulation tests (insulin, clonidine, arginine, L-dopa, glucagon) (Nejm 1988; 319:201)

Xray: Bone age is younger than chronologic age

Rx: (Nejm 1999;341:1206)

Replace HGH w recombinant HGH 0.3 mg/kg/wk im divided into qd doses, $20,000/yr, or less effective but cheaper GHRH; not for use in short children who are not GH deficient, Turner's syndrome, or chronic renal failure; $5000+/yr (Med Let 1999;41:2) but is being so used (Nejm 1999;340:502, 557). Adults may also be helped by replacement (Ann IM 1996;125:883; Nejm 1989;321:1797) w 6–25 μgm/kg. Adverse effects: edema, arthralgias; experimentally reverses some somatic aspects of aging in normal patients age >60 yr (Nejm 1990;323:1), but functional capacities are not improved (Ann IM 1996;124:708); may help some ICU pts (burns, trauma) but worsens others (Nejm 1999;341;785, 837)

PANHYPOPITUITARISM

Nejm 1994;330:1651

Cause:

- Neoplasms: polyendocrine adenomas including FSH-, LH-, and/or TSH-producing ones, which rarely secrete intact hormone (Nejm 1991;324:822), unlike (Nejm 1980;302:210) ACTH-, HGH-, and prolactin-producing ones (p 222); craniopharyngiomas; metastases especially from lung; neurofibromas
- Trauma
- Granulomas: Hans-Christian disease, sarcoid (often causes only prolactinemia) (Ann IM 1972;76:545), tuberculosis
- Vascular: carotid aneurysm, postpartum infarction (Sheehan's syndrome), diabetic vascular disease, prepartum in diabetics (Ann IM 1971;74:357)
- Late cmplc of extracranial head and neck tumor (Ann IM 1975; 83:771) or brain (Nejm 1993;328:87) irradiation
- Autoimmune (Ann IM 1981;95:166)
- Congenital

Epidem:

Pathophys: Order of most frequent hormonal defects w pituitary tumor: growth hormone > gonadotropins > TSH > ACTH. Prolactin may be autonomously produced by some pituitary tumors that cause hypopituitarism

Sx: Hypogonadism w amenorrhea w or w/o lactation; hypothyroidism; adrenal insufficiency; headaches; bitemporal visual field losses

Si: Findings of above

Crs:

Cmplc: r/o **"empty sella syndrome"** (Ann IM 1986;105:238), an incidental pickup of an enlarged sella on skull xray, usually but not always w normal pituitary function; **hypothalamic dysfunction,** seen w weight loss especially in anorexia nervosa

Lab:

Chem: Serum levels of HGH, T_3T_4, TSH after TRH, testosterone or estradiol, LH, FSH, ACTH, and cortisol all low

Hem: Anemia (Nejm 1971;284:479)

Xray: MRI, or CT if MRI not available, shows pituitary mass; w calcification in craniopharyngioma; plain skull films no longer done

Rx: Nejm 1991;324:1555

Replacement hormones: L-thyroxine, glucocorticoids, testosterone/ estrogen, and recombinant growth hormone (Nejm 1989;321: 1797), at least in children and perhaps in adults to preserve bone density (Ann IM 1996;883:932)

Surgical resection via transsphenoidal approach for documented adenomas; cmplc: diabetes insipidus

Bromocriptine (Pergolide) (Nejm 1983;309:704; Ann IM 1982;96:281) for prolactinoma

Radiation in some cases after surgery if residual tumor on MRI of galactorrhea/amenorrhea prolactinomas (p 222)

5.7 THYROID DISEASES

HYPOTHYROIDISM/MYXEDEMA/CRETINISM

Clin Ger Med 1995;11:252; Jama 1995;273:808

Cause:

- Immune: thyroid failure from atrophic or goitrous autoimmune (Hashimoto's) thyroiditis; transient TSH-inhibiting IgG in mother causing cretin children (Nejm 1980;303:739) or nonstimulating TSH receptor-binding IgG antibody (cf Graves'—Ann IM 1985; 103:26), these thyrotropin (TSH)-blocking antibodies often present in both atrophic and goitrous (Hashimoto's) types (Nejm 1992;326:513)
- Surgical excision
- Radiation: to neck for tumor, lymphoma, etc. (Nejm 1991;325: 599); or most commonly I^{131} rx (Ann IM 1972;76:721) of hyperthyroidism
- Dietary I_2 deficiency, eg, cretinism in Ecuador (Nejm 1969;280: 296) and China (Nejm 1994;331:1739), or in some patients w possibly underlying subclinical disease; excess iodine can precipitate hypothyroidism, eg, patients, or newborns of mothers on SSKI expectorants (Med Let 1970;12:61; Nejm 1969;281:816)
- Lithium rx acts like I_2 load, causes goiter in 10%, hypothyroidism in 1%

- Rarely secondary hypothryoidism from pituitary or hypothalamic failure, eg, post-brain irradiation (Nejm 1993;328:87)

Epidem: Associated w pernicious anemia and insulin-dependent diabetes through association of those w autoimmune Hashimoto's; phenytoin (Dilantin) and carbamazepine (Tegretol) may precipitate (Ann IM 1983;99:341)

Pathophys: Goiter, caused by edema lymphatic infiltration and hypertrophy

Sx: Hair loss, and coarseness; coarse skin; fatigue; swollen tongue w slurred speech; nonpitting edema; menorrhagia; feel cold; lactation from TRH stimulation of prolactin (Ann IM 1976;84:534); constipation; muscle cramps; mental dullness. Worsened or precipitated by smoking since that impairs thyroid hormone secretion and peripheral effect (Nejm 1995;333:969)

Si: Goiter; dry skin; hung-up reflexes (r/o hypothermia, β blockers, pregnancy, procainamide); diminished PMI from pericardial effusion (Nejm 1977;296:1); arthritis w synovial thickening and noninflammatory effusions (Nejm 1970;282:1172)

Crs: Very slowly progressive; insidious; 25% of atrophic type may revert (Nejm 1992;326:513)

Cmplc: Anemias from folate deficiency in 20%, hypoproliferative, Fe-deficient (Ann IM 1968;68:792); bleeding from diminished platelet stickiness (Ann IM 1974;82:342); cerebellar sx (30%); peripheral neuropathies (25%); coma, confusion, psychoses, seizures; hypothermia; hypoventilation, sleep apnea (Ann IM 1984;101:491); ASHD due to lipid as well as homocysteine elevations (Ann IM 2000;132:270; 1999;131:348)

  r/o **"euthyroid-sick syndrome"**: low T_3T_4, with normal or low TSH in presence of other severe illness (Nejm 1985;312:546); no specific rx required

Lab:

  Chem: TSH elevated in primary hypothyroidism, the earliest test to become abnormal, may be worth using as a screening test in the elderly (Ann IM 1990;112:840); if on thyroid and indications in doubt, may stop and check TSH, T_4 at 5 wk. Total T_3, free T_4, resin T_3 uptake (a measure of thyroid-binding globulins) all low. In secondary myxedema, TSH stimulation by TRH administration may be slow to respond w delayed peak (Nejm 1985;312:1085)

Cholesterol elevated >250 mg% in secondary not in primary types ("rapid TSH"); triglycerides elevated

CPK (MM) and liver enzymes often elevated

Xray: Chest may show incr heart size (pericardial effusion)

Rx: L-Thyroxine (Synthroid, Levoxyl, or generic, all the same—Jama 1997;277:1205) (Nejm 1994;331:174) 0.1–0.2 mg (100–200 μgm) qd po; 0.1 adequate for 2/3 of pts, 0.125 plenty for most (1.7 μgm/kg) (Ann IM 1986;105:11); monitor sensitive TSH (Ann IM 1990; 113:450) to keep ≥0.5 mIU/cc so hip fx risk minimized (Ann IM 2001;134:560). Some evidence that use of T_3 10–20 μgm qd w T_4 replacement may improve mood (Nejm 1999;340:424). Beware of concomitant rx w $FeSO_4$, which impairs absorption (Ann IM 1992;117:1010), as do calcium pills like Tums or Os-Cal (Jama 2000;283:2822), phenytoin (Dilantin), carbamazepine (Tegretol), rifampin, cholestyramine, sucralfate, and aluminum hydroxide antacids

in coma/confusion: 100–500 μgm iv/po qd, usually w concomitant stress steroid doses in case also hypoadrenal

in elderly, go very slowly, eg, 1/4 or less these doses, and work up slowly because normal T_3 half-life is several days and may be longer in the elderly, and T_4 half-life is nearly twice that of T_3

in pregnancy, dose requirements may increase, monitor with TSH (Nejm 1990;323:91)

in developing countries, I_2 in oil annually to all w euthyroid goiter? (Nejm 1992;326:236) and/or to pregnant women and babies in areas of endemic cretinism (Nejm 1986;315:791)

HYPERTHYROIDISM, THYROTOXICOSIS, AND STIMULATING AUTOIMMUNE THYROIDITIS (Graves' Disease)

Nejm 2000;343:1236; Jama 1995;273:808

Cause: Autoimmune stimulating antibody production, occasionally from *Yersinia enterocolitica* infection inducing cross-reacting antibodies (Ann IM 1976;85:735); or exogenous T_3T_4 ingestion; or thyroiditis (p 232); or hot nodule (p 234); or rarely, TSH-producing chorio- or testicular carcinomas, molar pregnancy (Ann IM 1975;83:307), or ovarian cancers, especially struma ovarii w ascites (Ann IM 1970; 72:883), and rare pituitary microadenoma (Ann IM 1989;111:827; Nejm 1987;317:12); organic iodine induction possible in any goiter patient (Nejm 1971;285:523), as is lithium or anti-retroviral therapy

Epidem: Graves'-associated positive family hx or at least often abnormal suppression tests in family members; pernicious anemia; mitral valve prolapse (Nejm 1981;305:497). Female:male = 4–6:1

Pathophys: In Graves', IgG thyroid-stimulating immunoglobin (TSI) antibody to TSH receptor (Ann IM 1978;88:379); ophthalmoplegia from immune-mediated periorbital inflammation, and ocular myopathy (Nejm 1993;329:1468)

Toxic si's and sx's from catechol facilitation, eg, lid lag from incr sympathetic tone, and/or primary uncoupling of oxidative phosphorylation w incr numbers of mitochondria (Nejm 1967; 276:110). Gynecomastia from incr estradiol (Nejm 1972;286:124)

Sx:

Thyrotoxic: palpitations; weight loss; amenorrhea; hyperactivity; hot, sweaty, smooth skin; prominent essential tremor; decr libido; frequent often diarrheal stools from steatorrhea, polyphagia of fat, and decr gi transit time (Ann IM 1973;78:669)

In Graves': above, plus goiter; diplopia and eye protrusion (proptosis); vitiligo, especially of extremities, often precedes toxicosis by years (Ann IM 1969;71:935)

Si:

Thyrotoxic: P >100 resting; "adrenergic stare," and lid lag; weight loss; apathetic depression, especially in elderly (Ann IM 1970; 72:679)

In Graves': above, plus ophthalmoplegias, especially convergence failure; exophthalmus, cornea >18 mm from lateral orbital rim, can be unilateral; goiter (97%) diffuse, firm (Ann IM 1968;69:1022); gynecomastia in men frequently; pretibial myxedema and localized dermopathy; onycholysis (nail separation); Plummer's nails (serrated) and clubbing; incr pigmentation (incr ACTH turnover); lymphadenopathy (10%)

Crs: Graves' is cyclic, worse in winter (daylight effects?); usually better in pregnancy from natural immune suppression (Nejm 1985;313:562)

Cmplc: Thyroid storm, especially w surgery or infection (Nejm 1974;291: 1396); cardiac (Nejm 1992;327:94) including myocarditis and CHF

(Nejm 1982;307:1165), atrial fibrillation, and angina precipitation; myopathies, plain, and hypokalemic (in Asians—Ann IM 1974;81: 332), myasthenia syndromes; osteoporosis (Ann IM 2001;134:560; 1999;130:750; 1994;120:8) incr 3× if TSH <0.1, reversible w rx ; newborn thyrotoxicosis from TSI at age 7–10 d when mother has been on suppressive medications prepartum, and fetal thyrotoxicosis in mothers w ablated thyroids (Nejm 1985;313:562)

Thoracic inlet obstruction w positive Pemberton si (p 234)

Lab:

Chem: Total T_4, free T_4, serum thyroglobulin (rules out surreptitious ingestion) all incr; sensitive TSH low (BMJ 1984;289:1334); TRH stimulation test w 250 μgm iv, draw TSH at 0 and 30 min, shows no rise, often the only abnormal test, especially in elderly w Afib

Alkaline phosphatase (bony) elevated in 50^+% Graves' pts (Ann IM 1979;90:164), parallels thyroid function if no liver disease. Calcium may be incr (in 10–25%) though PTH normal (Ann IM 1976;84: 668; Nejm 1976;294:431)

Hem: Atypical lymphs and lymphocytosis

Xray: RAIU elevated and useful to distinguish from I_2-induced and subacute thyroiditis types; usually not necessary, thyroid [131]I , ^{123}I, or technetium scan shows diffusely enhanced uptake

Rx: (Nejm 1994;330:1731; Ann IM 1994;121:281)

Propranolol 2–10 mg iv, or 20–80 mg po, or atenolol (Tenormin) 50–100 mg po qd to control sx; may not fully prevent storm (Nejm 1977;296:263); also will decrease hypercalcemia if symptomatic (Nejm 1976;294:431)

Antithyroid meds (Nejm 1984;311:1353): propylthiouracil (PTU) <100–200 mg po tid, or methimazole (Tapezole) 5–20 mg po qd; block organification of iodine to $T_3 T_4$ and autoantibody production by lymphocytes within the gland (Nejm 1987;316:15), rx × 6 mo, then immed start replacement; PTU may be preferred in pregnancy and during lactation; 40–50% failure rates, higher if high po iodine intake not controlled (Ann IM 1987;107:510; Nejm 1984;311:426). Adverse effects of both: rash, toxic hepatitis, and agranulocytosis (0.3%) though no point in screening CBCs

[131]I rx may be first choice under β-blocker protection, or used if fail 1 or more PTU courses; use w prednisone 0.5 mg/kg po qd × 1 mo,

then 2 mo taper to prevent transient worsening of opthalmopathy Nem 1998;338:73); β blockade may help sx and won't interfere w ^{131}I uptake. 76% become hypothyroid by 11 yr after rx even w most conservative dosing (Nejm 1984;311:426); ok in premenopausal women as long as not pregnant

Surgical thyroidectomy may be first choice, or if fail 2 or more PTU courses and judged unreliable to return if become myxedematous after ^{131}I, although >26% of surgical patients will be hypothyroid at 11 yr (Nejm 1984;311:426)

of storm: 1st β blockade, volume repalcement, and dexamethasone (peripheral T_4 to T_3 conversion blockade); then PTU ~1 gm initial dose, and possibly SSKI loading dose then 10–15 gtts po qid or lithium 300 mg tid

of ophthalmoplegia: stop smoking (Ann IM 1998;129:632); steroids as prednisone 0.5 mg/kg po qd for 1 mo then q 3 mo taper, clearly helpful, especially w radioactive iodine rx (Nejm 1989;321:1349); surgery (Nejm 1974;290:70); cyclophosphamide (Ann IM 1979;90: 921), or cyclosporine (Nejm 1989;321:1353)

of Graves' in pregnancy: low-dose PTU ok (Nejm 1986;315:24; 1981; 304:525,538), β blockers

of pretibial myxedema: topical steroids

of pituitary adenoma type: octreotide (Ann IM 1993;119:236)

NONSTIMULATING, AUTOIMMUNE THYROIDITIS (including Hashimoto's Thyroiditis)

Nejm 1996, 335:99; Ann IM 1986;104:219

Cause: Autoimmune

Epidem: Female:males 6–9:1; usually over age 40 yr. Associated w other autoimmune diseases including stimulating autoimmune thyroid disease and autoimmune ophthalmoplegia (Ann IM 1978;88:379); Turner's syndrome; Addison's disease; dermatitis herpetiformis (Ann IM 1985;102:194); mitral valve prolapse syndrome (present in 40% of Hashimoto's pts—Ann IM 1985;102:479); postpartum 2 wk–4 mo, perhaps due to peridelivery immunologic changes (Ann IM 1977;87:154)

Pathophys: A chronic destructive autoimmune thyroiditis or, if milder, simply autoimmune goiter-producing disease (silent subacute thyroiditis)

Sx: Hypothyroidism; rarely thyrotoxicosis; goiter; but generally few sx, unlike other thyroiditis; very rarely can be painful (Ann IM 1986; 104:355)

Si: As above; nontender gland

Crs: Half proceed on to myxedema over months to years

Cmplc: Myxedema; perhaps, rarely, lymphoma and leukemia (Nejm 1985; 312:601)

r/o much rarer Riedel's struma (fibrosis, increasing mass); post partum thyroiditis, usually transiently toxic then hypothyroid, then return to normal

Lab: (Ann IM 1978;88:383)

Chem: TSH elevated as become hypothyroid

Hem: ESR minimally elevated

Path: Thyroid bx shows lymphocytic infiltrate, if done, not necessary

Serol: Elevated antibodies against thyroperoxidase; or antithyroid microsomal antibodies, more specif and more sens (95%) than antithyroglobulin antibodies (60%) (J Lab Clin Med 1979;93:1035)

Xray: Thyroid ^{131}I, ^{123}I, or technetium scan shows no, or patchy, uptake; RAIU usually low, often 0

Rx: None, if radioactive iodine uptake is low, until are myxedematous; if RAIU is high, may have an organification defect from the auto-immune disease, or may have coincident Graves' and need rx for that (Nejm 1975;293:624)

SUBACUTE THYROIDITIS (Giant Cell, De Quervain's, or Pseudotubercular Thyroiditis)

Ann IM 1986;104:219

Cause: Viral?

Epidem: Epidemic pattern. Male:female = 1:4; 1/6 as common as nonstimulating autoimmune thyroid disease; 1/8 as common as stimulating autoimmune thyroid disease; 1/3 of cases follow a URI

Pathophys:

Sx: Many sx (in contrast to Hashimoto's) including fever, nervousness, tender painful neck

Si: Firm gland, usually tender, although 15% have no goiter or pain (Ann IM 1977;86:24)

Crs:

Months 1–2: Hyperthyroid with tender gland

Month 3: Transition with firm nontender gland

Months 4–6: Hypothyroid with firm gland becoming normal

Months 7+: Return to normal function and exam

Cmplc: r/o **acute pyogenic thyroiditis;** hemorrhage into thyroid nodule

Lab:

Hem: ESR 50–80 mm/h early in course

Serol: Occasionally (20%) positive antithyroid antibodies

Xray: Thyroid ^{131}I, ^{123}I, or technetium scan shows no uptake; low RAIU

Rx: Palliative, no effect on course, including: salicylates; short-term steroids, eg, prednisone 40 mg qd, taper to 20 mg qd over 2 wk; β blockers when toxic sx, replacement rx when hypo

MULTINODULAR GOITER (Nontoxic and Toxic)

Cause:

Nontoxic: Iodine deficiency; lithium, PAS, iodides, or phenylbutazone rx; genetic and/or autoimmune silent subacute thyroiditis (nonstimulating)?

Toxic: Progession from nontoxic

Epidem:

Nontoxic: Iodine deficiency especially in Ecuador (Nejm 1969; 280:296)

Toxic: Associated w elderly, CHF, AF, and angina

Pathophys:

Nontoxic: Unknown for most common type

Toxic: Autonomous function of 1 or more nodules

Sx:

Nontoxic: Goiter

Toxic: CHF sx, angina, palpitations

Multinodular Goiter, continued

Si:
   Nontoxic: Goiter
   Toxic: CHF, Afib, apathetic hyperthyroidism of elderly w ptsosis

Crs:
   Nontoxic: Slowly progressive

Cmplc:
   Both: Tracheal compression (Ann IM 1994;121:757); vague head and
      neck sx due to thoracic inlet compression manifest by positive
      Pemberton si = facial and head redness and suffusion w elevations
      of arms up to ears (Ann IM 1996;125:568)
   Both: r/o autoimmune thyroid disease

Lab:
   Chem:
   Nontoxic: Thyroid function tests normal
   Toxic: (Med Aud Dig 1983;30:18) T_4 incr or normal, r/o benign
      increase in 15% sick or psychotic patients; RAIU elevated;
      TRH/TSH test positive, better than T_3 suppression test; normal =
      TSH of 2–3 rises to 15[+]; abnormal = no increase in TSH w TRH
      stimulation

Xray: Thyroid ^{131}I, ^{123}I, or technetium scan; in nontoxic, shows large
   gland w diffuse patchy uptake; in toxic, shows hot nodule(s), rest of
   gland atrophic and cool

Rx: (Nejm 1998;338:1438)
   Nontoxic: Thyroid replacement? (p 228), but if any autonomous
      production, can lead to toxicity, especially in the elderly; ^{131}I or
      surgery especially if compressive sx (Ann IM 1994;1221:757)
   Toxic: [131]I rx; surgery

THYROID NODULE
Nejm 1998;338:1438; 1993;328:553

Cause: Neoplastic adenoma; or a nodule of multinodular goiter
   (Plummer's disease)

Epidem: Present in 4–8% of US adult population; up to 50% over age
   50 yr have one by ultrasound; in 20–30% of irradiated adult
   population 10–30 yr later, ~10% of which are malignant and 1/2 of

those detectable by physical exam (Ann IM 1981;94:176; Nejm 1976;294:1019). Male:female = 1:4

Pathophys: Only a small % will be "hot," producing T_3T_4 and toxic sx

Sx: Asx

Si: Thyroid nodule

Crs:

Cmplc: Cancer in 5–10% of cold nodules by biopsy studies; incr incidence in the young and males

Lab:

Chem: TSH to r/o thyrotoxicosis from toxic nodule

Path: Fine needle aspiration bx first to r/o cancer (Ann IM 1993;118: 282); <1% false positives, others report 80% sens/specif (Am J Med 1994;97:152)

Xray: [123]I scan only useful if aspiration cytology is suspicious/intermediate because can avoid surgery if nodule is hot (functioning)

Ultrasound especially to guide needle aspiration or f/u of neg nodules

Rx: Medical suppression w exogenous thyroid is controversial; some find that it prevents growth (Ann IM 1995;122:1) and decreases recurrence of benign nodules (both contradicted by Ann IM 1998; 128:386), but has no effect on malignancy incidence (Nejm 1989; 320:835); no better than placebo after 6 mo, would longer rx help? (Nejm 1987;317:70)

of hot nodule, ^{131}I rx to control hyperthyroid sx; but 25% develop myxedema at 5 yr and 20% stay as big or get bigger (Nejm 1983; 309:1473), so may need surgery eventually anyway

Surgery now rarely needed if aspiration bx done. See Fig. 5.7.1

THYROID PAPILLARY CARCINOMA

Nejm 1998;338:297; Ann IM 1991;115:133

Cause: Most cases occur as sporadic events in the population; incr incidence from irradiation under age 20, w risk thereafter peaking over 20 yrs then declining, eg, 1.7% at 20 yr after radiation rx of Hodgkin's (Nejm 1991;325:599); no increase after ^{131}I rx of Graves' disease (Nejm 1980;303:188)

Epidem: 75–90% of all thyroid cancers; mean age at dx is 45 yr. Female:male = 2–3:1

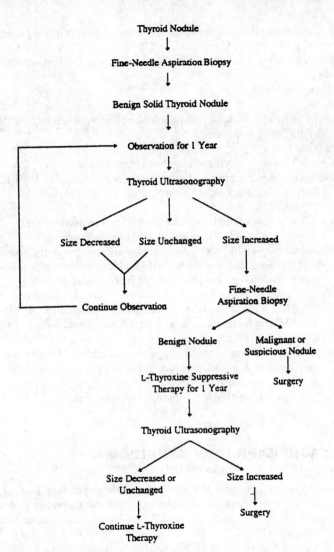

Figure 5.7.1 Decision making for treatment of patients with benign thyroid nodules. (Reproduced with permission from Ridgway EC. Medical treatment of benign thyroid nodules: have we defined a benefit. Ann IM 1998;128:404.)

Pathophys: Local invasion and metastases (primarily lymphatic), less often bloodborne metastases

Sx: Neck mass

Si: Thyroid mass (80%), 40% of the time in an abnormal gland from other thyroid disease

Stage at dx:

47% stage I, small intrathyroid

28% stage II, large intrathyroid

21% stage III, >4 cm and/or local extranodal invasion

4% stage IV, distant extranodal mets

Crs: Excellent, 90% >30 yr survival for stages I and II; worse if age >50 yr, >4 cm diameter, or local or distant metastases. Pts w positive lymph nodes may have equal survival to those w negative nodes

Radiation-induced cancers have same course as others (Ann IM 1986; 105:405)

Cmplc: r/o follicular, and undifferentiated carcinomas including giant cell, small cell, and medullary carcinoma (see below)

Lab:

Chem: No helpful pre op tests, post op is useful to follow thyroglobulin levels (>10 ngm/cc) as a tumor marker especially of mets

Path: Aspiration biopsy (p 235) and cytology; "rug fringe" effect, ie, papillae, but few mitoses; unlike well-formed follicles of follicular or anaplasia, w giant or small cells of undifferentiated types

Xray: Scan usually cold (Ann IM 1978;88:41)

Rx: Detect in irradiated patients w q 1 yr thyroid physical exam w bx of any nodules; debated if thryoid hormone suppression helps

Surgical thyroidectomy; lobectomy alone is inadequate even for stage I and II disease (4% vs 14% 30-yr recurrence); up to 14% get cmplc of surgery including hypoparathyroidism and recurrent laryngeal nerve injury. Postsurgical I^{131} rx (Ann IM 1998;129:622) w thyroid hormone suppression

Chemotherapy possible if metastases w adriamycin (Nejm 1974;290: 193), 5-FU, and cisplatin but none very good

MEDULLARY CARCINOMA OF THYROID
("Amyloid Struma")
Ann IM 1991;115:140; 1973;78:561

Cause: Neoplasia

Epidem: May be sporadic, familial, or associated w MEN type II (Sipple's syndrome): bilateral pheochromocytomas, gi mucosal neuromas (in 10%—Nejm 1976;295:1287), parathyroid adenomas (10%); inherited w autosomal dominant pattern w known detectable oncogene defects (Nejm 1996;335:947, Jama 1995;274:1149); contrast w MEN type I: ZE, parathyroid adenomas, and islet cell tumors (Nejm 1977;296:534)

Pathophys: Neoplasia of parafollicular thyroid cells, multicentric origin (Nejm 1973;289:437); characteristically produce CEA, and/or thyrocalcitonin, and/or serotonin, and other vasoactive substances; these cells are similar to pheochromocytoma cells, ie, of neural crest origin (Nejm 1973;289:545)

Sx: Diarrhea, flushing

Si: Thyroid mass

Crs: Long survivals despite anaplastic appearance

Cmplc: Local metastases; pheochromocytoma (30%); secondary Cushing's from ACTH; hyperparathyroidism (Nejm 1968;279:279) in MEN type II

Lab:

Chem: Thyrocalcitonin elevated by RIA (Nejm 1971;285:1115); CEA elevated

Path: Thyroid bx shows clumps of parafollicular cells surrounded by collagen ("amyloid struma")

Xray: Thyroid scan shows a cold mass, starts in upper poles. Plain films may show calcified metastases that can look like old tbc even w liver mets

Rx: Prevent cancer deaths in MEN II families w annual calcitonin stimulation tests (Nejm 1988;318:479)

Surgery w follow-up thyrocalcitonin/CEA levels as markers of residual tumor (Nejm 1974;290:1035)

Chemotherapy w adriamycin (Nejm 1974;290:193)

5.8 VITAMIN DISORDERS

VITAMIN A DEFICIENCY
Nejm 1984;310:1023

Cause: Deficiency of vitamin A, a fat-soluble vitamin

Epidem: Increased in low-income areas and developing countries

Pathophys: Necessary for visual pigment of eye; other tissue functions not known. Columnar epithelium changes to stratified squamous (keratinization) in trachea, urinary tract, conjunctiva. β-carotene and other carotenes are precursors

Sx: Poor growth in children; impaired vision day and night

Si: Keratinization of eye and Bitot spots on sclera (gray plaques); dryness of eyes and skin can be severe (Nejm 1994;330:994)

Crs:

Cmplc: Increased mortality and morbidity from most infections including measles (Nejm 1990;323:160)

Lab:

Chem: Low vit A levels

Rx: Vitamin A; given in small weekly doses reduces overall mortality by 50% in undernourished Indian children (Nejm 1990;323:929) probably by decreasing mortality from respiratory illness; given 10,000 U/lb po q 3 mo, it decreases diarrheal illness in HIV infected infants (Am J Publ Hlth 1995;85:1076)

VITAMIN A EXCESS
Nejm 1984;310:1023; Med Let 1980;22:19

Cause: Excessive ingestion by vitamin pill users

Epidem:

Pathophys: β-carotene and other carotenes are precursors; a fat-soluble vitamin

Sx: H/o >50,000 U qd ingestion for 1+ yr. Headache, lethargy, dry skin, sore mouth, fractures, and bone pain

Si: (Nejm 1976;294:805; Ann IM 1974;80:44) Clubbing, fractures (due to abnormal bone growth), desquamative dermatitis, pseudotumor cerebri

Vitamin A Excess, continued

Crs:
Cmplc: Cirrhosis (Nejm 1974;291:438); congenital malformations, esp. neural tube defects in infants exposed to ≥10,000 U/d of vit A (but not β-carotenes), esp. in 1st 7 wk of pregnancy (Nejm 1995; 333:1369)
Lab:
Rx: Stop intake

WERNICKE'S ENCEPHALOPATHY

Cause: Thiamine (B_1) deficiency + genetic enzyme abnormalities (Nejm 1977;297:1367)
Epidem: Most common in alcoholics; also in surgical patients on iv's × weeks w/o thiamine supplement; rarely, refed starving patients
Pathophys: Unknown
Sx:
Si:
- Ophthalmoplegia especially nystagmus (85%) progressing to paralysis of lateral gaze, ie, abducens palsies
- Global confusion
- Ataxia
- Hypothermia

Crs: May recover partially over 1 yr (Nejm 1985;312:16)
Cmplc: Korsakoff's psychosis (80%), confabulating responses
Lab:
  Path: Circummamillary body congestion and hemorrhage at base of brain on postmortem, and along floors of 3rd and 4th ventricles
Rx: Preventively put thiamine in all alcoholic drinks perhaps, especially wine (Nejm 1978;299:285)?
  Thiamine 100 mg im, iv (is safe—Jama 1995;274:562) or po qd × 3 d; always give 1st dose before start iv glucose

HOMOCYSTINURIA (Homocyst(e)inemia)

Cause: Genetic, autosomal recessive

Epidem: Heterozygote prevalence = 1/70 in general population. Elevations are present in ~20–30% of patients w premature (age <50 yr) ASCVD (Jama 1999;281:1817); overall prevalence similar in over-50 general population and levels correlate w increasing ASCVD risk (Ann IM 1999;131:321,387,352,363). Even secondary elevations w mild folate, pyridoxine, and vit B_{12} deficiencies are associated w incr ASCVD including arteriosclerotic heart (Jama 1996;275:1893; Nejm 1991;424:1149), peripheral, and CNS vascular disease.

In children, mental retardation, 1/200–300,000 (Nejm 1999;341:1572)

Pathophys: Accumulation of homocysteine in blood and urine due to blocked conversion of homocysteine to methionine. Vascular disease and emboli due to endothelial cell damage (Nejm 1998;338:1047). Homocysteine, the oxidized sulfide of the amino acid homocysteine, is the predominant form in blood and urine (Nejm 1995;333:325)

Sx: Of CNS and peripheral thromboembolic arterial and venous vascular disease (Ann IM 1995;123:747); 30% have had by age 20 yr, 60% by age 40 yr (Nejm 1985;313:709). Premature osteoporosis (Postgrad Med J 1977;53:488)

Si: "Marfanoid," arachnodactyly (Nejm 1982;307:781); myocardiopathy w aortic valve disease; mental retardation

Crs:

Cmplc: Lens dislocation, r/o Marfan's syndrome

Lab:
  Chem: Homocysteine level >10 μM/L (Rx Let 1999;6:8)

Rx: Newborn screening

  to prevent ASCVD in pts w or in whom mild homocysteinemia may be present (Nejm 1995;332:286); not yet proven in randomized trials

  • Folate (Nejm 1975;292:491), 0.5–1 mg po qd and follow homocysteine levels; 0.14 mg/100 gm cereal grain products now added in US to prevent neural tube defects but has the added benefit of reducing homocysteine levels (Nejm 1998;338:1009)

  • Betaine (Med Let 1997;39:12) 3–10 gm po bid, under age 3 start w 100 μgm/kg qd; a choline derivative; $150/180 gm

If folate alone doesn't decr homocysteine levels to normal (Nejm 2001;
344:1222):
- B_{12} supplements po
- Pyridoxine (B_6) (Nejm 1970;283:1206)

RICKETS (children) AND OSTEOMALACIA (adults)
Ann IM 1978;89:966

Cause:
- Vitamin D deficiency: dietary, esp in northern winters (p 309);
  malabsorption (Am J Med 2000;108:296) including biliary
  obstruction, steatorrhea, postgastrectomy (in 15%—Ann IM
  1971;75:220), post gastric stapling or bypass, Crohn's disease;
  relative deficiency, eg, rapid bone formation after
  parathyroidectomy
- Vitamin D resistance: hypophosphatasias from phosphate
  X-linked diabetes, renal tubular acidosis, all Fanconi syndromes
  including Wilson's, myeloma, old tetracycline, and heavy metals;
  renal insufficiency and aluminum depositions (Ann IM 1984;101:
  775) including premies on parenteral feeding (Nejm 1985;312:
  1337); chronic seizure medications like phenytoin and
  carbamazepine, via hepatic enzyme inductions (Nejm 1975;292:
  550; 1972;287:900)
- Calcium-deficient diet in tropical countries? (Nejm 1999;341:
  563,602)

Epidem: Rare in US

Pathophys: Disease all due to failure to calcify new bone matrix
Vit D functions:
- Increases gi calcium absorption (Nejm 1969;280:1396)
- Decreases urinary phosphate loss
- Increases reabsorp of bone
- Permissive action on PTH

Sx: Fractures, bone pain

Si: Rickets, includes severe bony distortions, frontal bossing, rachitic
rosary (costochondral junctions swollen), long bone bowing

Crs:

Cmplc:

Lab:

Chem: Ca^{2+} low or normal (low in renal insufficiency); PO_4^- low (due to PTH effect on bone and kidney) except in renal failure; alkaline phosphatase incr in all including RTA but not Fanconi and hypo-PO_4 types

Path: Bone bx shows incr number and size of osteoid seams; in children, noncalcification of epiphyseal cartilage

Urine: Ca^{2+} low in all w adequate PTH; glucose, amino acids present in RTA and Fanconi

Xray: Wide, thick epiphyseal cartilages in children; pseudocracks (Milkman's fractures) where vessels cross bone. Calcification of tendon insertions and capsules in 60% X-linked hypoPO_4 rickets (Nejm 1985;313:1)

Rx: Vitamin D as 25-hydroxy vit D 50,000–100,000 U qd; or 1,25-OH vit D (Rocaltrol), expensive and more easily causes hypercalcemia

Perhaps topical precursor to skin w UVB irradiation, gives slower and steadier levels, and is especially good in vit D-resistant types (Nejm 1980;303:349)

5.9 MISCELLANEOUS

Asx adrenal mass found incidentally on CT; w/u only if hypertension, sx of pheochomocytoma, hypoK^+, Cushingoid, or >5.6 cm (Ann IM 1999;130:759; Nejm 1990;323:1401)

Hypoglycemia, differential dx (Nejm 1995;332:1144):

Exogenous: (Nejm 1992;326:1020;1977;297:1029):
- Insulin; has lowest plasma C peptide levels
- Sulfonylureas; present in blood and urine
- Other medications (list—Ann IM 1993;118:536)

Fasting (Nejm 1992;326:1020; 1976;294:766):
- Pancreatic functioning tumor
- Nonpancreatic functioning tumor (Nejm 1981;305:1456)
- Liver disease, including:
  Acquired, especially from CHF

Congenital glycogen storage disease or galactosemia
Hepatoma
- Alcohol and/or poor nutrition, from decr gluconeogenesis; eg, in diarrheal disease in children (Nejm 1990;322:1358)
- Endocrine deficiencies, eg, Addison's, hypopituitarism, decr pancreatic α-cell function
- Normal physiologic responses in women and children (Nejm 1974;291:1275)

Reactive (postprandial); oral GTT no help, get blood glucose prn sx; ≤60 mg% is significant (Nejm 1989;321:1421):
- Rapid gastric emptying, rx w anticholinergics
- Fast absorption, rx w phenformin (Nejm 1973;288:1207), though now off the market because caused lactic acidosis
- Prediabetes
- Dumping syndrome
- Leucine sensitivity
- Hereditary fructose intolerance; autosomal recessive (Nejm 1982; 307:535)

Chapter 6
Gastroenterology

D. K. Onion

6.1 UPPER GI DISEASES

GASTROESOPHAGEAL REFLUX DISEASE (GERD)
Nejm 1997;336:924; Jama 1996;276:983; Nejm 1994;331:656; 1992;326:825

Cause: Mechanical reflux through incompetent sphincter

Epidem: Incr prevalence (Am J Med 1999;106:642) w age, obesity; in women, pregnancy, birth control pill use (progesterone effect—Ann IM 1982;97:93); scleroderma, smokers, drinkers, and those w family hx

Pathophys: Reflux of acid (rarely bile in achlorhydria) through transiently relaxing lower esophageal sphincter, plus inadequately neutralized acid from diminished saliva production; or diminished lower esophageal sphincter (LES) tone, which can be idiopathic from coffee (Nejm 1980;303:122), lowered intrinsic gastrin levels (Nejm 1973;289:182), or smoking (Nejm 1971;284:1136)

Hiatus hernia thought to have little to do w reflux, is present in 70% over age 70 yr, but as of 2000 began again to be thought to play some role. Diaphragmatic crura play some sphincter role too (Ann IM 1992;117:1051)

Sx: Substernal burning radiating upward, especially when recumbent or leaning over, and most often after meals, especially fatty ones

Si: Dental erosions, yellow (dentine) dished out areas on nonocclusal surfaces (Ann IM 1995;122:809)

Crs: Variable

Gastroesophageal Reflux Disease (GERD), continued

Cmplc: Stricture, Schatzki's lower esophageal ring; Barrett's esophagus (premalignant dysplasia) and adenocarcinoma (p 248); acid laryngitis, asthma w pulmonary aspirations

r/o **rumination syndrome** especially in retarded (Ann IM 1986; 105:573)

Lab: (Ann IM 1982;97:93) Test only if atypical hx or fails to respond to rx

Endo: Esophagoscopy, w bx if esophagitis present in immunocompromised; often normal despite reflux sx

Noninv: Manometry usually shows LES pressure <10 mm Hg; 24-h pH probe; continuous ambulatory esophageal pH monitoring is 80–90% sens/specif (Jama 1995;274:662)

Xray: Ba swallow of debatable help, since sx correlate w reflux, not presence of anatomic hiatus hernia; and radiologically induced reflux not clearly correlated w sx

Rx: Achieve ideal body weight; stop smoking and stop other ulcerogens like caffeine, aspirin, and alcohol; elevate the head of the bed; 2–4 h fast before going to bed; small meals; decrease fat

Medications:

1st:

- Antacids to both neutralize acid and increase LES pressure via gastrin (Ann IM 1971;74:223)
- H_2 blockers like cimetidine (Tagamet) 400–800 mg po bid, ranitidine (Zantac) 150 mg po bid then hs, famotidine (Pepcid) 20 mg po bid (Arch IM 1991;151:2394), or nizatidine (Axid) 150 mg po bid

2nd:

- Omeprazole (Prilosec) (Nejm 1990;323:1749) 20 mg po qd-bid, or other proton pump inhibitor (p 253); theoretically could cause B_{12} deficiency long term (Ann IM 1994;120:211), but can be used at doses of 10–20 mg po qd safely at least for 5–6 yr (Ann IM 1994; 121:161; Gastroenterol 1994;106:907; 1994;107:1305; Age Aging 1994;23:121; Gut 1994;35:590). 40 mg po qd × 7d can be used diagnostically if ablates sx (Am J Med 1999;107:219). But long term omeprazole in face of chronic *Helicobacter pylori* infection causes atrophic gastritis and presumably incr cancer risk unlike surgical fundal plication (Nejm 1996;334:1018)

3rd:

- Metoclopramide (Reglan) 10 mg po ac and hs (Ann IM 1983; 98:86; Nejm 1981;305:28; Med Let 1980;22:27), add to above

meds if refractory (Ann IM 1986;104:21). Adverse effects: in
10–30%, especially CNS, eg, confusion, tardive dyskinesia,
anxiety, and fatigue
- Bethanechol (Urecholine) 25 mg po qid; avoid in pregnancy, BPH,
COPD, peptic ulcer disease, heart disease (Ann IM 1980;93:805)
- Cisapride (Propulsid) 10–20 mg po qid; causes fatal arrythmias
(Rx Let 1999;6:42; 1998;5:43), often by drug interactions w long
QT drugs, 3/00 pulled from US market

Surgical: Nissen and other fundoplication procedures, probably
significant help for severe reflux but no better than omeprazole 40
mg bid (Surgery 2001;192:172); can be done laparoscopically; 10 yr
data (Jama 2001;285:2331) show inexplicably greater mortality in
surgically than medically treated pts, and no cancer prevention,
though need for medical rx diminished in 40%

ACHALASIA

Nejm 1997;336:924, Ann IM 1989;110:66

Cause:

Epidem: Primary type is most common; secondary is associated w cancer
of lung, stomach, and pancreas (Ann IM 1978;89:315).
Prevalence = 1/100,000

Pathophys: Debatable whether spasm leads to achalasia and whether both
are part of the same spectrum. Hyperactive esophageal spasm
present just in distal (lower) esophageal segment and sphincter
(LES) in achalasia, which is hypersensitive to gastrin (Nejm 1973;
289:182), while the upper esophageal segment is flaccid; all unlike
spasm w entire esophagous involved. Destruction of myenteric
plexus by autoantibodies

Sx: Sometimes h/o spasm; dysphagia; chest pain; weight loss

Si:

Crs:

Cmplc:

r/o:
- Cardiac pain
- Esophageal cancer since often confused w achalasia, so incidence
of cancer is high in 1st yr after diagnosis and overall incidence is

incr × 16 thereafter, but unclear that endoscopic screening improves survival (Jama 1995;274:1359)

- **Esophageal spasm:** associated w psychiatric illness in 84% (Nejm 1983;309:1337); solid and liquid dysphagia intermittently, associated w pain; manometry shows incr activity of whole esophagus in uncoordinated contractions, simultaneous contractions on at least 10% of wet swallows (Ann IM 1984; 100:242), can precipitate w 5 mg iv edrophonium (Tensilon) (Ann IM 1987;106:593); Ba swallow shows uncoordinated contractions; rx w dilatation w mercury bougies, nitrates and nitrites (Nejm 1973;289:23), nifedipine 10 mg t-qid po (Ann IM 1982;96:61), dicyclomine (Bentyl) 20 mg po t-qid pill or liquid, myotomy

Lab:

Noninv: Manometry shows spasm of lower esophageal sphincter, failure to relax high resting tone

Xray: Ba swallow shows no peristalsis, spasm of the LES, failure of the LES to relax with a swallow, dilated proximal, constricted distal esophageal segments; "rat tail deformity," r/o gastric cancer

Rx: (Gut 1999;44:231; Jama 1998;280:638)

Endoscopic dilatation, risk is of perforation; 50+% successful

Botulinum toxin by endoscopic injection of LES, lasts 6+ mo in 2/3 (Nejm 1995;332:774)

Surgical myotomy of lower esophageal sphincter, 90+% successful; cmplc: reflux and strictures.

ESOPHAGEAL CARCINOMA

Cause:

Epidem: Squamous cell types associated w smoking and alcoholism

Adenocarcinomas associated w obesity (Ann IM 1999;130:883), reflux sx (7 × risk) (Nejm 1999;340:825), which are also associated w achalasia, webs, and Barrett's esophagus (columnar epithelium-lined lower esophagus) (Nejm 1986;315:362) (30–60 × risk); rapidly incr rates since 1975 may be partly due to incr use of LES-relaxing meds

(Ann IM 2000;133:165) esp anticholinergics but also nitrates, theophyllines, and other bronchodilators

Pathophys: In adenocarcinoma type, malignant transformation (2% in 8 yr—Mayo; Nejm 1985;313:857) occurs in areas of chronic reflux, eg, in Barrett's esophagus, which is associated w strictures and ulcerations (Ann IM 1982;97:103) and occasionally familial (Ann IM 1985;103:52)

Sx: Dysphagia, weight loss

Si: Positive guaiac stools

Crs: 10% 5-yr survival w rx (Nejm 1996;335:462)

Cmplc: Other upper and lower airway cancers in smokers

Lab:

Endo: Esophagoscopy usually w gastroscopy and duodenoscopy as well (EGD), and biopsy

Path: Monoclonal antibody staining of lymph nodes predicts survival better than does routine microscopy (Nejm 1997;337:1188)

Xray: Ba swallow

Rx: Prevent w regular endoscopy of Barrett's (Ann IM 1987;106:902); but nothing works well, incidence is low, and there are no clear studies to show that screening works; would have to screen 1400 pts/yr to find 1 cancer if incidence = 20 × baseline (Nejm 1999;340:878)

All rx is basically palliative: surgery, then radiation and chemotherapy w cis-platinum + 5-FU (Nejm 1992;326:1593) or radiation + chemRx 1st then surgery (no—Nejm 1998;339:1979; vs yes—Nejm 1997;337:161; 1996;335:462,509) result in 40% 2-yr survival vs 10% for radiation alone, although the complication rate is higher

PEPTIC ULCER DISEASE (Gastric Ulcer [GU], Duodenal Ulcer [DU], Gastritis)

Nejm 1995;333:984 *(H. pylori);* 1990;322:909; Ann IM 1981;95:609

Cause: *H. pylori* infection (Can Med Assoc J 1994;150:177,189; Nejm 1989;321:1562; 1987;316:1557,1598; Ann IM 1988;108:70) in GU and DU but not gastritis (Arch IM 1998;158:1427)

Endogenous, nicotine, or NSAID-induced incr acid/pepsin secretion; and/or decr pancreatic or duodenal HCO_3 secretion (Nejm 1987; 316:374); or decrease in other gi defenses

Epidem: Duodenal ulcer, 90% assoc w chronic *H. pylori* infection often begins early in life, occurs in 10% of people, male:female = 4:1. Decreasing prevalence in developed world. *H. pylori* infection runs in families (Nejm 1990;322:359) probably because transmitted in emesis aerosols and diarrhea (Jama 1999;282:2240,2260). Only 15–20% of those chronically infected get duodenal or gastric ulcers.
Meckel's diverticulum in <1% of people, usually ulcerates in childhood.

Pathophys: Increased acid production in: Zollinger-Ellison syndrome; neurogenically incr secretion, eg, burn or CVA pts (Nejm 1970; 282:373); nicotine users (Nejm 1974;290:469); coffee users, but it's not the caffeine (Nejm 1970;283:897); TPN pts from the iv amino acids (Nejm 1978;298:27); hypersecretors, who can be divided into hypersecretors and hypergastrin responders (Ann IM 1980;93:540); NSAID and alcohol users (Gastroenterol 1997;112:683)
Diminished pancreatic secretions: 10% incidence in cystic fibrosis, may be first sx in heterozygote; perhaps w nicotine (Nejm 1972;286: 1212); perhaps w steroids (J Intern Med 1994;236:619; Nejm 1983; 309:21)
Impaired gi defenses: *H. pylori* infection, organism attaches to blood group O receptors on mucosal cells much like enteropathogenic *E. coli* attaches to bowel wall, tolerates high acid environment (Sci 1995;267:1621); aspirin and other NSAIDs (Ann IM 1991;114: 307) in elderly (Ann IM 1988;109:359) especially if concomitant steroid use (Ann IM 1991;114:735); alcohol ingestion causes incr permeability of mucosa to H^+ (Nejm 1971;285:716) and produces direct mucosal damage (Ann IM 1976;85:299); smoking inhibits duodenal HCO_3 secretion (Ann IM 1993;119:882)

Sx: Epigastric pain especially 1–2 h pc and 2 am; gi bleeding, occult, melena or hematemesis

Si: Epigastric tenderness; stool guaiac-positive

Crs: Before *H. pylori* rx, duodenal ulcer recurred in 10% except in smokers where 72% recur in 1 yr (Nejm 1984;311:689); gastric ulcer recurred in 50%; take ~8 wk to heal w rx (Ann IM 1985; 103:573)

H. pylori may be chronic, recurrent, and resistant to multiple rx attempts (Ann IM 1991;114:662) but 96% don't recur after cleared w antibiotic crs

r/o ZE if does recur, not a smoker, and no *H. pylori*

Cmplc: Persistent bleeding, perforation, obstruction, pain; possibly adenocarcinoma and non-Hodgkin's gastric lymphoma in pts w *H. pylori* (Nejm 1998;338:804; Jama 1996;275:937; Nejm 1994; 330:1267)

r/o cancer w all gastric ulcers, ie, endoscopically document healing; celiac artery compression/obstruction, which gives pc pain (abdominal angina) (Ann IM 1977;86:278); Zollinger-Ellison syndrome; (Nejm 1987;317:1201) if refractory

Lab:

Noninv:

- Urea breath test (UBT), radioactive labeled urea broken down to $NH_3 + C^{14}O_2$ in stomach if *H. pylori* present there and $C^{14}O_2$ in breath is measured; is very sens/specif except false negative within 4 wk of po antibiotics (Nejm 1995; 333:984); best for follow up test of cure, cost $60, 5–10% false neg. ^{13}C-urea blood test, 98% specif, 89% sens (Am J Gastroenterol 1999;94:1522)

- IgG- and IgA-specific antibodies in *H. pylori* type; 75–80+% sens/specif overall (Am J Gastroenterol 1999;94:1512), but over age 60 positivity increases to >50% (Ann IM 1988;109:11); used to f/u 1 yr after rx, an undetectable level indicates cure (100% sens) but some titer remains in 40% (60% specif) (Jama 1998;280:363)

Endo (EGD):

- Debatably best first test rather than empiric trial of H_2 blockers (Lancet 1994;343:811 vs Ann IM 1997;126:280); visible vessel ulcers bleed again within 24 h 50% of the time; other ulcers rarely do (Nejm 1981;305:915)

- "CLO test" (Med Let 1997) of biopsy specimens incubated × 4–24 h, gel incubation color change system that measures urea splitting by *H. pylori*

- Antral or ulcer bx giemsa or Warthin-Starry stain for *H. pylori* (Nejm 1990;322:359)

Xray: UGIS, but low sens for duodenal ulcer; KUB for subdiaphragmatic air if perforation

Rx: (Med Let 1997;39:1; Jama 1996;275:622)

Prevent w po vaccine? (Sci 1995;267:1621)

2nd: H$_2$ BLOCKER, histamine antagonists (Nejm 1990;323:1749); for all, double-dose hs as good as normal dose bid; prophylaxis w normal dose qd works for all; only cimetidine and ranitidine (slightly) alter cytochrome P450 enzyme systems; cimetidine and ranitidine generic available and cheap; action onset takes 1/2 h but lasts 6–10 h (Jama 1996;275:1428); renal excretion, lower dose if creatinine clearance <50 (Rx Let 2001;8:26)

- Cimetidine (Tagamet) 300–400 mg po bid or 800 mg hs better than split doses (BMJ 1984;289:1418) or iv q 6 h; decrease dose if BUN up; helps gastric ulcers too (Ann IM 1985;102:573; Nejm 1983;308:1319). Adverse effects: antiandrogen (Nejm 1989; 321:1012); confusion (Med Let 1978;20:77); drug interactions like incr levels of: lidocaine (Ann IM 1983;98:174), benzodiazepine (Nejm 1980;302:1012; Ann IM 1980;93:266), theophylline (Ann IM 1981;95:68), propranolol (Nejm 1981;304:692); and decr levels w concomitant antacids (Nejm 1982;307:400)
- Ranitidine (Zantac) 150 mg po bid or 300 mg hs (Med Let 1987; 29:17); 150–300 mg iv/24 h continuous drip better than bolus rx (Ann IM 1990;112:334); less CNS toxic than cimetidine
- Famotidine (Pepcid) 20 mg po bid or 40 mg hs; less CNS toxic than cimetidine (others disagree, say all equal—Ann IM 1991; 114:1027); works where cimetidine doesn't (Nejm 1983; 309:1368; 1982;306:20)
- Nizatidine (Axid) 150 mg bid or 300 mg hs (Med Let 1988;30:77)

3rd: PROTON PUMP INHIBITORS (Med Let 2000;42:65); better than H$_2$ blockers; some antibacterial action vs. *H. pylori*; especially good in reflux esophagitis and ZE ulcers; better healing of ulcers (~80%) in face of ongoing NSAID use than H$_2$ blockers (Nejm 1998;338:719). Adverse effects: B$_{12}$ deficiency w long-term use (Ann IM 1994;120:211), nocturnal erections, gynecomastia, anaphylaxis, and erythema multiforme; incr blood levels of phenytoin (Dilantin), diazepam, warfarin, digoxin, and disulfiram (Antabuse); $3–5/tab;

- Esomeprazole (Nexium) (Med Let 2001;43:36) 20–40 mg po qd; S-isomer of omeprazole
- Lansoprazole (Prevacid) (Med Let 1995;37:63) 30 mg po qd, 15 mg po qd to prophylact (Ann IM 1996;124:859); $116/mo
- Omeprazole (Prilosec) 20 mg po qd-bid (Nejm 1991;324:965); $125/mo, generic in 2001
- Rabeprazole (Aciphex) (Med Let 1999;41:110) 20 mg po qd, $111/mo

GASTROENTEROLOGY

- Pantoprazole (Protonix) 40 mg iv or po qd; none of the usual PPI drug interactions and few of the usual adv effects; $90/mo

4th: OTHERS

- Antacids, eg, Maalox or Mylanta 30 cc po 1 h pc and hs (Med Let 1982;24:61; Ann IM 1981;94:214); avoid ones w $CaCO_3$ because of acid rebound (Nejm 1973;288:923) although rapid onset (min) valuable (Jama 1996;275:1428)
- Propantheline (Pro-Banthine) 15 mg ac, works, potentiates cimetidine (Nejm 1977;297:1427)
- Sucralfate (Carafate) (Nejm 1991;325:1017) 1 gm po qid 1 h ac, benign, as good as cimetidine (Ann IM 1982;97:269) and same price; binds tetracycline, cimetidine, digoxin, warfarin

Surgical: Vagotomy and pyloroplasty (Nejm 1982;307:519); antrectomy and Billroth II, cmplc: dumping (Ann IM 1974;80:577), and retained antrum w high gastrin levels, or alkaline gastritis (rx with Roux-en-y, helps the bilious emesis—Ann IM 1985;103:178)

Prophylaxis

after an ulcer:

- Stopping smoking as good as any rx; if don't, 72% recur in 1 yr (Nejm 1984;311:689)
- H_2 blocker like cimetidine (Tagamet) 400 mg hs (Nejm 1984; 311:689), or ranitidine (Zantac) 150 mg po hs × years (Nejm 1994;330:382,428) but may increase infections by impairing gastric bacterial killing (Ann IM 1994;121:568)

w NSAID use (Rx Let 1999;6:5):

- Proton pump inhibitor; either omeprazole 20 mg po qd or lansoprazole better than H_2 blocker or misoprostol (Nejm 1998; 338:727)
- Misoprostol (Cytotec) (Ann IM 1991;114:307; Med Let 1989; 31:21) 100 μgm qid or 200 μgm b-tid (Ann IM 1995;123:344) po prevents NSAID-induced type ulcers debatably (Arch IM 1996; 156:2321; 1994;154:2020; Nejm 1992;327:1575 vs Ann IM 1995;123:241 [elderly]; 1993;119:257). Adverse effects: teratogenic in 1st trimester, causes Möbius' Syndrome (Nejm 1998; 338:1881)

in ICU patients, especially those w respiratory failure or coagulopathy (Nejm 1994;330:377, 428):

- Antacids or H_2 blockers like cimetidine 300 mg iv q 6 h (Ann IM 1987;106:562), or ranitidine 50 mg iv q 8h (Nejm 1998;338:791)
- Sucralfate 1 gm q 6 h (Nejm 1987;317:1376) and although not quite as good as antacids or ranitidine (10% bleed vs 4–6%), late pneumonia in ventilated pts is less (5% vs 16–20%) because acid killing of bacteria by stomach is preserved (Ann IM 1994; 120:653), others report no pneumonia difference (Nejm 1998; 338:791)

of bleeding (Nejm 1994;331:717), diagnostic endoscopy and occasionally endoscopic electrocoagulation or injection of visible vessel in ulcer crater decreases recurrent bleeding acutely from 50% to 20% (Gut 1992;33:456); and/or acute po omeprazole (Nejm 1997;336:1054); possibly octreotide (Ann IM 1997;127:1062)

of perforation, antibiotics, NG drainage and recheck in 12 h is as good as immediate surgery (Nejm 1989;320:970)

of obstruction: endoscopic balloon dilatation

CARCINOMA OF STOMACH (Stomach Cancer)
Nejm 1995;333:32

Cause: Neoplasia

Epidem: Decreasing incidence in US in past 50 yr, increasing incidence in Japan. Higher incidence in patients w blood type A (pernicious anemia predisposition in the same group).

Correlates w severe *H. pylori* gastritis (Nejm 2001;345:784) and gastric ulcers but not duodenal disease. Polyps do not predispose, but probably diet constituents of unknown type do (maybe nitrosamines from cured/fermented foods)

Pathophys: Low serum pepsinogen I correlates w metaplasia and development of "intestinal mixed/other" type cancer, that which occurs in Asians rather than the "diffuse," blood group A-associated type (Ann IM 1980;93:537). *H. pylori* infection clearly increases risk markedly 3–12 × (Sci 1995;267:1621)

Sx: Pain (51%), cachexia and weight loss (62%), hematemesis or melena (20%), dysphagia (26%)

Si: Acanthosis nigrans; when present in patient over age 40, patient has a high chance of having a gi adenocarcinoma; but acanthosis may be present in lymphoma, or benignly in hereditary ataxia telangiectasia, obese patients, children, or diabetics, especially insulin-resistant diabetics (Nejm 1978;298:1164; 1976;294:739)

Guaiac-positive stools

Crs: Rapidly downhill even w surgery; overall 5-yr survival: 10–15%; w surgery and negative nodes may be as high as 45%; better in Japan

Cmplc: Bleeding. Metastases to lung, especially via lymphatics and may appear as a diffuse pulmonary process; to ovaries, especially if signet ring cell type (Krukenberg's ovarian tumor); to bone, especially vertebrae

r/o gastric lymphoma (MALT: mucosa associated lymphoid tissue), low grade B-cell lymphoma associated w *H. pylori* infection and 50% cure rate w antibiotic rx of *H. pylori* (Ann IM 1999;131:88)

Lab:

Endo: Gastroscopy w 6$^+$ biopsies and brushings (Ann IM 1984; 101:550)

Xray: UGIS usually positive; failure of ulcer to project beyond normal margin of stomach suggests is malignant rather than benign

Rx: Prevention in future perhaps by *H. pylori* screening and rx (Nejm 2001;345:829)

Surgical, perhaps followed by local irradiation and chemRx (Nejm 2001;345:725)

Chemotherapy, palliative only, but multiple drug, eg, 5-FU, adriamycin, mitomycin C

6.2 PANCREATIC DISEASES

ACUTE PANCREATITIS

Nejm 1999;340:1412; 1994;330:1198; 1992;326:635

Cause:

- Gallstones (45–75%); in lower common duct (Nejm 1974; 290:484), or biliary sludge, half the time visible on ultrasound, probably the occult cause in 2/3 idiopathic types (Nejm 1992; 326:589)
- Alcohol (10–35%) possibly from sphincter of Oddi spasm
- Idiopathic (10–30%)

Table 6.1.1   Medications for *H. Pylori* Rx (Jama 1996;275:624; Med Let 1996; 38:51)

Drug	Dose	Cost/Wk
Amoxicillin (not ampicillin)	1 gm po bid or 500 mg qid w meals and hs	cheap
Bismuth subsalicylate (Peptobismol)	ii tab (120 mg) po qid w meals and hs	$3
Clarithromycin	500 mg po b-tid w meals	$50–$75(tid)
Metronidazole (Flagyl)	250 mg po qid w meals and hs, or 500 mg bid	$3
Omeprazole (Prilosec)	20 mg po bid ac	$50
Tetracycline (not doxycycline)	500 mg po qid w meals and hs	$3
Rifabutin (Mycobutin)	300 mg po qd w PPI + amox for failures (Rx Let 2001;8:21)	

of disease: stop tobacco, alcohol, NSAIDs, coffee; combined antibiotic
+ antisecretory rx w/o more w/u is most cost-efficient initial
strategy (Ann IM 1995;123:260)
Medications:
1st: ANTIBIOTIC rx of *H. pylori* × 1–2 wk (see Tables 6.1.1 and 6.1.2
below). Only helps if ulcer present (Nejm 1999;341:1106)

Table 6.1.2   Cure Rates and Costs of Various Combinations to Rx *H. Pylori*
(Jama 1996;275:624; Med Let 1996;38:51)

Combination	Cure Rate, 95% Cls	Cost
Bismuth/metronidazole/tetracycline × 1 wk	86–90%	<$10
Bismuth/metronidazole/tetracycline × 2 wk	88–90%	<$10
Bismuth/metronidazole/tetracycline/ omeprazole × 1 wk	94–98%	$60
Bismuth/metronidazole/amoxicillin × 1 wk	75–81%	<$15
Bismuth/metronidazole/amoxicillin × 2 wk	80–86%	<$15
Metronidazole/clarithromycin/omeprazole × 1 wk	87–91%	$200
Amoxicillin/clarithromycine/omeprazole × 1 wk	86–91%	$200
Metronidazole/amoxicillin/omeprazole × 1–2 wk	77–83%	$50–$100 (2wk)
Amoxicillin/clarithromycin/lansoprazole (PrevPac) (Rx Let 1998;5:15) × 2 wk	84–90%	$200

- Hereditary types I and V hyperlipidemia
- Other, rare causes (10%): posterior duodenal ulcer; trauma, accidental or at operation; hyperparathyroidism w calcium stone formation; infectious, eg, mumps, coxsackie, many viruses including HIV as well as ascariasis and clonorchiasis in developing countries; cancer of duodenum, pancreas, or ampulla; choledochal cysts, duodenal diverticula; pancreas divisum; pregnancy; protein starvation (Ann IM 1971;74:270); vasculitis; drugs such as thiazides, steroids, sulfasalazine (Azulfidine) and other sulfas, furosemide, azathioprine (Nejm 1973;289:357); postpump after bypass surgery, probably from the iv CaCl given (Nejm 1991; 325:382)

Epidem: Male:female = 2:1; incidence ~400/million/yr, but in AIDS, 5–20/100/yr

Pathophys: Enzyme (trypsin and lipase) activation and retention in pancreatic substance leads to autodigestion

Hypocalcemia from calcium soap formation? (Nejm 1986;315:496) or glucagon-induced? (Nejm 1976;294:512)

Sx: Epigastric abdominal pain relieved by leaning forward, radiates to back/flank; abdominal distension, nausea, and vomiting

Si: Ileus; guarding; fever, or hypothermia sometimes; erythema nodosum-like lesions due to focal fat necrosis; Grey-Turner si = flank ecchymoses w retroperitoneal bleeding

Crs: 50–80% never recur. See Table 6.2.1

Cmplc: ARDS; ATN; tetany w hypocalcemia; shock; pancreatic abscess (4%) (Nejm 1972;287:1234); **pancreatic pseudocyst** formation, which can result in infection or rupture into peritoneal cavity, spleen or dissection along body planes (Nejm 1972;287:72); gi bleeding and splenomegaly from splenic vein thrombosis rare (Ann IM 1971;75:903)

Lab:

Chem: Amylase: serum levels up for 3 d, >225 IU, 95% sens, 98% specif (Ann IM 1985;102:576); higher in gallstone (often >1000) than alcoholic type; r/o false neg w elevated triglyceride; false pos w renal failure, macroglobulin binding (Nejm 1967;277:94), and salivary source (Ann IM 1979;91:200)

Glucose may be up from transient glucagon release (Ann IM 1975; 83:774)

Calcium reaches nadir at 2 d (Ann IM 1975;83:185)

GASTROENTEROLOGY

Table 6.2.1 Ranson Criteria (Am J Gastroent 1982;77:633) Risk Factors: Mortality <1% if ²2 Risk Factors, 16% if 3–4, 100% if 7 or More

	Risk Factors	
	If Not Gallstone Induced	If Gallstone Induced
on admission	age > 55	age > 70
	WBC > 16 000	WBC > 18 000
	glucose > 200 mg%	glucose > 220 mg%
	LDH > 350 IU	LDH > 400
	AST (SGOT) > 250	AST (SGOT) > 250
within 48 hr of admission	hct drops > 10 pts	hct drops > 10 pts
	BUN increased > 5 mg%	BUN increases > 2 mg%
	Ca < 8 mg%	Ca < 8 mg%
	pO_2 < 60 mmHg	
	acidotic	acidotic
	>6 L volume depleted	>4 L volume depleted

Lipase stays up longer than amylase, peaks at 4–7 d, correlates w hypertriglyceridemia that follows acute attacks

Isoamylase equally as good as lipase as a confirmation test (Ann IM 1985;102:576)

Alanine aminotransferase ≥3 normal indicates gall stone etiology w 95% certainty (Am J Gastroenterol 1994;89:1863)

Paracentesis fluid has elevated amylase (>100 U) and polys but no bacteria, helps r/o bowel strangulation

Amylase/creatinine clearance ratio probably not useful

Urine: Trypsinogen-2 dipstick positive (92% sens/specif) (Nejm 1997; 336:1788)

Hem: Crit may be >60% due to plasma loss; white count may be >25,000/mm³

Xray: Lytic bone lesions (fat necrosis); calcifications in pancreas; gallbladder ultrasound 2–3 wk after acute episode; CT w contrast if very ill

Rx: ICU care even if look stable initially w TPN

ERCP perhaps early (within 24–72 h) w sphincterotomy only if obstructive jaundice or cholangitis (Nejm 1997;336:237)

Opiates usually necessary although may worsen

Surgery substantially increases mortality; rarely needed if ERCP available; perhaps debridement late if massive necrosis or infected phlegmon

NG suction or cimetidine to decrease acid stimulation of pancreas via secretin debated, but neither shown to help (Ann IM 1985;103:86) but usually needed for ileus anyway

Antibiotics, eg, imipenem usually used × 2–4 wks, debatable help; more clearly helpful if gallstone induced

Peritoneal lavage no help (Nejm 1985;312:399)

CHRONIC PANCREATITIS AND PANCREATIC INSUFFICIENCY

Nejm 1995;332:1482

Cause: Recurrent acute attacks; chronic alcohol use (70%), damage precedes first attack of acute pancreatitis (p 256); surgical resection; cystic fibrosis, sometimes as the only manifestation of a CF gene mutation (Nejm 1998;339:645,653,687); hyperparathyroidism; sclerosing pancreatitis (Nejm 2001;344:732)

Epidem:

Pathophys: Sx from impairment of exo- and endocrine function. B_{12} deficiency from pancreatic intrinsic factor deficiency, restorable w pancreatic extract po (Nejm 1971;284:627). >90% destruction necessary before exocrine and/or endocrine function is impaired (Nejm 1972;287:813)

Sx: Recurrent acute attacks or abdominal pain; steatorrhea; weight loss

Si: Cachexia

Crs: 50% 20-yr mortality

Cmplc: Malabsorption and maldigestion including B_{12} deficiency, vit K deficiency, etc (p 285), diabetes; night blindness from vit A malabsorption (Nejm 1979;300:942); pancreatic duct obstruction into "chain of lakes"; pseudocyst formation (Nejm 1972;287:72); slightly (2–4%) incr incidence of pancreatic carcinoma after 10–20 yr (Nejm 1993;328:1433); biliary obstruction w reversible hepatic fibrosis (Nejm 2001;344:418)

Lab:

Chem: Amylase and lipase normal or mildly elevated because no more pancreatic tissue to release

Chronic Pancreatitis and Pancreatic Insufficiency, continued

Noninv: Maldigestion tests (p 285)
ERCP to evaluate duct if not clear on CT or KUB
Stool: Qualitative and quantitative elevations of fat by Sudan stains
Xray: Ultrasound, especially for cysts, 85% sens/specif; CT/MRI,
especially for tumors and cancer
KUB: pancreatic calcifications (30%)
Rx: Avoidance of alcohol may prevent recurrent pain but fibrosis can still
progress
Pancreatic enzymes 6–12 gm qd po w meals or q 1 h w antacids (Nejm
1977;296:1318; 1969;281:201), eg, pancrelipase (Viokase) 6 tab po
qid helps pain; microspheres now available, eg, Creon; in children
at least, must keep daily lipase dose <1000 U/kg to avoid fibrosing
colonopathy (Nejm 1997;336:1283)
Cimetidine 300 mg po 1/2 h ac can speed enzyme transit through
stomach and thus help po enzymes work better (Nejm 1977; 297:
854; 1977;299:995)
Surgically or endoscopically drain cysts, sphincterotomies, occasionally
pancreatectomies (Nejm 1968;279:570) and
pancreaticojejunostomies
of pain, celiac blocks, octreotide 200 mgm sc tid

PANCREATIC CARCINOMA
Nejm 1992;326:455

Cause: Neoplasia
Epidem: Incidence = 9/100,000/yr; incr in smokers, obesity (Jama 2001;
286:921, 967), gasoline/naphthalene/benzidine workers, pts after
partial gastrectomy, and perhaps cholecystectomy pts and diabetics
(Jama 2000;283:2552 vs Nejm 1994;331:83).
Pathophys: Si and sx produced by compression of adjacent tissues,
especially in head, and invasive replacement of pancreatic tissue
Stage I: Intrapancreatic
Stage II: Adjacent organs w/o nodes
Stage III: Node involvement
Stage IV: Diffusely metastatic
>75% are in head of pancreas, rest are in body and tail. See Table 6.2.2

Table 6.2.2

	Head %	Tail %		Head %	Tail %
Sx:					
weight loss	92	100	weakness	35	43
jaundice	90	7	pruritus	24	0
pain	90	90	diarrhea	18	3
anorexia	62	33	melena	12	17
nausea	45	43	hematemesis	3	17
vomiting	37	37	abdominal distension	8	17
Si:					
icterus	87	13	palpable gallbladder	29	0
big liver	83	33	tenderness	26	27
ascites	14	20	abdominal mass	13	23

Crs: 20% 1-yr, 3% 5-yr survival, lowest of all cancers

Cmplc: Diabetes (80%), from islet amyloid polypeptide secretion, hence reversible w resection (Nejm 1994;330:313); duodenal obstruction (10%)

r/o ampullary or distal bile duct cancer (Nejm 1999;341:1368), which has a 50% 5-yr survival w resection

Lab: Jaundice workup

Path: Needle aspiration cytology is 60–90% sensitive but causes seeding; ultrasonographic endoscopic fine needle aspiration, 90% sens, 95% specif (Ann IM 2001;134:459)

Serol: Ca 19-9 antibody elevated >70 U/cc; 70% sens, 87% specific (Ann IM 1989;110:704); useful to follow postop like CEA in colon cancer, not diagnostically, but useful if elevated in a nonoperative candidate w a mass on CT

Xray: Ultrasound, 36% false neg, usually done first to distinguish obstructive from nonobstructive jaundice, done endoscopically nearly 100% sens (Gastrointest Endosc 1991;37:347); CT scan 25% false neg (do first—Ann IM 1985;102:212). ERCP if any of the above positive (Mayo—Nejm 1977;297:737; rv of all—Nejm 1973;288:506); 7% false neg; scan w labeled VIP (Nejm 1994; 331:1116)

Rx: Surgical Whipple procedure or less if stage I, maybe if stage II, not if stage III or IV. This means only 5–10% are eligible; 10% operative mortality; 5–15% 5-yr survival

Palliative biliary and/or gastrojejunal bypass for younger, or ERCP stenting for elderly or sick; increase survival from 6 mo to nearly a year in some; chemotherapy w 5-FU + intra- and post-op radiation as adjuvant rx, or gemcitabine (Gemzar) (p 264)

6.3 BILIARY DISEASES

CHOLECYSTITIS AND BILIARY COLIC

Nejm 1993;328:412

Cause: Cholelithiasis (gallstones), often w secondary bacterial infection w common gi organisms. Possibly biliary sludge (Ann IM 1999;130: 301) but also seen reversibly in pregnancy, prolonged starvation/fasting, TPN (100% have sludge at 6 wk), ceftriaxone and octreotide therapy

Epidem: Female:male = 2:1; stones present in 10% of adult women in US, 70% in southwestern Native American women (Nejm 1970; 282:53). Higher incidence of stones with: increasing age, multiple pregnancies (Nejm 1980;302:362), during pregnancy but later reverting to normal (Ann IM 1993;119:116), chronic thiazide rx (debated—Nejm 1980;303:546 vs 1981;304:954), hemolytic disease, bcp (Nejm 1974;290:15) and marginally w ERT (Ann IM 2001;135:493), alcoholism, cirrhosis (45%), vagotomy, lower exercise levels (Nejm 1999;341:777), obesity especially during weight loss (Ann IM 1999;130:471; 1993;119:1029), ileal disease, elevated triglycerides

Lower risk w coffee (Jama 1999;281:2106), statin rx (Ann IM 2001; 135:493)

Pathophys: Stones are usually mucin protein + cholesterol (75%), less often w bilirubin and calcium (Hepatol 1982;2:879). Cholecystitis is inflammation/infection of gallbladder; colic is caused by an obstructed gallbladder

Sx: Colic, steady (thus colic is a misnomer), epigastric or right upper quadrant pain that subsides over several hours, radiates to right scapula; nausea and vomiting, w temporary partial relief after vomiting

Cholecystitis, persistent steady pain over days, first periumbilical, radiating to right upper quadrant as parietal peritoneum involved

Si: Fever; Murphy's si (tender subcostally on deep inspiration)

Crs: (Ann IM 1993;119:606) 10–20% chance of sx w stones over 20–30 yr (Nejm 1982;307:798), 2%/yr × 5 yr then diminishes; after first sx, 50% will recur over 20 yr, 25–50% get complications vs 1/3 will recur in 2 yr, 70% in 5 yr (Ann IM 1984;101:171)

Cmplc: Pancreatitis; common duct stone w biliary obstruction; **cholangitis,** infection of obstructed biliary collecting system; hydrops and/or empyema of gallbladder; perforation and peritonitis; rarely gallstone "ileus," a small bowel obstruction usually at ileocecal valve from stone that has eroded through gallbladder into duodenum or stomach; perhaps gallbladder cancer (Nejm 1979; 301:704), though stones may be effect rather than cause

Lab: Cholestasis/jaundice w/u (rv—Nejm 1983;308:1515); acute right upper quadrant pain w/u—Ann IM 1988;109:752, 722)

Chem: If stones in common duct or severe edema, usual pattern is obstructive LFTs including bilirubin, GGTP, and alkaline phosphatase elevation, usually higher than >AST (SGOT) or ALT (SGPT) elevations, though sometimes reversed

Urine: Urobilinogen elevated if bacterial infection in biliary tree is breaking down bile, eg, recently relieved obstruction, improving hepatitis, or ascending cholangitis

Xray: KUB may show calcified stones (20%); air in duodenal cap next to inflamed gallbladder (sentinel loop); or air in biliary tree, if cholangitis from gas formers or fistula formation; "porcelain gallbladder," ie, wall calcified, associated w cancer of gallbladder ~50% of the time

Gallbladder ultrasound (Ann IM 1988;109:722; Nejm 1980;302:1277) 5–10% false neg, 2–6% false pos, 1% indeterminant; sens/specif = 95%

HIDA scan, if doubt after ultrasound in acute, or occasionally as first test in acute (96% sens, 94% specif); no visualization of gallbladder indicates cholecystitis, no tracer into duodenum indicates common duct obstruction

Percutaneous cholangiography or ERCP if common duct obstruction

Perhaps biliary scintiscan (99% sens/specif) (Br J Surg 2000;87:181), or MR cholangiography (Gastroenterol 1996;110:589)

Rx: Prevention of stones w ursodeoxycholic acid 600 mg po qd in weight loss programs, NNT-4mo = 5 (Ann IM 1995;122:899)

of asx stone rarely indicated (Ann IM 1993;119:606,620); but maybe for people away from medical care, typhoid carriers, "porcelain gallbladders" (cancer risk), long-term TPN, and questionably in diabetics due to high operative mortality, especially if nonfunctioning, but not statistically demonstrable (Ann IM 1988; 109:913) and in other patients w predictably deteriorating health

of cholecystitis, cholecystectomy usually acutely; occasionally wait 1–2 wk for it to cool down

of symptomatic gallstones, even though ~30% won't recur (Ann IM 1993;119:606,620), usually open minilap vs laparoscopic cholecystectomy w ERCP 1st if suspect common duct stones that cannot get laparoscopically; laparoscopic technique shortens stay w less pain (Nejm 1991;324:1075; Med Let 1990;32:115) and lower mortality, being done at higher rate than opens were done (Nejm 1994;330:403; Lancet 1994;343:135). Adverse effects: **postcholecystectomy "cholecystitis" pain syndrome** due to obstruction of sphincter of Oddi, can rx w ERCP sphincterotomy (Nejm 1989;320:82) but that has a 21% cmplc rate (Nejm 1996;335:909). Rarely lithotripsy plus po rx with ursodeoxycholic acid (Ursodiol) (Ann IM 1994;121:207; Nejm 1990;323:1239)

PRIMARY BILIARY CIRRHOSIS

Nejm 1996;335:1570

Cause: Autoimmunity (Nejm 1974;290:63); associated w HLA-DR$_w$8 (Nejm 1990;322:1842). Impaired hepatic sulfoxidation (Nejm 1988;318:1089)

Epidem: Middle-aged women predominantly; female:male = 10:1; all races; incidence, 10/million/yr, 1000 × higher in members of affected families

Pathophys: Circulating immune complexes may be picked up by the liver and cause complement fixation and liver damage (Nejm 1979;300:274); damage also due to intracellular toxic bile acid deposition (Nejm 1991;324:1548). Pruritus of this and other causes of cholestasis probably induced via central opioid system (Ann IM 1995;123:161)

Sx: Chronic pruritus, most frequent initial sx along w fatigue, w subsequent insidious onset of jaundice; frequently also picked up by finding asx elevations of alkaline phosphatase. Diarrhea due to fat malabsorption/digestion

Si: Xanthomata (40%) in late disease; hepatomegaly initially, later small liver; splenomegaly in ?35% at time of dx, more later

Crs: Median survival 13 yr if asx, 7 yr if sx at time of dx; bilirubin levels are a rough predictor of course, consider transplant when become jaundiced

Cmplc: CREST syndrome, scleroderma, Sjögren's, primary hypothyroidism (20%), osteoporosis in most perhaps due to toxic impairment of osteoblast function (Ann IM 1985;103:855) w consequent fractures. No increase in ASHD despite elevated lipids (Ann IM 1975;82:227)

r/o sarcoid overlap disease (Nejm 1983;308:572); cholestatic drug reactions; mechanical obstruction by ultrasound, ERCP, or CT; primary sclerosing cholangitis (p 266)

Lab:

Chem: Alkaline phos and GGTP elevations $\gg$ bilirubin elevation (obstructive picture)

Cholesterol total and HDL elevated (50%), occasionally >1000 mg%

Path: Liver biopsy shows cirrhosis, elevated copper content, sometimes as high as in Wilson's disease (Ann IM 1972;76:62), bile duct dropout and granulomas (r/o sarcoid etc.—Nejm 1972;287:1284), small cell infiltrates in portal areas; staging predicts crs

Serol: Complement levels depressed (Ann IM 1979;90:72)

Antimitochondrial antibodies elevated in 90–95% (Ann IM 1972;77:533), but may be falsely positive in chronic (>3 mo) extrahepatic obstruction (Nejm 1972;286:1400); M_2 fraction is specif

IgM levels elevated

Rx: Supportive: cholestyramine or colestipol may help pruritus as can rifampin (Dig Dis Sci 1991;36:216); vit D and calcium to prevent osteoporosis; vitamins K, E, and A

Primary Biliary Cirrhosis, continued

Medical: ursodeoxycholic acid (Ursodiol) 13–15 mg/kg qd by RCT (Nejm 1994;330:1342 vs Lancet 1999;354:1053)

Methotrexate 5 mg po q 12 h × 3 q 1 wk (Ann IM 1997;126:682)

Colchicine 0.6 mg po bid prophylaxis helps decrease mortality and improve LFTs but not biopsy appearance (Nejm 1986;315:1448)

Surgical: liver transplant (Nejm 1990;322:1419; 1989;320:1709) can produce a 70% 5-yr survival; disease may recur? (Nejm 1982;306:1 vs Nejm 1985;312:1055)

PRIMARY SCLEROSING CHOLANGITIS

Nejm 1995;332:924

Cause: Genetic, plus viral precipitation?; HLA DR_w52a present in all, and HLA C_w7 present in 86% (Nejm 1990;322:1842)

Epidem: Associated w inflammatory bowel disease often (70%), especially ulcerative colitis, and retroperitoneal/mediastinal fibrosis; highest incidence in young men; 70% males; 70% under age 45 yr

Pathophys: Ongoing inflammation, destruction, and fibrosis of intra- and extrahepatic bile ducts, possibly from toxic bacterial products of the gut?

Sx: Insidious (≥ 1 yr) onset, fatigue, pruritus, jaundice; attacks of RUQ pain and chills

Si: Jaundice, big liver, big spleen (one or more present upon dx in 75%)

Crs: Many fatal within 10 yr w/o early detection and rx, but many cases much more benign

Cmplc: Cirrhosis and portal hypertension

r/o primary biliary cirrhosis (p 264), chronic active hepatitis (p 275), and idiopathic biliary ductopenia (Nejm 1997;336:835)

Lab:

Chem: Alkaline phosphatase $\geq 2\times$ normal, ceruloplasmin and other copper studies elevated (75%), bilirubin elevated in 50%

Noninv: ERCP is diagnostic, showing narrowings and dilatations of ducts

Path: Liver biopsy shows cholangitis/portal hepatitis, and later periportal hepatic fibrosis w bridging and eventual biliary cirrhosis

Xray: Cholangiograms show strictures, irregular tortuosity of intra- and extrahepatic bile ducts; extrahepatic duct involvement distinguishes from primary biliary cirrhosis

Rx: None short of liver transplant; 70% 1-yr survival w transplant
Antibiotics for acute bouts of pain
Ursodiol (ursodeoxycholic acid) (Nejm 1997;336:691; Hepatol 1992; 16:707); plus perhaps immunosuppressants (Ann IM 1999;131:943) like azathioprine, prednisone, and/or methotrexate (Gastroenterol 1994;106:494 vs Ann IM 1987;106:231), all may help LFTs but no effect on cr

6.4 HEPATIC DISEASES

GILBERT'S DISEASE (Familial Nonhemolytic Jaundice)

Ann IM 1972;77:527; Nejm 1967;277:1108

Cause: Genetic, autosomal recessive, but positive family hx in 40% because so common; defect is in the promoter region of the gene so less glucuronyl transferase produced although what is made is normal (Nejm 1995;333:1171)

Epidem: Male:female = 2:1; common explanation of mild elevations of unconjugated bilirubin found serendipitously on chem screens. Prevalence = 3–10%

Pathophys: Diminished hepatocyte uptake of circulating unconjugated bilirubin and decr glucuronyl transferase activity; some studies show 50% decrease in rbc survival but others subsequently show no incr in hemolysis (Ann IM 1975;82:552)

Sx: Jaundice especially w starvation (>24 h), infection, alcohol, exercise. Hepatic tenderness often present w onset but probably because this is a nonspecific sx that brings attention to the jaundice

Si: Scleral icterus in otherwise healthy person

Crs: Benign, does not appear before age 10 yr

Cmplc: None

Lab:

Chem: Bilirubin = 1–3 mg %, predominantly indirect; unnecessary usually to confirm by checking fasting (<300 cal/d) levels, which rise to 6 mg% over 3 d. Other LFTs normal

Hem: CBC normal
Path: Liver bx, which should not be done, will be normal
Rx: None (phenobarb has been given for questionable sx of malaise, probably unrelated)

ALCOHOLIC HEPATITIS
Nejm 1988;319:1639

Cause: Ethanol and poor nutrition

Epidem: Perhaps an unusual metabolism in predisposed people, hotly debated (Nejm 1976;294:9); but something genetically and metabolically different since twins raised apart and sons of alcoholic fathers raised apart have incr incidence (Science 1984;225:1493)

Pathophys: (rv of ethanol metabolism—Nejm 1970;283:24,71) Acute and chronic complications of alcohol occur more often in women than men due not to size differences but to differences in gastric mucosa alcohol dehydrogenase activity (Nejm 1990;322:95)

Sx: Those of hepatitis

Si: Fever
Dupuytren's contractures; parotid enlargement

Crs:

Cmplc: Laënnec's cirrhosis; hepatic failure (p 280)

Lab:
Chem: AST (SGOT) incr > ALT (SGPT), usually
Hem: Depressed platelets, smaller than average size, indicates direct alcohol suppression of synthesis
Path: Liver bx shows fatty liver infiltration (r/o fatty infiltration of pregnancy (p 616), and other non-alcoholic steatohepatitises w abnormal LFTs as in obesity (Ann IM 2000;132:112), diabetes, tetracycline in high doses, CCl_4, steroid rx, starvation, and hyperlipidemias (Am J Med 1999;107:450; Ann IM 1997;126:136); usually alcoholic hyaline distinguishes it from viral hepatitis

Rx: Propylthiouracil 150 mg po bid decreases damage and mortality (Nejm 1987;317:1421); may help other toxic exposure damage too, like Tylenol overdose

Prednisone 40 mg qd × 28 d, possibly helpful in severe acute alcoholic hepatitis (Ann IM 1990;113:299; 1989;110:685 vs Gut 1995; 37:113)

Pentoxifylline (Trental) (Gastroenterol 2000;119:1637) 400 mg po tid × 4wk may be better than prednisone

Androgens (oxandrolone) × 30 d may be helpful (Nejm 1984; 311:1464)

of cirrhosis, perhaps colchicine 1 mg po qd (Nejm 1988;318:1709)

AUTOIMMUNE HEPATITIS

Nejm 1996;334:897; 1995;333:958,1004

Cause: Autoimmunity to HLA IB8, IIDR3, and DR52a loci

Epidem: F >>M; overlap w primary biliary cirrhosis, primary sclerosing cholangitis, chronic hepatitis C (Ann IM 1996;125:588)

Pathophys:

Sx: Malaise, jaundice

Si: Of chronic liver disease, eg spiders, jaundice, splenomegaly

Crs:

Cmplc: Cirrhosis/liver failure, reversible w rx (Ann IM 1997;127:981)

Lab:

Chem: ALT (SGPT), AST (SGOT), bilirubin all elevated

Serol: Globulins incr, esp γ globulins; autoantibodies, esp ANA, anti-smooth muscle, and anti-actin antibodies at titers >1/40 (Nejm 1995;333:958,1004)

Rx: Steroids + azathioprine help 85+%

HEPATITIS A (Infectious Hepatitis)

Nejm 1985;313:1059

Cause: Hepatitis A virus, a pico-RNA enterovirus

Epidem: Fecal/oral contact w infected persons for up to a year after clinical disease (Jama 1958;200:365); occasionally parenteral; higher incidence in parents of daycare center children, children are often asx (Nejm 1980;302:1222)

In developing countries, 3/1000/mo incidence for first class hotel users, 20/1000/mo for community living guests; thus is most frequent preventable infection in travelers (Jama 1994;272:885)

Pathophys: Only in humans; because it is an enterovirus, incidence up in late summer and early winter; 45% of adults have had it (Nejm 1976;95:755); incr incidence in gay males (Nejm 1980;302:438)

Sx: 15–40 d incubation period (Am J Med 5/62)

In children, only 5–15% get sx

Malaise (48% in children/63% in adults), anorexia (41%/42%), abdominal pain (48%/37%), fever and/or chills (41%/32%), jaundice (65%/88%), diarrhea (58%/18%), dark urine (58%/68%), light stools (58%/58%), nausea and vomiting (65%/26%)

Si: Jaundice, though anicteric form also common and more benign

Crs: Benign, 15% morbidity and rare (0.3%) mortality (Ann IM 1998; 128:111); sx peak 2 wk after onset and take about 4 wk to clear; relapse in 6% at 1–3 mo (Ann IM 1987;106:221)

Cmplc: Fulminant hepatitis, relapsing hepatitis, no chronic active hepatitis (Eric Mast, CDC 11/95)

r/o Q fever, mononucleosis, CMV, toxoplasmosis, Fitzhugh-Curtis syndrome, psittacosis, and other viral hepatitis (p 275), esp hepatitis E, which is spread via water sources esp. in equatorial areas (Virol 1993;4:273) and in pregnant women, who have a 25% mortality (Eric Mast, CDC 11/95)

Lab:

Chem: Typical hepatitis enzyme picture w ALT (SGPT) > AST (SGOT) > LDH > alkaline phos levels

Serol: Hepatitis A IgM antibody present when first sx present (Ann IM 1982;96:193); later IgM goes negative and IgG appears and stays

Rx: (Ann IM 1985;103:391)

Prevent by: avoiding fecal contamination

Vaccine, inactivated (Havrix, or Vaqta) (Nejm 1997;336:197; Med Let 1995;37:51; Jama 1995;273:906; 1994;272:885; Nejm 1992;327:453) 2-shot (1 cc w 1440 ELU im) series for adults 6–12 mo apart, 3-shot (0.55 cc, 720 ELU im) series for children at 0, 1 mo, and 6–12 mo; 100% effective, no need to screen titers if born after 1945, may be useful post exposure (80% efficacy) (Lancet 1999;353:1136) but not clearly better than IgG (ACP J Club 1999;131:45), how often will need to boost still unclear; cost, $55/dose

Prophylax w IgG 0.02 cc/kg up to 2 cc im if exposed
of disease, bed rest probably no benefit (Nejm 1969;281:193)

HEPATITIS B

Nejm 1997;337:1733, Ann IM 1980;93:165

Cause: Hepatitis B virus; genetic susceptibility at least for carrier states?
(Nejm 1973;289:1162)

Epidem: Primarily spread venereally or via blood and blood products
(transfusion risk = 1/63,000—Nejm 1996;334:1685), fresh, dry, or
frozen (Nejm 1978;298:637), eg, communal autolet in hospitals
(Nejm 1992;326:721). Transmitted by mucous membranes but not
by urine and feces (Nejm 1969;281:1375); and via eczematous skin
(Ann IM 1976;85:573). Reactivated in HBsAg carriers w
chemotherapy (Ann IM 1982;96:447)

Increased incidence in medical personnel, gay males (Ann IM 1982;
96:170), renal dialysis units (Nejm 1969;281:571), narcotic addicts
(Nejm 1967;276:703)

Pathophys: Sometimes viral DNA incorporated into liver genome, then
less hepatitis, but still can produce HBsAg, associated w carcinoma
more often? (Nejm 1986;315:1187)

Sx: 60–160 d incubation period; arthralgias/arthritis (Ann IM 1971;74:
207; 1971;75:29; Nejm 1978;298:185), cryoglobulins (Ann IM
1977;87:287), urticaria and other rashes (Ann IM 1978;89:34)

Si: Many cases anicteric

Crs: Acute hepatitis, leads to:
- Benign course, recover or have relapsing, or portal mild
  hepatitis; or
- Acute liver necrosis; all pts die w/o transplant; or
- Submassive hepatic necrosis (bridging); 60% of pts die or go on to
  postnecrotic cirrhosis, the balance recover completely; or
- Chronic active hepatitis, usually with a progressive downhill
  course over 5–10 yr; or
- Asx carrier state in ~90% newborns, 20% school age children,
  <1% young healthy adults (WWII vaccine epidemic—Nejm 1987;
  316:965)

Cmplc: Hepatoma, 2% over 10 yr (Ann IM 2001;135:759); chronic
active hepatitis (10%) (p 275); delta (δ) agent infection (hepatitis D),

an RNA viral parasite of hep B virus, only can replicate if hep B around, leads to acute hepatitis itself or severe chronic active hepatitis (Nejm 1987;317:1256), hep B carriers get it from subsequent transfusions (Nejm 1985;312:1488,1515); fasting hypoglycemia (Nejm 1972;286:1436); serum sickness (20%), polyarteritis, nephritis (Bull Rheum Dis 1983;33:16) especially membranous GN (Nejm 1991;324:1457)

Lab:

Chem: Typical hepatitis enzyme picture w ALT (SGPT) > AST (SGOT) > LDH > alkaline phos levels; get CPK to r/o myopathy if LDH > AST (SGOT) > ALT (SGPT)

Path: Liver bx, consider if not improving in 2–3 wk

Serol: Core IgM antibody always up by time of first sx (Nejm 1978; 298:1379); HBsAg (Ann IM 1982;96:193) elevated; e-antigen elevation correlates w infectivity; anti-HBsAg appears shortly after sx develop, but there may be a window of infectivity when HBsAg and antibody is negative but core (c) antibody is positive which, if IgM, can be distinguished from remote infection w attenuation of all but IgG core antibody (S. Sears 11/95). See Fig. 6.4.1

Rx: (Ann IM 1985;103:391)

Prevention:

- Body fluid precautions including wearing gloves (Ann IM 1981; 95:133)
- Monitor hep B pos health workers but let work unless surgeons doing high exposure surgery, then should not work if HBeAg positive or documented transmissions (Nejm 1997;336:178)
- Screen all pregnant women for HBsAg (Ann IM 1987;107:412) so can prophylax and immunize their infants
- Hep B immune globulin (HBIG) prophylaxis 0.05 cc/kg × 2, 30 d apart within 24–72 h of exposure, $160/dose (Nejm 1980;303: 833; Med Let 1978;20:9); for newborns of HBsAg pos mothers 0.5 cc within 12 h of birth (Nejm 1985;313:1398) along w vaccine
- Immunization w recombinant vaccine (Nejm 1997 336:196; Med Let 1985;27:118; Ann IM 1982;97:379,362); cmplc: rare post-vaccine alopecia (Jama 1997;278:1176), no incr in later MS (Nejm 2001;344:319,327), perhaps other autoimmune diseases (RA?) (Rx Let 1998;5:72)

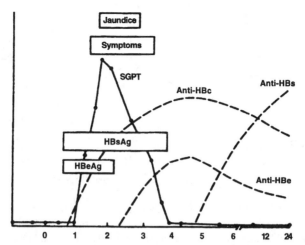

Figure 6.4.1 Course of hepatitis B serologies. (Reproduced with permission from Modern Medicine 1983;51:53. Copyright by Advanstar Communications, Inc.)

Adults/children w 20 μgm q 1 mo × 2 then 3rd dose in 6–12 mo like
   dT, or q 1 yr × 3 doses also works (Rx Let 1999;6:38); $100; boost
   w 2 μgm q 3 yr? (Ann IM 1988;108:185), q 10 yr (S. Sears 11/95);
   less effective in gay males (Nejm 1986;315:209); neither vaccine nor
   HBIG necessary if anti-HBc present, but are needed if only
   anti-HBsAg (Ann IM 1985;103:21,201)
Newborns, all w 10 μgm at birth, 1 and 6 mo (Jama 1995;
   274:1201) esp to SE Asian children to prevent 7% incid of
   child-to-child transmisssion (Jama 1996;276:906; Nejm 1989;
   321:1301); for newborns of HBsAg pos mothers (Med Let 1992;
   34:69), vaccinate and give HBIG as above. Vaccination has halved
   Taiwan rate of childhood hepatoma (Nejm 1997;336:1855)
of disease, to prevent cirrhosis progression and/or hepatoma:
Interferon-α-2a or -2b × 4–6 mo may permanently help 30–40% if
   given early on, certainly for chronic δ-agent infection (Nejm 1994;
   330:88), and for chronic hep B (Nejm 1994;330:137), esp if
   e-antigen pos (Nejm 1996;334:1422; Ann IM 1995;122:664)

Lamivudine (3TC) 100$^+$ mg po qd × 1 yr (Nejm 1999;341:1256; 1998;339:61, 114), but resistance develops so multidrug regimens being explored (Ann IM 2000;132:723)

No steroids (Nejm 1976;294:722)

HEPATITIS C

Nejm 2001;345:41; Jama 1997;277:1268; Ann IM 2000;132:296

Cause: Hepatitis C RNA virus, several genotypes, 1a and 1b most common in US

Epidem: 1.8% prevalence of antibodies in the US, 4 million infected (Nejm 1999;341:556), but up to 5$^+$% in Africa and Middle East

Over 50% of cases due to iv drug use; 50–80% of iv drug users contract within first yr of use; 97% of post-transfusion hepatitis in US (Nejm 1991;325:1325)

Transfusions, incidence = 1/100,000 transfusions using screened blood (Nejm 1996;334:1685), 18/10,000 using unscreened blood (Nejm 1992;327:369)

Post-organ transplant, eg, renal (Nejm 1992;326:454)

Sexual transmission rates are low but real, eg, 2–3% annual incidence in wives of infected hemophiliacs (Ann IM 1994;120:748; 1991; 115:764)

Neonatal transmission rate low, 2.5% (Ann IM 1992;117:881,887) to 5% (Nejm 1994;330:744) as is intrafamilial rate (Jama 1995;274: 1459)

Chronic carrier state develops in 85$^+$% after acute infection and lasts years even w normal LFTs (Nejm 1992;327:1899); 75–90% w hep C antibody have viremia (Nejm 1990;323:1107)

Pathophys: No protective antibody response develops

Sx: 2–20 wk incubation, 6–7 wk average; 80% are anicteric

Si:

Crs: 17$^+$ yr after infection, 80$^+$% had fatigue, all had at least mild inflammation on bx, 55% had pos enzymes, but only 2% had cirrhosis (Jama 2000;284:450; Nejm 1999;340:1228); vs 11% of HCV pos army recruits eventually got liver disease over 45 yr (Ann IM 2000;132:105)

Cmplc: Mixed cryoglobulinemia (p 382)

Chronic active hepatitis in 80% over 10^+ yr, 20–35% of whom go on to cirrhosis over 20^+ yr; hepatocellular carcinoma 1–4%/yr after onset of cirrhosis; get CPK, especially if LDH > AST (SGOT) > ALT (SGPT) to r/o myopathy; liver bx (do if sx beyond 6–12 mo or worsening) shows fibrosis w bridging between hepatic lobules but pathologic picture waxes and wanes

Vasculitis of various types

r/o other causes of chronically elevated LFTs: hemochromatosis, Wilson's disease, α_1-antitrypsin deficiency (Nejm 1981;304:558), drug-induced hepatitis from various drugs including α methyldopa and oxyphenisatin laxatives (Nejm 1971;285:813), NSAIDs (Med Let 1983;25:15), primary biliary cirrhosis (p 264), alcohol and other toxins, diabetes, myxedema, myopathies

r/o other non-A non-B hepatitis like: **hepatitis E** virus infection, an enterovirus that causes only acute mild hepatitis like hep A (Nejm 1997;336:795); and **hepatitis G,** rare, benign, blood-borne (Nejm 1997;336:741,747,795; Ann IM 1997;126:874), and may impair HIV virulence (Nejm 2001;345:707,715,761)

Lab:

Chem: Elevated LFTs, esp SGPT (ALT), but not 100% sens (Ann IM 1995;123:330)

Serol: Anti hep C virus IgG antibody levels (ELISA w RIBA f/u) first detectable 10–50 wk after exposure and 4–50 wk after LFT elevations appear; hep C viral RNA correlates w infectivity and persistence as chronic active hepatitis (Nejm 1991;325:98), tested for by PCR method or more inconsistent branched-chain DNA PCR assay (Ann IM 1995;123:321). Cryoglobulins in 50%

Path: Liver bx

Rx: (Mmwr 1998;47:RR-19)

Prevent by avoiding high risk behaviors (iv drugs, sexual promiscuity), body fluid precautions, and by screening donors for anti-HCV levels will prevent 60% (Nejm 1990;323:1107) to 85% of cases; a small % of donors will be infectious but won't yet be antibody positive

Prophylaxis w immune globulin is ineffective

of disease (Ann IM 2000;133:665) (elevated ALT, viremia and cirrhosis on bx); decreases incidence of hepatoma (Ann IM 1998;129:94); much more effective in the 25% w a susceptibility gene (Nejm 1996; 334:77); NIH CDC suggests checking ALT and RNA levels after 6 mo rx and stopping if not markedly improved (Ann IM 1997;

127:855,866,918; Hepatol 1996;24:778). May decr cancer incidence 50[+]% (Ann IM 1999;131:174); can reverse cirrhotic fibrosis (Ann IM 2000;132:517) w

- interferon α-2a (Roferon-A), or α-2b (Intron-A) sc tiw × 24–52 wk; or better, prolonged release form, peg α-2a (Peg-Intron) (Med Let 2001;43:54) q 1 wk (Nejm 2000;343:1667,1673,1723), $1000/mo, combined w
- Ribavirin (Med Let 1999;41:53; Am J Med 1999;107:112; Lancet 1998;352:1426) (sold w interferon α-2b as Rebetron; ways to give w peg α-2a available soon) × 6–12 mos, many side effects and $8000/6 mo, but helps over 50% cost effectively (Am J Med 2000; 108:366);

Other options: liver transplant; lamivudine (3TC) possibly at 100[+] mg pq qd (Nejm 1995;333:1657); hep A vaccination if not immune already, to prevent frequently fatal hep A infection of chronic hep C hepatitis (Nejm 1998;338:286)

WILSON'S DISEASE

Ann IM 1991;115:720; Nejm 1978;298:1347

Cause: Genetic, autosomal recessive, on chromosome #13

Epidem: Onset age 6–50 yr; usually late childhood; hepatitis sx usually appear before age 30, CNS sx usually after 30. Heterozygote (single gene) prevalence = 1/200; disease prevalence = 1/30,000

Pathophys: A chronic hepatitis. Defective Cu metabolism/excretion w deposition in liver and basal ganglia; ceruloplasm binding defect from diminished ceruloplasmin synthesis, a chromosome #13 gene. Either hepatic or neurologic sx may predominate or exist alone

Sx: Tremulousness (50% at time of dx); abdominal pain (42% at dx); dystonia (36% at dx), especially loss of fine hand motor function, eg, writing or piano playing; excessive salivation and drooling; psychiatric sx; hepatic failure sx

Si: Kaiser-Fleischner ring (68%), brownish opacity around edge of cornea, usually seen by slit lamp only early (Ann IM 1977;86:285); hepatomegaly (50%); splenomegaly (50%); neurologic si's like resting and intention tremors (50%), dysarthria (50%) and drooling

(12%), ataxia (32%), rigidity, and major psychiatric si (12%); blue
nail lunulae

Crs: Chronic illness leading to death before age 30 yr if no rx

Cmplc: Portal hypertension, hypersplenism; hemolytic anemia (Ann IM
1970;73:413); proximal tubule Fanconi-like syndrome (Ann IM
1968;68:770)

Lab:

Chem: Ceruloplasmin < 20 μgm%, 7% false negative, falsely positive
in heterozygotes 10% of the time and in babies age <6 mo, or w
estrogen rx (Ann IM 1977;86:285; Nejm 1968;278:352)

Uric acid decr due to poor proximal tubule reabsorption, r/o ASA rx,
Fanconi syndrome, and other renal tubular syndromes (Ann IM
1974;80:42)

Hem: Thrombocytopenia (22%)

Path: Liver bx shows chronic active hepatitis histology or biliary
cirrhosis (Nejm 1982;306:319) and Cu content >100 μgm or 3.9
mmol/gm dry liver, falsely positive in primary biliary cirrhosis and
heterozygotes; >250 μgm/gm dry liver, falsely positive only in
babies age <6 mo (Nejm 1968;278:352)

Urine: Cu excretion/24 h >100 μgm in later stages; aminoaciduria

Rx: Prevent by screening family members for ceruloplasmin and copper
levels, or by PCR analysis (Ann IM 1997;127:21)

of disease:

1st: D-penicillamine po daily; probably reasonable to rx asx people;
questionable if children can be on it safely (Nejm 1975;
293:1300). Adverse effects: rash and renal tubular damage

2nd: Trientine qd divided between meals; increase q 6 mo to get Cu
<20 μgm% (Nejm 1987;317:209; Med Let 1986;28:67)

3rd: Zinc, po (Ann IM 1983;99:314), which inhibits gi Cu
absorption

HEMOCHROMATOSIS

Nejm 1999;341:1986; Jama 1998;280:172; Ann IM 1980;93:519 (35
cases)

Cause: Genetic (Ann IM 1999;130:953), most are autosomal recessive
HFE gene mutation C282Y on chromosome #6 (Nejm 1999;341:

718,755), 50^+% manifestation in homozygotes; but a small % are H63D mutations of the same gene (Jama 2001;285:2216)

Iron overload, eg, in thalassemia major patients (Ann IM 1983;99:450), or dietary overload in African genetically predisposed (Nejm 1992;326:95). Heterozygous state may have some reproductive advantage to women by preventing iron deficiency (Nejm 1996;335:1799)

Epidem: Usually in pts age >40 yr; women usually older than men since menstruation protects (Ann IM 1997;127:105). Gene frequency ~1/15, 1/250 are homozygotes (Nejm 1999;341:718,755; 1988; 318:1355). Many homozygous pts have asx or unreported cmplc and go undetected (Nejm 2000;343:1529)

Pathophys: A chronic hepatitis; hemosiderin deposition especially in pancreas, skin, liver, testes, heart, kidneys

Sx: Increased skin pigmentation (iron stimulation of melanin production); weakness/fatigue (70%); abdominal pain (60%); arthritis (often first sx in 40–60%); diabetic sx's

Si: Skin pigmentation (75%), diabetic si's (60%); cardiac failure

Crs: Normal life expectancy w phlebotomies if no cirrhosis (Nejm 1985; 313:1256); heterozygotes have mildly elevated iron levels but no iron overload cmplc (Nejm 1996;335:1799)

Cmplc: Hepatic cirrhosis (60%), hepatoma (10%); pituitary impotence (30%), reversible w rx (Ann IM 1984;101:629); CHF from myocardiopathy w a rapidly downhill course; diabetes, usually insulin dependent

Lab:

Chem: α-Fetoglobulin elevated (r/o hepatoma); cirrhotic LFTs
- Ferritin >250 μgm/L (women), >350 μgm/L (men) (99.5% sens, 94% specif) (Ann IM 1998;128:338) or less (Ann IM 2000; 133:329)
- Iron/TIBC % saturations >60% (Nejm 1982;307:1702) in men, >50% in women (98% sens, 94% specif) (Ann IM 1998;128:338) or less (Ann IM 2000;133:329)
- Genetic analysis for C282Y mutation of HFE gene (Ann IM 2000; 132:261)

Path: Bx of liver, synovium, marrow, rectal mucosa all show incr iron deposition and, in liver, cirrhosis w periportal concentrations

Rx: Prevent by screening all adults w Fe and TIBC for homozygous state by above iron level criteria (Ann IM 1998;128:338); or pt and family members for C282Y mutation of HFE gene, useful and cheap ($95) (Ann IM 2000;132:261)

of disease:

   1st: Phlebotomy of 1 U q 3–7 d to keep ferritin <50 μgm/L, may take 1^+ yr, then 3–4x/yr to keep there; rapid, effective, and safer than deferoxamine (Clem Finch, 1972)

   2nd: Deferoxamine iv or sc (Nejm 1977;297:418); 12-h sc pump best, especially for Fe overload patients, eg, thalassemia major (Ann IM 1983;99:450). Adverse effects: deafness and blindness (Nejm 1986;314:869). Or L_1, an iron chelator, oral as effective as parenteral (Clin Pharmacol Ther 1991;50:294)

HEPATOMA, HEPATOCELLULAR CARCINOMA
Ann IM 1988;108:390

Cause: Idiopathic neoplasia; or associated w hep B virus chronic carrier state, although HBsAg may be undetectable (Nejm 1990;323:80), or hep C (Ann IM 1991;115:644) because of the cirrhosis it causes (Ann IM 1992;116:97)

Epidem: Higher incidence in hep B carriers, postnecrotic cirrhosis (probably all hep B), and hemochromatosis (iron overload patients w hep B or C?). Increasing incidence associated w hep C in Japan (Nejm 1993;328:1797,1802) and in US now 2.5/100,000 (Nejm 1999;340:745)

Pathophys: Hep B causes hepatoma somehow by viral genome incorporation into liver cell DNA

Sx: Failure to thrive; worsening ascites or liver failure

Si: Abdominal mass; cachexia

Crs: <5% 5 yr survival (Nejm 1999;340:745)

Cmplc: Polycythemia (Lancet 1967;2:1276), gynecomastia due to HCG production, hypercalcemia due to incr PTH (Nejm 1970;282:704), dysfibrinogenemia bleeding, 2nd primary hepatoma in 45% at 3 yr (Nejm 1996;334:1561)

   r/o birth control pill-induced pedunculated liver tumors (Ann IM 1975; 83:301), can regress off pill (Ann IM 1977;86:180)

Lab:
  Chem: Alkaline phos elevated more than bilirubin
  B_{12} incr 10–100× normal in adolescent group only due to binding
    protein (Nejm 1973;289:1053)
  α-Fetoprotein/protein ratio incr (a nonfunctioning fibrinogen—Nejm
    1978;299:221); 50% false neg, 1% false pos (Nejm 1968;278:984);
    but r/o embryonal cell testicular and gastric cancers (Nejm 1971;
    285:1058), and low level elevations in ataxia telangiectasia and
    5–10% of viral hepatitis
  Hem: Increased abnormal prothrombin (Nejm 1984;310:1427);
    polycythemia in 10%
Xray: Cold mass by routine liver scan/ultrasound, CT, or MRI; hot by
  gallium
Rx: Prevent by screening cirrhotics w α-fetoprotein levels and
  ultrasounds? (Nejm 1991;325:675)
  Surgical lobectomy sometimes possible (Nejm 1994;331:1547)
    followed by interferon rx if bhep C caused (Ann IM 2001;134:963),
    or total hepatectomy w liver transplant (Ann IM 1998;129:643;
    Nejm 1996;334:693)
  Percutaneous ethanol injection of tumor, or surgical extirpation w f/u
    vit A analog po qd decreases rate of 2nd primary tumors (Nejm
    1996;334:1561)
  Chemoembolization no help (Nejm 1995;332:1256)

HEPATIC FAILURE: ASCITES
  Nejm 1994;330:337; 1993;329:1862; Ann IM 1986;105:573

Cause: Multiple etiologies result in end-stage hepatic failure, which has
  four major complications: ascites, hemorrhage, renal failure, and
  encephalopathy
Pathophys: Ascites underfill theory is that postsinusoidal block raises
  portal vein pressure, which causes capsular weeping, which causes
  decr blood volume and incr aldosterone and ADH, which causes
  more extracellular fluid and/or ascites; or underfill may be due to
  vasodilatation of splanchnic bed (cf pregnancy—Nejm 1988;319:
  1127) and caused by excess nitric oxide production by endothelial

cells (Nejm 1998;339:533); others support a comparable overfill theory w incr sympathetic activity (Ann IM 1991;114:373).

Budd-Chiari hepatic vein occlusion occurs (75% of cases) w occult myeloproliferative disease especially in young adult females (Ann IM 1985;103:329)

Sx: Abdominal swelling/edema

Si: Increased abdominal girth; fluid wave, shifting dullness, spiders, hepatosplenomegaly

Crs: 50% 2-yr mortality

Cmplc: Pleural effusions, usually on R side from ascites leakage into chest (Am J Med 1999;107:262). Spontaneous bacterial peritonitis (Nejm 1999;341:403), present in 20% of those admitted w ascites; dx by peritoneal fluid WBC counts >250 and cultures; rx w cefotaxime plus iv albumen to prevent hepatorenal syndrome;

r/o **Meig's syndrome** of ovarian carcinoma and peritoneal mesothelioma

Lab:

Ascitic fluid: Transudate (serum albumin level $\geq$1.1 gm% greater than ascitic albumin level) (Ann IM 1992;117:215), contrasts w malignant ascites (Am J Med 1984;77:83)

Bact: Ascitic fluid w pH <7.31 suggests peritonitis; if poly count >250/mm^3, take cultures in blood culture medium flasks

Chem: Hyponatremia in ascitics from hypovolemia-induced ADH (Ann IM 1982;96:413)

Rx: Prophylaxis of SBP (GE 1991;100:477) w norfloxacin

of nontense ascites: Na restriction + spironolactone working up to 400 mg qd w furosemide to achieve 1 kg/d loss if edema present, 0.3 kg qd if not (Nejm 1970;282:1391)

of tense ascites:

- Transjugular intrahepatic portosystemic stent (TIPS) shunt placement works like other shunting procedures w a 5% significant bleeding cmplc rate and 25% encephalopathy induction rate; used for both bleeding and intractable ascites (Nejm 1995; 332:1192,1994;330:165,182; Ann IM 1995;122:816; Jama 1995; 273:1824); better than large volume taps? (Nejm 2000;342:1701 vs 1745); or

- 4–6 L paracentesis w or w/o optional 6–8 gm albumin iv (GE 1996;111:1002) Ann IM 1990;112:889) or dextran (J Clin Gastroenterol 1992;14:31); then repeated outpt taps; or

- Peritoneal/venous LaVeen shunt (Nejm 1991;325:829; 1989; 321:1632); or
- Perhaps extracorporeal ultrafiltration and iv reinfusion; or
- Liver transplant

HEPATIC FAILURE: HEMORRHAGE
Nejm 2001;345:669; 1993;329:1862; 1989;320:1393,1469

Cause: Multiple etiologies result in end-stage hepatic failure, which has four major complications: ascites, hemorrhage, renal failure, and encephalopathy

Pathophys: Variceal bleeding and/or gastritis/ulcers; depressed prothrombin and fibrinogen; depressed platelets from bleeding and hypersplenism; perhaps diminished platelet adhesiveness from incr BUN (Nejm 1969;280:677); incr plasminogen activators due to diminished hepatic filtration

Sx: Hematemesis, melena

Si:

Crs: Cause of death in 20% of cirrhotics (Nejm 1966;275:61)

Cmplc:

Lab:

Hem: Clotting studies, serial hemoglobin/hematocrit

Rx: Preventive maneuvers (Ann IM 1992;117:59; Nejm 1987;317:893)
- Propranolol or other β blocker to pulse <60, decreases recurrent bleeding and first bleeds, and increases survival by 5–10% (Nejm 1999;340:1033 vs 988; 1991;324:1532)
- Isosorbide (Isordil) 20–40 mg po bid as good (GE 1993;104: 1460), or used w β blocker is better than scleroRx (Lancet 1996;348:1677; Nejm 1996;334:1624); and then endoscopic ligation (Nejm 2001;345:648)
- TIPS shunt placement works like other shunting procedures w a 5% significant bleeding cmplc rate and 25% encephalopathy induction rate; used for both bleeding and intractable ascites (Jama 1995;273:1824; Nejm 1994; 330:165,182)
- Surgical shunt for recurrent bleeding, not prophylactically (Ann IM 1969;70:675)

of acute bleeding:

- Somatostatin analogs like: octreotide 25 mgm/h iv continuous drip (Nejm 1995;333:555 vs BMJ 1995;10:310); or valpreotide 50 μgm iv bolus then drip/hour (Nejm 2001;344:23), prior to endoscopy to help decr acute bleeding but no incr in survival
- Vasopressin or terlipressin
- Sengstaaken tube w accessory NG tube (GE 1971;61:291) until can get endoscopy
- Endoscopic ligation (Ann IM 1995;123:280; Nejm 1992;326: 1527) as good as surgery (which has a 50% survival), better than medical rx after a bleed but not used prophylactically if has never bled (Nejm 1991;324:1779), is better than sclerosis (Ann IM 1993; 119:1).
- Sclerosis of varices directly via gastroscope (Nejm 1987;316:11); also useful preventively after a bleed (Ann IM 1997;126:849,858)
- Open esophageal stapling if sclero rx fails (Nejm 1989;321:857).

HEPATIC FAILURE: HEPATORENAL SYNDROME
Nejm 1993;329:1862

Cause: Multiple etiologies result in end-stage hepatic failure, which has four major complications: ascites, hemorrhage, renal failure, and encephalopathy

Epidem:

Pathophys: Unknown etiology, but acts like ATN, although ATN is not present in biopsies, and damage is reversible since one can transplant hepatorenal kidneys successfully to other patients (Nejm 1969;280:1367)

Sx: Of renal failure (p 750)

Si:

Crs: 20% of patients w hepatic failure die from renal failure

Cmplc: Of renal failure (p 750)

Lab:

Chem: Elevated BUN and creatinine; low urinary Na

Rx: Supportive care including dialysis, perhaps TIPS (Alliment Pharmacol Ther 2000;14:515; Gastroenterol 1999;116:1264)

HEPATIC FAILURE: HEPATIC COMA/ENCEPHALOPATHY

Nejm 1993;329:1862; 1985;313:865; Ann IM 1989;110:532

Cause: Multiple etiologies result in end-stage hepatic failure, which has four major complications: ascites, hemorrhage, renal failure, and encephalopathy

Epidem:

Pathophys: Nitrogen-induced types, by blood in gut or protein-containing food ingestion; and non-nitrogen-induced types by drugs and hypokalemia (Nejm 1969;280:1). Lactulose helps nitrogen-induced types producing H^+ in bowel, which traps NH_3, and by causing diarrhea. Increased GABA in the brain by an endogenous benzodiazepine? (Nejm 1991;325:473)

Sx: Organic brain syndrome/delirium (p 573)

Si: Spectrum from mild flap (asterixis) and constructional apraxia, all the way to decorticate/decerebrate coma (Nejm 1968;278:876)

Crs: 33% of pts w hepatic failure die from coma

Cmplc:

Lab:

Chem: Blood NH_3 elevated, although degree of elevation does not correlate w severity but may be useful to follow individual patient. R/o other causes of ammonia elevations like: ureterosigmoidostomy or atonic bladder causing UTI and hence systemic NH_3 absorption (Nejm 1981;304:766); or **orotic aciduria,** sex-linked w coma in men and postpartum women who are carriers (Nejm 1990; 322:1641,1652); or **ornithine transcaramylase deficiency** (Nejm 1996;335:855)

Rx: (Nejm 1997;337:473)

1st: Low-protein diet

2nd: Lactulose 30–60 gm qd po to produce 2–4 acidic (pH <6) stools qd helps all types, can cause osmotic diarrhea and hypernatremia

3rd: Neomycin 6 gm qd; or metronidazole (Flagyl) 800 mg po qd; or rifaximin 1200 mg po qd; or ampicillin; or L-dopa (Ann IM 1975; 83:677); or bromocriptine po hs (Nejm 1977;296:793); or debatably ornithine salts of branched chain amino acids (Ann IM 1980;93:545 vs Med Let 1983;25:72) like ornithine aspartate 9 gm po tid

6.5 SMALL BOWEL DISEASES

MALABSORPTION AND MALDIGESTION

Nejm 1969;281:1111

Cause:

Failures of digestion:

- Blind loops, strictures, diverticula, and inadequate mixing syndromes, eg, postsurgery or associated with disorders of motility w secondary bacterial overgrowth causing bile salt breakdown, poor lipase stimulation, and poor absorption especially of fats (Nejm 1967;276:1393)
- Zollinger-Ellison syndrome, high duodenal pH inactivates pancreatic enzymes
- Pancreatic, either disease destroying >90% of the organ (Nejm 1972;287:813) like cystic fibrosis, alcoholic pancreatitis, or postgastrectomy lack of cholecystokinin stimulation of pancreas

Inadequate absorption length:

- Gross lesions, eg, >50% small bowel resection, gastric acid often overwhelms the residual bowel, but can rx w cimetidine (Nejm 1979;300:79)
- Specific lesions, eg, ileal and/or proximal colon resection causing loss of enterohepatic circulation and hence of bile salts, which causes fat malabsorption
- Relative, ie, rapid transport syndromes
- Mesenteric arterial insufficiency
- Lymphatic obstruction impairing fatty acid and TG absorption as in tumor or Whipple's disease

Enteropathies:

- Inflammatory, like sprue, regional enteritis, tbc, amyloid, sarcoid, milk allergy (Nejm 1967;276:761), giardia, coccidiosis (Nejm 1970;283:1306)
- Biochemical and/or genetic disorders like hypoparathyroidism; defects in carbohydrate, fat, and protein absorption

Sx: Weight loss, steatorrhea, abdominal distension

Si: Cachexia

Crs: Depends on etiology

Cmplc: Tetany from vit D deficiency and calcium salt precipitation; bleeding from vit K malabsorption; anemia from B_{12} deficiency and bleeding; vit E deficiency (Nejm 1983;308:1063) w secondary spinocerebellar dysfunction w progressive ataxia, r/o rare α-tocopherol transfer protein deficiency (Nejm 1995;333:1313); drug absorption will be abnormal w malabsorption but not maldigestion (Nejm 1971;285:1531)

Lab: (Nejm 1971;285:1358)

Chem: Carotene low (25% false neg), worth doing?

Specific malabsorption vs maldigestion tests like:

- Schilling test: first load w im B_{12}, then 3 h later, give hot B_{12} po and measure excretion in 24–48-h urine sample; normal >15%; then repeat w intrinsic factor to see if corrects
- Gly-1-C^{14}: give hot cholate po, and if $C^{14}O_2$ in breath in 3 h, means poor ileal absorption of bile salts or bacteria in small bowel (Nejm 1971;285:656)
- Xylose tolerance test: 25 gm po; w malabsorption, ≥5 gm in urine in 5 h; bacterial overgrowth or ascites will cause false pos

Path: Intestinal bx

Stool: Sudan stain for qualitative fat positive; 72-h stool fat

Rx: Cholestyramine 16 gm po qd for ileal resection diarrhea if mild (<20 gm fat qd)

Medium chain triglycerides (Nejm 1969;280:1045)

Pancreatic enzymes (Nejm 1969;281:201); can enhance absorption w omeprazole rx (Ann IM 1991;114:200)

Vitamins D, B_{12}, and K

DISACCHARIDASE DEFICIENCIES

Nejm 1984;310:42

Cause: Genetic

Epidem: Lactase deficiency discovered in Holland during WWII when babies w it improved during milk shortages; present in 80% blacks (Nejm 1975;292:1156), 10% whites (Nejm 1967;276:1283), 100% Asians, in 25% of US adults, 75% of all other adults (Nejm 1995; 333:1).

Sucrase-isomaltase deficiency (Nejm 1987;316:1306) in 0.2% of US population, 10% of Greenland Eskimos

Pathophys: Mucosal cell deficiency of invertases lactase and sucrase-isomaltase. Diarrhea from osmotic effect, bacterial degradation of these sugars to lactic acid, and steatorrhea

Sx: Osmotic diarrhea; sucrose or milk intolerance causes bloating and cramps; most common cause of recurrent abdominal pain in children (Nejm 1979;300:1449)

Si:

Crs: Decreasing tolerance as patient ages from 1–11 yr (Nejm 1967; 276:1283)

Cmplc: r/o milk allergy (p 666)

Lab:

Chem: Lactose tolerance by breath test; or by giving 50 gm lactose po and do w hourly blood sugars over 3 h; a normal person should increase blood sugar by 20 mg% if not diabetic

Stool: Elevated lactic acid, lowered pH (test after a milk shake)

Rx: Withhold milk and/or malt and/or sucrose, or prepare food w or add lactase to milk before feeding (Med Let 1981;23:67) although 250 cc (8 oz) milk qd is generally tolerated (Nejm 1995;333:1); yogurt may be tolerated because of autodigestion (Nejm 1984;310:42). Baker's yeast po w sucrose decrease sx (Nejm 1987;316:1306)

WHIPPLE'S DISEASE

Nejm 1992;327:293,346

Cause: *Tropheryma whippelii,* Whipple's bacillus

Epidem: Males > females; peak incidence in middle age. Incidence = 10/yr worldwide

Pathophys: Infection of small intestinal mucosal layer causes lymphatic blockage, which in turn causes fatty acid malabsorption, probably at lamina propria level

Sx: Diarrhea, steatorrhea, and malabsorption (not always—Ann IM 1978; 89:65); postprandial pain; polyserositis including arthritis in 70%, frequently the presenting sx; fever, weight loss; lymphadenopathy; hyperpigmentation of skin; blurred vision from uveitis, may be only sx (Nejm 1995;332:363)

Si: As above

Crs:

Cmplc: Myocarditis and aortic insufficiency (Nejm 1981;305:995); CNS, including gaze paresis, nystagmus, myoclonus, polydipsia, hypersomnolence, all of which may be a continuing problem if primary sx are treated w an antibiotic that doesn't cross blood-brain barrier (Nejm 1979;300:907)

Lab:

Bact: Gram-pos bacillus of actinomycetes group; identifiable by PCR; and culturable now (Nejm 2000;342:620)

Hem: CBC peripheral smear may show red stippled rbc's (organisms in the red cells) (Nejm 1994;331:1343)

Path: Intestinal bx shows diagnostic changes of enlarged villi; foamy, carbohydrate-filled macrophages staining positive w PAS; and fat in mucosa, lacteals, and lymph nodes (Nejm 1971;285:1470); r/o AIDS or *Mycobacterium avium* intestinal infection; and, if has noncaseating granulomata, sarcoid

Rx: (Nejm 1996;335:26) Procaine penicillin 1.2 million U im qd × 14 d + streptomycin 1 gm im qd × 14 d + Tm/S bid prophylaxis continuously

CELIAC DISEASE (Nontropical Sprue)

Nejm 1991;325:1709

Cause: Ingestion of gluten, a protein in rye, barley, wheat. Genetic component, HLA 1 and 8 linked (Nejm 1973;288:704)

Epidem: Associated w dermatitis herpetiformis (p 134) and insulin-dependent diabetes (Nejm 1983;308:816). Seen in whites, not blacks or Asians 1/300–1/1000

Pathophys: Perhaps an enzyme deficiency, perhaps large peptide toxicity, perhaps immunologic. Iron deficiency occurs from both malabsorption and occult gi bleeding (Nejm 1996;334:1163)

Sx: Malabsorptive, including diarrhea, flatulence, weight loss, and fatigue

Si: Of malabsorption; iron or folate deficiency anemias; osteoporosis

Crs: Nearly normal prognosis on gluten-free diet

Cmplc: Those of malabsorption; ulceration, perforation can cause death even in remission (Nejm 1967;276:996); incr incidence of foregut tumors of esophagus, pharynx and stomach, and lymphomas r/o IgA deficiency causing sprue sx but biopsy negative (Nejm 1968; 279:1327)

Lab:
Chem: If do xylose tolerance test, use 5 gm rather than 25 gm to avoid causing severe diarrhea

Path: Per oral or endoscopic biopsy of duodenum for dx (Nejm 1971; 285:1470)

Serol: Anti-endomysial antibodies, most sens/specif; also anti-gliadin IgA and IgG antibodies, 46% sens and 98% specif in high-likelihood populations but do not obviate need for bx (Scand J Gastroenterol 1994;29:148)

Xray: Small bowel follow through

Rx: Gluten-free diet; rice, corn (maize), and oats ok (Nejm 1995;333: 1033); if fails, consider lactose deficiency or giardiasis coincident w disease; initiate diet in hospital to ensure compliance; most improve in <10 d if they are going to; if diet fails, consider steroid use (Nejm 1976;295:131); cyclosporine? (Ann IM 1994;119:1014)

REGIONAL ENTERITIS (Crohn's Disease and Granulomatous Colitis)

Nejm 1991;325:928,1008; Gastroenterology 1979;77:847

Cause: Probably genetic (HLA-linked) component in some types (Ann IM 1980;93:424) from autoimmune antibodies to intestinal epithelium (Ann IM 1989;110:786)

Epidem: Males = females; incr in Jews

Pathophys: Excess T_4 helper lymphocytes in lungs as in sarcoid; a variant of the same disease? (Ann IM 1986;104:17)

Sx: Onset age 11–35 yr (75%). Cramps, partly relieved by bowel movement; diarrhea, although constipation may also intermittently predominate and may be bloody, although less often than in ulcerative colitis

Si: Inflammatory mass. Extraintestinal manifestations: iritis; erythema nodosum; sclerosing cholangitis (p 264); pyoderma gangrenosum; clubbing and arthritis (20%), especially of knee, ankle, PIP joints, and may even develop clear-cut ankylosing spondylitis (Bull Rheum Dis 1987;37(1):1)

Crs: Teenagers get the most malignant form of ileocolitis, older people more often have a more localized disease. 90% recurrence in 20 yr (Nejm 1975;293:685). Cancer risks? (Nejm 1978;298:1099; 1972; 287:111)

Cmplc: Abscesses; strictures and fistulas; malabsorption; small bowel obstruction; anemias; renal stones, usually oxalate for unclear reasons (Nejm 1973;289:172; 1972;286:1370); small bowel cancer rarely (Nejm 1970;283:136); gallstones; colon cancer (see above); hepatic disease from portal bacteremia in 90% (Ann IM 1971;74: 518) or autoimmune (sclerosing cholangitis) (p 266); stress and depression result, do not cause (Ann IM 1991;114:381); rare avascular necrosis of femoral head (Nejm 1993;329:1314)

In pregnancy, moderate increase in spontaneous abortions, otherwise healthy babies and no significant increase in risk for mother even if need surgery, steroids, or sulfa (Nejm 1985;312:1616)

r/o bile salt diarrhea, rx w cholestyramine; *Yersinia* (Nejm 1990; 323:113)

Lab:

Path: Small bowel or colonic bx may show noncaseating granulomas and distorted glandular architecture

Noninv: Endoscopy (colonoscopy) may demonstrate diagnostic findings

Xray: UGIS and small bowel follow through show segmental involvement ("string sign"). BE shows ileitis w reflux into ileum and/or proximal colon; disease characterized by "step ladder" mucosal edema pattern and longitudinal intramural fistulas (Nejm 1970;283:1080)

Rx: (Nejm 1996;334:84, Ann IM 1990;112:50)

Medical of acute disease/flare:

- Mesalamine (Asacol) (5-ASA) 800–1600 mg po t-qid
- Steroids like prednisolone 40 mg po qd × 2 wk, then taper 5 mg qd over 6 wk (Nejm 1994;331:842); or budesonide LA (Entocort-CIR) 9 mg po qd × 8 wk, induces remissions in 50–60% vs 20% in controls and 36% w mesalamine alone (Nejm 1998;339:370; 1994;331:836)
- Azathioprine (Imuran) or 6-MP (Ann IM 1995;123:132) adjusted by CBC and platelets, helps heal fistulas over 2–4 mo (Ann IM 1989;111:641; Nejm 1980;302:981), induces and maintains remissions

- Methotrexate 25 mg im q 1 wk (Nejm 1995;332:292);
- Infliximab (Remicade) (Med Let 1999;41:19), a monoclonal antibody to TNF-α (Nejm 1997;337:1029) 5 mg/kg iv infusion at week 0, 2, and 6 helps >50% within 1 month when given to pts w refractory fistula producing disease (Nejm 1999;340:1398)
- Metronidazole (Flagyl) 250 mg b-qid × 2–4 mo helps perianal and colonic disease
- Human growth hormone (Nejm 2000;342:1633) 5 mg sc qd × 1 wk, then 1.5mg sc qd
- Cyclosporine debatably (Nejm 1994;330:1846 vs 1989;321:845)

Medical remission maintenance: (steroids not worth the risk—ACP J Club 1999;130(2):36)

- Methotrexate 15 mg im q 1 wk, esp if induced w mtx (Nejm 2000; 342:1627)
- Mesalamine (Pentasa) 500 mg po qid given chronically (GE 1993; 104:435), or Asacol 800 mg po tid
- Fish oil caps perhaps, enteric coated n-3 fatty acid (Nejm 1996; 334:1557,1599)

Surgical: ~40% require reoperation within 15 yr (Nejm 1981;304: 1586). Big debate about appendectomy performance. Colectomy may cure if isolated there (debated—Nejm 1972;287:111; 1970; 282:582)

TPN (Nejm 1977;297:1104) or enteral elemental diet like Vivonex (Sci Am Text Med 1984), important adjuncts in severe disease

CARCINOID TUMOR (Argentaffinoma)

Nejm 1999;340:858

Cause: Neoplasia

Epidem: 1–2/100;000/yr in US

Pathophys: Derived from argentaffin cells in primitive foregut (Ann IM 1972;77:53). Syndrome develops only after metastases. Symptoms related to secreted serotonin (Nejm 1967;277:1103), kallikrein (Ann IM 1969;71:763; Nejm 1967;277:406), gastrin (Nejm 1978; 299:1053), histamine, dopamine, substance P, prostaglandins, et al.

Also arise in stomach w ZE or atrophic gastritis and sometimes pernicious anemia due to excessive gastrin stimulation (Nejm 1997; 336:866), lungs, ovary, or pancreas (Ann IM 1972;77:53); or gi tract; those originating in appendix are rarely malignant and rarely metastasize, while those of small bowel origin become malignant (20%), many metastasize; rectal ones small and without sx

Sx: Diarrhea, wheezing/asthma, red/violaceous flushes inducible by alcohol

Si: Right-sided heart murmurs, due to right heart scarring; fundi during flush show decr blood flow and lesions of macular area (Nejm 1967; 277:406); plastic induration of penis (Nejm 1973;289:844)

Crs: Very low-grade malignancy, can live years even with mets

Cmplc: r/o mastocytosis (p 142)

Lab:

Chem: 24-h urine shows 5-HIAA (a serotonin degradation product) elevated, 86% sens, 100% specif (D. Oppenheim, 11/93) but can get false positives w glycerol guaiacolate expectorants, bananas, phenothiazines, caffeine, acetaminophen (Tylenol)

Path: Biopsy positive on silver stains

Provocative tests: Epinephrine 0.5–1 mg iv reproduces sx, no false positives w mast cell tumors (Ann IM 1971;74:711). Pentagastrin also causes a flush (Nejm 1978;299:1055)

Xray: Scan w labeled octreotide (somatostatin analog) to pick up primary (12/13) and mets (Nejm 1990;323:1246)

Rx: Cimetidine (Tagamet) + diphenhydramine (Benadryl) (or any other H_2 + H_1 blocker combination) decrease flush sx (Nejm 1979;300: 236)

Somatostatin analog (octreotide) sc q 8–12 h controls flushing and diarrhea sx (Med Let 1989;31:66; Nejm 1986;315:663; Ann IM 1985;103:362) by blocking somatostatin receptors on the tumor (Nejm 1990;323:1246)

Streptozocin and 5-FU or cyclophosphamide for malignant types (Nejm 1975;292:941)

Surgical of appendiceal types, simple appendectomy if <2 cm or elderly; right colectomy if >2 cm irrespective of degree of wall or other invasion (Nejm 1987;317:1699)

of metastatic disease, hepatic artery occlusion followed by 2-drug chemotherapy (Ann IM 1994;120:302); perhaps liver transplant

SMALL BOWEL ISCHEMIA/INFARCTION

Cause: Thrombosis, embolism, hypotension associated w atherosclerosis, hypercoagulable states

Epidem: Embolic associated w Afib or MI. Thrombosis associated w atherosclerosis, low flow hypotensive states, rarely bcp's (Nejm 1968;279:1213)

Pathophys: Superior mesenteric artery or vein (Nejm 1997;336:567) thrombosis

Sx: Acute: sudden onset, pain disproportionate to physical findings
Chronic: h/o weight loss, pc abdominal pain for days to weeks; pain, often radiating to back; abdominal distension within 24 h

Si: Decreased bowel tones; stool guaiac-positive

Crs: In acute ischemia, w/o surgery, nearly all die (Nejm 1969;281:309); some survive w surgery, especially those that are embolic in origin

Cmplc: r/o mesenteric venous thrombosis (Nejm 2001;345:1683)

Lab:
Hem: Elevated wbc
Paracentesis: Rbc's, wbc's; and bacteria late in course

Xray: Mesenteric arteriogram

Rx: of acute syndrome: endarterectomy and limited bowel resection
of abdominal angina, frequent small feedings; surgery, preferably in anginal stage before infarction

---

6.6 LARGE BOWEL DISEASES

APPENDICITIS

Jama 1996;276:1589; Nejm 1986;315:1546

Cause: Obstructed appendix from fecolith, lymphoid hyperplasia from viral illness

Epidem: 7% lifetime risk; incid in ER pts w abdominal pain under age 60 = 25%, over age 60 = 4%

Pathophys:

Sx: Nausea, anorexia; pain, periumbilical at first, then migrates to right lower quadrant; <72 h duration; sensation of constipation and urge to defecate

Si: Fever 99.5°–101.3°F (37.5–38.5°C); <101°F (<38.3°C). Right lower quadrant guarding and rebound tenderness; tenderness may only be on pelvic/rectal exam or w heel pounding; later rigidity and diminished bowel sounds; mass; any or all may be absent especially in the elderly

Crs: 12–24 h

Cmplc: Perforation (20–25%) w peritonitis; perforation increases prevalence of infertility × 5 (Nejm 1986;315:1506)

r/o PID; intussusception in children < age 4 yr; mesenteric adenitis including *Yersinia* pseudoappendicular syndrome (p 418) (Nejm 1989;321:16); diverticulitis; typhilitis, a cecal colitis seen w aggressive chemoRx of leukemia

Lab:

Hem: CBC not sens or specif, but usually wbc about 10,000–13,000 w some left shift

Urinalysis: Often shows hematuria, suggesting ureteral impingement

Xray: KUB not helpful

Ultrasound, 25% false neg, 0% false pos? (Nejm 1987;317:666)

Helical CT after Gastrografin enema (Nejm 1998;338:141); or CT w rectal contrast, which combined w US in children has 94% sens and specif (Jama 1999;282:1041)

Rx: Surgery; w prophylactic cefoxitin perioperatively if perforation likely? Neg pathology in 15–20% overall despite current diagnostics (Jama 2001;286:1748), and in 45% of young women

ISCHEMIC COLITIS

Ann IM 1965;63:535

Cause: Atherosclerotic disease w low flow states; embolic

Epidem:

Pathophys: Partial or full inferior mesenteric artery occlusion

Sx: Crampy and often bloody diarrhea

Si: Guaiac-positive stool

Crs: After initial acute illness, gradual scarring w lumen narrowing, which gradually improves but not always

Cmplc: Strictures sometimes, although most heal

Lab:

Noninv: Endoscopy w bx quite specif

Xray: Ba enema has classic "thumbprints" in colon wall that represent mucosal hemorrhages

Rx: Surgery usually not necessary; watch for stricture later

ULCERATIVE COLITIS

Nejm 1991;325:928,1008

Cause: Genetic component (Ann IM 1989;110:786)

Epidem: Onset age 20–40 yr, occasionally younger (Nejm 1971;285:17). Lower incidence in smokers and other nicotine users! (Nejm 1983; 308:361) and in pts s/p appendectomy before age 20 (Nejm 2001; 344:808)

Pathophys: Strictures from muscularis mucosal hypertrophy, not fibrosis, in left colon (Nejm 1969;281:290)

Sx: Bloody diarrhea; cramps, poorly relieved w bowel movement; arthritis (20%), especially of hip, knee, ankle, pip joints, and full ankylosing spondylitis syndrome (Bull Rheum Dis 1973;24:750); fever and weight loss

Si: Friable rectal mucosa (positive "wipe test," ie, when bowel wall is wiped punctate bleeding sites seen; now, w flexible sigmoidoscope, usually manifests simply as more than usual "scope trauma"); clubbing; erythema nodosum; uveitis, though less common than in regional enteritis

Crs: 80% recur in 1 yr; 100% within 17 yr

Cmplc:
- Carcinoma (Nejm 1990;323:1228), especially if diffuse disease; risk is double normal when disease is left-sided, but even higher when pancolitis exists or the disease starts under age 15 yr; at 35 years of disease, risk is 30% for pancolitis, and 40% if started under age 15; 0% at 5 yr unless over age 40, then is 5%. May be more malignant than usual colon cancer since it has a 25% 5-yr mortality
- Strictures
- Perforation and peritonitis, and/or megacolon
- Esophagitis (Ann IM 1969;70:971)
- Hepatitis (10%), chronic active, cirrhosis, and sclerosing cholangitis (p 266)(Ann IM 1985;102:581)

- Stress and depression result, but do not cause (Ann IM 1991; 114:381)
- Pyoderma gangrenosum in <5% toxic patients, may occur even when bowel quiescent

In pregnancy, some increase in spontaneous abortions but no other adverse effects on baby or mother even if need surgery, steroids or sulfa (Nejm 1985;312:1616)

r/o other causes of acute diarrhea: clostridial colitis (p 426) (Nejm 1979;301:414); ulcerative proctitis, similar disease isolated to rectum, can get above it on sigmoidoscopy, rx w steroid enemas and mesalamine (Rowasa) 500 mg pr bid (Gut 1998;42:195); postcolostomy diversion colitis in empty colorectal segments, rx w instillation of short-chain fatty acids (Nejm 1989;320:23)

Lab:

Serol: Ameba titers to r/o before starting steroids? (Nejm 1975;292: 262); will be pos only if extra-gi disease (S. Sears 1/93)

Xray: BE shows distal colonic involvement progressing proximally without skip areas; pseudopolyps; and when chronic, smooth wall, "lead pipe" colon. Ba can result in false-negative ova and parasite exams for amebae.

KUB to r/o megacolon (6–8 cm diameter)

Rx: (Nejm 1996;334:841; Ann IM 1990;112:51)

Screening and surveillance for Ca:

Colonoscopic (Gastrointest Endosc Clin N Am 1997;7:1:129); perhaps q 1–2 yr with q 10 cm biopsies for dysplasia after 8–10 yr of pancolitis (efficacy disputed—Nejm 1987;316:1654) vs q 5–10 yr unless sx change

Ursodiol, esp if primary sclerosing cholangitis, may markedly (80%) reduce colon Ca risk long term (Ann IM 2001;134:89)

of disease:

Sulfasalazine (Azulfidine) as 500-mg tabs, 2–4 gm po qd (Ann IM 1984;101:377) or more up to 12 gm qd, active metabolite is 5-aminosalicylic acid (5-ASA) (Nejm 1980;303:1499); used prophylactically it keeps disease in remission (25% recur/yr—Lancet 1992;339:1279); as good as and much cheaper than 5-ASA meds except in allergic pts (Ann IM 1993;118:540). Adverse effects (incr when >4 gm qd in slow acetylators—Nejm 1973;289:491): allergic worsening of sx (Nejm 1982;306:409); rash, can be desensitized w increasing doses (Ann IM 1984;100:512)

5-Aminosalicylic acid (5-ASA) (Med Let 1992;34:80) as coated mesalamine (Asacol) (Ann IM 1991;115:350) 400 mg po t-qid very effective (Nejm 1987;317:1625) and works moderately well at 400 mg po b-qid to prevent recurrence (Ann IM 1996;124:205), or as 500 mg Pentasa; or 4 gm hs in 60-cc retention enema to help left-sided disease (Med Let 1988;30:53); or as 5-ASA dimer, olsalazine (Dipentum) 500 mg po bid up to 1 gm bid. Adverse effects: diarrhea (Med Let 1990;32:103); cost $25/wk; or as precursor balsalazide (Colaxel) (Med Let 2001;43:62) 2.25 gm po tid

Steroid enemas or systemically, eg, prednisone 60–80 mg po qd, or ACTH 120 U/24 h iv for severe flare; chronically try to get off entirely, at least <10 mg po qd to avoid adverse effects (p 788)

Ciprofloxacin? (Gastroent 1998;115:1072) 500–750 mg po bid × 6 mos for resistant flares

6MP if can't get off steroids; some small cancer risk as well as reversible problems (Ann IM 1989;111:642); cyclosporine 4 mg/kg iv qd helps 80% within 1 wk of those who fail iv steroids for a week when flaring (Nejm 1994;330:1841)

Nicotine 14^{+} mg patch qd helps many (Ann IM 1997;126:364; Nejm 1994;330:811,856) during acute phase only, does not prevent recurrences (Nejm 1995;332:988)

Surgical colectomy w ileostomy usually cures, although when this should be done is debatable; but for recurrent flares, must do if both iv steroid and iv cyclosporine fail (Nejm 1994;330:1841)

DIVERTICULITIS/DIVERTICULOSIS

Nejm 1998;338:1521

Cause: Diverticulosis, which may be congenital but is usually acquired

Epidem: Diverticulosis prevalence = 5–10% over age 45, 80% over age 85. Right sided disease more common in Asians. Diverticulitis occurs in 20% of those w divertiuclosis; 20% of pts w divertiuclitis are <50

Pathophys: (Nejm 1975;293:83) Low-residue diet leads to incr intracolonic pressures causing outpocketings (diverticula); diverticulitis caused by micro and macro perforations

GASTROENTEROLOGY

Sx: Left lower quadrant pain usually, though may be anywhere; fever; diarrhea intially often, then constipation

Si: Tenderness, mass in left lower quadrant; fever

Crs: Variable; under age 50, 33% recur over 10 yr, higher recurrence in older pts

Cmplc: Perforation; partial obstruction; abscess; fistulas; bleeding from diverticulosis alone, dx by colonoscopy acutely (Nejm 2000; 342:78), r/o right-sided angiodysplasia of the colon, often seen in elderly and associated w aortic stenosis

Lab:
   Hem: elevated wbc and L shift

Xray: CT scan; ultrasonography; tagged red cell scan or angiography (Nejm 1972;286:450) to localize diverticular bleeding

Rx: Prevent w high-fiber diet; avoid opiates

   Antibiotics for acute disease, eg ciprofloxacin + metronidazole × 7–10 d po, or iv ampicillin + gentamicin + metronidazole

   CT guided percutaneous drainage if abscess > 5 cm diameter

   Surgical staged colonic resection w temporary colostomy for perforation/abscess

IRRITABLE BOWEL SYNDROME

   Nejm 2001;344:1846; Ann IM 1995;123:688; 1992;116:1001,1009

Cause: Unknown, perhaps bowel motility deficits, perhaps psychiatric/ stress

Epidem: 10–20% prevalence; female > male; associated w sexual abuse in women; and w other functional gi disorders (Ann IM 1995;123:688)

Pathophys: Probably a heterogeneous mix of disorders, psychiatric dx's seem to increase reporting of sx but not disease prevalence

Sx: Alternating constipation and diarrhea; and/or abdominal pain × 12+ wk, w mucus stools but no blood; bloating and sense of incomplete emptying; in women, irritable bowel or dyspeptic sx are associated w a h/o sexual abuse in over 50% (Ann IM 1991;114:828)

Si: Usually normal exam

Crs:

Cmplc: r/o *Giardia,* IBD, colon cancer, bowel ischemia, impaction, laxative abuse, malabsorption

Lab:

Chem: TSH, chemistry profile

Endo: Flexible sigmoidoscopy

Hem: CBC, ESR

Stool: NaOH drops added to stool to test for phenolphthalein and commercial screens to r/o laxative abuse; O + P; Sudan stain for fat; leukocytes

Rx: Bran or other bulking agents, Al(OH)$_3$ antacids; psychiatric care (GE 1991;100:450) including antidepressants like tricyclics if diarrhea, SSRIs if constipation; not alosetron (Lotronex) (Med Let 2000; 42:53, Rx Let 2000;7:69), pulled from mkt in 2000 due to ischemic colitis

For pain, antispasmodics; for diarrhea, loperamide (Imodium) 2–4 mg po qid or diphenoxylate (Lomotil). If sx still persist, get *Giardia* antigen on stool and consider bile-salt binding

COLON POLYPS AND CANCER

Nejm 2000;342:1960

Cause: Neoplasia; at least 20% are clearly genetic (Nejm 1985;312:1540), autosomal dominant, and maybe all are (Ann IM 1990;113:779)

Epidem: After lung, 2nd most common cancer in US; 6% lifetime risk, 130,000 incidence/yr in US, 60,000 die/yr in US. Most arise from adenomatous polyps over years and decades (Ann IM 1993;118:91) and occasionally from villous adenomas, but not from hyperplastic polyps (Ann IM 1990;113:760), although hyperplastic polyps still are assoc w an incr cancer risk (?—Nejm 2000;343:162,169). Adenomatous polyps themselves are associated w high-animal-fat, low-fiber diets (Ann IM 1993;118:91); lower adenoma/cancer rates w incr dietary fiber (Nejm 1999;340:169,223) but such a diet does not decr recurrence after 1st polyp removed (Nejm 2000;342:1149, 1156)

Associated w family h/o cancer or adenomatous polyps (Ann IM 1998; 128:900; Nejm 1996;334:82) in a 1st degree relative, 2–5 × (5 ×, under age 45) baseline rate if one such relative, 3–5× baseline rate if ≥2, but by age 60 family hx effect gone (Nejm 1994;331:1669);

autosomal dominant multiple gi polyposis syndromes (adenomatous, hamartomatous, or nonpolyposis syndromes) (Nejm 1994;331:1694; Ann IM 1990;113:779): **familial colonic polyposis** and **Turcot** (colonic polyps and CNS tumors—Nejm 1995;332:839) **syndromes** (gene defects on chomosome #5—Nejm 1993;329:1982; 1990;322:904); **Gardner's syndrome** with pigmented retinal lesions (Nejm 1987;316:661); and **Peutz-Jegher syndrome** of hamartomas throughout the gi tract, pigmented spots on lips, w gi bleeding, and gi, breast, and gyn cancers developing in >50% (Ann IM 1998;128:896; Nejm 1987;316:1511); **Lynch syndrome,** hereditary nonpolyposis colon cancer and cancer of endometrium, ovary, stomach, small bowel, biliary tree (Jama 1997;277:915). Polyposis syndromes are generally associated w distal cancers, whereas nonpolyposis genetic types are associated w proximal cancers and other cancers (esp endometrial) in the same patient and 1st degree relatives and have defects in DNA repair genes (Nejm 1998;338:1481)

Also associated w *Streptococcus bovis* septicemia, cancer is present 85% of the time (Ann IM 1979;91:560); ulcerative colitis sx >10 yr (p 295); elevated cholesterol in men (Ann IM 1993;118:481)

Not associated w inguinal hernia as often claimed (Nejm 1971; 284:369)

Lower colon cancer mortality w ASA use >16 tab qd, due to earlier detection vs direct cancer suppression? (Nejm 1991;325:1593)

Sx: Change in bowel habits; blood in stool or on toilet paper (ask in ROS, positive response assoc w 24% prevalence of significant pathology—Jama 1997;277:44); abdominal cramps and other obstructive sx early w left-sided tumor, late w right-sided tumor

Si: Acanthosis nigrans (see gastric cancer for differential dx); palpable rectal or abdominal mass; blood in stool, gross or by guaiac

Crs: Good prognosis correlates w low or absent CEA antigen (Jama 1972; 221:31)

Duke's Stage A(I): Confined to submucosal area, 90% 5-yr survival w surgery

Stage B(II)$_1$: Through muscularis mucosa, 60–80% 5-yr survival

Stage B(II)$_2$: Through serosa, 45–70% 5-yr survival

Stage C(III)$_1$: <5 pos nodes, 30–40% 5-yr survival

Stage C(III)$_2$: >5 pos nodes, 25% 5-yr survival

Stage D(IV): Widely metastatic, 0% 5-yr survival

Cmplc: Metastases; CEA-antibody complex-induced nephrotic syndrome (Nejm 1973;289:520); *S. bovis* endocarditis (Ann IM 1979;91:560; Nejm 1977;297:800)

r/o anal canal cancer (Nem 2000;342:792) caused by HPV, rx'd w radiation and chemRx

Lab:

Endo: Sigmoidoscopy or colonoscopy for primary prevention (p 676) Colonoscopy q 3–5 yr in patients who have had an adenomatous polyp removed (Nejm 1993;328:901) whether large or small, since 30% will have proximal neoplasia (Nejm 1997;336:8). Screen if one or more 1st degree relatives had colon cancer or adenomatous polyps (Ann IM 1998;128:900), start at age 40 (ACS, and Nejm 1994; 331:1669)

Path: Histologic staging as above, each worse if blood vessel invasion Adenomatous and/or villous polyps deserve full bowel w/u (Jama 1999;281:1611), but not single tubular adenomas under 5 mm in low risk pts (Ann IM 1998;129:273), and not hyperplastic polyps

Serol: CEA to monitor for recurrence and perhaps preop estimate of prognosis (Nejm 1978;299:448), but in neither case does it result in significant change in survival (Ann IM 1986;104:66)

Stool: Screening occult blood testing (p 677)

Xray: Air contrast barium enema; possibly scan w labeled VIP (Nejm 1994;331:1116); "virtual colonoscopy" CT can detect most polyps >6mm (Nejm 1999;341:1496)

Rx:

Prevent w:

- ASA or other NSAIDs like ibuprofen tiw-qd (Gastroenterol 1998; 114:441; Nejm 1995;333:609; Ann IM 1994;121:241) vs no help (Ann IM 1998;128:713); sulindac (Clinoril), continuous rx causes polyp regression in multiple polyposis syndromes (Ann IM 1991; 115:952) but incompletely (Nejm 1993;328:1313); probably work by inhibiting cyclo-oxygenase (COX-2) found in aggressive colon Ca (Nejm 2000;342:1960; Jama 1999;282:1254), hence COX-2 drugs like celcoxib 400 mg po bid induce regression of adenomas at least in familial polyposis syndrome (Nejm 2000;342: 1946)

- ERT decreases the risk by 30–40% if cont'd (Ann IM 1998;128: 705)

GASTROENTEROLOGY

- Calcium qd in low fat dairy products (Nejm 1999;340:101; Jama 1998;280:1074) or as $CaCO_3$ to decrease fatty acid irritation (Nejm 1985;313:1381)
- Folate qd × yrs may reduce absolute risk × 30% after 15 yr (NNT-15 = 3) (Ann IM 1998;129;517); perhaps genetic screening for adenomatous polyposis coli gene if pos fam hx (Nejm 1997; 336:823). Vits E, C, and A (β-carotene) do not prevent (Nejm 1994;331:141)

Surgical excision by laparotomy or colonoscopy; prophylactic removal of adenomatous polyps, even those <1 cm (Nejm 1993;329:1977) decreases cancer rate by 90%

Chemotherapy (Nejm 1994;330:1136) postop for stage C(III) w adjuvant 5-FU and levamisole + radiation + maybe Me-CCNU (Ann IM 1995;122:321; FDA Bull 1990;20(2):4; Med Let 1990; 31:89; Nejm 1990;322:352); rectal cancers helped by adjuvant radiation and 5-FU more than colonic, but trade prolongation of life for toxicity (Nejm 1994;331:502; 1991;324:709); of advanced disease, 5-FU + leucovorin iv qd × 5 d q 4–5 wk; or irinotecan (Camptosar) (Nejm 2000;343:905) iv weekly ($1000/dose—Med Let 1997;38:8)

of liver mets: resection then hepatic artery chemoRx (Nejm 1999; 341:2039)

in rectal cancer, preop radiation (Jama 2000;284:1008; Nejm 1997; 336:980) and AP resection but latter has postop sexual dysfunction in 1/3; 1/3 of these improve after 2 yr (Dis Colon Rectum 1983;26:785)

GROIN HERNIAS (Femoral, Indirect and Direct Inguinal)

Jama 1997;277:663

Cause: Indirect is usually due to congenital failure to close processus vaginalis combined w incr intra-abdominal pressure, eg, from coughing or something else; direct from a defect in transversalis fascia

Epidem: Male:female = 25:1

Pathophys: Direct inguinal protrudes anteriorly, often bilateral
Indirect goes down inguinal canal, can go to scrotum
Femoral (3%)
Sx: Fullness, bulge, pain
Si: Hernia present, at least w straining when standing
Crs:
Cmplc: Strangulation, most often in 1st 3 mo; most often w femoral type
(>50%)
Lab:
Xray:
Rx: Trusses for direct and indirect types help some
Various surgical repairs; open or laparoscopic repairs, which result in
faster recovery and lower recurrence rates (3% at 2 yr) (Br J Surg
1999;86:316; Nejm 1997;336:1541); vs 3 yr 23% recurrence rate w
mesh repair, but 42% recurrence w suture repair!? (Dutch—Nejm
2000;343:392)

6.7 MISCELLANEOUS

Abdominal pain, nonsurgical causes of: Angioedema, hereditary and
acquired; porphyria and lead poisoning; familial Mediterranean fever;
thrombotic thrombocytopenic purpura; sickle cell crisis; paroxysmal
hemoglobinuria (PNH); anaphylactoid purpura and other vasculitides;
urticaria pigmentosa and all causes of urticaria; abdominal epilepsy?

Anal fissure (Nejm 1998;338:257)
Epidem: Common, >10% of rectal complaints
Pathophys: Once started, perpetuated by firm bowel movements. Assoc w
and perpetuated by spasm of internal (not external) anal sphincter
(Nejm 1999;341:65)
Sx: Rectal pain
Si: Posterior (90%) fissure/ulcer between anal verge and dentate line; skin
tag at anal verge; prominent proximal papilla
Cmplc: r/o inflammatory bowel disease, especially if not posterior
Rx: (Nejm 1999;341:65)

1st: Nitroglycerine 0.2% ointment (nitropaste diluted × 10) bid ×
6 wk; 60% cure; adv effects: headache
2nd: Botulinum toxin injections (Nejm 1998;338:217; Lancet 1997;
349:11) 20 U in each side of anal sphincter, 96% cure
3rd: Surgical lateral internal sphincterotomy; 90–95% cure; cmplc:
permanent weakness of anal sphincter w gas, mucus, and rarely
stool leakage

Colonic distention, acute nonobstructive (Ogilivie's syndrome), pseudo-obstruction

Epidem: Hospitalized pts
Crs: 40% recur
Cmplc: 3% perforate and have 50% mortality
Xray: KUB shows colon diameter >10 cm
Rx: Colonoscopic decompression helps 70%
Neostigmine 2 mg iv (Nejm 1999;341:137) helps 90%

Constipation (Ann IM 1994;121:520)
Cause: Drugs, diet, colon lesions, hypothyroid, autonomic neuropathies
Sx: Abdominal cramps
Si: Abdominal mass from stool
Cmplc: Fecal impaction (Nejm 1989;321:658) w fever, dyspnea,
encopresis (diarrhea around a fecal impaction) (Peds Rv 1998;19:
22; Ped Clin N Am 1996;43:279; Clin Peds 1991;30:669) especially
in children age 3–5
r/o hypothyroidism, Hirschsprung's in children (rarely have fecal
incontinence)
Xray: Try to avoid BE
Rx: Laxatives:
1st: Fiber
2nd: Psyllium (Metamucil etc.)
3rd: Sorbitol 70% soln, 30–60 cc po hs, as effective as:
- Lactulose (p 284), w fewer side effects and cheaper (Am J Med
1990;89:597)
- Polyethylene glycol (PEG) (Miralax, Colyte, GoLytely) tbsp/8oz
water qd (Rx Let 1999;6:28)
- Emollients like dioctyl Na succinate (Colace, Surfak)
- Lubricants like mineral oil
- Mg compounds like Milk of Magnesia
- Stimulants/irritants like cascara, senna, and castor oil

of **encopresis:** Bisacodyl (Dulcolax) ii tabs po qd w mineral oil; enemas if football-sized stool

Fecal incontinence (Nejm 1992;326:1002)

Cause: Diarrhea; overflow from impactions (encopresis—see above); rectal neoplasms; neurologic, eg, myelomeningocele, MS, dementia, CVA, neuropathy, cord lesions; abnormal pelvic floor, eg, congenital and trauma especially from ob, aging, and pelvic floor denervation

Epidem: Especially common in the elderly

Rx: 1st, high-fiber diet, loperamide (Imodium), diphenoxylate (Lomotil), enemas if impacted; 2nd, biofeedback; 3rd, surgery

Hiccoughs

Cause: Lower esophageal obstruction as in achalasia or stricture (Ann IM 1991;115:711)

Rx: 1 tsp dry sugar (Nejm 1971;285:1489)

Liver bx techniques (Nejm 2001;344:495; 1970;283:582[Menghini]); place in w/u of elevated LFTs (Ann IM 1989;111:472)

Liver function test abnormalities: Differential dx and w/u (Nejm 2000;342:1266; Mayo Clin Proc 1996;71:1093):

Nausea and vomiting (rv of all causes—Ann IM 1984;101:211)
- Vagal stimulation directly: gagging or stomach distension >20 mm Hg; uterine, bladder, renal distension; elevated CNS pressure

Rx: Diphenhydramine (Benadryl) 25–50 mg po q 6 h, since both antihistamine and anticholinergic effects
- Labyrinthine stimulation causing cerebellar nausea, eg, motion sickness and all diseases affecting middle ear

Rx: Dimenhydrinate (Dramamine) best (Med Let 1981;23:89); scopolamine patch (Transderm V—Med Let 1981;23:89); or meclizine (Antivert) 25 mg po bid
- Medullary chemoreceptor trigger zone stimulation by morphine, digoxin, tetracycline, oncologic chemRx, disulfiram (Antabuse), estrogens, uremia, radiation, cancer, toxins, anesthetics

Rx: Prochlorperazine (Compazine) 10 mg iv/im, better than promethazine (Phenergan) (Ann Emerg Med 2000;36:89); chlorpromazine (Thorazine); metoclopramide (Reglan) iv helps during cisplatin rx (Nejm 1981;305:905); marijuana (Nejm 1975;293:795);

GASTROENTEROLOGY

tetrahydrocannabinol po or smoked (Ann IM 1979;91:819), better
than Compazine? (Nejm 1980;302:135 vs Ann IM 1979;91:825);
nabilone 2 mg po q 6–8 h (Nejm 1979;300:1295); ginger? (Lancet
3/20/82:655); ondansetron, a serotonin antagonist (Nejm
1990;322:810, 816), better than metoclopramide

Peritonitis
Sx: Pain w cough (78% sens/specif—BMJ 1994;308:1336)
Si: Rebound, pain w pelvic shake, heel percussion pain

Diarrhea
Acute (gastroenteritis causes and w/u—Am J Med 1999;106:670;
Nejm 1991;325:252, 327):
Following list grouped by fever and fecal leukocyte findings (see
individual diseases on each cause as well); work it up if: fever, fecal
blood, fecal leukocytes, sx >5 d, known exposures (Ann IM
1986;105:785), HIV positive or otherwise impaired host, traveler
on return home, severe volume depletion, or a community outbreak
If fever and/or fecal leukocytes present, consider empiric rx (Med Let
1998;40:47) on day 1 w ciprofloxacin 500 mg po × 1 dose (Lancet
1994;334:1537) or bid × 3d, or Tm/S (Septra) DS bid × 3–5 d (Ann
IM 1987;106:216; Nejm 1982;307:84) + loperamide (Imodium) ii
2 mg tabs, then i/stool up to 8 pills qd, lower doses for children
(Ann IM 1991;114:731, safe in all adults—Ann IM 1993;118:377);
unless it might be due to O157:H *E. coli* where both antibiotic and
antimotility rx worsens disease (Rx Let 2000;7:45)
If no fever, blood or mucus: loperamide as above w simethicone
250 mg/dose (Arch Fam Med 1999;8:243)
Rehydration and supportive care for all, like oral rehydration solution
(p 739); bismuth subsalicylate (Pepto-Bismol) 60 cc in adults or
1.14 cc/kg (100 mg/kg) in children helps speed recovery (Nejm
1993;328:1635, Pediatrics 1991;87:18), as does zinc gluconate
20 mg po qd within 1st 3 d in 3rd world children (Nejm 1995;333:
839); perhaps racecadotril 1.5 mg/kg po q 8 h in children (Nejm
2000;343:463)
Chronic (>4wk) (Nejm 1995;332:725)
Cause: In order of frequency: chronic infection, IBD, steatorrhea,
carbohydrate malabsorption, medications/food additives, previous
surgery w bacterial overgrowth, endocrine (adrenal insufficiency,
hyper/hypothyroidism, diabetes mellitus), laxative abuse, ischemic

bowel, radiation enteritis, colon cancer, idiopathic/functional, microscopic colitis (Am J Med 2000;108:416) from either collagenous or lymphocytic colitis, which presents as chronic watery diarrhea, have a normal appearing mucosa on endoscopy but abnl pathlogy on bx

Pathophys: Bacterial gut wall invasion; enterotoxin production; bacterial adherence to epithelial cell membrane cytotoxin production; unabsorbed solutes causing osmotic diarrhea; deconjugated bile salts and hydroxylated fatty acids; congenital/familial absorptive/ secretory abnormalities; Zollinger-Ellison syndrome, vasoactive intestinal peptide, calcitonin, carcinoid tumors; diabetic autonomic neuropathy; factitious from laxative use, eg, phenolphthalein, or water dilution of stool (Nejm 1994;330:1418)

Crs: Of idiopathic diarrhea, if w/u neg, is benign and resolves in <4 yr (Nejm 1992;327:1849)

Lab:

Chem: Lytes, BUN/creat, TSH, T4, gastrin, VIP if >1 L/d

Hem: CBC, ESR

Endo: Sigmoid/colonoscopy w bx

Stool: For fecal leukocytes, O + P × 3 before Ba studies, pH, 24 h weight, 72 h fat

Xray: KUB, UGIS and SBFT, BE

Rx: Somatostatin analog octreotide (Ann IM 1991;115:705); verapamil; loperamide (Imodium) 2 mg tabs up to 8 qd in adults; cholestyramine; antibiotics

GASTROENTEROLOGY

Chapter 7
Geriatrics

D. K. Onion and K. Gershman

7.1 DISEASES/DYSFUNCTION

DYSFUNCTION IN THE ELDERLY

Cause: Loss of physical, mental, and social function, excessive family burden (Gerontol 1980;20:649) usually caused by a mixture of geriatric syndromes including sensory changes (vision and hearing), affect changes (depression), delirium, falls, and incontinence; latter 2 are associated w impairments of upper and lower extremities (Jama 1995;273:1348)

Epidem: In 1985, 20% of elderly were disabled; by 2060, 30% will be disabled (J Gerontol 1992;47:S253); 40% visual impairment/blindness prevalence in nursing homes (Nejm 1995;332:1205)

Pathophys: Causes of geriatric failure to thrive (Ann IM 1996;124:1075)

Sx: Loss of self-care/independent living skills

Si: Inability to read; inability to answer short, whispered question such as "what is your name?"; urinary incontinence; weight below acceptable range for height; inability to recall 3 objects after 1 min; often sad or depressed; can't get out of bed, make own meals, do own shopping; trouble w stairs, bathtubs, rugs, lighting; doesn't know where to call in emergency or if ill (Ann IM 1990;112:699); inability to touch back of head w both hands, touch back of waist, or contralateral hip; inability to sit and touch toe of shoe; no grip strength (J Fam Pract 1993;17:429)

Activities of daily living (ADLs): Katz functional assessment (Gerontol 1970;10:20) records loss of independence in 6 skills (BATHING, DRESSING, TOILETING, TRANSFERRING, CONTINENCE,

FEEDING) in the order in which they are usually lost, and regained in reverse order; assess actual capacity, not reported performance (J Gerontol 1983;38:385). Speed and pain in performing ADLs in arthritis pts (J Chronic Dis 1978;31:557); rehab for ADLs (Arch Phys Med Rehab 1988;69:337)

Instrumental activities of daily living (IADLs), more complex activities like shopping, seeking transportation, preparing food, climbing stairs, and managing finances, housework, telephone, medications, and job (Fillenbaum IADLs—J Am Ger Soc 1985;33:698). Other IADL scales: home assessment (Clin Ger Med 1991;7:677); nutrition (Am Fam Phys 1993;48:1395); driving (Clin Ger Med 1993;9:349)

Crs: For every 5 adults w 5–6 limitations in ADLs, one may be expected to improve in 2 yr (Millbank Q 1990;68:445). Shorter time to dependence if functioning patients report difficulty performing some ADLs (Ann IM 1998;128:96)

Cmplc: Nursing home placement; Medicaid eligibility for NH admission requires a medical or behavioral dx, plus 2 impaired ADLs

Caregiver burnout: 70% of primary caregivers are middle-aged, married women, 30% are elderly themselves (Gerontol 1987; 27:616); prevalence of depression among caregivers is 30–50% (J Gerontol 1990;45:181)

Lab:

Rx: Prevent w annual geriatric evaluation unit eval (Nejm 1995;333:184)

Rehab; change medical regimen so as not to inhibit function; solicit community services; OT evaluation (Jama 1997;278:1321)

OSTEOPOROSIS

Ann IM 1995;123:452(men); Nejm 1992;327:620; Bull Rheum Dis 1988;38(2):1

Cause: (D. Spratt 9/95) See Table 7.1.1

Epidem: More in female smokers from changes in estrogen metabolism (Nejm 1994;330:387; 1985;313:973); less frequent in blacks and Polynesians because they start with higher adolescent bone densities (Nejm 1991;325:1597)

Pathophys: (Nejm 1988;318:818) Perhaps from incr prolactin premenopausally (Nejm 1980;303:1571) and/or simple estrogen

Osteoporosis, continued

Table 7.1.1 Causes of Osteoporosis

Acromegaly
Alcoholism
Anorexia (Ann IM 2000;133:790)
Cushing's disease/syndrome (even 10 mg prednisone qd enough), including chronic
   steroid use even inhaled in asthmatics (Nejm 2001;345:941) and rheumatoid
   arthritis (Ann IM 1993;119:963)
Diabetes, type I
Estrogen deficiency in postmenopausal women or amenorrheic athletes (Nejm 1984;
   311:277); hypogonadotrophic hypogonadism in men
Homocystinuria
Hyperparathyroidism
Hyperthyroidism
Idiopathic, at least some of which is genetic in structure of bone matrix protein
   (Nejm 1998;338:1016)
Malabsorption
Myeloma
Puberty, late onset, at least in men (Nejm 1992;326:600)
Renal calcium leak (rx'd w thiazides)
Scurvy
Vitamin A chronic excessive intake (Ann IM 1998;129:770)
Vitamin D winter time deficiency (Jama 1995;274:1683)
Vitamin D antagonist meds like phenytoin

---

deficiency postmenopausally; in athletes and other younger women,
the problem is either the estrogen and/or progesterone deficiency
from short or absent luteal phase, whether patient is athlete or not
(Nejm 1990;323:1221)

Sx: Bone pain, especially vertebral; fractures
Si: Decreased height/kyphosis from vertebral compression fractures
Crs: Chronic, slowly progressive
Cmplc: Rib and vertebral fractures (Nejm 1983;309:265)
   r/o causes listed above when premature, ie, in men under 70 and
   women under 60
   r/o **osteogenesis imperfecta** in young pts especially children; genetic;
   prevalence 1/20,000; genetic defect in collagen matrix (Nejm 1992;
   326:540); w blue sclerae (picture—Nejm 1998;339:966), deafness,
   double jointedness, cardiac valve degeneration (Nejm 1993;329:
   1406); fractures decrease w puberty, increase w menopause (Nejm

1984;310:1694); rx w pamindronate 7 mg/kg iv q 6 mo (Nejm 1998;339:947)

Lab:

Chem: PTH, serum and urine calciums to r/o hyperparathyroid and renal calcium leak in asx postmenopausal type (D. Spratt 9/95)

Xray: Osteopenic bones and fractures

Screening debatable (NIH/CDC—Jama 2001;285:785) using:
- Densitometry (Nejm 1991;324:1105; 1987;316:212) w dual xray absorptiometry (Med Let 1996;38:103), T scores (standard deviation from mean density of 30 yr old woman), $>1 - <2.5$ SDs = osteopenia, >2.5 SDs = osteoporosis and has a $5\times$ incr risk of fx; Z score is SD's from same age group; scores may take 2 yr to change w rx (Jama 2000;283:1318); cost = \$50
- Quantitative CT scan or
- Debatably femoral neck cortical thickness

Rx: (Med Let 2000;42:97; Nejm 1998;338:736) All preventive or instituted to slow the progression (Med Let 1992;34:101) and work to prevent the steroid-induced type as well (Nejm 1993;329:1406)

Weight-bearing exercise (Nejm 1996;124:187, Ann IM 1988;108:824)

Smoking cessation; helps exercise and allows protective effect of estrogens (Ann IM 1992;116:716)

Calcium replacement therapy (Med Let 2000;42:29), as $CaCO_3$, 1–1.5 gm of elemental Ca^{2+}/d; milk has 300 mg Ca^{2+}/cup; chewable Tums, 200 or 500 mg/tab; Oscal, 500 mg/tab (Med Let 1989;31:101); Ca citrate (Citracal) 315 mg/tab, but absorbed better especially in achlorhydrics/elderly (Nejm 1985;313:70); all come w 200 IU vit D/500 mg of Ca^{2+}; \$5–7/mo. Substantial effect even without estrogen (Ann IM 1994;120:97), eg, 50% less loss/yr (Nejm 1993;328:460)

Bisphosphonates; all around \$55/mo
- Alendronate (Fosamax) (Med Let 2001;43:26; Nejm 1995;333:1437) 10 mg po qd or 70 mg q 1 wk clearly helps prevent progression over 3 yr, NNT-3 = 10–30 (Lancet 1996;348:1535), or 5 mg po qd or 35 mg q 1 wk for prevention in high-risk women (eg, on steroids) or women who can't take ERT (Ann IM 1998;128:253,313; Nejm 1998;339:292; 338:485; Rx Let 1997;4:21). Adverse effects: various gi sx, rarely chemical esophagitis esp if

not taken w lots of fluids and pill sits on esophageal mucosa
(Nejm 1996;335:1016)
- Risedronate (Actonel) (Jama 1999;282:1344) 2.5–5 mg po qd (Rx
  Let 2000;7:26); decr hip fx in elderly women, NNT-3 = 90 (Nejm
  2001;344:333)
- Etidronate (Didronel) (Nejm 1997;337:382)
- Pamidronate (Aredia), esp if on steroid or leuprolide (Nejm 2001;
  345:948) rx; 60 mg iv q 3–4 mo
- Zolendronate (Zometa) (Med Let 2001;43:110) 2–4 mg iv over
  only 15 min (unlike Pamidronate); $850/4 mg like Pamidronate

Vitamin D as 225–400 IU qd (400 IU in multivitamins) or calcitriol
(D_3) 0.25 μgm po bid markedly decreases fractures without
producing stones by preventing incr PTH of winter at least (Nejm
1993;327:1637; 1992;326:357; 1989;321:1777; Ann IM 1991;
115:505); one RCT finds no effect? (Ann IM 1996;124:400)

Estrogen replacement therapy (p 624), decreases fracture rates by 2/3
(wrist, hip, other), start soon after menopause and continue (Ann
IM 1995;122:9), may take 10^+ yr to begin to make measurable
difference (HERS Study—S. Cummings 1999) and debatably helpful
if not started until fx's develop and/or over age 60 (Jama 2001;285:
2891,2909); or selective estrogen receptor modulators (p 624) like
raloxifene (Evista) (Med Let 1998;40:29) 60 mg po qd; or androgens
in men if hypogonad

Calcitonin (Cibacalcin) 100 IU sc/im or 200 IU nasally qd; also relieves
acute fx pain possibly via opiate effect (J Fam Pract 1992;35:93),
not as good as alendronate (J Clin Endocrinol Metab 2000;85:
1783); nasal $60/mo, sc/im $225/mo

Statin drug rx of incr cholesterol also helps slow osteoporosis? (Jama
2000;283:3205,3211,3255 vs 285:1850)

Thiazides help bone density and fx rate? (Ann IM 2000;133:516;
1996;124:187; 1993;118:657,666; Nejm 1990;322:286 vs Nejm
1991;325:1)

NaF in slow release form 25 mg po bid (Med Let 1996;38:3) or 20 mg
qd, 12 mo on, 2 off, appears to decrease fx rates in spine when
given w 1000^+ mg Ca (Ann IM 1998;129:1; 1995;123:401, 466),
but is controversial

Parathormone SC daily, experimental; NNT=10 (Nejm 2001;
344:1434)

FALLS IN THE ELDERLY

Ann IM 1994;121:442; Nejm 1994;331:821

Cause: (J Am Ger Soc 1988;36:266)

Accidents especially in home (37%), weakness/balance/gait problems (12%), drop attacks (11%), unknown (8%), dizziness or vertigo (7%), orthostatic hypotension (5%), CNS events (1%), syncope (1%); and (combined = 18%) acute illnesses, confusional states, visual impairments (Nejm 1991;324:1326), and drugs (>4 medications a risk factor) such as long-acting benzodiazepines (J Am Ger Soc 2000;48:682), tricyclics, and phenothiazines (Nejm 1987;316:363) as well as other psychoactive drugs (J Am Ger Soc 1999;47:30) especially in nursing homes (Nejm 1992;327:168), trazodone and SSRIs only slightly less risky than TCAs (Nejm 1998;339:875); and paradoxically incr by restraints (J Am Ger Soc 1999;47:1202; Ann IM 1992;116:369)

Epidem: 30% of elderly >65, 50% of those >80 living in the community fall each year (Nejm 1997;337:1279), 10% of those sustain serious injury, 6% fracture something. Over 50% of all NH pts fall during their stay (J Am Ger Soc 1995;43:1257) because of greater frailty and better reliability of reporting (J Am Ger Soc 1988;36:266); in nursing homes, higher rates at shift change and w lower staffing ratios (Primary Care 1989;16:377; J Am Ger Soc 1987;35:503)

Majority occur during mild-moderate activity, especially in bedroom or bathroom, walking, stepping up or down, or changing position; 70% at home; 10% on stairs, descending worse than ascending (Age Aging 1979;8:251); >50% accidents are due to environmental hazards: cords, furniture, small objects, optical patterns on escalators, stairs, floors (Clin Ger Med 1985;1:555)

Females > males, whites > blacks

Active elderly at greater risk of injury than frail elderly? (J Am Ger Soc 1991;39:46)

Pathophys: Fx risk from falls incr in elderly because of decr energy absorption capability of tissue and impaired protective responses like reaction time, muscle strength, level of alertness, cognition (J Gerontol 1991;46:M164)

Sx: H/o hypotensive sx posturally, postprandially, on micturation; may have h/o PAT, SSS, AS, hemiplegia, neuropathy, seizures, anemia, hypothyroidism, poor nutritional status, alcohol abuse, intercurrent illness (UTI, pneumonia, CHF); or medications (use of

GERIATRICS

antihypertensives, antidepressants, sedatives, hypoglycemics, phenothiazines, or carbamazepine)

Si: Evaluate environment: stairs, floors (slippery from urine, highly polished linoleum, thick pile rugs), low-lying furniture, pets, shower, lighting, stairway handrails, toilet grab bars, footwear/slippers

Inability to balance on 1 leg correlates w markedly incr risk of fall (J Am Ger Soc 1997;45:735)

Tinetti Gait/Balance Assessment

Crs:

Cmplc: Hip fx (p 315)

Falls are the 6th leading cause of death in elderly (Ann Rev Pub Hlth 1992;13:489); clustering of falls associated w high 6-mo mortality (Age Aging 1977;6:201); 1% result in hip fx, 5% other fx, 5% serious soft tissue injury (Nejm 1988;319:1701)

Prolonged lies waiting for help (<10% of falls), if >1 h may cause dehydration, pressure sores, rhabdomyolysis, pneumonia (J Gerontol 1991;146:M164)

25% of fallers subsequently avoid ADLs and IADLs for fear of falling again (J Gerontol 1994;49:M140; Nejm 1988;319:1701)

NH admissions (Nejm 1997;337:1279; Am J Pub Hlth 1992;82:395); incr use of health care services (Med Care 1992;30:587); ~50% pts hospitalized for falls are discharged to NHs (Emerg Med Clin N Am 1990;8:309)

Lab: Routine w/u: CBC w diff, UA, chem screen, stool guaiac, sTSH, B_{12} and ESR (to r/o PMR), EKG, CXR, and/or CT as history indicates

Noninv: No need to Holter monitor; prevalence of ventricular arrhythmia is 82% in both fallers and nonfallers; no sx reported w these arrhythmias (J Am Ger Soc 1989;37:430)

Rx: Prevent; fall reduction programs reduce falls by $\geq 1/3$ (Jama 1997; 278:557; Nejm 1994;331:821); pt education handouts (Am Fam Phys 1997;56:1815)

- Assessing falls in elderly (J Am Ger Soc 1993;41:309,315,479)
- Minimizing number and doses of medications
- Treating osteoporosis w estrogen replacement (Nejm 1993;329: 1141; Am J Med 1993;95:75S)
- Exercise programs to increase muscle strength and flexibility (J Am Ger Soc 2001;49:10; Jama 1995;273:1341); balance and gait training especially getting in and out of chairs, turning

around; NH standard PT is of moderate benefit (J Am Ger Soc 1996;44:513; Jama 1994;271:519)

- Assistive aids: walker use s/p hip fx by advancing 20–30 cm, then moving weak leg first; front-wheeled walker for Parkinson's, which avoids retropulsion and tripping. Cane use s/p hip fx only if ipsilateral upper extremities and contralateral lower extremities are strong, <25% of pt's weight should be placed on cane; when going up or down stairs keep good leg up higher, ie, "up with good, down with bad." Trochanteric pads decrease hip fx's (Jama 1994;271:128)
- Proper shoes
- Chairs should have arm rests
- Obstacle-free, glare-free, adequately lit environment
- Avoid physical and pharmacologic restraints (Ann IM 1992;116: 369; Jama 1991;265:468); alternatives: special areas for walking, lower beds, floor pads, alarm systems (Am Fam Phys 1992;45:763), surveillance by staff; hospital alternatives: use of family visitors, professional sitters, lower beds, "functional" ICUs

HIP FRACTURE
Nejm 1996;334:1519

Cause: Falls + osteoporosis

Epidem: Rates lower in blacks; rates incr by thinness, (Nejm 1995;332: 767) pos family hx, alcohol use, CVA hx (Nejm 1994;330:1555), smoking (Nejm 1987;316:404), hyperthyroidism, inactivity, caffeine use, visual impairment (Nejm 1991;324:1326), and drugs such as long-acting benzodiazepines (J Am Ger Soc 2000;48:682), tricyclics, SSRIs (Lancet 1998;351:1303) and phenothiazines (Nejm 1987;316: 363) as well as other psychoactive drugs especially in nursing homes (Nejm 1992;327:168); and paradoxically maybe also incr by restraints (Ann IM 1992;116:369). Assoc w being on feet <4% of the day, higher pulse rates (Nejm 1995;332:767)

Pathophys: 45% femoral neck (intracapsular), 45% intertrochanteric (good blood supply), 10% subtrochanteric

Falls and fractures occur in the elderly because:
- Slow gait results in more falls on hips rather than other body parts
- Diminished protective responses

GERIATRICS

- Less fat/muscle protection
- Diminished strength (J Gerontol 1989;44:M107)

Sx: H/o fall; hip pain, but may be vague in the elderly

Si: External rotation of the leg w shortening; pain w motion

Crs: 25% of fall-induced hip fractures result in death within 6 mo, 25% in subsequent functional dependence; 50% are walking independently 1 yr postfracture (Am J Pub Hlth 1987;79:279). Usually fatal unless repaired. Prefracture mental status and physical functional level are best predictor of eventual outcome (J Am Ger Soc 1992;40:861)

Cmplc: After fx, frequently develop in hospital (J Gen IM 1987;2:78): confusion (49%), UTI (33%), arrhythmia (26%), pneumonia (19%), depression (15%), CHF (7%), DVT

r/o, if xrays neg, stress fx, pubic ramus fx, acetabular fx, greater trochanteric fx, and trochanteric bursitis or contusion

Lab:

Xray: Plain films, AP and lateral or AP w 15–20° internal rotation show fx, often subtle, especially if impacted; after 72 hr, bone scan or MRI if dx still in doubt

Rx: Prevent first episode or recurrence w rx of osteoporosis (p 309) (Nejm 1992;327:1637) w:
- Hip protectors in high risk pts (Nejm 2000;343:1506,1562; Lancet 1993;341:11); worn in special underpants, 30% refuse to use but when do, 60% reduction in hip fx's, NNT-5 = 8
- Statin drugs? (Jama 2000;283:3211; Lancet 2000;355:2185 vs Jama 2001;285:1850)
- Thiazides? (Ann IM 2000;133:516; 1996;124:187; 1993;118:657, 666; Nejm 1990;322:286 vs Nejm 1991;325:1)
- Avoid use of slippery throw rugs in the home and restraints (Ann IM 1992;116:369)

Surgical reduction, pinning/fixation, or arthroplasty if badly displaced intracapsular; within 48 hr if possible w 48 hr periop antibiotics

Postsurgery consider heparin, low molecular wgt heparin 12 hr preop and 1 mo post op (Nejm 1996;335:696), warfarin DVT prophylaxis (p 36), or perhaps hirudin 30 min preop (Nejm 1997;337:1329); as well as compression stockings (Arch IM 1994;154:67); weight bearing in 1–2 d and early rehab in hospital, rehab unit, or NH (Jama 1998;279:847; 1997;277:396)

7.2 DEMENTIAS

ALZHEIMER'S DEMENTIA (Dementia, Alzheimer's Type) (DAT)

Nejm 1999;341:1670; Clin Ger Med 1994;10:239

Cause: Unclear (see Jama 1997;277:775–840), but several genes implicated, on chromosomes #1, #14 (Nejm 1995;333:1283), #12 (Jama 1997;278:1237), and amyloid A4 protein deposition (Lancet 1992;340:467; Ann Neurol 1992;32:157) gene on chomosome #21 (Nejm 1989;320:1446)

Early onset (<60):
- Amyloid precursor protein gene on chromosome #21
- Presenilin single gene
- Presenilin two gene type

Late onset (>60):
- Apolipoprotein-E gene, E4 allele hetero- and homozygotes on chromosome #19 (Nejm 2000;343:450)
- Chromosome #12 gene (Jama 1997;278:1237)

Epidem: Prevalence = 5% at age 70, 20% at 80, 50% at 90 (Jama 1995; 273:1354) vs 40% of population at age 85 yr (Nejm 1999;341: 1670) but varies 10× depending on which criteria used (Nejm 1997;327:1667); 20–50% incidence in family members of late-onset Alzheimer's patients (Ger 2000;55:34; Ann IM 1991;115:601); males = females; 100% of Down's syndrome pts age >35 yr (Science 1992;258:668; Ann IM 1985;103:526)

40$^+$% of elderly dementia is Alzheimer's, the rest is vascular multi-infarct type predominantly (Nejm 1993;328:153)

Pathophys: (Nejm 1991;325:1849)

Neuronal dropout; decr acetylcholine synthesis (Nejm 1985;313:7), hence anticholinergics worsen (Nejm 1985;313:7)

E4 allele of apolipoprotein E (Nejm 1996;334:752, 791; Jama 1995; 273:1274) facilitates β amyloid protein deposition in neurofibrillary tangles (Nejm 1995;333:1242), concentrations of which correlate w cognitive decline (Jama 2000;283:1571)

Sx: Loss of social skills and memory usually unacknowledged by patient

Si: Abnormal mental status (Psych Clin N Am 1991;14:309; 1-page test—Ann IM 1977;86:40) w memory loss >6 mo + ≥1 other cognitive function impairments (DSM-IV; Am Psychiatr Assoc 1994;142; Neurol 1984;34:939)

- Memory deficits: recent much worse than remote; including orientation to time (day, mo, yr) (day of week is 53% sens, 92% specif—Ann IM 1991;115:122); recall 3 items
- Construction deficits: perceptive/spatial disorientation, eg, answers to "how do you get there from here?"; clock face drawing; copy interlocking pentagons, gets lost
- Language impairments: anomias/paraphasias/aphasias, which often result in neologisms or circumlocutions
- Abstraction impairments: "what does it mean to give someone the cold shoulder?", categorization, calculations
- Praxis impairments: Inability to perform complex movements necessary for behaviors like writing, meal preparation, dressing
- Prosody defects: trouble conveying and reading facial expressions of emotions, affect changes
- Executive function problems (Lancet 1999;354:1921): frontal lobe difficulty creating and executing complicated goal-directed behaviors. Test w ability to draw (not copy) a clock showing 2:10 (impaired person draws hands to 2 and 10 rather than 2 and 2), and other tests

Pupillary dilatation >20% within 30 min to 1/100 diluted tropicamide gtts, even 1 yr before measurable DAT, 95% sens/specif (Sci 1994; 266:1051) vs not helpful and not being used clinically (Arch Neurol 1997;54:165)

Crs: Slowly progressive; mean survival from first sx = 10 yr, shorter the more severe it is (Ann IM 1990;113:429). Stages (Am J Psych 1982; 139:1136) 1 and 2, forget familiar names and places; stage 3, coworkers aware; stage 4, difficulty w finances; stage 5, need assistance dressing; stage 6, incontinence, delusional; stage 7, grunting, nonambulatory

Cmplc: r/o: Reversible causes (Adams—Nejm 1986;314:1111):
- Delirium (p 573), if <1 mo, in which alertness may fluctuate from fear, lethargy to hypervigilance, delusions and distortions, easily distracted because attention span is most prominent deficit; test by serial 7's; serial digits up to 7, eg, phone numbers; spell "world" or do days of week backward
- Depression pseudodementia (p 323); more "I-don't-know" answers than the guesses of DAT; often both occur together; language

Mini Mental Status Exam

Test	Content	Points
Time orientation	Year/month/day of week/season/date	5
Place orientation	State/city/part of city/building/floor	5
Registration	3 objects (table, hat, apple)	3
Concentration	serial 7's, or spell world backwards	5
Recall	recall above 3 objects	3
Naming	name 2 objects (watch, pen)	2
Repetition	repeat "no ifs, ands, or buts"	1
Command	3 part command (L hand to R ear and close eyes	3
Written command	sign that says "close your eyes"	1
Composition	write a sentence	1
Spatial orientation	copy interlocking pentagons	1
Total		30

Normal: 23-26 for uneducated; 29+ for college educated; impaired <23

Figure 7.2.1

preserved; psychomotor retardation. If mini-mental status exam score ≥ 21, they are more responsive to antidepressants
- Drugs, single or multiple (6/100)
- Myxedema (4/100)
- Toxins like occult solvent/paint exposure, lead, arsenic, mercury, manganese, thallium, carbon monoxide
- Subdural hematoma (2/100)
- Frontal/temporal tumor
- Tertiary syphilis
- AIDS
- B_{12} deficiency
- Wernicke-Korsakoff w antegrade memory loss, alcohol hx; may recover partially over 1 yr (Nejm 1985;312:16)

Nonreversible causes (Ann IM 1984;100:417):
- Frontal/subcortical (type 2) dementias (J Am Ger Soc 1998;46:98), which show loss of executive control function, forgetfulness, and motor findings 1st (Arch Neurol 1993;50:873), unlike amnesia and language deficits in DAT; eg, Parkinson's, Huntington's, Wilson's, olivopontine degeneration, and normal pressure

GERIATRICS

hydrocephalus (may be partially reversible), as well as many of the above reversible causes
- Multi-infarct dementia when stepwise crs, young, emotional lability prominent, and h/o HT, CVA, or ASHD
- **Pick's disease,** which is similar but w less memory impairment and more behavioral change, is rare and anatomic changes are isolated to frontal and temporal lobes
- Lewy body disease (J Am Ger Soc 1998;46:1449; Neurol 1996;47: 111) w attention deficits, hallucinations, and extrapyramidal si's

Lab:

Chem: $T_3 T_4$, chemistry panel, lytes if acute, perhaps B_{12} level

Hem: CBC

Noninv: EEG occasionally helpful to distinguish DAT (slow waves) from depression (normal)

Path: Brain histology at postmortem shows neurofibrillary tangles, senile plaques w eosinophilic amyloid; experimental apo-E genotyping 65% sens/specif (Nejm 1998;338:506)

Serol: VDRL, perhaps HIV antibody if young

Xray: Head CT or MRI distinguishes from multi-infarct dementia (Neurol 1993;43:250), only if si's of subdural or rapid onset (Ann IM 1984;100:417); in all possibly? (Nejm 1986;314:964); very low yield of reversible disease, eg, <1/250 (Ann IM 1994;120:856)

Rx:

Preventive:
- Statin rx of incr cholesterol may prevent or slow onset (Arch Neurol 2000;57:1410,1439; Lancet 2000;356:1627)
- ERT may help (Lancet 1996;348:429) but conflicting evidence (Nejm 2001;344:1207; Jama 2001;285:1489; 1998;279:688) and does not slow progression once started (Jama 2000;283:1007)
- Apolipoprotein E screening not appropriate (1997;277:832; Jama 1995;274:1627)
- NSAIDs (not ASA or acetaminophen) may decr risk (Jama 1998;279:688; Neurol 1997;48:626) if taken $\times$ 2$^+$ yr (NNT=16) (Nejm 2001;345:1515,1567)
- Screening/preventive rx of other diseases must be truncated to acount for overall prognosis and risk benefits (Jama 2000;283:3230)

Memory meds (Nejm 1999;341:1672):
- Acetylcholinesterase inhibitors (like physostigmine); all cost $130/mo
- Donepezil (Aricept) (Arch IM 1998;158:1021; ACP J Club 1998;129(3):68; Med Let 1997;39:53) 5–10 mg po hs; no long term effects on crs, no help w behavioral sx; cmplc: NV+D, agitation/ insomnia, myalgias, unlike galantamine and rivastigmine (Clin Ger Med 2001;17:346); metabolism slowed by paroxetine (Paxil) (Rx Let 2000;7:10)
- Galantamine (Reminyl) (Med Let 2001;43:53) 4 mg po bid, incr to 8–12 mg bid; adv effects like donepezil
- Rivastigmine (Exelon) (Med Let 2000;42:93) 1.5–6 mg po bid; minimal drug interactions w p 450 drugs like phenytoin, carbamazepine, ketoconazole; adv effects: NV+D, wgt loss
- Tacrine (tetrahydroaminoacridine, THA) (Cognex) 10–40 mg po qid (Jama 1994;271:985; Med Let 1993;35:87) may help cognition? (Jama 1998;280:1777; Nejm 1992;327:1253,1306; vs Nejm 1990;322:1272; 1991;323:349); cmplc: hepatitis in 25–50%
- *Ginko biloba* extract 40 mg po tid helps modestly over 1 yr by DBCT (Jama 1997;278:1327) but others (Med Let 1998;40:63) skeptical of study design and results; adv effects: coma when used w trazodone (Rx Let 2000;7:53)
- Selegiline 10 mg po qd (Nejm 1997;336:1216), can prolong independent living
- Vitamin E 2000 IU po qd (Nejm 1997;336:1216)
- Vasodilators like ergoloid mesylates (Hydergine) 2 mg tid × 6 mo (Arch Neurol 1994;51:787; Ann IM 1984;100:896; no use—Nejm 1990;323:445)

of agitated behavior:
 1st: Carbamazepine (Tegretol) 25 mg po bid up to 200 tid to a level of 6–7 mg % following CBC and LFTs (J Clin Psych Neurol 1990;51:115)
 Gabapentin (Neurontin) (Rx Let 1998;5:64)
 2nd: Respirodone (Respirdal) 1–3 mg po bid; or olanzapine (Zyprexa); or quetiapine (Seroquel)
Other options depending on predominant sx, in decreasing order of desirability:
- Clozapine avoids extrapyramidal sx but causes agranulocytosis, hypotension, and seizures (J Ger Psych Neurol 1994;7:129)

- Phenothiazines (p 690) in order of increasing extrapyramidal and decreasing sedation/anticholinergic/hypotensive effects. Haloperidol (Haldol) 1–3 mg/d is effective for psychosis and disruptive behavior (Am J Psych 1998;155:1512) but tardive dyskinesia 3–5× higher in the elderly compared to younger pts
- Trazodone 50 mg po b-qid (J Clin Psych 1986;47:4)
- Benzodiazepines such as oxazepam (Serax) 10 mg po tid, or lorazepam (Ativan), but diminished effect after several months
- Propranolol 60–600 mg po qd (Can J Psych 1992;37:651; Psych Ann 1990;20:446)
- Estrogen perhaps for sexual aggression in men? (J Am Ger Soc 1991;39:1110)

In NH, wandering can also be managed by "wandering areas," sign posts, pictures of residents on resident room doors, tape barriers, half-doors, coded locks

Driving issues (Jama 1997;45:949; 1995;273:1360; J Am Ger Sioc 1996;44:85); not at night, not in traffic, informally test regularly

of inanition: tube feedings no help and risky (Nejm 2000;342:206; Jama 1999;282:1365)

NORMAL PRESSURE HYDROCEPHALUS
Nejm 1985;312:1255

Cause: Idiopathic, or postsurgical, trauma, or infection
Epidem:
Pathophys: A "communicating hydrocephalus" (in contrast to foraminal or aqueductalstenosis) and obstruction is therefore at cisterna. Hence, 4th ventricle may dilate, causing cerebellar si's
Sx: First, trouble walking (ataxia) and may remain as only sx; or may then develop progressive dementia and incontinence
Si: Horizontal nystagmus, normal discs, spasticity, frontal lobe si's
Crs: Progressive dementia
Cmplc:
Lab:
  CSF: Transient improvement w removal of 50 cc (Acta Neurol Scand 1987;75:566) 1–3 × in 1 wk; some neurosurgeons now not doing shunt unless see improvement with this first

Xray: CT scan shows big ventricles (100%); cisternogram shows delayed or no movement of dye out over hemispheres, but there are false negatives

Rx: Surgical shunt, 80% success (Jama 1996;44:445, Nejm 1985;312: 1255); cmplc: infections in 3–5%

DEPRESSION IN THE ELDERLY

Nejm 1989;320:164

Cause: Often situational; hypothalamic/pituitary/adrenal axis and circadian rhythm disruption; drugs including alcohol, amantadine, antipsychotics, cimetidine, clonidine, cytotoxic agents, digoxin, α-methyldopa, propranolol, sedatives, steroids, reserpine (M.A. Jenike, Ger Psych and Psychopharm, St Louis: Mosby Yearbook 1989)

Epidem: Prevalence is 10–15% in the geriatric population

Pathophys: MAO activity is incr in brains of elderly (Am J Psych 1984; 141:1276)

Sx: Major depression has 5/8 of the following × 2 wks unless recent major loss:
- Impaired sleep, often w early morning awakening
- Diminished interest (anhedonia)
- Diminished energy
- Impaired concentration and/or appetite
- Feelings of guilt
- Agitation
- Psychomotor retardation
- Diminished self-esteem (J Am Ger Soc 1986;34:215)

Masked depression may present as somatization syndrome

Si: Depression scales (Clin Gerontol 1986;5:165); weight loss

Crs:

Cmplc: Suicide, 20% fatal

r/o grief reaction, dysthymia, schizophrenia, drug reactions

Lab:

Chem: TSH, B_{12} level

Hem: CBC

Rx:
Medications: tricyclics (p 692), generally use 1/3 usual adult doses
(demethylation is decr in the elderly); beware drug interactions
- SSRIs like sertraline (Zoloft) 25–50$^+$ mg po qd; paroxetine (Paxil)
  10–20$^+$ mg po qd (DBRCT—Jama 2000;284:1519); citalopram
  (Celexa) 10–40 mg po qd
- Trazodone (Desyrel) up to 150 mg po qd; soporific
- Desipramine (Norpramin) 25–150 mg po qd; useful if sleeping too
  much
- Imipramine (Tofranil) up to 150 mg po qd; especially if also has
  urge incontinence
- Nortriptyline (Pamelor, Avantyl) 10–35$^+$ mg po qd
- Amoxapine (Asendin), especially good to get eating, cf. Ritalin
- Mirtazapine (Remeron) 15–45 mg q hs; sedates, incr appetite
- Bupropion (Wellbutrin) 50 mg po bid
- Enhancers: L-thyroxine 0.025 mg po qd, methylphenidate
  (Ritalin) 5–10 mg po q am and noon (Am J Psych 1995;152:929),
  or lithium up to 300 mg po tid following 12 h postdose levels
Electroshock therapy very effective in the elderly (Nejm 1984;311:163)

7.3 MISCELLANEOUS

Abuse of elderly, detection and rx (Nejm 1995;332:437)

ASHD rx in the elderly
HT rx of pressures >140/90, even though prevalence >50%, helps
  prevent MIs and CVAs, NNT-5 = 18 (Jama 1994;272:1932); lifestyle
  changes, then thiazides, then β blockers? (Jama 1994;272:842; HT
  1994;23:275)

Albumin levels <3.5 gm% predict >50% 5-yr mortality vs 10–20% if
  >4 gm% (Jama 1994;272:1037)

Code status: Durable power-of-attorney applications; mail to pts age
  >65 yr after hospitalization (Nejm 1994;271:209). CPR in elderly age
  >70 yr success so low not worth it? (Ann IM 1989;111:193, 199 vs

Jama 1990;264:2109). Prior competent choice vs best interest standard is moving focus to pts' subjective experience at time of therapy (J Am Ger Soc 1998;46:922)

Driving by elderly (>72 year old) (Ann IM 1995;122:842); accident risk incr from 6–50% as go from 0/3 to 3/3 correct answers to following: (1) ability to copy interlocking pentagons, (2) walk >1 block qd, and (3) 2^+ structural abnormalities of feet. Visual tracking techniques can also help stratify cognitively impaired pts (J Am Ger Soc 1998;46:556; 1997;45:949)

Incontinence (AHCPR Public #92-0039 US Pub Hlth Svc 1992; Nejm 1989;320:1; 1985;313:800)
Innervations: bladder, parasympathetic (cholinergic); sphincter, α-sympathetic

• Urge incontinence
Cause: Decreased CNS inhibition, eg, dementia, Parkinson's, CVA; or parasympathomimetic drugs such as bethanechol (Urecholine); or irritation from cystitis, prostatitis, BPH, bladder tumor
Pathopys: Detrusor instability w or w/o impaired contractility
Lab: Cystometrics show spastic contractions
Rx: Antibiotics for any infection only if recent change in incontinence pattern or other evidence of symptomatic UTI (Ann IM 1995;122:749)
  Anticholinergics (parasympathetic inhibition):
  Antimuscarinics (all cause dry mouth sx)
  • Imipramine 25–50 mg po hs
  • Propantheline 7.5–30 mg po tid
  • Oxybutynin (Ditropan) 2.5–5 mg po tid; long-acting forms not as effective (Med Let 2001;43:28)
  Muscarinic receptor antagonists (much less dry mouth)
  • Tolterodine (Detrol) (Med Let 1998;40:101; Rx Let 1998;5:26) 1–2 mg po bid; long-acting forms not as effective (Med Let 2001;43:28); $75/mo
  • Flavoxate (Urispas)
  Biofeedback (Ann IM 1985;103:507) and behavioral training (Kegel anal sphincter contraction w abd muscle relaxation); better than medications (J Am Ger Soc 2000;48:370; Jama 1998;280:1995) vs

GERIATRICS

no clear benefit (Cochrane Library metanalysis ACP J Club 1999;130:67)

- **Overflow incontinence**

Cause: Bladder outlet obstruction, eg, BPH, uterine prolapse, constipation, α-stimulant drugs, neuropathy (impaired sensory input to sacral micturation center); or diminished detrusor strength (flaccid due to lower motor neuron disease or meds such as anticholinergics, calcium channel blockers, smooth muscle relaxants)

Sx: Obstructive w diminished urinary stream, frequency; if neuropathic, will have no sensation of bladder fullness

Lab: Postvoid residuum >100 cc; cystometrics show no contractions w 400$^+$ cc when due to diminished sensation

Rx: Self-catheterization (J Am Ger Soc 1990;38:364)

Stool softeners for constipation

Rx prolapse or BPH

Increase detrusor strength w bethanechol (Urecholine) 10$^+$ mg po tid, or phenoxybenzamine (Dibenzyline) 10 mg po qd (parasympathomimetics)

Block sphincter constriction (α blockade) w prazosin (Minipres) 1–2 mg po tid or terazosin (Hytrin)

- **Stress incontinence** (Urol Clin NA 1998;25:625; Am Fam Phys 1998;57:2675)

Cause: Estrogen deficiency effect on urethral mucosa; or pelvic relaxation after childbirth or urologic surgery; neuropathies; α-blocking meds

Pathophys: Sphincter insufficiency

Sx: Loss of urine w cough, sneeze, laugh

Si: Cystocele on physical exam if due to pelvic relaxation

Rx: Estrogen vaginal ring better than po systemic rx (J Am Ger Soc 1999;47:1383); Kegel exercises qid (J Am Ger Soc 1983;31:476); pessaries (Am Fam Phys 2000;61:2723); surgery (A/P repair, sphincter repairs)

of neuropathic types, imipramine 25$^+$ mg hs (α stimulation, parasympathetic inhibition); or biofeedback (Ann IM 1985;103:507)

• Functional incontinence

Cause: Can't get to toilet

Si: All normal

Rx: Schedules plus reinforcement, if oriented × 1 and can identify 1 of 2 objects, prompting can decrease incontinence from 25% to 6–9% (Jama 1995;273:1366)

MI, acute, aggressive rx w angiography, angioplasty, and CABG of minimal benefit (Jama 1994;272:859,891)

GERIATRICS

Chapter 8
Hematology/Oncology

D. K. Onion

8.1 CHEMOTHERAPY

MANAGING CANCER AND CHEMOTHERAPY

Cachexia/wasting syndromes (Nejm 1999;340:1740):
Assess diet; r/o other disease; if testosterone deficient, replace w
testosterone enanthate 300 mg im q 3 wk (Ann IM 1998;129:18), not
scrotal patch (Am J Med 1999;107:130)
Other possible aids:
- Androgens: nandrolone (Jama 1999;281:1275) 100 mg im q 1 wk,
  in renal failure; oxandrolone (Jama 1999;281:1282) 20 mg qd po
  in AIDS
- Growth hormones possibly in AIDS (Ann IM 1996;125:865,873,
  932), but cost $1000/wk
- Marijuana, marinol
- Megestrol (Megace) (a progestin) 40 mg po qid or liquid 40 mg/cc
  up to 800 mg qd, stimulates appetite and weight gain (Ann IM
  1994;121:393,400)
- Thalidomide? (Am J Med 2000;108;487; Rx Let 1997;4:66)
- TPN during chemotherapy of questionable (Ann IM
  1984;101:303) or no (Ann IM 1989;110:734) benefit

Fetal damage: None in oncology nurses (Nejm 1985;313:1173); no
increase in cancer (Nejm 1998;338:1339) or anomalies (Nejm
1991;325:141) in offspring conceived by pts later in life after
chemotherapy, except maybe anomalies after dactinomycin

Fevers: Require stat w/u and rx (p 363)

Nausea and vomiting prophylaxis (eg, with some emetogenic drugs like
cisplatinum) and rx (Nejm 1993;329:1790; Med Let 1993;35:124)
- 1st: Dexamethasone, 8–20 mg iv 30 min before, then 4 mg po bid (Nejm
  2000;342:1554), or 10 mg qid × 24 h (Nejm 1984;311:549; 1981;305:
  520); or 10 mg iv before chemotherapy with metaclopramide 10 mg po
  qid afterward is better than ondansetron (Nejm 1993;328:1076)
- 2nd: Ondansetron (Zofran) (Med Let 1991;33:63), 0.15 mg/kg iv over
  15 min once ($200) then 8 mg po bid (Nejm 2000;342:1554), or 4 mg
  po tid (Ann IM 1993;118:407); start 1/2 h before chemotherapy; better
  w dexamethasone w 1st dose; or 8 mg po b-tid (Nejm 1993;328:1081),
  with metopimazine (a phenothiazine) 30 mg po qid (Nejm 1993;328:
  1076); twice as good as metaclopramide (Ann IM 1991;114:834)
  Adverse effects: headaches, constipation, elevated LFTs all limit use
  (ACP J Club 1997;127(3):65)
- Dolasetron (Anzemet) (Med Let 1998;40:53) similar to ondansetron, a
  5-HT antagonist; 100 mg iv or po × 1; $150/dose
- Granisetron 3 mg iv, similar to ondansetron, also a 5-HT antagonist
  (Nejm 1995;332:1)
- Hypnotic desensitization (Nejm 1982;307:1476)
- Marijuana (Ann IM 1983;99:106; Med Let 1980;22:41); dronabinol
  (Marinol = tetrahydrocannabinol) 10–20 mg po q 4–6 h (Ann IM 1997;
  126:791; Med Let 1985;27:98) or nabilone (Cesamet—Med Let 1987;
  29:2)
- Prochlorperazine 5–20 mg po, pr, im, or occasionally iv
- Acupuncture w or w/o electrostimulation qd reduces emesis × 2/3 in
  DBCT (Jama 2000;284:2755)

Pain (Nejm 1996;335:1124; Med Let 1982;24:95):
WHO analgesic ladder (dosing, p 783)
  1st, NSAID
  2nd, add opiate (codeine, oxycodone)
  3rd, add stronger opiate (morphine, oxycodone, fentanyl) + tricyclic
  or anticonvulsant

Thrombocytopenia prophylactically rx w interleukin–1a (Nejm 1993;
328:756)

(Listed by tumor type and toxicities—Med Let 2000;42:83)

Generally administered under the direction of an oncologist and used in combination with each other in complex regimens, not as single agents; doses adjusted for each cycle depending on the other agents being used and patient response

ALKYLATING AGENTS

Several increase leukemia risk by 6–20× up to 8 yr after treatment ends; risk is incr by splenectomy and minimally affected by radiation rx; but overall fewer than 2% get leukemia after chemotherapy (Nejm 1990; 322:1,7)

- Busulfan (Myleran); adverse effects: marrow suppression, pulmonary fibrosis, some alopecia
- Chlorambucil (Leukeran) po; adverse effects: marrow suppression, pulmonary fibrosis
- Cyclophosphamide (Cytoxan); or analog ifosfamide (Ifex). Adverse effects: marrow suppression; alopecia; pulmonary fibrosis; hemorrhagic cystitis, and bladder cancer risk = 5% at 10 yr, 10% at 12 yr, 16% at 15 yr after rx (Ann IM 1996;124:477; Nejm 1988;318:1028), give with mesna to detoxify urine so bladder spared (Med Let 1989;31:98)
- Melphalan (Alkeran); adverse effects: marrow suppression, especially of platelets; leukemia risk 10× more than for cyclophosphamide (Nejm 1992;326:1745; Ann IM 1986;105:360)
- N-mustard; adverse effects: marrow suppression, some alopecia
- Thiotepa; adverse effects: marrow suppression

ANTIMETABOLITES

- Azathioprine (Imuran) and 6-MP po, but absorption erratic (Nejm 1983; 308:1005). Adverse effects: marrow suppression, gi ulcerations, cholestasis, incr effect with allopurinol, excessive toxicity in the 1/300 homozygous for catabolic enzyme deficiency (Ann IM 1997;126:608)
- Cytosine arabinoside (Cytarabine); adverse effects: marrow suppression
- 5-FU iv, po no good; adverse effects: marrow suppression, gi ulcerations (Nejm 1978;299:1049)
- Gemcitabine (Gemzar) (Med Let 1996;38:102) iv weekly; for pancreatic Ca where it improves pain and functional status and marginally

prolongs life, also in breast, bladder, and pulmonary small cell Ca; cmplc: marrow suppression, NV+D; cost $600/wk

- Methotrexate (Nejm 1983;309:1094) po or intrathecal. Adverse effects: marrow suppression, gi ulcerations, aspirin increases effect (protein binding is decreased), in rheumatoid arthritis EBV lymphomas, which regress w withdrawal of the mtx (Ann IM 1993;328:1317), reversible pneumonitis
- Thioquanine; adverse effects: marrow suppression, excessive toxicity in the 1/300 homozygous for catabolic enzyme deficiency (Ann IM 1997; 126:608)

ANTHRACYCLINES

- Daunorubicin (Daunomycin) (Med Let 1980;22:34; Ann IM 1979; 91:710). Adverse effects: marrow suppression; red urine; alopecia; cardiotoxicity (Nejm 1998;339:900) especially at doses >40 mg/kg, age-related, decr by 2–4 d infusions (Ann IM 1982;96:133); in children, long-term adverse cardiac effects (Ann IM 1996;125:47; Nejm 1991; 324:808)
- Doxorubicin (Adriamycin) iv. Adverse effects: marrow suppression; cardiotoxicity at all doses (Ann IM 1996;125:47) especially those >350 mg/m^2 total (Nejm 1979;300:278) preventable w dexrazoxane (Med Let 1991;33:85)
- Epirubicin (Ellence) (Med Let 2000;42:12), analog of doxorubicin used for breast Ca, less cardiotoxic, more expensive
- Idarubicin (Idamycin); similar to daunorubicin for AML (Med Let 1991; 33:84)

ARABINES (Purine Analog)

- Cladribine (Leustatin) (Ann IM 1994;120:784); for hairy cell leukemia, CLL, and T-cell lymphomas
- Fludarabine (Fludara) iv for CLL (Med Let 1991;33:84)
- Vidarabine

EPIPODOPHYLLOTOXINS
Nejm 1991;325:1682

- Etoposide (a podophyllin) (Med Let 1983;25:48); for testicular cancer, small cell, ALL, etc. Adverse effects: marrow suppression; AML in 4–12%, especially if given weekly
- Teniposide; for ALL; adverse effects: AML in 4–12% especially if given weekly

OTHER

- Asparaginase (Med Let 1978;20:103) iv; adverse effects: hemorrhagic pancreatitis, hepatitis, anaphylaxis, transient decrease of thyroid-binding globulin (Nejm 1979;301:251)
- BCG (Nejm 1974;290:1413); mainly for superficial bladder cancer
- Bleomycin (Ann IM 1979;90:945); adverse effects: pneumonitis and fibrosis
- Carboplatin (Med Let 1989;31:83); for ovarian cancer after cisplatinum fails or as first drug
- Carmustine (BCNU) iv. Adverse effects: pulmonary fibrosis, most manifest within the first 3 years after rx but may not appear for up to 15 yr (Nejm 1990;323:378); delayed suppression of polys and platelets
- Cisplatin (Ann IM 1984;100:704; Nejm 1979;300:289) iv or intraperitoneal (Ann IM 1982;97:845); for testicular cancer cures and in combination rx of oat cell, head and neck, ovarian, and cervical cancers. Adverse effects: renal damage (Ann IM 1988;108:21); neuropathy, prevent with ACTH analog (Nejm 1990;322:89); pulmonary fibrosis; low Mg^{2+} (Ann IM 1981;95:628); MIs and CVAs (Ann IM 1986;105:48); rarely leukemia (Nejm 1999;340:351)
- Cyclosporine (Nejm 1989;321:1725) for immunosuppression in organ transplants; use w diltiazem or ketoconazole to reduce cyclosporine dose costs (Nejm 1995;333:628). Adverse effects: lymphomas develop in 13% (Nejm 1984;310:477); nephropathy, severe and progressive when dose ≥5 mg/kg/d, or is continued in face of increasing creatinine, or age >30 (Nejm 1992;326:1654; Ann IM 1992;117:578); incr uric acid and gout (Nejm 1989;321:287); hypertension (Nejm 1990;323:693); levels incr by grapefruit (Rx Let 1997;4:21)
- Dacarbazine (DTIC); adverse effects: marrow suppression
- Dactinomycin (Actinomycin D); adverse effects: marrow suppression, mucous membrane ulcerations
- Heat (Nejm 1981;304:583; Ann IM 1979;90:317), with anesthesia, core temperature brought to >113°F (>45°C) for several hours
- Hydroxyurea; adverse effects: marrow suppression, leg ulcers (Ann IM 1998;128:29)
- Imatinib (Gleevec) (Med Let 2001;43:49) tyrosine kinase inhibitor used in CML
- Mithramycin (Plicamycin) iv; for testicular Ca, hypercalcemia; with hydroxyurea for CML blast crisis (Nejm 1986;315:1433). Adverse effects: marrow suppression, especially of platelets, causing bleeding

- Mitomycin; adverse effects: marrow suppression
- Mitoxantrone (Med Let 1988;30:67); adverse effects: marrow suppression, cardiotoxic, blue urine and nails
- Mycophenolate mofetil (CellCept) (Med Let 1995;37:84) used w cyclosporine instead of azathioprine for organ transplant
- Paclitaxel (Taxol) (Nejm 1995;332:1004) and similar docetaxel (Taxotere) (Med Let 1996;38:87) iv q 3 wk; used vs breast and ovarian cancers for palliation; adverse effects: neutropenia, hypersensitivity reactions, peripheral neuropathies; cost: $1200–2000/dose
- Pegascargase (Oncaspar), a polyethylene glycol-conjugated asparagenase, which makes it less sensitizing (Med Let 1995;37:23)
- Procarbazine (Matulane) (Ann IM 1974;81:796); adverse effects: marrow suppression, crosses blood-brain barrier, an MAO inhibitor
- Retinoic acid, 13-cis, po; for epithelial cancers? (Nejm 1980;303:560)
- Semustine (Lomustine, methyl-CCNU); adverse effects: delayed suppression of polys and platelets
- Sirolimus (Rapamune) (Med Let 2000;42:13), immunosuppressant like cyclosporine, used in transplant pts w steroids and cyclosporine
- Tacrolimus iv/po; immunosuppressant like cyclosporine; used w steroids, eg, for liver transplant (Nejm 1994;331:1110)
- Topotecan (Hycamtin) used in late ovarian Ca (Med Let 1996;38:96)
- Vinblastine (Velban) weekly iv; adverse effects: marrow suppression
- Vincristine (Oncovin) (Ann IM 1974;80:733) weekly iv; adverse effects: peripheral neuropathy (rx to loss of reflexes), constipation

BIOLOGIC RESPONSE MODIFIERS; CYTOKINES

- Interferons; for multiple, rapidly expanding tumors, eg, α-interferon for Kaposi's sarcoma in AIDS (Ann IM 1990;112:812) and macrophage activation (Nejm 1991;324:509). Adverse effects: various autoimmune diseases (Ann IM 1991;115:178), depression helped by preventive SSRI rx (Nejm 2001;344:961)
- Interleukin 2 with or without lymphocyte-activated killer cells for metastatic melanoma and renal cell cancer; adverse effects: sepsis due to impaired granulocytic chemotaxis (Nejm 1990;322:959)
- Tumor necrosis factor
- Granulocyte colony-stimulating factors: filgrastim (Neupogen) and sargramostin (Leukin); use after chemotherapy to increase polys and decrease infections (Ann IM 1994;121:492; Med Let 1991;33:61)

HEMATOLOGY/ONCOLOGY

- Gemtuzumab (Mylotarg) (Med Let 2000;42:67) for AML, currently approved for pts >60 in 1st relapse; a recombinant human monoclonal antibody directed type

8.2 VITAMIN DEFICIENCY ANEMIAS

B₁₂ DEFICIENCY ANEMIA

Nejm 1997;337:1441; 1966;275:978

Cause:
- S/p gastric resection, even yrs later may develop, probably the most common cause now (Ann IM 1996;124:469), or post gastric bypass or even plication
- Pernicious anemia (PA) with no intrinsic factor (IF): congenital juvenile type (Nejm 1972;287:425), and adult autosomal dominant, atrophic gastritis type; both genetic but unrelated (Ann IM 1974;81:372)
- *Diphylobothrium latum* competition for gut B_{12}
- Dietary deficiency, very rare, perhaps only in strict non-ovolacto vegetarians (Nejm 1978;299:317)
- Distal small bowel absorptive defect, limited to as little as 10–20 cm in some patients
- Blind loop bacterial consumption (Ann IM 1977;87:546)
- Drugs: PAS, neomycin, colchicine (Nejm 1968;279:845)
- "Pancreatic intrinsic factor" deficiency of enzyme to break down salivary protein-B_{12} complex so can bind IF in stomach (Nejm 1971;284:627)

Epidem: PA incr in Scandinavians and blood group A people; prevalence in all races in US ~0.1% (Nejm 1978;298:647; Ann IM 1971; 74:448), 1.9% over age 60

Pathophys: B_{12} is a crucial coenzyme for ribonucleotide reductase (RNA to DNA) and propionic acid catabolism, lack of which may cause CNS demyelination first in posterior, then in lateral columns. In PA, antigastric parietal cell (where IF made), as well as H^+/K^+-ATPase antibodies

Sx: Of anemia, sore mouth; mean age of onset of PA = 60; 20% of PA pts have pos family hx; diarrhea and other malabsorptions sx

Si: Anemia, glossitis, stomatitis, fair complexion, vitiligo

Crs: Sx onset after 2 yr of total deficiency

Cmplc: CHF due to profound anemia; thrombocytopenic purpura; stomach cancer with adult PA; subacute combined degeneration of cortex and posterior and lateral (corticospinal) columns of spinal cord w sx of distal paresthesias and numbness, paraplegia, vibratory sense and position sense loss, pos Rhomberg, psychiatric sx and dementia, and peripheral neuropathy, seen even without macrocytosis (Nejm 1988;318:1752); carcinoid secreting tumor due to chronic gastrin stimulation (Nejm 1997;336:866)

r/o (Nejm 1973;288:764) other macrocytic anemias: folate deficiency, orotic aciduria (Nejm 1990;322:1641,1652), di Guglielmo's syndrome, anti-DNA drugs

Lab:

Chem: Hgb F and A_2 incr; B_{12} by RIA <100 pgm/cc; incr LDH, Fe, bilirubin, gastrin levels sky high (no acid inhibition since acid-secreting cells hit harder than gastrin secretors—Nejm 1970;282:358); serum homocysteine levels elevated before overt B_{12} deficiency (Ann IM 1996;124:469)

Gastric: Aspirate shows no acid, no false negatives?

Hem: Macrocytic anemia, neutropenia, and hypersegmented polys, normal or sometimes low platelets (ineffective production) unlike Fe deficiency

Path: Marrow is megaloblastic with red cell precursor nuclei still open, ie, not pyknotic in late normoblastic stage, Howell-Jolly bodies, giant "C" metamyelocytes. Small bowel shows decr growth and size of villi (Nejm 1967;277:553). In PA, stomach shows lymphatic infiltration early; CNS shows multifocal myelin degeneration with microcavities and glial scar

Schilling test: First load with im B_{12}, then 3 h later give hot B_{12} po and measure excretion in 24–48 h urine sample, normal >15%; then repeat with intrinsic factor to see if corrects

Rx: B_{12} 1000 μgm im qd loading dose × 7 d, or nasal spray (Nascobal) 500 μgm q 1 wk (8 doses/bottle) (Rx Let 1997;4:64); then 100 μgm/mo im maintenance

Consider gastroscopy at least at diagnosis, maybe regularly to pick up cancer in situ, which has an 85% 5-yr survival

HEMATOLOGY/ONCOLOGY

FOLIC ACID DEFICIENCY

V. Herbert, Trans Assoc Am Phys 1962;75:307

Cause:
- Dietary: poor, pregnant (18% Boston City Hospital pregnant females—Nejm 1967;276:776) and/or alcoholic
- Inadequate absorption: small bowel disease, throughout length, eg, sprue, blind loop
- Antifolate drugs, most of which inhibit deconjugase in gut mucosa since only monoglutamic folate readily absorbed (Nejm 1969;280:985): alcohol, Dilantin, mysoline, birth control pills (Nejm 1970;282:858), triamterine (Ann IM 1970;73:414), pyramethamine, chemotherapy especially with methotrexate

Epidem:

Pathophys: Minimum daily requirement is 50 μgm/d in adults and children; 400 μgm/d in pregnancy. Reserves last 3–6 mo. Polyglutamic folic acid is present in meat, eggs, cow's (not goat's) milk products, vegetables (prolonged steaming will leach out); necessary for thymidylate synthesis (the important one), histidine catabolism (FIGLU an intermediate), methionine synthesis, and two steps in purine metabolism

Sx: Of anemia; sore tongue and mouth, diarrhea

Si: Glossitis, stomatitis, hemolytic jaundice

Crs: Anemia in 20 weeks after intake becomes zero; megaloblasts and some anemia after 40–60 d (R. Hillman, Nejm 1971;284:933)

Cmplc: Bleeding in pregnancy (Nejm 1967;276:776); incr MI and other ASCVD risk even w/o anemia, probably via incr homocysteine (Jama 1996;275;1893)

r/o other megaloblastic anemias (Nejm 1973;288:764): B_{12} deficiency, orotic aciduria (Nejm 1990;322:1641, 1652), di Guglielmo's syndrome, anti-DNA drugs

Lab:

Chem: Serum folate level by radioimmunoassay (Nejm 1972;286:764)

Hem: Anemia, macrocytic with macro-ovalocytes; neutropenia and hypersegmented polys; platelets normal or low unlike Fe deficiency

Path: Marrow is megaloblastic with giant "C" metamyelocytes (bands); macrocytic cells elsewhere too, eg, gut mucosa (Nejm 1970;282:859)

Rx: Additive in cereal products to decr congenital spinal abnormalities and for possible beneficial effects on heterozygous homocystinemia

Monoglutamic folic acid 1 mg po qd is twice the adequate replacement dose; BEWARE, doses of 15 mg qd will reverse B_{12} anemia but not the neurologic deficits (Arch IM 1960;105:372)

IRON DEFICIENCY ANEMIA

Nejm 1999;341:1986; in infancy and childhood—Nejm 1993;329:190

Cause: Insufficient Fe for heme and related coenzyme synthesis because of gi blood loss from cancers, benign diseases like ulcers, eg, chronic *Helicobacter pylori* gastritis (Jama 1997;277:1135); or in runners (Ann IM 1984;100:843); or from cow's milk-induced GI bleeding in infants <1 yr old; or because of absorptive defects in mucosa, as in sprue

Epidem: Prevalence in US (Jama 1997;277:973): children age 1–2 = 3%, adolescent girls = 2%, childbearing women = 5%

Increased prevalence in

- Areas of low dietary Fe (eg, Maritime Provinces)
- Children in first year of life with Fe-deficient mother and/or diet
- Adult women with heavy menses, pregnancy, nursing, or dieting
- Adult men with occult gi bleed, especially cancers
- Pica, since starch, clay, etc. absorb Fe
- Post-gastric surgery, 50% at 10 yr due to rapid transit and absent H^+, which is necessary for Fe absorption
- Any patient with colon, esophageal, or other gi cancer

Pathophys: Fe absorption is a balance between the reticuloendothelial system storage and gi mucosal cells shedding of ferritin, a storage form (Nejm 1971;284:1413)

Sx: Of anemia; sore mouth or tongue; pica (cause or effect? Ann IM 1968;69:435)

Si: Angular stomatitis, glossitis, nail spooning (r/o hyperthyroidism)

Crs: With rx, reticulocytes increase in 5 d, hgb increases 0.2 gm/d

Cmplc: Plummer-Vinson syndrome, seen in women, with esophageal webbing between cricoid and arch of aorta causing dysphagia. In children, Fe % saturations <10% w anemia, even if corrected, correlate w poor later school performance (Nejm 1991;325:687)

r/o COLON CANCER ALWAYS, w colonoscopy or air contrast BE unless UGI sx, in which case w EGD 1st; hypoproliferative normochromic normocytic **anemia of chronic disease** caused by depressed erythropoietin (Nejm 1990;322:1689) and treatable w po Fe and erythropoeitin 150 U sc biw (Nejm 1996;334:619); also other microcytic anemias: thalassemia, lead intoxication, inherited hemoglobin E, paroxysmal nocturnal hemoglobinuria

Lab:

Chem: Serum iron <120 mg %, TIBC >340 mg %, % saturation <8% (between 8% and 20% may be hypoproliferative low reticuloendothelial system Fe release). Ferritin decrease (reflects marrow Fe but can be falsely elevated with inflammation)

Hem: Anemia w hgb <11%, hct <32%; diagnostic trial of iron should lead to normal crit in <2 mo

Platelets incr (Nejm 1970;282:492)

Polys decr in severe disease

Rbc's show microcytes, hypochromia, targets, pencil forms; indices show MCHC <30 mg %, decr MCH and MCV (r/o β thalassemia, hemoglobin C or D disease, spherocytosis, lead poisoning, and chronic aluminum toxicity (Nejm 1997;336:1556)

Path: Marrow shows no intracellular iron

Rx: FeSO$_4$ or ferrous gluconate 300 mg tid po, or qd if no rush; use elixir if rapid transit causes poor absorption; with vitamin C to increase absorption in elderly or unusual, especially achlorhydric, conditions; avoid taking w tea, which decreases absorption by 75%

Fe dextran iv only (not im), rarely need

8.3 HEMOGLOBINOPATHIES

HEMOGLOBIN C DISEASE

Cause: Genetic, autosomal recessive (trait may manifest if coincident with sickle trait)

Epidem: In black Africans, perhaps up to 15% with disease in some areas; 3% of US black population

Pathophys: Single amino acid alteration in β chain of hgb A

Sx:

Si: Splenomegaly; compensated hemolytic anemia

Crs:

Cmplc: Increased thrombotic disease; proliferative peripheral retinopathy r/o hemoglobin D disease, similar but rarer

Lab:

Hem: Hemolytic anemia with elevated reticulocytes and bilirubin, and erythroid hyperplasia in marrow; peripheral smear shows targets, microcytes; hgb electrophoresis shows characteristic hgb C

Rx: Transfusions for crisis; folic acid

SICKLE CELL ANEMIA

Nejm 1999;340:1021; 1997;337:762

Cause: Genetic, autosomal

Epidem: In US blacks, 7% are trait, 0.5% homozygous. Genetic distribution in world correlates with history, geography, and malaria (Ann IM 1973;79:258)

Pathophys: Val substituted for Glut in β chain leading to hgb S, unstable at low O_2, which causes polymer precipitation, which in turn sickles cells. These sickled cells stick to vessel walls, thus cause clots and infarctions. Splenic infarcts produce diminished antibody formation, which leads to incr infections. Hgb F ($\alpha_2\gamma_2$) may persist as survival mechanism into adult life. Heterozygous cells sickle only in severe hypoxia or if hgb C or D present. Renal damage to medulla causes decr concentrating ability, K^+ loss, papillary necrosis, etc. α-Thalassemia trait protects and vice versa (Nejm 1982;307:1441)

Sx: Painful crises in 60%; frequency correlates w worse prognosis (Nejm 1991;325:11)

Si: Retarded growth and sexual maturation (Nejm 1984;311:7); frontal bossing; skin ulcers, especially lower legs; angioid streaking of fundi indicates neovascularization (r/o Paget's, pseudoxanthoma elasticum)

Crs: 50% live to age 45 yr, longer if fetal hgb >8.6% (Nejm 1994;330:1639); heterozygotes have no clinical disease

Cmplc:

- Acute chest pain syndrome (Nejm 2000;342:1854); most common cause of death; includes hypoxia, ARDS, and pneumonia
- Aplastic crises associated w parvovirus B19 infection in children, and with severe pain

- Pneumococcal and *Salmonella* sepsis/infections, especially osteomyelitis (Nejm 1973;289:803)
- CVAs, which may be predictable by intracranial Doppler studies, then perhaps prevent with transfusions (Nejm 1992;326:605)
- Renal failure, 25% have proteinuria that may progress to renal failure (Nejm 1992;326:910)
- Bony infarcts, necrosis
- Gout (incr uric acid production)
- Gallstones
- Sudden death rate with heavy exertion incr to 32/10,000 in heterozygotes in contrast to 1/100,000 in whites (Nejm 1987; 317:781)
- Myonecrosis and myofibrosis (Ann IM 1991;115:99)

Lab:

Hem: ESR low, sickled cells in peripheral smear; hemoglobin electrophoresis shows hgb S + incr hgb F (Nejm 1978;299:1428)

Urine: UA w hematuria, low specific gravity due to inability to concentrate even in heterozygotes

Xray: Long bone infarcts/necrosis, "hair on end" skull, step fractures of vertebrae

Rx: Preventive maneuvers:

- Amniocentesis and abortion of affected fetuses (Nejm 1983; 309:831)
- Penicillin prophylactically until age 5
- Pneumococcal vaccine (Nejm 1977;297:897); or phenoxymethyl penicillin 125 mg bid works age 4 mo–3 yr? (Nejm 1986; 314:1593)
- Preop exchange transfusion helps (Nejm 1990;322:1666), but prophylactic transfusion in pregnancy does not work (Nejm 1988; 319:1447)
- Vitamin E 450 IU qd increases rbc survival (Nejm 1980;303:454)
- Hydroxyurea (Jama 2001;286:2099; Nejm 1995;332:1317) 10–25 mg/kg/d gradually incr to just start suppressing polys; stimulates fetal hgb production (Nejm 1990;322:1037); if used with erythropoietin, no benefit (Nejm 1990;323:367), but may be if used w iron (Nejm 1993;328:73). Butyrate (short chain FA) is ineffective (Nejm 1995;332:1606)

of surgical crisis: transfuse to normal hematocrit (Nejm 1995;333:206)
of anemia:
- Transfusions, but rx limited by sensitization, less with black blood donors (Nejm 1990;322:1617)
- Marrow transplant perhaps worth the risk because it works if patient survives (Nejm 1996;335:369,426); 90% w compatible donor survive

of nephropathy: ACE inhibitors to prevent progression (Nejm 1992; 326:910)

of sepsis: ceftriaxone im in children as outpts (Nejm 1993;329:472)

of crisis: iv fluids, NSAIDs, narcotics; possibly steroids (Nejm 1994; 330:733)

of stroke: transcranial doppler ulstrasound and transfusions (plain or exchange) (Nejm 1998;339:5)

α-THALASSEMIA
Nejm 1976;295:710

Cause: Genetic

Epidem: Increased prevalence in Asians, Shiite Arabs (Nejm 1980;303: 1383), and all populations exposed to malaria because heterozygous individuals have some resistance

Pathophys: Impaired α-hgb chain synthesis, absolute or qualitative, and often associated with mental retardation (gene linkage) or fetal hydrops (Nejm 1981;305:607,638). Thus homozygote unable to make hgb A ($\alpha_2\beta_2$), hgb A$_2$ ($\alpha_2\delta_2$), or hgb F ($\alpha_2\gamma_2$).

Sx:
Homozygotes: Severe disease at birth with hydrops fetalis, ie, anasarca due to anemia
Heterozygotes: None or mild anemia

Si:
Homozygotes: Splenomegaly, increased marrow proliferation and space

Crs:
Homozygotes: Perinatal death

Cmplc:
Heterozygotes: Severe disease when combined with another hemoglobin abnormality; hemosiderosis/iron overload

Lab:

Hem: In both homo- and heterozygotes, peripheral smear shows rbc
stippling (RNA and mitochondria), siderocytes, targets, rbc
"ghosts," and bizarre forms

In heterozygote, MCV <73 m^3, hgb A$_2$ <3.5%; iron levels normal
(Nejm 1973;288:351); normal hgb proportions, or hgb H (β$_4$) incr
(r/o acquired hgb H, rarely in erythroleukemics—Nejm 1971;
285:1271)

In homozygote, hgb electrophoresis shows no hgb A, A$_2$, or F; hgb
Barts (γ$_4$) (Nejm 1990;323:179) and/or hgb H may be present; both
the latter are incompetent O$_2$ carriers

Rx: Transfusions, beware of iron overload

β-THALASSEMIA

Nejm 1999;341:99; Ann IM 1979;91:883

Cause: Genetic, autosomal. Homozygote = thalassemia major, Cooley's
anemia. Heterozygote = thalassemia minor or thalassemia trait

Epidem: Whites, especially Mediterraneans, eg, Greeks and Italians, up to
60% gene prevalence in some villages. Blacks, 1% of US black
population carries. Southeast Asians, 2–10% gene prevalence
(Found Blood Res 10/86). Sustained by partial malaria resistance in
heterozygotes

Pathophys: β-Hemoglobin chain synthesis blocked in homozygotes so
they are unable to make hgb A (α$_2$β$_2$) but can make hgb A$_2$ and hgb
F. Heterozygote has some decr β-chain synthesis

α/β-Thalassemia interaction: in β-thal, β/α = 0.5, but can be >0.5
toward 1 if concomitant α-thalassemia gene as well, since this
decreases inclusion production and thus ineffective intramedullary
rbc production, leaving only a hypochromic, microcytic pattern
(Nejm 1972;286:586)

Sx:

Thal major: Onset age 3–6 mo when hgb A replaces hgb F
Thal minor: Asx unless α precipitants (Nejm 1974;290:939)

Si:

Thal major: Skull bossing (marrow proliferation)

Thal minor: Splenomegaly

Crs:

Cmplc:

Thal major: Hemochromatosis/siderosis with transfusions leading to diabetes, insulin resistance (Nejm 1988;318:809), and hypopituitarism with impaired puberty and 2° amenorrhea; prevented with Fe binding rx begun before age 10 (Nejm 1990;323: 713); r/o thal trait plus hgb E, which looks like thal homozygote, **hemoglobin E** is present in 40% of Southeast Asians (Found Blood Res 10/86); B_{12}; folate deficiency

Thal minor: sickle/thal disease (1/4 as common as SS disease). Fe deficiency decreases α chain production which in turn worsens the disease (Nejm 1985;313:1402). B_{12}, folate deficiency. Most commonly presents as a mild microcytic anemia so r/o other causes (p 338)

Lab:

Amniotic fluid: To detect affected fetus, DNA probes work 85% of time, no false pos or neg (Nejm 1983;309:384; 1983;308:1054)

Chem: In thal major, iron and % saturation both incr; bilirubin, urine, and stool urobilinogen all increased

Path: Liver bx to monitor iron load (Nejm 2000;343:327)

Hem: In both MCV <79 m^3, rbc stippling (RNA and mitochondria); siderocytes (hemosiderin-laden) in peripheral blood; targets; rbc "ghosts"; teardrops if spleen still in, vacuoles if not (Nejm 1972;286:589)

Hgb electrophoresis: in thal minor, hgb A_2 ($\alpha_2\delta_2$) persists at $\geq 2\times$ normal %; >3.5% is diagnostic (Nejm 1973;288:351). In thal major, no significant hgb A; hgb F may persist

Xray: Skull films show "hair-on-end" evidence of marrow space increase

Rx: Genetic counseling to prevent

of thal major: splenectomy and transfusions to keep hgb >10 and thus diminish bone fragility (Nejm 1972;286:586); marrow transplant, 25% mortality (Nejm 1990;322:417), but only ~6% if transplanted early in course before liver damage (Nejm 1993;329:840); 5-azacytidine iv over 4 d q 1 mo increases hgb F (Nejm 1993;329: 845) as does hydroxyurea and butyrate iv qd (Nejm 1993;328:81)

of Fe overload: AVOID FE RX; tetracycline po to decrease gi absorption (Nejm 1979;300:5); deferoxamine sc with pump hs decreases diabetes, late liver and heart disease (Nejm 1994;331:567, 574), but can cause dose-dependent deafness and blindness (Nejm 1985;313:869); or possibly deferiprone po (Nejm 1998;339:417; 1995;332:918), but not effective, and adverse effects: agranulocytosis, hepatic fibrosis

8.4 PORPHYRIAS

HEPATIC PORPHYRIAS (Acute Intermittent Porphyria, Variegate Porphyria, Porphyria Cutanea Tarda)

Nejm 1991;324:1432; Ann IM 1978;89:238; Nejm 1972;286:279

Cause: All 3 are genetic, autosomal dominant (VP—Nejm 1978;298:358)

Epidem:

Acute intermittent porphyria: (AIP) more women than men. *Variegate porphyria* (VP): incr in South African whites and in alcoholics (Nejm 1978;298:358). *Porphyria cutanea tarda* (PCT): incr in cirrhotics and hepatoma pts

Pathophys: Generally excess porphyrins cause skin sensitization; and excess ALA and porphobilinogen (PBG). Impaired mitochondrial enzyme systems: succinyl CoA + glycine (with ALA synthetase, the rate-limiting enzyme) → ALA → PBG → UroPG I-III → CoproPG III → ProtoPG III → ProtoPorph → heme (pathways—Nejm 1970; 283:955). In AIP, drug/diet induces ALA synthetase increase and deficiency of UroPG synthetase (PBG deaminase) causing incr ALA and PBG, in turn causing demyelination and perhaps pain. In VP, defect unclear but decr conversion PPG → PP (Nejm 1980;302:765). In PCT, decr conversion UPG → CPG in rbc (Nejm 1978;299:1095) and liver (Nejm 1982;306:766); skin damage from UV and/or traumatic activation of complement (Nejm 1981;304:213)

Sx: Precipitated by barbiturates, sulfas, griseofulvin, alcohol (even in mouthwashes—Nejm 1975;292:1115), estrogens and pregnancy, infections, weight reduction (Nejm 1967;277:350)

AIP: Onset age 20–40, abdominal colic, vomiting, constipation, urine becomes brown on standing after voiding; no skin involvement at all

VP: Onset age 11–30, abdominal colic, rash like PCT

PCT: Dermal sensitivity with bullae and scars, hyperpigmentation, red urine

Si:

AIP alone: Hypertension, tachycardia, low-grade fevers

AIP and VP: Peripheral motor and sensory neuropathy, psychoses, and neuroses

PCT: Rashes, hirsutism, scarring, vitiligo, milia especially on hands

Crs:

AIP: 25% 5-yr mortality after first attack; worse in younger patients

Cmplc:

AIP: Respiratory paralysis, infections

VP and PCT: r/o scleroderma; congenital erythropoietic porphyria (Nejm 1986;314:1029); protoporphyria (Nejm 1991;324:1432); naprosyn, tetracycline, or nalidixic acid photosensitization or similar skin changes seen with hemodialysis, and in all of which urine tests will be neg

Lab:

Hem: In PCT: hgb, Fe, and TIBC incr often

Urine:

   In AIP: Red brown on standing (pyrroles condense to porphyrins); Watson-Schwartz test, Hoechst test (2 gtts urine turns red immediately), or 24 hr urine PBG level >2× normal during acute attack (Am J Med 1999;107:621); urine porphyrins between attacks less helpful

   In VP Watson-Schwartz, Hoechst, or other tests for precursors (ALA and PBG) positive in acute attacks; chromatography is positive in acute attacks only; urine fluoresces red under Wood's lamp

   In PCT Watson-Schwartz test negative or faintly positive; chromatography shows incr UPG and CPG in urine; urine fluoresces red under Wood's lamp after acidification

Rx: Prevent attacks of AIP and VP by avoiding weight loss, infections, and drugs; test relatives; warn about pregnancy and oral contraceptives. In VP and PCT, avoid skin changes with protective clothing

for VP: Phlebotomy (Nejm 1978;298:358)

for PCT: Phlebotomize 500 cc q 2 wk; unknown mechanism perhaps via hepatic Fe metabolism (Nejm 1968;279:1301). Chloroquine 250–500 mg qd × 5–8 d, exacerbates, then long remissions (Jama 1980;223:515) *of AIP attacks:* iv glucose. Hematin iv inhibits ALA synthetase (Med Let 1984;26:42); can use perimenstrually (FDA Drug Bull 1983; 13:26); can cause DIC if spoils (Nejm 1986;315:235). Luteinizing hormone analog qd for perimenstrual exacerbations (Nejm 1984; 311:683)

8.5 HEMOLYTIC ANEMIAS

APLASTIC ANEMIA

Nejm 1997;336:1365; Ann IM 1981;95:477

Cause: A stem cell disease. Autoimmune via drugs, infectious agent, or chronic immune disease, eg, quinidine (Nejm 1979;301:621), phenylbutazone, chloramphenicol, gold salts; viral hepatitis, EBV (Ann IM 1988;109:695), parvo B19 virus (Ann IM 1990;113:926; Nejm 1989;321:484,519,536); thymomas, rheumatoid arthritis (Ann IM 1984;100:202), SLE, myasthenia gravis, myxedema, viral hepatitis (Nejm 1997;336:1059)

Epidem:

Pathophys: Sudden insult to stem cell from autoantibody or lymphocytic immune response (Nejm 1979;301:621); rarely folate-responsive in adult type (Nejm 1978;298:469); perhaps antibody to erythropoietin in some cases

Sx: Recent PNH (15%); petechiae, infection, anemia

Si:

Crs:

Cmplc: Hematologic and solid tumors after marrow transplant or immunization (Nejm 1993;329:1152); PNH (Ann IM 1999;131: 401, 467) in 25% of immunologically mediated aplastic anemias

Lab:

Hem: Pancytopenia, ncnc anemia, retics <2%, nucleated rbc's, normal Fe and TIBC

Path: Marrow shows marked decrease in rbc precursors, E/M ratio ≪1:3

Serol: B19 parvovirus IgM and IgG titers (p 508); or by DNA hybridization studies of serum if immunosuppressed (Ann IM 1990;113:926)

Rx: (Nejm 1991;324:1297)
- Marrow transplant if young and compatible donor, 69% 15 yr survival (Ann IM 1997;126:107)
- High dose cyclophosphamide 50 mg/kg iv qd × 4d; 65% complete remission (Ann IM 2001;135:477)
- Antilymphocyte globulin (Nejm 1983;308:113) + prednisone + cyclosporine (Nejm 1991;324:1297), 38% 15 yr survival (Ann IM 1997;126:107); same response in older pts though mortality higher (Ann IM 1999;130:193)
- Transfusions; use irradiated blood to prevent graft vs host disease from transfused lymphocytes
- Androgens (Nejm 1973;289:72), probably only help when hypoplasia not aplasia, eg, stanozolol 2 mg qd, works perhaps via incr 2–3 DPG effect (Nejm 1972;287:381); try others if one doesn't work
- Perhaps biologic response modifiers like growth-stimulating factors; plasmapheresis? (Nejm 1981;304:1334)

IMMUNE HEMOLYTIC ANEMIA

Cause: Autoimmune in one of several different ways (see below) via drugs, cold agglutinins, idiopathic immune globulins
Epidem:
Pathophys:
  Types:
- Autoimmune: perhaps spontaneously, perhaps induced by unknown agents
- Drug induced: how?, perhaps via suppressor T cell inhibition (Nejm 1980;302:825); eg, methyldopa (antibodies are vs Rh antigens, 20% have positive Coombs' after 5 mo rx, dose-related but much lesser % of hemolysis because of coincident RES impairment—Nejm 1985;313:596), procainamide (20%—Nejm 1984;311:809)
- Hapten type: drug or virus (Nejm 1971;284:1250) attaches to rbc and antibody is directed against this combination; eg, penicillin, especially high-dose iv (Nejm 1972;287:1322); possibly tetracycline (Nejm 1985;312:840)

- "Innocent bystander": agent/drug loosely attaches to rbc, antibody + C' attaches to rbc antigen-agent combination, agent/drug falls off, leaving antibody + C'-coated rbc, which is then picked up and lysed by RES rather than intravascularly; occasionally similar coincident platelet injury; eg, penicillin (ibid), tetracycline (ibid), cephalothins (Ann IM 1977;86:64), quinine, quinidine, sulfas (Nejm 1970;283:900)
  - Cold agglutinin disease: usually IgM, unlike above, which are usually IgG (Ann IM 1987;106:238)

Sx: Of anemia

Si: Splenomegaly, jaundice

Crs: Drug types resolve with drug withdrawal; others respond to rx of primary disease, splenectomy, and steroids

Cmplc: Pulmonary emboli are most common cause of death; infections

Lab:

Chem: Bilirubin incr

Hem: Smear shows spherocytes, "too many to be congenital spherocytosis"; retics incr; Coombs' often positive, though can be negative if antibody pulled off rbc by test serum; anti-C'3 Coombs' positive; in innocent bystander type, incr osmotic fragility; IgG coating of rbc, 35–200 molecules/rbc too few to give positive Coombs' but can be detected (Nejm 1971;285:254), debate about what number is significant and what false-pos/neg rate at each level, may be useful to follow autoimmune and drug-induced types

Rx: Steroids (often relapse on moderate doses); cyclophosphamide (Nejm 1976;295:1522); androgens like danazol 600–800 mg qd until better, then 200–400 mg qd maintenance (Ann IM 1985;102:298)

Splenectomy, 50% permanent remission, though Coombs' may remain positive; takes 3 wk to help, unlike rbc-defective hemolytic anemias, probably because needs time for antibody levels to diminish

8.6 CLOTTING DISORDERS

SCREENING TESTS OF CLOTTING FUNCTION

- **Activation Sequences**:

  Stage 1 (intrinsic system): $XII \rightarrow XI \rightarrow IX* \xrightarrow{VIII} X*$ activation (VIII acts as an enzymatic enhancer of $IX \rightarrow X$)

  Stage 1 (extrinsic system): $VII* +$ tissue thromboplastin $\rightarrow X*$ activation

  Stage 2: $X* \xrightarrow{V} II*$ (prothrombin) activation (V acts as an enzymatic enhancer of $X \rightarrow II$)

  Stage 3: $II* \rightarrow I$ (fibrinogen) $+ XIII$ activation

  (* = vitamin K-dependent factors)

- Tourniquet test: BP cuff at 100 mm Hg × 5 min, normal is no petechiae; tests vessels and platelets (Nejm 1970;283:186)
- Bleeding time (BT), Ivy (Nejm 1972;287:155, plus rv of all platelet function tests—Nejm 1990;324:27): normal = ~4 min; tests vessels and platelets (ibid); a linear function of platelet numbers between 10,000 and 100,000; NSAIDs and aspirin (by far the worst) prolong via platelet effect that lasts platelet lifetime (3 d half-life—Nejm 1969;280:453) ASA tolerance test: normal result is BT still <15 min; greater elevation probably reflects underlying clotting disorder
- Clotting time: normal = <10 min; tests primarily stage 1 but stage 2 changes will also increase it
- Prothrombin time (PT): normal = 11–14 sec, tests extrinsic system and stages 2 and 3
- Fibrinogen level: normal = >200 mg %
- Activated partial thromboplastin time (aPTT): normal = 30–40 sec; tests stages 1–3 without VII or platelets; stage 1 if PT ok
- Fibrin split products

CLASSIC HEMOPHILIA (Hemophilia A)

Nejm 1994;330:38

Cause: Genetic, sex-linked recessive causing factor VIII deficiency

Epidem: 80% of all patients with lifelong bleeding diathesis (Ann IM 1966;65:782); 1/7000–10,000 male births, only 1/3 have complete VIII deficiency

Classic Hemophilia, continued

Pathophys: Intrinsic system defect (p 349) caused by deficiency of functioning factor VIII, although present in plasma immunologically (defective protein). Factor VIII is synthesized in blood vessel endothelial cells, circulates complexed to vonW protein, which enhances VIII synthesis, protects it from proteolysis, and concentrates it at sites of active hemostasis

Sx: Male; positive family hx in 2/3 (1/3 are due to new mutations). Wide spectrum from postsurgical bleeding to chronic bruising, joint bleeds, and crippling arthritis; gu bleeding (usually insignificant); no bleeding after minor cuts

Si: Bleeding after trauma. Spontaneous hemarthroses only in severe disease

Crs: Lifelong, 1995 prognosis nearly comparable to normal population if don't get HIV or hep B (Ann IM 1995;123:823)

Cmplc: Psychiatric conditions related to chronic illness; hep B (Ann IM 1977;86:703) and C; AIDS; flexion contractures of joints; intracranial bleeding, the cause of death in 25%

Lab:

Hem: Prolonged PTT but normal PT and platelet count; r/o factor VIII autoantibody inhibitor, factor XI deficiency, antiphospholipid antibodies, lupus anticoagulants, or factor XII deficiency

Factor VIII levels: none detectable = severe disease, 1–4% of normal = moderate disease, 5–25% of normal = mild disease

Rx: Preventively avoid ASA and other NSAIDs; prenatal dx and abortion (Nejm 1979;300:937), in first trimester with DNA probe (Nejm 1985;312:682); detect female carriers by recombinant DNA techniques (Nejm 1985;313:842)

Comprehensive outpatient programs save money and lives (Nejm 1982;306:575); try to keep VIII >15% w recombinant DNA VIII, no viral contamination risks (Nejm 1993;328:453; Med Let 1993; 35:51), cost $20,000–100,000/yr

of VIII antibody formation (IgG), in 10%; rx with activated prothrombin concentrates (Konyne, proplex—Nejm 1981;305:717; 1980;303:421; 1974;291:164); or big doses of VIII; can also use plasmapheresis, steroids, and cyclophosphamide; not yet clear if will be an issue with recombinant VIII (Nejm 1993;328:453)

Desmopressin (DDAVP) (Nejm 1998;339:245) 0.3 μgm/kg over 30 min iv, or 150 μgm in children, 300 μgm in adults via nasal spray (Ann IM 1991;114:563) increases VIII transiently, eg, perisurgically or after trauma (Ann IM 1985;103:228; Med Let 1984;26:82). Adequate alone in 80% (Ann IM 1985;103:6)

VON WILLEBRAND'S DISEASE (Pseudohemophilia)

Cause: Genetic, autosomal dominant; or acquired, eg, with lymphoma (Nejm 1978;298:988)

Epidem: Prevalence = 1/25,000. Associated with mitral valve prolapse and Marfan's, both inherited connective tissue defects (Nejm 1981; 305:131)

Pathophys: VonW protein normally complexes and circulates with factor VIII, which enhances synthesis of VIII, protects it from proteolysis, and concentrates it at sites of active homeostasis (Nejm 1994; 330:38)

Platelets have decr adhesiveness, probably due to a coenzyme deficiency, normally provided by factor VIII. No factor VIII inhibitors develop

Types (Nejm 1983;309:816): I = decrease in VIII protein; IIA and IIC = decr ability to form large VIII multimers; IIB = incr removal rate of large multimers

Sx: Bleeding, some menstrual and/or birth-related bleeding despite normal increase in VIII during pregnancy

Si: Severe bleeding from abrasions, mucous membranes, postsurgery; rarely into joints like true hemophiliacs

Crs: Much less morbidity than hemophiliacs with similar VIII levels

Cmplc: Blood loss, spontaneous CNS or abdominal bleeding

r/o associated mitral valve prolapse syndrome (Nejm 1981;305:130)

Lab:

Hem: VIII deficiency by levels and clot workup (p 349); antigen/function ratio $\leq$1, unlike hemophilia (Ann IM 1978;88:403)

Clotting studies: normal PT and platelets normal; PTT prolonged; bleeding time may be normal, but not after ASA when BT >15 min reliably, normals don't (D. Deykin, 1978); ristocetin test shows abnormal platelet function

Immunol: Deficient vonW factor by immunoassay, also called "factor VIII antigen"

Rx: Avoid ASA, indomethacin, phenylbutazone, and other NSAIDs

Desmopressin (DDAVP) (vasopressin analog) (p 350 for dosing), for types I and IIA only, worsens other types through platelet aggregation (Ann IM 1985;103:228; Med Let 1984;26:82; Nejm 1983;309:816); via nasal spray also effective (Ann IM 1991;114:563); adequate alone in 80% (Ann IM 1985;103:6); even helps non-vonW pts, eg, normals having cardiopulmonary bypass (Nejm 1986;314:1402)

Factor VIII w vonW factor content, eg Humate-P

8.7 PURPURA AND PLATELET DISORDERS

DISSEMINATED INTRAVASCULAR COAGULATION (DIC)

Nejm 1999;341:586

Cause: 2 requirements: (1) reticuloendothelial system blockade by pregnancy, endotoxin, radiation, steroids, colloid, and (2) clotting system activated by:
- Thromboplastin releaser, eg, frozen tissue, placenta, tumors, trypsin, snake venom (Nejm 1975;292:505), open brain trauma (Nejm 1974;290:1043), renal transplant rejection (Nejm 1970; 283:383); or
- Defibrination agent, eg, amniotic fluid; or
- Platelet factor 3 (phospholipid) release, eg, platelet clot, hemolysis, fat embolism, immune reaction; or
- Activation of factor XII, eg, by exo- or endotoxin from sepsis

Epidem: More common than TTP. Increased incidence in OB especially with septic abortions, abruptio, eclampsia, mole, amniotic fluid embolus, missed abortion, retained dead fetus, fatty liver of pregnancy (Ann IM 1983;98:330); leukemias, cancers, and all cases of severe tissue damage; freshwater drownings; gram-negative sepsis

Pathophys: Fibrinogen is low due to consumption and rapid lysis; tissue damage especially in CNS, lung, and kidneys from thrombotic ischemia

Sx: Bleeding, coma; fever only if there is a secondary cause of fever, unlike TTP

Si: Palpable purpuric rash (r/o allergic vasculitis); shock, hypotension; oozing/bleeding at all sites

Crs: Acute, hours to days; rarely chronic (Nejm 1968;278:815)

Cmplc: Renal cortical necrosis, ATN, Sheehan's syndrome, acute cor pulmonale, adrenal insufficiency (rarely fatal)

r/o other microangiopathic anemias: TTP, HELP, HUS, malignant HT, and chemoRx induced types

Lab:

Hem: Smear shows microangiopathic anemia with helmets and other fragments. Platelets <100,000. ESR = 0 (afibrinogenemia). PT, very sensitive (R. Hillman 3/86), and PTT prolonged. Fibrinogen <40 mg %; low levels of II (hence PT long), VIII, V (<50% is diagnostic). Fibrin split products (D-dimers) markedly elevated; prolonged thrombin time. Elevated antithrombin III (Hillman 3/86)

Urine: Hematuria, isosmolar anuria late when ATN develops

Rx: Treat primary problem; replace factors, eg, fresh-frozen plasma and platelets; perhaps heparinize at low doses like 300–400 U/hr or w LMW heparin, possibly antithrombin III, to break the consumption cycle; never do so in face of liver disease, and only as a last resort if chronic cause and uncontrollable bleeding

THROMBOTIC THROMBOCYTOPENIC PURPURA (TTP)

Nejm 1991;325:427

Cause: VonW factor cleaving protease IgG inhibitor (acquired type) or deficiency (familial type) (Nejm 1998;339:1578,1585,1629)

Epidem: Incidence is 4/million; 1/1000 autopsies, male:female = 2:3. Associated with IgG platelet antibodies in Graves' and Hashimoto's diseases (Ann IM 1981;94:27); with *E. coli* O157:H7 infections (Ann IM 1995;123:698); occasionally w drugs, eg, ticlopidine rx (Jama 1999;281:806; Ann IM 2000;132:794), or rarely clopidogrel (Plavix) (Nejm 2000;342:1766)

Pathophys: VonW factor multimers build up due to lack of cleaving protease, cause platelet aggregation/consumption and fibrin arteriolar plugging (Nejm 1998;339:1578,1585,1629; 1982; 307:1432)

Sx: Fever, abdominal pain, bleeding especially in urine and gi tract, syncope (95%), headaches (34%), visual changes (8%) from retinal hemorrhages, seizures (8%)

Si: Fever usually (80%) <102°F (<38.9°C); purpura; retinal hemorrhages; neurologic si's in 90% (Curr Concepts Cerebro Dis 1977;12:17); coma (31%), mental changes (26%), paresis (20%), aphasia (11%), dysarthria (7%)

Crs: <90 d in 80%, 90–365 d in 13%, >1 yr in 7%. Mortality ~90% without rx, 10% with rx (Nejm 1991;325:398); nearly 20% of cases are recurrent, 36% recurrence over 10 yr (Ann IM 1995;122:569)

Cmplc: Renal failure; occasionally Stokes-Adams attacks due to bundle of His degeneration, seen also in Doberman dogs (Ann IM 1979; 91:359)

Lab:

Chem: Bilirubin (85%) and BUN (90%) elevated

Hem: Smear shows microangiopathic anemia with red cell fragments, burr cells, helmets, and nucleated rbc's. Hgb <10.4 gm. Retics incr a lot, eg, ~20%. Platelets <120,000 (97%). WBC ~4000–5000 or less. Clot studies normal except mildly incr fibrin breakdown products. VonW factor cleaving protease deficiency or inhibitor present (unlike HUS)

Noninv: EKG and EEG, both may be nonspecifically abnormal

Path: Gingival biopsy may show fibrin plugs; 60% false neg, 0% false pos (Ann IM 1978;89:500). Marrow shows incr megakaryocyte numbers

Urine: Active nephritic sediment with protein, rbc's, wbc's, casts

Rx: (Nejm 1991;325:398)

Plasma (which has vonW factor cleaving protease) as FFP, cryosupernatant, solvent treated plasma, or plasma exchange (Am J Med 1999;107:573; Nejm 1985;312:985)

Immunosuppression to inhibit IgG antibody to vonW factor-clearing protease, w:

• Steroids iv, eg, 200 mg prednisone qd

• Splenectomy perhaps for recurrence (Ann IM 1996;125:294)

HEMOLYTIC-UREMIC SYNDROME

Nejm 1990;323:1161; 1985;312:117

Cause:

- *Classic:* Possibly viral via endotoxin or allergy; or post-chemotherapy or quinine po (Ann IM 1993;119:215) in adults
- *Post-infectious or post-partum* (Nejm 1985;312:1556) via endotoxin; verotoxin produced by: *E. coli* O157:H7 (Ann IM 1995;123:698; Nejm 1995;333:364; 1987;317:1496) infection from hamburger and milk results in HUS in 6% of those children infected, and also causes TTP; also caused by other *E. coli* (Nejm 1996;335:635), *Shigella,* pneumococcus, *Salmonella*
- *Genetic:* Autosomal, both recessive and dominant types

Epidem: Increasing incidence; most under age 5 where now incidence = 6/100,000; day care clusters. 65% of all types are postinfectious

Pathophys: Very similar to TTP but predominant renal involvement (Nejm 1991;325:426). All types show a shiga toxin-induced vasculitis, possibly allergic, with 4 systems involved: kidney, skin, joints, bowel. Plasminogen activator is elevated, cause or effect? (Nejm 1993;327:755)

Classic: Glomerular thrombotic microangiopathy

Postinfectious: More diffuse thrombotic microangiopathy

Genetic: Arterial thrombotic microangiopathy

Sx: Diarrhea (86%), vomiting (75%), bloody diarrhea (59%), abdominal cramps (50%), fever (49%), seizures (17%)

Postinfectious type may have a h/o viral or bacterial infection 1–2 wk before

Si: As above

Crs: 2 wk average; <5% mortality if supported; ie, is self-limited

Cmplc: Renal failure (47% require dialysis temporarily), shock, cardiac arrest, blindness, CVAs

Lab:

Chem: Elevated BUN and creatinine

Hem: Crit <30%; microangiopathic picture with red cell fragments, platelets <150,000; if wbc's >15,000, prognosis worse. VonW factor-cleaving protease function normal (unlike TTP) (Nejm 1998; 379:1578)

Urine: Hematuria, proteinuria

Rx: (Nejm 1991;325:398)

Prevent by avoiding antibiotic rx of *E. coli* O157:H7 diarrhea (Nejm 2000;342:1930)

Supportive; steroids may help by decreasing edema; plasma exchange transfusions help (Am J Med 1999;107:573; Nejm 1985;312:984); antihistamines no help

HENOCH-SCHÖNLEIN OR ANAPHYLACTOID PURPURA

Nejm 1997;337:1512; Semin Arth Rheum 1991;21:103; Arth Rheum 1990;33:1114

Cause: Perhaps an IgA immune complex disease precipitated by URIs, strep throat, medications, or food allergies; but none of these is clearly associated

Epidem: Mostly in children, but up to 30% in adult? (Med Clin N Am 1986;70:355)

Pathophys: A small vessel IgA immune complex vasculitis, with 4 systems involved: renal focal proliferative GN, skin purpura, joint arthritis, bowel edema and bleeding

Sx: H/o viral or bacterial infection 1–2 wk before (65%). Diffuse extensive purpura; abdominal pain, with nausea and vomiting often as first si, gi bleeding; hematuria; joint pain and swelling; fever

Si: Purpuric rash, palpable in 85%, especially over legs, arms, and buttocks; in adults, the rash blisters and ulcerates more, and more often involves the trunk; joint swelling

Crs: Usually benign and self-limited; <10% recurrence. In adults, morbidity and mortality may be higher, all from renal disease (Clin Nephrol 1989;311:60); others find outcomes similar in adults and children (Semin Arth Rheum 1991;21:103)

Cmplc: Bowel obstruction due to intussusception, may look like appendicitis; glomerular nephitis, nephrotic syndrome, and end stage renal disease (5%)

r/o other small vessel vasculitis (p 834)

Lab:

Chem: BUN and creatinine incr in 10–20%

Hem: Platelets normal

Path: Polys around, but usually not in small arteriole walls; this finding helps distinguish it from **leukocytoclastic vasculitis,** which is seen in most systemic small vessel vasculitis (p 834)

Stool: Guaiac-positive

Urine: Hematuria and proteinuria in 50%

Rx: Steroids w azathioprine may help; antihistamines no help. Plasma exchange transfusions may help when rapidly progressive GN

IDIOPATHIC THROMBOCYTOPENIC PURPURA (ITP)

Ann IM 1997;126:319, Nejm 1994;331:1207; 1981;304:1135

Cause:

- Autoimmune direct antiplatelet antibodies; part of hemolytic anemia spectrum (Nejm 1977;297:517), SLE, lymphoma, CLL, cancer (Ann IM 1983;99:471); a type II direct cytotoxic antibody (p 63, Nejm 1985;313:1375)
- Hapten type and innocent bystander immune reactions (type III, IgG immune complexes—Nejm 1985;313:1375; 1984;311:635) involving: transfusions (Nejm 1972;287:291); drugs like gold (Ann IM 1981;95:178), heparin (Nejm 1976;295:237), quinidine, thiazides, sulfas; perhaps transient viral infections

Epidem: Chronic form, 70% women, 70% <age 40 yr; childhood type usually abrupt onset, remits, M = F

Pathophys: Spleen produces IgG, which coats platelets, decreases half-life from 3–5 d to <0.5 d because macrophages gobble up; delayed (type IV) hypersensitivity reaction may also play some role

Sx: Easy or spontaneous bruising

Si: Petechiae, purpura

Crs: Remission spontaneously in 85% children, 10% adults

Cmplc: Spontaneous bleeding only when platelet counts <10,000–20,000 (Nejm 1997;337:1870); in pregnant patients, follow antibody levels and platelet counts (Nejm 1990;323:229,264)

r/o other causes of thrombocytopenia:

- Impairments of production: hypoproliferative, eg, pernicious anemia, PNH; or ineffective production, eg, alcoholics

- Impairments of distribution, eg, splenic pooling
- Consumption, eg, immune destruction (ITP) or vascular (DIC)

Lab:

Chem: Plasma glycocalicin incr (50–250% of normal range), a fragment of platelet membranes, incr in all consumptive thrombocytopenias (Nejm 1987;317:1037)

Hem: Platelets decr in number, incr in size (immature). Bleeding time unnecessary but will be normal because, though numbers decr, stickiness is increased. Coombs' test may often be positive since low-grade hemolytic anemia is often present as well (Nejm 1977; 297:517); this constitutes Evan's syndrome, seen in SLE, pregnancy. Platelet-radiolabeled Coombs' test (Nejm 1983;309:459)

Path: Marrow shows incr megakaryocytes

Rx: Consider when platelet counts consistently <30,000/cc (Ann IM 1997;126:307; Nejm 1993;328:1226)

1st: Prednisone, ~100 mg po qd × 1–2 wk or to response then taper; or, in resistant cases, dexamethasone 40 mg po daily × 4 d q 28 d helped 10/10 perfectly with 15–20% long-term remission (Nejm 1994;330:1560)

2nd: Splenectomy works in 75% (60% complete and 15% partial remissions) (but only 14% of SLE—Ann IM 1985;102:325); response is predicted by response to high dose iv IgG (1 gm/kg iv qd × 2) (Nejm 1997;336:1494); must balance against later fear and risk of sepsis (death in 1–2% lifelong before pneumovax, unknown what it is now)

3rd: Chemotherapy with cytoxan, azathioprine, colchicine, vincristine, vinblastine; or MOPP (mustard, Oncovin [vincristine], procarbazine, prednisone), or CMOPP regimens

4th: Danazol 200 mg po qid (Nejm 1983;308:1396) or 50 mg qd after induce remission (Ann IM 1987;107:177) and/or vinblastine, both work by decreasing Fc fragment receptors on monos and macrophages, not by decreasing IgG (Nejm 1987;316:503)

5th: Immunoglobulin rx w plasmapheresis transient help; or IgG, high-dose iv, will overwhelm RES and produce transient remission, eg, for surgery, very expensive (Nejm 1982;306:1254) $3000–4000/dose; or iv anti-Rh(D) IG, which costs 1/2 as much and, in Rh positive pts, saturates spleen w coated rbc's so can't consume platelets (Med Let 1996;38:6); Fc receptor monoclonal IgG (Nejm 1986;314:1236)

In pregnancy, steroids iv, IgG, and cesarean section all potentially useful but only justified if sx in mother (Nejm 1990;323:229,264)

8.8 MYELOPROLIFERATIVE DISORDERS

THROMBOCYTHEMIA

Cause: A myeloproliferative disease; perhaps viral (doubtful—Nejm 1968; 278:1185), perhaps from irradiation, perhaps from hydrocarbons

Epidem: Possible association by debatable interconversion with others in myeloproliferative spectrum including polycythemia vera, CML, and myelofibrosis

Pathophys: Excess production of defective platelets (Nejm 1969;280:453)

Sx: Bruises, melena, hematemesis, etc.

Si: Purpura, bleeding

Crs: Benign in young

Cmplc: CVA and seizures (Ann IM 1984;100:513); **erythromelalgia** = attacks of redness and burning of extremities relieved for days by one aspirin, a platelet microvascular disorder (Ann IM 1985;102:466)
r/o other causes of elevated platelets but no effect on clotting in any: stress, malignancy (30–40% of all with elevated platelets), Fe deficiency, s/p splenectomy

Lab:
Chem: Pseudohyperkalemia, acid phosphatase, and LDH elevated; plasma levels normal but incr in test tube due to platelet contraction
Hem: Platelets incr usually >1 million but function may be diminished, eg, by thromboplastin generation test or response to epinephrine (Ann IM 1975;82:506); levels between 400,000 and 1 million are usually reactive in etiology
Basophils incr >40/mm^3. Marrow shows incr megakaryocyte size, inappropriately large for platelet count, unlike CML and secondary causes of elevated platelets (C. Finch, 1971)

Rx: In young, ASA and dipyridamole only
of sx like recurrent thrombosis or abnormal clotting studies and surgery planned: hydroxyurea though leukemia risk present (Nejm 1995;332:1132); alkylating agents, eg, busulfan, melphalan, but

leukemia risk; radioactive ^{32}P; irradiation perhaps; anagrelide 1–1.5 mg po q 6 h × 5–12 d until platelets decrease to normal, then 1.5–4 mg po qd (Nejm 1988;318:1292)

POLYCYTHEMIA VERA

Ann IM 1981;95:71 (UCLA rv of all polycythemias)

Cause: A myeloproliferative disease; monoclonal stem cell proliferation (P. Fialkow proved with women with 2 kinds of G6PD—Nejm 1976; 295:913)

Epidem: Male > female; perhaps associated with other myeloproliferative diseases because they may interconvert (controversial—Ann IM 1975;83:820; 1970;72:285)

Pathophys: Caused by loss of Bcl-X$_L$ apoptosis regulator genes dependence on erythropoietin (Nejm 1998;338;564,572,613). Excessive production of rbc's causes elevated crit, sludging at crits >60% only (Nejm 1970;283:183); incr cellular breakdown, causing gout; venous distension and headache; incr atherosclerosis, why?

Sx: Headache, dizziness, warm bath-induced pruritus (Nejm 1972; 286:845)

Si: Splenomegaly (75%), hepatomegaly, red sclerae (r/o conjunctivitis), plethora

Crs: 3% annual mortality, 3.5%/yr incidence of thrombotic events (Ann IM 1995;123:656)

Cmplc: Gout; erythromelalgia (p 359), Budd-Chiari due to hepatic venous occlusion even in occult myeloproliferative disease, ie, may be first sx especially in young female (Ann IM 1985;103:329)

r/o other etiologies of high crit:

- Hypovolemia: pheochromocytoma, Addison's, stress
- Increased erythropoietin causes (can rx all by adenosine receptor inhibition of erythropoietin effect by theophylline—Nejm 1990; 323:86):

  Hgb abnormalities with incr O$_2$ affinity, eg, hgb Rainier, Chesapeake, Kempsey, Yakima, M.

  Hypoxia due to lung disease etc. = 95% of polycythemics; may be diurnal; in smokers (Nejm 1978;298:6)

Tumor producing erythropoietin, eg, of posterior fossa of brain, hepatoma, renal, uterine fibroid

Renal transplant

Lab:

Hem:

- White count incr to 30,000 with incr or normal LAP activity
- B_{12} high due to incr binding protein in all myeloproliferative diseases and some leukemoid reactions (Ann IM 1971;765:809; 1969;71:285,719)
- Platelets elevated (80%)
- Basophils, elevated >40/mm^3 is diagnostic of myeloproliferative disease though some false negs (Clem Finch, 1972)
- Erythropoietin levels; low to normal = 3–5 U/d in 24-h urine; elevate to 30 U/d in anemia or secondary polycythemia; useful in 2nd stage w/u of polycythemia (Nejm 1986;315:283)
- Plasma volume incr in 60% of p. vera (decr in stress polycythemia)
- Rbc volume incr in p. vera and secondary causes, normal in stress polycythemia
- Hgb electrophoresis or blood gases at 98.6°F (37°C) (graph—Ann IM 1976;84:518) to r/o abnormal hgb
- Carboxy hgb level to r/o smoking cause (Nejm 1978;298:6)
- Marrow shows larger megakaryocytes, unlike CML and secondary causes of elevated platelets (Finch); erythroid hyperplasia; no fat; no Fe

Rx: Maintain crit <45% with phlebotomies

Possibly interferon α-2b sc tiw (Ann IM 1993;119:1091)

ChemoRx worsens prognosis by increasing neoplasms (Ann IM 1995; 123:656)

MYELOFIBROSIS WITH MYELOID METAPLASIA

Nejm 2000;342:1255

Cause: Unknown

Epidem: Older people (age >50); most common cause of splenomegaly in this age group. May interconvert with p. vera, debatable (p 360)

Pathophys: Hematopoiesis moves to liver and spleen as marrow fibroses; a clonal stem cell disorder causes ineffective erythropoiesis, dysplastic megakaryocytes, immature granulocytes, and reactive myelofibrosis

Sx: Bleeding, bruising; abdominal masses; failure to thrive
Si: Hepatosplenomegaly, anemia, purpura/ecchymoses, hypermetabolic cachexia in later stages
Crs: Slow, median survival 3–6 yr
Cmplc: Gout, renal stones, and failure
Lab:
  Hem: Anemia; smear shows bizarre rbc's, droplet forms diagnostic (r/o other infiltrative disease of marrow, eg, metastatic cancer), immature granulocytes, nucleated rbc's
  WBC incr to <50,000, terminally can be ≥100,000
  LAP normal to elevated
  Platelets often incr with giant forms and megakaryocytes on peripheral smear
Rx: of pain or hypersplenism: perhaps splenectomy, or irradiation, and hope that liver and marrow can take over, but danger of thrombocytosis post-splenectomy
  of anemia: transfusions, androgens
  of leukocytosis: hydroxyurea, interferon α

CHRONIC MYELOGENOUS LEUKEMIA (CML)
Nejm 1999;340:1330, 341:164; Ann IM 1999;131:207

Cause:
Epidem: Median age of onset = 53, but wide range down to childhood; incid = 1–2/100,000/yr; 15% of adult leukemia. 95% are due to a Philadelphia (Ph) chromosome (#22 from #9 crossover, opening up oncogene—Nejm 1985;313:1429); also incr incidence in Down syndrome trisomy #21, and with atom bomb or ^{32}P exposure
Pathophys: Unregulated signal tranduction by a tyrosine kinase formed as a result of a chromosome #22 and #9 translocation. Marrow invasion, leads to decr rbc's, platelets, and wbc's. Single-cell origin suggested by G6PD type A or B enzyme exclusively in Ph-positive cells (Nejm 1973;289:307)
Sx: Fatigue, anorexia/wgt loss, purpura, hives, and pruritus (histamine release); but 40% are asx when found on CBC

Si: Splenomegaly (50%), anemia, purpura, swollen gums (cellular infiltrate); no lymphadenopathy; "chloroma," red-brown skin papule becomes green when blood squeezed out of it (Nejm 1998;338:969)

Crs: Median survival ~40 mo; then acute blastic crisis develops; w rx, 50% 5-yr, 30% 10-yr survival

Cmplc: Pulmonary and endocardial fibrosis with eosinophilic variety. Lymphoid blast crisis (B or T cells; suggests primary defect in a very pluripotential stem cell—Nejm 1979;301:144)

Lab:

Chem: Serum B$_{12}$ markedly incr, often >1000 pgm/cc, r/o cancer if >20,000 pgm/cc (Nejm 1974;290:282). Uric acid increased

Hem:

- Smear not diagnostic, may have elevated wbc's; wbc = 50,000–250,000, mostly myelocytes; idiopathic, moderate elevation of wbc's may persist for years and be benign (Ann IM 1971;75:193). Blastic phase = 30^{+}% blasts; 2/3 AML type, 1/3 ALL type, which determines rx choices and prognosis
- Basophils elevated >40/mm^3, marrow mast cells also incr (Ann IM 1978;88:753)
- Platelets incr in number though function impaired
- LAP decr even when in relapse, r/o infectious mono, PNH, and slight decrease in sickle cell disease (Nejm 1975;293:918)
- Marrow has positive Ph chromosome prep in all (C. Finch, 1971); all erythroid and myeloid elements increased; even erythroblasts have Ph chromosome

Rx:

- Marrow transplant (Ann IM 1997;127:1080; Nejm 1998; 338:962), potentially curative in young pts so 1st choice there; 50–75% 5-yr survival
- Antimetabolites like cytosine arabinose
- Imatinib (Gleevec) (Med Let 2001;43:49)
- Interferon α (Nejm 1997;337:223; 1994;330:820; Ann IM 1996; 125:541) im qd × 28 d then tiw (Ann IM 1994;121:736); or w cytarabine

8.9 WHITE CELL DISORDERS/ LYMPHOMAS/LEUKEMIAS

AGRANULOCYTOSIS

Nejm 1983;308:1141

Cause:
- Allergic directly as with chloramphenicol or via lupus, eg, from procainamide (Ann IM 1984;100:197)
- Autoimmune antibodies and occasionally, perhaps, killer T cells (Ann IM 1985;103:357); idiopathic usually; ibuprofen induced, reversible (Nejm 1986;314:624)
- Direct toxic drug effect from chemotherapy, chloramphenicol

Epidem: Autoimmune type associated with rheumatoid Felty's syndrome

Pathophys:

Allergic type: delayed hypersensitivity T-cells kill in marrow; drugs can act as hapten to induce (Sci Am Text Med 1986)

Autoimmune type: antibodies especially to HLA surface antigens

Sx: Malaise, sore throat

Si: Pharyngitis, recurrent infections

Crs: Idiopathic autoimmune type very benign (Nejm 1980;302:908)

Cmplc: Sepsis

r/o genetic cyclic neutropenia (Nejm 1989;320:1306)

Lab:

Hem: Polys <500/mm^3

Rx: to prevent sepsis:
- Protective isolation, probably no benefit (Nejm 1981;304:448), but at least eliminate salads (Nejm 1981;304:433)
- Antibiotic prophylaxis, with Tm/S (Ann IM 1980;93:358); or fluoroquinolone + penicillin (Jama 1994;272:183); or ofloxacin + rifampin (Ann IM 1996;125:183); but now deaths from resistant organisms (Nejm 1982;306:16, 43)
- Granulocyte colony-stimulating factor (Nejm 1992;327:99), eg, filgrastim (Neupogen) or sargramostim (Leukin) (Med Let 1991; 33:61); but, at least in chemotherapy-induced type, no practical clinical benefit (Nejm 1997;336:1776,1781)
- Lithium po increases production of polys; level 0.7–1.4 decreases infections and increases survival (Nejm 1980;302:257)
- Transfusions of polys no help even with documented infection (Ann IM 1982;97:509)

of allergic type: steroids, cyclophosphamide

of autoimmune type: splenectomy helps, 70% by decreasing IgG (Nejm 1981;304:580; Ann IM 1981;94:623)

of direct toxic type: stop offending medication

of fever/sepsis (Med Let 1996;38:25; Nejm 1993;328:1323): ceftazidime (Ann IM 1994;120:834) or imipenem alone; or with aminoglycoside (Nejm 1987;317:1692; 1986;315:552,580), eg, amikacin qd (Ann IM 1993;119:584); or aztreonam + vancomycin. Oral Augmentin w or w/o ciprofloxacin as good or better than iv regimens (Nejm 1999;341:305,312,362) at least when is short lived during cancer chemoRx. If not better in 4+ days, add antifungal rx like amphotericin (Nejm 1993;328:1323), or less toxic fluconazole (Am J Med 2000;108:282) or itraconazole (Ann IM 2001;135:412)

ACUTE NONLYMPHOCYTIC LEUKEMIA (Including Myeloblastic [AML] and Monoblastic)

AML—Nejm 1999;341:1051

Cause:

Epidem: Increased incidence in patients treated for Hodgkins, multiple myeloma, Waldenström's, and ovarian cancers treated with radiation, MOPP (4% at 10 yr get it—Ann IM 1970;72:693), and alkylating agents like melphalan, chlorambucil, thiotepa, and cyclophosphamide (Nejm 1990;322:1,7); may be preceded by a myelodysplastic syndrome assoc w somatic chromosomal deletions. 2.4 cases/100,000/yr in US; 12.6/100,000/yr > age 65

Pathophys: Perhaps a defect in a maturation stimulator so cells don't die as normally would (Nejm 1971;284:1225)

Sx: Weakness, bleeding, fever, infections

Si: Anemia; petechiae and ecchymoses (83%); sternal tenderness, lymphadenopathy, hepatosplenomegaly; testicular, skin, meningeal, gum, and perianal infiltration, especially with monocytic types

Crs: Grim; grimmer if alkylating agent-induced (Ann IM 1980;93:133), preceded by myelodysplasia, or if monomyelocytic

Cmplc: CNS involved (7%); sepsis always; significant bleeding

Lab:

Chem: Elevated B_{12}, uric acid, phosphate; low calcium with rx due to PO_4 released by dead cells (Nejm 1973;289:1335)

Hem: Anemia; decr platelets; smear shows blasts, if >200,000 needs leukophoresis. Marrow shows blasts >30%; Auer rods sometimes and nucleoli in myeloblasts

Immunol: Circulating immune complexes correlate with worse prognosis (Nejm 1982;307:1174)

Rx: (Nejm 1994;331:896)

Induction w cytarabine + daunorubicin; if decide to do, takes 1 mo in hospital, makes aplastic and septic usually, 65% chance of inducing 6–14-mo remission. In a small subset (10%) (promyelocytic), tretinoin (all-trans-retinoic acid) matures the leukemic clone (Nejm 1997;337:1021; 1993;329:177; 1991;324:1385)

Maintenance: marrow transplant (Ann IM 1985;102:285) with autologous marrow, or HLA-matched sibling (Nejm 1980;302:1041), or unrelated donor, as good as (44% >4 yr-survival) continued intensive chemotherapy? (Nejm 1998;339:1649 vs 1995;332:217)

ACUTE LYMPHOCYTIC (-blastic) LEUKEMIA (ALL)

Nejm 1998;339:605

Cause: 2 types, child and adult. Adult type is probably genetic, HLA-linked, autosomal recessive (Ann IM 1978;89:173)

Epidem: Adult type represents 15% of adult leukemia. Incidence of childhood type is 32/million/yr (Nejm 1991;325:1330); no incr incidence near power lines (Nejm 1997;337:1)

Pathophys: CNS involvement more common (40%) than in AML (7%) 78% are of B cells; 17% are T-cell types; 5% have no monoclonal antibody markers (Nejm 1991;324:800); some also have myeloid antigens that correlate with worse prognosis (ibid)

Associated with chromosome #9 deletion that has interferon-α and -β genes (Nejm 1990;322:77)

Sx: Malaise, fever (1/3 due to sepsis, 2/3 due to tumor)

Si: Pallor; hepatosplenomegaly

Crs: In children, now much higher cure rates, 70+% 5-yr survivals (Nejm 1993;329:1289; 1991;325:1330) unless Ph chromosome positive (Nejm 2000;342:998). In adults prognosis is much worse than in children; T-cell types have worst prognosis, rest susceptible to rx (Ann IM 1979;91:759); 30–40% cure currently

Cmplc: Varicella zoster disease with 7% mortality (Nejm 1980;303:355); 6% recurrence in testes, prevent with irradiation, which decreases testosterone later (Nejm 1983;309:25); *Pneumocystis carinii*; CMV, progressive multifocal leukoencephalopathy; AML after chemotherapy in 4% (Nejm 1989;321:136), 2nd primaries in 0.5% of children (Nejm 1991;325:1330); sterility (Nejm 1989;321:143)

Lab:

Hem: CBC shows anemia, low platelets, incr wbc's

Marrow shows invasion; tissue cultures of treated patients predict relapse if grow blasts with original tumor surface markers (Nejm 1986;315:538)

Lymphocyte terminal deoxynucleotidyltransferase, a primitive lymph enzyme normally present in thymus, is present in childhood and T-cell ALL, and occasionally in blast crisis of CML

Flow cytometry to tell B from T cell and the subtypes

Rx: (Ann IM 1980;93:17,133; Nejm 1979;300:1189)

Induction: prednisone, vincristine, asparaginase (or its less-sensitizing conjugate, pegaspargase [Oncaspar] Med Let 1995;37:23), daunorubicin (hard on children's hearts—Nejm 1991;324:808) + mtx >80% remission

CNS (asx) rx: irradiate + intrathecal mtx after in remission (Nejm 1983; 308:477)

Maintenance: w mtx, teniposide, and cytarabine (Nejm 1998;338:499); can stop after in remission × 3 yr

Marrow transplant (allogenic or autologous) in 2nd remission if recurs, 50% work (Nejm 1994;331:1253) or more aggressive chemoRx (Nejm 1986;315:273)

CHRONIC LYMPHOCYTIC LEUKEMIA (CLL)

Nejm 1995;333:1052

Cause: Perhaps viral, irradiation, genetic?

Epidem: Adults, M > F, 90% age 50+ yr, median age at onset = 65 yr (case report in asx child—Nejm 1971;284:431); very rare in Asians

Pathophys: Usually CD5$^+$ B-cell leukemia, often associated with trisomy of chromosome #12 (Nejm 1986;314:865). The rare T-cell types, often associated with retrovirus infections (Nejm 1995;332:1744, 1749), or chromosome #14 inversion (Nejm 1986;314:865), are systemically spread (Ann IM 1980;93:223) but are the only types that involve the skin (Ann IM 1974;80:685), then called SŽzary syndrome

Platelets decr due both to autoimmune and splenomegaly mechanisms

Sx: Onset insidious, asx for years; rash and/or ulcer; no fever from tumor unless infected (M. Turck 1/69)

Si:

Stage 0: Lymphocytosis >15,000

Stage I: Above + adenopathy

Stage II: Above + hepato- and/or splenomegaly

Stage III: Above + anemia

Stage IV: Above + depressed platelets (purpura)

Crs: Correlates with abnormal karyotypes (Nejm 2000;343:1910). See Table 8.9.1

Table 8.9.1 Rai Staging (Nejm 1998;338:1506)

Stage	0	I	II	III	IV
At presentation (%)	31%	35	26	6	2
Median survival (yr)	10+	9	5	6	2

Cmplc: 2nd malignancy; sepsis especially with encapsulated organisms like H. flu and pneumococcus; ichthyosis; cardiac involvement (25%) rarely diagnosed pre-mortem

Lab:

Chem: Elevated uric acid

Hem: Ncnc anemia in 2/3; Coombs'-positive, steroid-responsive anemia in 1/3 (C. Finch, 1969); thrombocytopenia; wbc's >15,000, by definition, usually >100,000 with 75–90% lymphs, prolymphocytic variant may have up to 54% prolymphocytes but if more than that is prolymphocytic CLL w a bad prognosis; marrow shows monotonous lymphocytic infiltration. Flow cytometry to id monoclonal surface markers. CD5 markers on cells identify B-cell CLL and r/o reactive lymphocytosis

Rx: Only if sx or progression beyond stage I or II
  Prophylactic iv IgG q 3 wk decreases bacterial infections × 1/2 (Nejm 1988; 319:902) but no prolongation of survival
  Chemotherapy (Med Let 1991;33:89) for stage II⁺–III⁺ only, no help for stages 0, I and II unless progressive (Nejm 2000;343:1799;1998; 338:1506); usually with fludarabine (Nejm 2000;343:1750) or chlorambucil + prednisone, which gives a 60–80% response, but <10% are complete and overall survival is not improved. Then try 2-chlorodeoxyadenosine (Nejm 1994;330:319 says not effective, earlier references say it is, eg, Nejm 1992;327:1056; 1990;322: 1116), busulfan, cyclophosphamide, vincristine; interferon α often w AZT especially for T-cell types (Nejm 1995;332:1744,1749); 70% response rate
  Radiation, total body; 50% response but less toxic than above

NON-HODGKIN'S LYMPHOMA (Including diffuse histiocytic, hairy cell, lymphosarcoma; gastric type p 256)
  Nejm 1993;328:1023; Ann IM 1981;94:218

Cause: Perhaps hep C virus induces B-cell type (Ann IM 1997;127:423). Distinctive chromosomal changes associated with the different cellular subtypes (Nejm 1982;307:1231)

Epidem: 35,000/yr in US. Occurs in older (less tolerant of rx) pts than Hodgkin's and is otherwise a totally differently acting tumor (Nejm 1978;299:1446), although does represent 7% of all childhood/adolescent tumors (500/yr in US)
  Increased incidence in patients with diminished immune responses: AIDS (Nejm 1984;311:565), Sjögren's syndrome (Ann IM 1978;89: 888), sarcoid, malaria, celiac disease, radiation + chemoRx-treated Hodgkin's pts (Nejm 1979;300:452)

Pathophys: 80% are B-cell types and include all those associated with Sjögren's (Nejm 1978;299:1215; Ann IM 1978;89:318)

Sx: Adenopathy

Si: Splenomegaly, adenopathy

Crs: 5-yr survival = 32–83% depending on age, stage (like Hodgkin's staging), LDH, functional status, and cell type. Indolent lymphomas have long survivals but no cures, aggressive lymphomas the opposite

Cmplc: Leukemia
   r/o **bovine babesiosis** in splenectomized patients (Ann IM 1981;94:
     326); cutaneous T-cell lymphomas (p 153)

Lab: Stage like Hodgkin's
   Chem: Marked increase in LDH, unlike myeloma (Ann IM 1989;
     110:521)
   Hem: Ncnc anemia
   Path: Low grade
     • Small lymphocyte (CLL)
     • Follicular small cleaved cell
     • Follicular mixed cell
   Intermediate grade
     • Follicular large cell
     • Diffuse small cleaved cell
     • Diffuse mixed cell
     • Diffuse large cell
   High grade
     • Immunoblastic
     • Lymphoblastic (ALL)
     • Small noncleaved (Burkitt's etc.)
   Serol: M spike, or κ or λ chains in a small % (Nejm 1978;298:481)

Rx: (in children—Nejm 1983;308:559)
     • Observation alone is an option for low-grade asx types until or
       unless sx or progress
     • Chemotherapy with:
       1st: CHOP (cyclophosphamide, doxorubicin
         [hydroxydaunorubicin], vincristine [Oncovin], prednisone
         (Nejm 1993;328:1002; 1992;327:1342)
       2nd: Interferon α w COPA (same as CHOP) for low and
         intermediate grades (Nejm 1993;329:1608; 1992;327:1330);
         especially good for cutaneous T-helper cell types like Sézary's
         syndrome and mycosis fungoides (Ann IM 1984;101:484)
     • Immunotherapy with anti-idiotype antibodies for B-cell
       lymphomas (Nejm 1989;321:851), eg rituximab (Rituxan) (Med
       Let 1998;40:65) iv q 1 wk × 4; $11,000; ie, after remission
       induced, immunize w im injections of the specific portion of the
       IgG specific to that tumor class (Nejm 1992;327:1209)

- Marrow transplantation (Nejm 1987;316:1493,1499) w chemotherapy for recurrence improves 5-yr event-free survival from 12% to 50% (Nejm 1995;335:1540)
- Irradiation, total body or involved field combined w CHOP (Nejm 1998;339:21) of hairy cell type leukemia: 2 chlorodeoxyadenosine (2-eda); or interferon α

BURKITT'S LYMPHOMA
Nejm 1981;305:735

Cause: Epstein-Barr virus in B lymphocytes (Nejm 1976;295:685)

Epidem: Endemic in Africa and New Guinea; less frequent in US and England

Pathophys: A subtype of non-Hodgkin's lymphoma; malignant lymphoma of undifferentiated B lymphocytes; solid extranodal growth, no leukemia; a phytohemagglutinin type of transformation of lymphocytes

Sx: Jaw mass (50% of African cases); abdominal tumors (most common presentation in US, 2nd after jaw in Africa)

Si:

Stage I: Single tumor mass

Stage II: 2 or more masses

Stage III: Intrathoracic, abdominal or osseous (excluding facial bones) involvement

Stage IV: CNS and/or marrow invasion

Crs: Rapid onset and progression without rx

Stages I and II remit with rx in 80%

Stages III and IV remit with rx in 50%

Cure possible, perhaps 50% overall

Cmplc: Marrow invasion (50% in US, 10% in Africa); leukemia (<1% in Africa, 10% in US)

r/o developing country **immunoproliferative small bowel disease** and subsequent "Mediterranean" lymphoma (Nejm 1983;308:1401)

r/o **angioimmunoblastic lymphadenopathy** (Ann IM 1988;108:575) rare autoimmune lymphoproliferative disorder with fatigue, weight loss, fever, nodes, hepatosplenomegaly, and rash; 30% 2-yr survival; rx with steroids + cyclophosphamide

HEMATOLOGY/ONCOLOGY

Burkitt's Lymphoma, continued

Lab:
  Bact: EBV isolatable
  Path: "Starry sky" pattern = macrophages interspersed among undifferentiated tumor cells
  Serol: Diminished primary antibody responses, incr IgG, decr IgM. Normal delayed hypersensitivity. Increased antibody titers to EBV
Rx: "World's fastest growing tumor"; start rx within 48 h
  Surgical debulking very important
  Chemotherapy with cyclophosphamide, methotrexate including intrathecally, or cytosine arabinoside intrathecally

HODGKIN'S DISEASE
  Nejm 1992;326:678

Cause: Neoplasia w genetic predisposition precipitated by unknown viral infection (Nejm 1995;332:413); EBV associated, is it the cause or an innocent bystander? (Nejm 1989;320:502,689)

Epidem: Pattern like polio virus; incr in wealthy, small families, etc. Perhaps patient-to-patient contacts, or shared contacts; extensively examined in NY school studies (Nejm 1973;289:499,532) but questioned (Nejm 1979;300:1006). Male:female = 2:1; 3200 die/yr in US; bimodal age incidence, peaks at age 15–30 yr and ~50 yr

Pathophys: Possibly a retroviral infection or other perturbation of T and/or B cells, which become a Reed-Sternberg line arising in lymph nodes and spreading in contiguous groups of nodes

Sx: Fever (classic Pel-Epstein fever = 2 wk on, 2 wk off, occurs in 15%), night sweats or weight loss (any of these 3 make it stage B), nodes, pruritus

Si: Lymphadenopathy (painless, firm and rubbery), fever, 25% are stage I or II when present
  Stage I: Limited to 1 anatomic area
  Stage II: 2 contiguous anatomical areas, 1 side of diaphragm
  Stage III: 2 or more contiguous areas on 2 sides of diaphragm but involving only nodes and spleen
  Stage IV: Extranodal sites, diffuse infiltrations, eg, of liver

Crs: Overall 1992 cure rate = 75% with current w/u and rx

In 1982 with MOPP + ABVD, 85% of stage IV's were disease-free at 5 yr (Nejm 1982;306:770)

Cmplc:

- Leukemia or non-Hodgkin's lymphoma after rx, 1%/yr but plateaus after 15 yr, although solid tumor rate remains steady (Nejm 1988;318:76) and may even increase for breast Ca especially if rx'd as a child (Nejm 1996;334:745,792)
- Thyroid disease, especially myxedema after radiation rx (Nejm 1991;325:599)
- Sepsis, especially if had staging splenectomy (10% get—Nejm 1977; 297:245), and stages III and IV are unresponsive to pneumovax (Nejm 1978;299:442)

r/o toxoplasmosis, phenytoin (Dilantin) syndrome, other lymphomas, immunoblastic lymphadenopathy, AIDS

Lab:

Hem: ESR >30 mm/h before and especially after rx predicts (50%) relapse within 18 mo (Ann IM 1991;114:361). Bone marrow to look for infiltration

Path: Node bx shows Reed-Sternberg cells, aberrant macrophages (Nejm 1978;299:1208), multilobed dark nuclei with inclusions

Xray: CT of abdomen and thorax, lymphography of legs

Rx: Preventively immunize with 23-valent pneumococcal vaccine, H. flu vaccine, and tetravalent meningococcal vaccine 10 d before rx if can, otherwise after rx completed (Ann IM 1995;123:828, 1986;104:467)

Chemotherapy (Nejm 1993;328:560) with 6+ cycles of ABVD (Adriamycin, bleomycin, vinblastine, dacarbazine) (Nejm 1993;327:1478), or the former gold standard, MOPP. Other regimens being tried alternating with MOPP to further increase survival and cures: ABVD (Adriamycin, bleomycin, vinblastine, dacarbazine) or BCVPP (Ann IM 1984;101:447). Adverse effects: sterility and decr testosterone in males (Nejm 1978;299:12); female productivity affected less (Nejm 1981;304:1377); leukemia risk w MOPP

Radiation, 3000–4000 rads over 4 wk, for stage Ia and some II's. Cardiac function impaired 10 yr later (Nejm 1983;308:569); radiation pneumonitis especially when later withdraw steroids (Ann IM 1974;80:593)

HEMATOLOGY/ONCOLOGY

8.10 IMMUNOLOGIC DISEASES

Jama 1997;278(22)

MULTIPLE MYELOMA

Nejm 1997;336:1657; 1994;330:484; Br J Hem 1969;16:599

Cause: Neoplastic B cells

Epidem: 10,000 deaths/yr in US; incidence in blacks twice that in whites. Older patients, peak incidence in 50–60-yr age group; benzene workers (Nejm 1987;316:1044)

Pathophys: Immunoglobulin structure; see Fig. 8.10.1

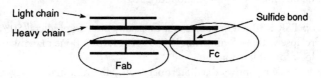

Figure 8.10.1

Of all M-protein disease: 50% IgG (60% with Bence-Jones protein), 24% IgA (70% with BJ), BJ only (21%), IgD (3%), no M protein (1.5%), IgM + Waldenström's (0.5%)

IgG and IgA have specific heavy chains and common light (λ and κ) chains. M-protein is a homogeneous protein electrophoresis spike. Myelomas with a specific antigen to which the M component is directed (eg, ASLO, RA, cold agglutinin anti-I, etc.) raise interesting questions of pathogenesis (Nejm 1971;284:831)

Sx: Recurrent infections; skeletal pain and pathologic fractures; Raynaud's if M component is an IgG cryoprotein; arthritis, first sx in 5% (R. Ritchie 1975)

Si: Bone pain (infiltration), hepatosplenomegaly

POEMS syndrome seen with myeloma and plasmacytomas: Polyneuropathy; Organomegaly, especially adenopathy, splenomegaly, and hepatomegaly; Endocrinopathy, including hypogonadism and hypothyroidism; Monoclonal gammopathy; Skin changes including hyperpigmentation and thickening

Crs: Die in <2 yr of diagnosis; probably takes 5–10 yr for isolated lesion to spread and kill. With rx, 30 mo mean survival, 2% 10-yr survival (Nejm 1983;308:314)

Cmplc:

- Sepsis especially with H. flu and pneumococcus, at least with IgG type
- Anemia
- Pancytopenia
- Renal failure: ATN often precipitated by IVP, RTA, Fanconi's syndrome, urate deposition, amyloid
- Hypercalcemia
- Amyloidosis (10%)
- Neuropathy due to myelin antibodies (Nejm 1980;303:618)
- Leukemia in 15% at 4 yr after rx (Nejm 1979;301:743)
- Hyperviscosity (9% of IgGs) correlates with Sia water test (Ann IM 1972;77:853)
- Angioneurotic edema due to autoantibody against M component, consumes C'1 inhibitor (Nejm 1985;312:534) (p 172)

Lab:

Chem: Anion gap low, cationic proteins increased (Nejm 1977; 296:858)

Hem: Anemia with decr rbc half-life due to IgG coating; peripheral smear shows plasma cells (5%). Marrow shows >10% atypical plasma cells in 90%, usually immature. ESR incr in most, though may be temperature-dependent if cryoprecipitate and hence low at room temperature

Serol: (Bull Rheum Dis 1975;25:810):

SPEP shows >3 gm monoclonal protein; false pos in 0.1% at age 40 yr, 5% at age 80 yr; spurious spikes from aggregated IgG after standing, fibrinogen or bacterial or hgb contamination in β area, hyperlipidemia in α_2 area.

Urine protein electrophoresis: monoclonal light chain (κ or λ), Bence-Jones protein; either this or SPEP is positive in 99% (r/o amyloid, malignant lymphomas, occasionally benign)

Xray: Skull, spine show osteolytic (punched out) lesions (half heal during remissions—Ann IM 1972;76:551) and/or diffuse osteoporosis

Rx: Irradiation for sx relief or if suspect an isolated plasmacytoma, especially IgA type

Chemotherapy only if anemia, elevated creatinine or calcium, or bone lesions (Nejm 1980;302:1347); use melphalan + prednisone, or

HEMATOLOGY/ONCOLOGY

cyclophosphamide + carmustine (Nejm 1982;306:743); or, 2nd
choice, VAD (vincristine, Adriamycin, dexamethasone) cycled rx
(Nejm 1984;310:1353). Coincident monthly pamidronate infusion
prevents pathologic fx's (Nejm 1996;334:488). Maintenance after
induction with interferon α (Ann IM 1996;124:212; Nejm 1990;
322:1430). Thalidomide helps 30% of refractory cases (Nejm 1999;
341:1565)

Marrow transplant (Nejm 1991;325:1267) after high dose chemoRx
(Nejm 1996;335:91); or, perhaps better, transfusion of placental
stem cells w less graft vs host disease despite ≥2 HLA mismatches
(Nejm 1996;335:157,167,199)

IgG iv prophylactically may prevent infection (Lancet 1994;343:1059)
but costs $25,000/yr (Ann IM 1994;121; suppl 2:32)

of anemia: erythropoietin tiw helps (Nejm 1990;322:1693)

of bone pain and hypercalcemia, and perhaps w initiation of chemoRx:
pamidronate iv (Nejm 1996;335:1836) or other bisphosphonate
(Ann IM 2000;132:734)

AGAMMAGLOBULINEMIAS

Ann IM 1993;118:720 (acquired); Nejm 1984;311:235,300

Cause:

Acquired common variable immunodeficiency (Nejm 1995;333:434):
primary, or secondary to protein loss via malnutrition nephrotic
syndrome, exfoliative dermatitis, or enteropathy

Congenital (Nejm 1995;333:431): Genetic, X-linked mutation in
Bruton tyrosine kinase gene; occasionally autosomal recessive from
MU heavy chain gene mutation on chromosome #14 (Nejm 1996;
335:1486)

Epidem:

Acquired: M > F, family h/o SLE, ITP, IgA deficiency

Congenital: Sx at age 5–6 mo

Pathophys:

Acquired: Absent B lymphs, a few have activated suppressor T cells
(Nejm 1980;303:372)

Congenital: Defect in B cell development (Nejm 1987;316:427) from a cytoplasmic signal-induced molecule mutation

Sx:

Acquired: Onset age 8⁺ yr; recurrent purulent infections, especially sinus and lung, and ECHO virus of CNS (Nejm 1977;296:1485); sprue syndrome and *Giardia*

Congenital: Onset age 6–12 mo, rarely as late as 4 yr; RA-like sx often 1st (mycoplasma-induced); recurrent purulent sepsis, leads to bronchiectasis; sprue syndrome and *Giardia*

Si:

Acquired: Lymphadenopathy, hepatosplenomegaly, eczema

Congenital: Lymphadenopathy in older pts, hepatosplenomegaly, *P. carinii,* hypoplastic tonsils

Crs:

Cmplc:

Acquired: Pernicious anemia (33%), ITP, hemolytic anemia, neutropenia, noncaseating granulomas (Ann IM 1997;127:613), gi tumors, gastric cancer, mycoplasma RA syndromes, bronchiectasis, pneumocystis infections (Nejm 1992;326:999)

Congenital: Bronchiectasis, incr neoplasias, polio from live viruses

r/o severe combined immunodeficiency (Nejm 1995;333:435) rx'd w marrow transplant (Nejm 2000;342:1325), X-linked Wiskott-Aldrich syndrome (Nejm 1998;338:291; 1995;333:437), DiGeorge syndrome which rx w thymus transplant (Nejm 1999;341:1180), and hereditary thymic aplasia and dysplasia (Nejm 1984;311:235, 300; 1980;302:892)

Lab:

Path: No plasma cells in marrow or RES

Serol: Diminished or absent IgG (<100 mg%) and absent IgA, and IgM

Xray:

Congenital: Lateral neck shows diminished lymphoid tissue

Rx: Prevention: carrier detection by recombinant DNA probes of B cells can work (Nejm 1987;316:427)

IgG 300–600 mg/kg in adults, 400–800 in children iv q 4 wk (Ann IM 2001;135:165) can result in nearly normal life; beware of IgE antibodies to IgA, which can cause anaphylaxis (Nejm 1986; 314:560)

in acquired, cimetidine helps some by suppressing suppressor T cells (Nejm 1985;312:198); interleukin-2 weekly sc (Nejm 1994;331:918)

8.11 MISCELLANEOUS

HEMATOLOGY

Anemia w/u in primary care
1st: CBC, w indices, peripheral smear exam, and retic count
2nd: Folateand B_{12} and/or iron and TIBC if indicated by #1
3rd: Bone marrow aspiration and bx

Eosinophilia (Nejm 1998;338:1592)
Cause: Allergic, helminth parasitic infections, malignancy, vasculitis, idiopathic, drug allergy usually reversible except for tryptophan-induced eosinophilia/myalgia syndrome (Ann IM 1990;112:85) (p 804); interleukin-5-producing T cell clones (Nejm 1999;341:1112)
Pathophys: (Nejm 1991;324:1110)
Lab:
  Hem: >350/mm^3 is abnormal, >1500/mm^3 needs w/u and rx
Rx: of idiopathic type with counts >1500/mm^3 to prevent heart disease (Ann IM 1982;97:78) w steroids, hydroxyurea, vincristine, or interferon α (Ann IM 1994;121:648)

Erythrocyte sedimentation rate: Methods and rare utility (Ann IM 1986;104:515); acute phase reactants probably better measured by C-reactive protein elevations (>10 mg/L) (Nejm 1999;340:448)

Erythropoetin (Epogen, Procrit) (Med Let 2001;43:40) 50–150 U/kg iv/sc tiw; or darbepoetin (Avenesp) (Med Let 2001;43:109) sc/iv qwk; helps in renal failure, cancer chemoRx, HIV disease, pre-surgical (see below)

Methemoglobinemia, acquired (Nejm 2000;343:337)
Epidem: Rare, induced by oxidizing drugs like benzocaine, dapsone, nitrates, sulfonamides
Sx: SOB
Si: Ashen pallor
Lab: O_2 sat decr; brown serum
Rx: Methylene blue 2mg/kg iv or po

Normal marrow ratios: Marrow:fat = 1:1, erythroid:myeloid (granulocytic) series = 1:3

Platelet transfusions: Leukocyte reduction and UVB irradiation decr antibody formation and incr survival (Nem 1997;337:1861); as does crossmatch before, can do with HLA typing or simply serum and platelet xmatch in aggregometer (Nejm 1975;292:130); can freeze and keep longterm now like rbc's, eg, draw when well, transfuse when on chemotherapy (Nejm 1978;299:7)

Red blood cell indices: Calculations: MCV = hct/rbc MCH = hgb/rbc MCHC = hgb/hct

Transfusions of RBCs

At what hgb level? RCT shows keeping >7 gm% better than higher levels in critically ill pts (Nejm 1999;340:409,467)

Of autologous red cells: draw 1 U q 1 wk, can harvest 4–6 U in 3 wk for elective surgery using supplemental recombinant erythropoietin rx if initial hct <39% (Nejm 1997;336:933), especially helpful in women and children (Nejm 1989;321:1162) but risks may not warrant unless odds of needing tfx high (Nejm 1999;340:525); or 4 wk prior to surgery, weekly erythropoietin + iron polysaccharide complex 150 mg po tid, w/o banking units also helpful (Ann IM 2000;133:845)

Viral infection risk (Nejm 1999;340:438) = 1/34,000+ U w screened blood, 88% of risk is for hep B, and rest is HIV risk (1/676,000)

2,3-DPG:

Increases with incr pH and decr pO_2, and causes easier O_2 dissociation, hence compensates for anemia (Nejm 1970;283:165); Hgb F binds 2,3-DPG poorly relative to HgbA, which explains incr O_2 binding by fetal blood (Nejm 1971;285:589)

ONCOLOGY

Cancer epidemiology 1950–1985 in US, incidence and prevalence (Nejm 1986;314:1226)

Cancer induction by:

• Oncogenes (clear reviews—Nejm 1994;330:328; Ann IM 1984;101:223), viral (v-onc) and cellular (c-onc); tumor suppressor gene

mutations correlate especially w sarcomas (Nejm 1992;326:1301,1309); retinoblastoma gene is on chromosome #13 (Nejm 1991;324:212)
• Dioxin, perhaps in low levels (Nejm 1991;324:212)

Marrow cellular component stimulation:
PMNLs, w granulocyte colony stimulating factor
Rbcs w recombinant erythropoietin
Platelets w recombinant thrombopoietin (Ann IM 1997;126:673)

Marrow transplant (Nejm 1994;330:827)
HLA-matched (Nejm 1990;322:485; Ann IM 1989;110:51). Useful for various conditions: Wiskott-Aldrich syndrome, aplastic anemia, combined immunodeficiency (even non-HLA matched works—Nejm 1999;340:528), Fanconi's anemia, Hurler's disease, possibly thalassemia major (40–50% survival), possibly sickle cell disease, hematologic cancers, some solid tumors like breast, ovarian, melanoma, and glioma. Costs $150,000–500,000 and for some diseases may be no better than standard rx
Placental/cordblood source more available and often better w less GVH disease (Nejm 2001;344: 1818; 2000;342:1846), 75% success (Nejm 1998;339:1565; Med Let 1996;38:71)
Peripheral blood stem cells from a donor after filgrastim (granulocyte colony stimulating factor) are better source for transplant (Nejm 2001; 344:175; Ann IM 1997;126:600)
Cmplc:
   • Rejection: use methotrexate + prednisone + antithymocyte globulin (Nejm 1982;306:392); avoid transfusion of blood or platelets beforehand, which diminishes success from 75% to 25% (Ann IM 1986;104:461)
   • Graft vs host disease (rv—Nejm 1991;324:667) including bronchitis (Nejm 1978;299:1030), skin, gi tract, and liver (venoocclusive disease—Ann IM 1979;90:158), latter prevented w ursodiol prophylaxis (Ann IM 1998;128:975)
   • B-cell lymphoproliferative syndromes from "mono" to lymphoma (Nejm 1991;324:1451)
   • Solid tumors (melanoma, squamous cell, thyroid, bony, CNS) all incr × 2.5–4, 5–10 yr out (Ann IM 1999;131:738; Nejm 1997; 336:897)
Rx: Prophylactic pneumovax against incr pneumococcal disease (Ann IM 1979;91:835); acyclovir against herpes simplex (Nejm 1981;305:63);

CMV immune plasma against CMV (Ann IM 1982;97:11). Weekly IgG no help (Ann IM 1993;118:937)

Filgrastim, a granulocyte-stimulating factor, can reinduce transplanted marrow growth (Nejm 1993;329:757)

Metastatic cancer, unknown origin
Ultimate diagnoses and rx options (Nejm 1993;329:257)

Detection at molecular level in lymph nodes possible by PCR and may be used to better stage pts (colon Ca—Nejm 1998;339:223,264)

Surgical cancer survival
Better in/w hospitals/surgeons w higher volume where surgery is major and complex, eg esophagectomy, pelvic exenteration, hepatectomy, pancreatectomy, pneumonectomy (Jama 1998;280:1747)

Vitamin prevention of cancer: No diminished cancer rate with:
• Vitamin A or β-carotene (Nejm 1996;334:1145,1150), although possibly low dietary vitamin A intake may increase breast cancer rate and po A may help in that small way (Nejm 1993;329:257); with vitamin E (Nejm 1994;330:1029)
• Vitamin C rx by Pauling (Nejm 1985;312:137)

IMMUNOLOGY

Allergy testing (rv—Ann IM 1989;110:304)
• Skin prick testing for wheal/flare mediated by IgE; easiest and best first test to up to 30 allergens; if patient intolerant, use RAST tests
• Intradermal tests if above neg; problem is false positives
• Total IgE levels somewhat helpful if extreme, eg, if <50 μgm/L then atopic disease excluded, if >900 μgm/L then likely
• Provocation tests, eg, bronchial or oral occasionally helpful
• Skin patch testing for DHS contact dermatitis helpful if substance is not irritating
• IgG levels only useful to measure antivenom blocking antibody

Chemical sensitivity to multiple agents not immunologic, rather apparently psych in origin (Ann IM 1993;119:97)

HEMATOLOGY/ONCOLOGY

Cold agglutinins (rv—Nejm 1977;297:538, 583)

Cryoglobulinemia (Nejm 1997;337:1512)
Cause: 98% have hep C (p 275) as the cause (Ann IM 1992;117:573) if no clear other cause like SBE, HIV in 23% (Ann IM 1999;130:226), or leprosy. Both types II and III are associated w hep B and C, Sjögren's, and Waldenström's (Nejm 1992;327:1490)
Pathophys: Immune complex small vessel vasculitis
Sx: Arthralgias
Si: Purpura, neuropathic weakness (Ann IM 1977;87:287)
Cmplc: Membranoproliferative glomerulonephritis, and porphyria cutanea tarda (Ann IM 1995;123:615,625; 1992;117:573; Nejm 1993;328:465); debatably Sjögren's/sicca syndrome, polyarteritis
Lab:
  Type I: Monoclonal IgG, usually assoc w malignancy
  Type II: Mixed, polyclonal IgG and monoclonal IgM rheumatoid factor
  Type III: Mixed polyclonal IgG and IgM rheumatoid factor
  Complement: C_4 very low but normal C_3
Rx: NSAIDs, steroids, cyclophosphamide; if systemic disease, possibly interferon α-2a helps esp in hep C types (Nejm 1994;330:751)

Hypersensitivity reactions:
Type I: Anaphylactic, IgE on mast cells, eg, anaphylaxis from bee sting
Type II: Cytotoxic, antigen contained in or on cell surface; eg, Rh hemolysis
Type III: Immune complex, eg, serum sickness
Type IV: Delayed hypersensitivity (DHS), eg, IPPD tubercular skin test

Plasmapheresis: Expensive and not clearly beneficial in many situations for which promoted (Nejm 1984;310:762); may help chronic but not acute (Guillain-Barré) inflammatory demyelination polyradiculoneuropathy (Nejm 1986;314:461)

Protective isolation: No benefit for granulocytopenias (Nejm 1981;304:448) (p 364)

Zinc deficiency induces decr DHS by suppressing T lymphs (Ann IM 1981;95:155)

Chapter 9
Infectious Disease: Bacteriology

D. K. Onion and S. Sears

9.1 ANTIBIOTICS

Antibiotic of choice (Med Let 2001;43:69); doses of all in renal failure
(West J Med 1992;156:633). Drug prices are average wholesale
prices quoted in Med Let (1998;40:33, 85, et al) for generic type if
available; current retail prices may vary widely.

PENICILLINS

- Amoxicillin 250–500 mg po bid adequate (Rx Let 1999;6:33); less
diarrhea than ampicillin; cheap
- Amoxicillin + clavulanic acid (Augmentin) po 250 mg/125 mg or
500/125 tid; spectrum includes β-lactamase organisms, ie, is resistant to
penicillinase, thus used against H. flu, staph, *Bacillus fragilis, Escherichia
coli;* for OM, UTIs, sinusitis, and for animal and human bites. OK in
pregnancy; not effective vs *Pseudomonas* spp, *Enterobacter* spp, *Serratia
marcesans;* adverse effects: diarrhea; $100/10 d for 500 mg tid
- Ampicillin 250 mg qid po or 1–2 gm q 2–6 h iv; penicillinase-sensitive;
very cheap
- Ampicillin + sulbactam (Unasyn) 2 gm po or 1 gm iv q 6 h; $47/d
- Penicillin G po/iv/im; if parenteral form in short supply, can substitute
ampicillin
- Phenoxymethyl penicillin (Pen V) po; gastric acid-resistant; $2–5/10d

PENICILLINASE-RESISTANT ANTISTAPH PENICILLINS

- Nafcillin iv; resistant to penicillinase. Adverse effects: ASA-like platelet impairment (Nejm 1974;291:265); dose-dependent neutropenia; glucose and alkali increase its degradation, so give it in saline (Nejm 1970;283: 118); adv effects: hard on veins
- Oxacillin po or iv/cloxacillin 500 mg qid po; resistant to penicillinase. Adverse effects: hepatitis, reversible, anicteric, occurs at >1 gm qd (Ann IM 1978;89:497); hard on veins. $23/10 d po
- Dicloxacillin 250 mg po qid. $8/10 d

ANTI-PSEUDOMONAL/EXTENDED SPECTRUM PENICILLINS

- Carbenicillin (Ann IM 1982;97:755) 4 gm daily divided qid po; spectrum includes *Pseudomonas* spp and *Proteus vulgaris* (indole +); is synergistic w aminoglycosides. Adverse effects: Na content = 65 mEq/10 gm, AST (SGOT) elevations, won't cross blood-brain barrier; rarely used now
- Piperacillin (Med Let 1982;24:48) 2–5 gm q 4 h, iv/im; cost = $430/7 d
- Piperacillin + tazobactam (Zosyn) (Med Let 1994;36:7) 3 gm/375 mg iv q 6 h; spectrum and cost like Timentin
- Ticarcillin (Med Let 1985;27:69) + clavulanic acid (Timentin) (Med Let 1986;28:32); spectrum includes staph, gram-negs, and anaerobes; $60/d

1ST-GENERATION CEPHALOSPORINS

Some resistance developing but generally all are good vs *E. coli, Klebsiella* spp, *Proteus mirabilis,* gram-positive cocci except methicillin-resistant staph and *Enterococcus* spp; MIC vs staph <0.5 mgm/cc

- Cefadroxil (Duricef) 1–2 gm/d po divided bid; $30–70/10 d
- Cefazolin (Ancef) 1–8 gm/d iv divided q 8 h
- Cephalexin (Keflex) 1–4 gm/d po divided qid; cost: trade = $80/10 d, generic = $5
- Cephalothin (Keflin) 2–12 gm/d iv divided q 6 h, im is painful; $400/10 d iv
- Cefradine (Velosef) 1–4 gm/d po divided; $12/10 d generic

2ND-GENERATION CEPHALOSPORINS

MIC vs staph = 1–2 μgm/cc

- Cefaclor (Ceclor) 1–4 gm/d po; vs H. flu; not as effective as other 2nd generation ones and higher incidence of hypersensitivity reactions; $42/10 d for 500 mg tid

- Cefmetazole (Zefazone) (Med Let 1990;32:65); 2 gm iv tid; adverse effects: prolonged PT; $35/d
- Cefotetan (Cefotan) (Med Let 1986;28:70) iv q 12 h; vs anaerobes, *Neisseria* spp, gram-positives and negatives, but not *Listeria* or *Enterococcus.* Adverse effects: rare vitamin K-reversible increase in protime; $41/d
- Cefoxitin (Mefoxin) (Ann IM 1985;103:70) 3–12 gm/d iv; spectrum includes gc, anaerobes (80%); $500/10 d iv
- Cefprozil (Cefzil) (Med Let 1992;34:63) 250 mg po q 12 h; 2nd or 3rd choice for otitis media or bronchitis; $122/10 d for 500 mg bid
- Cefuroxime (Zinacef) 0.75–3 gm q 8 h iv, or 125 mg po bid (as Ceftin); spectrum includes penicillin-resistant gc, H. flu and *Moraxella catarrhalis;* $350/10 d iv; $136/10 d for 500 mg bid
- Loracarbef (Lorabid) (Med Let 1992;34:87) 200 mg po q 12 h; no better than others; $60/10 d

3RD-GENERATION CEPHALOSPORINS

All good vs gc, *M. catarrhalis,* H. flu; ok vs *Klebsiella, E. coli;* miss anaerobes, *Listeria, Pseudomonas,* enterococci, atypicals (*Legionella, Mycoplasma,* chlamydia). MIC vs staph = $\sim 5^+$ μgm/cc for all except for ceftriaxone, which is lower. All $50–70/d
- Cefdinir (Omnicef) (Med Let 1998;40:85) 300 mg or 7 mg/kg po bid; similar spectrum to cefpodoxime; $67/10d
- Cefepime (Maxipime) (Med Let 1996;38:84) no advantages over others
- Cefixime (Suprax) (Med Let 1989;31:73) 400 mg po × 1; ok vs gonorrhea (Nejm 1991;325:1337), but no good vs *Pseudomonas,* staph, or anaerobes; $7/d
- Cefoperazone (Cefobid); biliary excretion hence for biliary infections; q 8–12 h
- Cefotaxime (Claforan) 2–12 gm iv/im qd divided
- Cefpodoxime (Vantin) (Med Let 1992;34:107) 100–400 mg po bid; good vs methicillin-sens staph and intermediately penicillin-sens pneumococcus, for gc (single dose), 2nd choice for OM/sinusitis (R. Holmberg 9/93); $76/10 d 200 mg bid
- Ceftazidime (Fortaz); good vs *Pseudomonas* but high MIC for staph so not reliable for it
- Ceftibuten (Cedax) (Med Let 1996;38:23) 400 mg po qid; poor vs staph and pneumococcus (Med Let 1998;40:85), no advantages over others; $68/10 d

ID: BACTERIOLOGY

- Ceftizoxime (Cefizox) iv q 8–12 h
- Ceftriaxone (Rocephin) iv/im qd-bid; good CSF penetration hence best for blind rx of childhood meningitis (Nejm 1990;322:141), can be used for penicillin-sens strep SBE, useful outpt drug (Jama 1992;267:264). Adverse effects: pseudocholecystitis and true gallstones (Ann IM 1991; 115:712)

AMINOGLYCOSIDES
(Ann IM 1983;98:813; in renal failure Ann IM 1981;94:343)

Work well vs gram-negative bacilli; some activity against staph, penicillin-resistant diphtheroids, enterococci w a penicillin. All renal and vestibular toxic. Once daily dosing reasonable and perhaps less toxic (BMJ 1996;312:338; Ann IM 1996;124:717; 1992;117:693)
- Amikacin 24 mg/kg/24 h (Ann IM 1981;95:328); useful for resistant gram-negs
- Gentamicin 3–5 mg/kg/24 h iv or q 2 half-lives (half-life = 4 × creatinine in mg%); get peak, half hr after dose, 6–9 μgm/cc; and get trough, half h before dose, <2 μgm/cc. Better vs *Serratia* than tobramycin. Vestibular toxicity is worse than auditory nerve toxicity
- Tobramycin; same dosing as gentamicin; $60/gm, 10 × gentamicin cost; less renal toxicity (Nejm 1980;302:1106), monitor levels w goal = 5–10 μgm/cc (J Inf Dis 1984;149:443); better than gentamicin for *Pseudomonas*

CARBAPENEMS
- Imipenem + cilastatin (Primaxin) (Med Let 1986;28:29) 0.5–1 gm iv q 6 h; resistant to penicillinase; broader spectrum than 3rd-generation cephalosporins, good vs strep, staph, anaerobes, resistant gc and H. flu, most gram-negs, gets into CSF; *Pseudomonas* resistance develops, inadequate vs methicillin-resistent staph, *Enterococcus, Mycoplasma,* chlamydia. Adverse effects: seizures. $100/d
- Meropenem (Merrem) (Med Let 1996;38:88) 1 gm iv q 8 hr; similar to imipenem/cilastin but a little better vs gm negs and a little less good vs gm pos organisms, ok vs *Listeria;* renal excretion; cost $150/d

FLUOROQUINOLONES

(Nejm 1991;324:384) Avoid all in pregnant women and children under 18 (cartilage damage)

1st Generation:

- Nalidixic acid (closely related quinolone but not a fluoro-quinolone); po; rapid resistance develops
- Norfloxacin (Ann IM 1988;108:238); 200–400 mg bid po; for UTIs and gc; $60/10 d

2nd Generation:

- Ciprofloxacin (Med Let 1988;30:11) 250–750 mg po bid, or 400 mg iv q 12 h (Med Let 1991;33:75); no good vs anaerobes, *Enterococcus,* chlamydia, staph (resistance develops quickly—Ann IM 1991;114:424), or strep, but gets all else including gonorrhea and other gram-negatives including *Pseudomonas aeruginosa* in UTIs, sputa of cystic fibrosis patients and chronic external otitis; as prophylaxis in leukemias (Ann IM 1987;106:1,7). Adverse effects: causes increases in theophylline levels. $61/10 d po
- Ofloxacin (Floxin) (Med Let 1992;34:58; 1991;33:71) 400 mg po ×1 for gc, or 400 mg po bid × 1$^+$ wk; good vs gc, all H. flu, gi pathogens except *Clostridium difficile,* mycoplasma, and chlamydia; no good vs anaerobes or pseudomonas, iffy vs staph and strep; $3/400-mg pill

3rd Generation: (mainly for resistant pneumococcus)

- Gatifloxacin (Tequin) (Med Let 2000;42:15); 400 mg po or iv qd; like levofloxacin, covers atypicals, resistant pneumococcus, H. flu, and moraxella, but not as good as cipro vs gm negs; may prolong QT; $70/crs po, $115/3d crs iv
- Grepafloxacin (Raxar) withdrawn from mkt 11/99 due to long QT syndrome arrhythmias
- Levofloxacin (Levaquin) (Med Let 1997;39:41) 500 mg po/iv qd; like others, is active isomer component of ofloxacin, better than cipro vs gram-pos cocci, covers atypicals, resistant pneumococcus, H flu, and *Moraxella,* but not as good as cipro vs gm negs; $77/10 d
- Moxifloxacin (Avelox) (Med Let 2000;42:15) 400 mg po qd, like levofloxacin, covers atypicals, resistant pneumococcus, H. flu, and *Moraxella,* but not as good as cipro vs gm negs; can prolong QT interval; $90/crs

ID: BACTERIOLOGY

- Sparfloxacin (Med Let 1997;39:41) 400 mg po load then 200 mg po qd; longer 1/2 life. Adverse effects: QT prolongation, sun sensitivity so may be w/drawn from mkt. Cost $75/10 d
- Trovofloxacin (Trovan) (Rx Let 1998;5:8; Med Let 1998;40:30) 100–200 mg po qd or 300 mg iv qd, or 100 mg po × 1 for UTI; effective vs gram positives including resistant pneumococcus, as well as vs anaerobes (only quinolone w such coverage). Adverse effects: fatal allergic hepatitis and pancreatitis, esp if > 21 d use (Rx Let 1999;6:37; 1998;5:67), which has caused FDA to severly restrict use

IMMUNOLOGIC AGENTS

- Immune globulin (Nejm 1991;325:110, 123); 100+ mg/kg/mo im to keep trough IgG >400 mg%; used for IgG deficiencies, in AIDS children (Nejm 1991;325:73), Kawasaki's disease, ITP, immune neutropenia, and sometimes in CLL (Nejm 1991;325:81) but may not be worth it; $100–1000 per dose
- Interferon α-2a; for hepatitis B and C disease. Adverse effects: marrow suppression, flu-like illness, depression, sometimes irreversible autoimmune disorders like thyroiditis (1–2%)
- Interferon γ; adjunct in atypical tbc, leprosy, toxoplasmosis, leishmaniasis (Nejm 1994;330:1348), and other persistent intracellular infections as well as chronic granulomatous disease (Ann IM 1995;123:216)

MACROLIDES
(Med Let 1992;34:45)

Beware cardiotoxic effects (long QT, p 79) when given w terfenadine and other nonsedating antihistamines (Jama 1996;275:1339), or alone esp in women (Jama 1998;280:1774)
- Azithromycin (Zithromax) po or iv, 500 mg or 10 mg/kg × 1, then 250 mg or 5 mg/kg po qd × 4 d; or 1–2 gm po × 1 for chlamydial cervicitis and urethritis (Nejm 1992;327:921), *Mycobacterium avium, Legionella,* gonorrhea; also available iv; less gi sx than erythromycin; less good than erythromycin for staph and strep; $40/course
- Clarithromycin (Biaxin) 250–500 mg po bid, also available as qd XL though levels lower (Rx Let 2000;7:18); spectrum like erythromycin; fewer gi sx; $65/10 d for 250 mg bid
- Dirithromycin (Dynabec) (Med Let 1995;37:109) 500 mg po qd. Adverse effects: gi intolerance, probable interactions w nonsedating antihistamines like other macrolides. $27/7 d

- Erythromycin 250–500 mg po/iv qid. Adverse effects: increased digoxin, theophylline, warfarin, and carbamazepine levels (Med Let 1985;27:1) $7.50/10 d

MONOBACTAMS

- Aztreonam (Med Let 1987;29:45) used vs aerobic gram negs; $50/d

OXAZOLIDINONES

- Linezolid (Zyvox) (Med Let 2000;42:45) 600 mg po or iv bid; vs MRSA and other vancomycin resistant organisms. Adverse effects: NV+D, avoid w tyramine foods and several antidepressants. $100–150/d

SULFAS

- Sulfisoxazole (Gantrisin) 8 gm in 24-h load, then 4 gm qd maintenance po divided; vs UTIs. Adverse effects: allergies, migrating pulmonary infiltrates
- Trimethoprim/sulfa (Septra, Bactrim) po, iv (Med Let 1981;23:102). Adverse effects: resistance develops in gi tract organisms w prophylactic use (Nejm 1982;306:130), decreased polys w azathioprine (Imuran) due to folate metabolism interference (Ann IM 1980;93:560); hyperkalemia at high doses (Ann IM 1993;119:291, 296) or even standard doses (20% have K >5.5 mEq/L) especially if renal failure (Ann IM 1996;124:316). Cheap

MISCELLANEOUS

- Chloramphenicol 3 gm qd iv/im [im as good as iv (Nejm 1985;313:410)] or 100 mg/kg/24 h divided, eg 150 mg qid; vs anaerobes, *E. coli, Salmonella, Rickettsia;* liver excretion. Adverse effects: sideroblastic marrow aplasia, dose-related or allergic. $21/d
- Clindamycin; vs anaerobes, especially w gentamicin, as well as soft tissue and bone infections w staph and strep. Adverse effects: *C. difficile* colitis
- Dapsone; a sulfone used for dermatitis herpetiformis, leprosy, or w Tm/S for pneumocystisosis
- Doxycycline 100 mg po bid. Adverse effects: similar to tetracycline
- Fosfomycin (Monurol) (Med Let 1997;39:66; Rx Let 1997;4:21) 3 gm po in water × 1; no better than Tm/S or cipro for UTI
- Metronidazole (Flagyl) (Nejm 1980;303:1213); 500 mg po as good as iv (Nejm 1981;305:1569) or topically as gel 5 gm bid × 5d; vs *Trichomonas, Giardia,* amoebic abscess, most anaerobes especially

ID: BACTERIOLOGY

B. fragilis (Med Let 1981;23:13). Adverse effects: Antabuse effect, decreased warfarin metabolism
- Minocycline (Ann IM 1993;119:16) 100 mg po qd; adverse effects: similar to tetracycline, gi intolerance, rare allergic pneumonitis (Ann IM 1992;117:476), vestibular sx
- Mupirocin (Bactroban) topically tid for impetigo; as good as po antibiotics; $10/15 gm tube (Med Let 1988;30:55)
- Quinupristin/dalfopristin (Synercid) (Med Let 2000;42:45; 1999;41:109), iv, active vs MRSA and vanco-resistant enterococci; lots of drug interactions; cost $3000/10 d
- Rifabutin (Med Let 1993;35:36) 300 mg po qd; used to prophylact AIDS pts vs *M. avium*
- Rifampin (Ann IM 1976;85:82) 600 mg qd/bid; vs tbc, meningococcal carrier. Adverse effects: elevated liver function tests, depressed white count, hearing loss, tbc resistance, increased warfarin metabolism
- Spectinomycin; vs gc in penicillin-allergic patients
- Tetracycline 250–500 mg po qid. Adverse effects: photosensitivity, discolors children's teeth, fatty liver in pregnancy (Ann IM 1987;106:703), adsorbed by milk, antacids, and po iron; gi intolerance; cheap
- Vancomycin (Med Let 1986;28:121) 1 gm iv q 12 h or 125–500 mg po qid; vs clostridium enterocolitis, *Streptococcus viridans* SBE if penicillin-allergic, methicillin resistant staph, ok alone vs *Enterococcus;* $800/10 d iv, $20/d po

9.2 GRAM-POSITIVE ORGANISMS

ANTHRAX
Nejm 2001;345:1607,1621; Nejm 1999;341:815

Cause: *Bacillus anthracis*
Epidem: Soil organism w long-lived endospores. Biologic weapon
Pathophys: Infected by skin contact, inhalation of spores, or contact w infected animals or their meat. Endospores germinate and multiply in macrophages, leading to septicemia w exotoxin production including "edema toxin"
Sx: No sore throat and no rhinorhea. Painless skin papule at contact site, then black eschar and edema

(r/o brown recluse spider bite, erythema gangrenosum in neutropenic pts w Pseudomonas aeruginosa bacteremia, furuncle, ecthyma)

Si: GI ulcerations and edema; fulminant pneumonits and mediastinitis (Jama 2001;286:2549,2554) after 5–10 d incubation

Crs: Skin, 80–90% benign resolution w antibiotics; GI disease resolves in 10–14 d; pulmonary, fatal

Cmplc: Meningitis; skin scarring; GI perforation

Lab:

Bacti: Gram pos rods in long chains ("bamboo"); grows like *Bacillus cereus;* lab may call it a contaminant unless warned

Skin tests: 82% pos 1–3 d after sx; 99% by 4 wk

Rx: (Med Let 2001;43:87,91) Vaccine 0.5 cc sc at 0, 2 and 4 wk; then 6, 12, and 18 mo; then q 1 yr

Prophylaxis after exposure w doxycycline 100 mg po bid, amoxicillin or Pen V 500 mg po tid, or ciprofloxacin 500 mg po bid × 4 wk if vaccinated at the same time, or 60 d otherwise

of disease: penicillin and doxycycline; if pen allergic, chloramphenicol, erythromycin, + cipro

DIPHTHERIA (Membranous Croup)

Ann IM 1989;111:71; Nejm 1988;318:12, 41

Cause: *Corynebacterium diphtheria,* gravis and midas strains lysogenic for a specific phage (other species are opportunistics in debilitated pts) (Ann IM 1969;70:919)

Epidem: Epidemically present in US still, and resurging in Russia; immunization of >50% of population begins to decrease incidence; peak incidence at age 15–39 yr; female:male = 2:1. Big Seattle epidemic (>1100 cases) in alcoholics (Ann IM 1989;111:71). Human carriers are reservoirs; acutely ill patients are communicable only ~2 wk. Skin lesions can also be both portal of entry and source of carrier state (Nejm 1969;280:135)

Pathophys: Exotoxin produced by phage hits conducting cells, eg, heart and nerves. Resulting anatomic changes in heart increase incidence of arrhythmias and failure years later. Gravis strain causes more lymphadenopathy, especially in pharynx, and hits heart more often

Sx: Weakness, slight sore throat (90%), low-grade fever (85%), dysphagia and nausea (25%), headache (18%)

Diphtheria, continued

Si:

- Fever
- Membrane: exudate flows over tonsils where thickens in 2–3 d to classic fibrin pharyngeal waxy material, blue-white bleeds when peeled, but has minimal inflammation
- Edema of neck (18%)
- Conjunctivitis. Infected skin lesions

Crs: 2–5 d incubation period

Cmplc:

- Airway obstruction, especially w midas strain
- Cardiac arrhythmias and myocarditis especially w gravis strain; EKG abnormal in 65%; 10% fatality rate from cardiac arrest
- Neuropathies: peripheral (15%); rarely palatal motor impairment in first days of illness; cranial nerves III, VI, VII, IX, and × motor in 2–3 wk; Guillain-Barré rarely months later

r/o mononucleosis, which can mimic membrane (L. Weinstein 3/85)

Lab:

Bact: Smear shows club-shaped, nonmotile gram-pos bacilli, close to actinomycetes; culture on Loeffler's slant can detect within 12 h if holding rx; if already treated w penicillin, may grow in 1 wk on tellurite slant, sharply selective

Rx: Prevent w active immunization of infants w toxoid in DPT 4-shot series, booster at school age, or over age 7 with 3-shot dT series; 80% of US population now immunized; no deaths in patients w at least 1 immunization; q 10 yr thereafter w tetanus as dT (rv CDC—Ann IM 1985;103:896); some now argue boost in adults unnecessary (Lancet 1985;1:1089)

for carrier state: penicillin as Bicillin × 1, or erythromycin (resistance developed in Seattle) 250 mg qid × 7 d (89% effective), or clindamycin 150 mg qid × 7 d

for active disease: penicillin or erythromycin (resistance developed in Seattle), of questionable help (L. Weinstein 3/85); antitoxin ineffective

if given >48 h after onset (Weinstein) and probably not worth complication risk anyway but can be done w 50,000 U antitoxin for acute gravis in first 24 h and repeated in 24 h × 1

LISTERIAL INFECTIONS

Nejm 1996;334:770

Cause: *Listeria* spp

Epidem: Present in most soils, animal gi tracts, and raw milk from infected cows, though it can occur even if pasteurized (Nejm 1997;336:100; 1985;312:404), or cheese (Mexican cheese epidemic in Calif—Nejm 1988;319:823)

Increased in pregnant women, elderly, neonates (Nejm 1971;285:599), and immunocompromised (Ann IM 1992;117:466)

Pathophys: Intracellular pathogenesis, usually picked up by gut macrophages and spread from there

Sx: Of sepsis, meningitis (p 416)

Si: Sepsis, meningitis esp in children age < 6 mo (p 416)

Crs:

Cmplc: Meningitis, sepsis, spontaneous abortion

Lab:

CSF: Gram-positive rods, tumbling motility; often <80% polys

Rx: Ampicillin first choice; Tm/S a second choice or used w ampicillin

ENTEROCOCCAL INFECTIONS

Cause: *Enterococcus faecalis* and *E. faecium,* a group D strep

Epidem: Fecal organism; increasing resistance

Pathophys: In mixed infections, often "selected out" by cephalosporins

Sx: Abscesses, cellulitis, septic arthritis, UTIs

Si:

Cmplc: SBE

Lab:

Bact: Gram-positive cocci

Rx: Aminoglycoside plus a penicillin essential for synergy; many β-lactamase-producing, gentamicin-resistant strains are appearing now, treatable w vancomycin or ampicillin/sulbactam (Unasyn) (Ann IM 1992;116:285), though resistance a major continuing problem (Inf Contr Hosp Epidem 1992;13:695; Am J Med 1989; 110:515), even vancomycin resistance (Nejm 2000;342:710) where can use quinupristin/dalfopristin (Synercid) or linezolid (Zyvox)

STAPH FOOD POISONING

Nejm 1984;310:1368,1437

Cause: *Staphylococcus aureus*

Epidem: Most common type of food poisoning

Pathophys: Heat-stable enterotoxin produced by staph in food after preparation, eg, potato salad. Lack of fever indicates a toxin disease

Sx: 8-h incubation period. Nausea, vomiting, and some diarrhea without fever. Excess nausea and vomiting relative to diarrhea suggests staph rather than others

Si:

Crs:

Cmplc: r/o clostridial and *B. cereus* food poisonings, both of which also lack fever

Lab: None unless need to work up for public health reasons, then Gram stain and culture the food

Rx: Symptomatic

STAPH TISSUE INFECTIONS

Nejm 1998;338:520

Cause: *S. aureus*

Epidem: Normal inhabitant of skin and upper respiratory track; 90% resistant to penicillin

Pathophys: Multiple exotoxins increase its pathogenicity including β-lactamase, coagulase, hyaluronidase, other proteases, leukocidin, lipases, staphylokinase. Hair follicles infected because fibrin restrains spread but retards healing

Sx: Pain, swelling, may have fever

Si: Abscesses, carbuncle, furuncle, pneumonia, and empyema; acute endocarditis involving healthy valves; osteomyelitis, usually metaphyseal; septicemia

Crs: Bacteremia mortality = 11–43%

Cmplc: DIC, endocarditis including R-sided especially in drug users, metastatic infections

Lab:

> *Bact:* Gram-positive cocci clusters, coagulase-positive; methicillin resistance present in over 50% in some ICUs (Nejm 1998;339:520)

Rx: Surgical drainage

β-Lactamase-resistant drug like nafcillin/oxacillin iv, later go to po cloxacillin or diclox. Cephalosporin, clindamycin, Tm/S, erythromycin.

of methicillin-resistant staph (Nejm 1989;320:1188): 1st, vancomycin w or w/o rifampin, although time to bacteremic clearing in SBE may be up to 2 wk (Ann IM 1991;115:674), and rare resistance now appearing (Nejm 1999;340:493,517); or 2nd, Tm/S (Ann IM 1992;117:390), minocycline, fluoroquinolones, clindamycin

of vancomycin resistant staph, linezolid (Zyvox) or Synercid

of recurrent abscesses: prevent w rifampin 600 mg bid × 5 d (Nejm 1986;315:91) + vancomycin or Tm/S (Ann IM 1982;97:317); topical antibiotics, especially mupirocin to the anterior nares to eliminate carrier states especially of methicillin-resistant staph (Ann IM 1991;14:101,107)

of infected orthopedic appliances: pencillinase resistant penicillin + rifampin × 2 wks then quinolone + rifampin f/u rx × 3–6 mo (Jama 1998;279:1537)

TOXIC SHOCK SYNDROME

Nejm 1998;339:527; Ann IM 1982;96(2)—whole issue is rv; 1982;97:608

Cause: *S. aureus;* occasionally strep-induced (Nejm 1987;317:146) by group A *Streptococcus pyogenes,* which produces scarlet fever toxin A (Nejm 1991;325:783; 1989;321:1)

Epidem: Initially 97% cases were associated w tampon use during menses, now none is w change in tampon manufacture, but some cases still assoc w menstruation. Associated w influenza (Jama 1987;257:1053)

Pathophys: Enterotoxins produced at any body site

Sx: Diarrhea (98%), vomiting (92%), headache and sore throat (77%), myalgias

Si: Fever (87%), hypotension, scarletiniform rash that later desquamates

Crs: 10–15% mortality

Cmplc: Hepatitis and renal failure. Recurrent (25%). Chronic headache and memory changes (Ann IM 1982;96:865)

r/o Kawasaki's disease (p 657)

Lab:
   Bact: S. aureus in cultures of infected site, blood cultures usually
     negative
Rx: Fluids, staph antibiotics like clindamycin that shut down toxin
    production; perhaps steroids, perhaps gamma globulin

STAPH EPIDERMIDIS INFECTIONS
   Ann IM 1989;110:9

Cause: *Staphylococcus epidermidis* (coagulase-negative staph)
Epidem: Normal skin inhabitant. Most common cause of
    hospital-acquired bacteremia; often catheter-, prosthesis-, or
    vascular graft-associated
Pathophys: Enmeshes in glycocalyx coating of catheters and prosthetics
Sx:
Si: Infections of implanted prosthetics
Crs:
Cmplc: 30% mortality w bacteremia
Lab:
   Bact: Culture, coagulase-negative staph. r/o *Staphylococcus
    saprophyticus,* also a pathogen, at least in urinary tract
Rx: (Ann IM 1983;98:447)
   >60% are methicillin-resistant; 1st vancomycin (Ann IM 1982;
    97:503), but resistance appearing (Nejm 1987;316:927); rifampin;
    gentamicin

GROUP B STREP INFECTIONS
   Nejm 2000;343:175,209; 1990;322:1857

Cause: *Streptococcus agalactiae,* a group B strep
Epidem: 0.6/1000 births; 2000/yr in US; 15–40% of pregnant women are
    colonized. Increasing incidence of serious (21% mortality) infections
    in nonpregnant adults as well as pregnant women, a minority of

group B strep infections in the US now are in infants. Affects elderly and/or sick adults (Nejm 1993;328:1807,1843), especially diabetics

Pathophys: Vaginal colonization leads to newborn and maternal infections

Sx: Floppy baby

Si: Newborn sepsis, and maternal chorioamnionitis, endometritis, and post-C/S wound infections

Crs:

Cmplc: r/o *E. coli, Listeria, S. epidermidis*

Lab:

  Bact: Gram-positive cocci in chains; usually β-hemolytic; PCR assay 45 min test now possible at presentation in labor (Nejm 2000;343: 175,209)

Rx: Prevent perhaps someday by immunization w group B polysaccharide vaccine (Nejm 1988;319:1180), but pneumovax to mothers doesn't help (Nejm 1980;303:173)

  Ampicillin iv (Nejm 2000;342:15; 1986;314:1665) intrapartum and to baby, in women w 35–37 wk prenatal positive vaginal/rectal cultures, AND fever, and/or premature labor (<37 wk), and/or prolonged (>12 h) ruptured membranes

PNEUMOCOCCAL INFECTIONS

Cause: *Streptococcus pneumoniae* especially types 3 and 6 (most virulent)

Epidem: Population carriers disseminate to pts w diminished resistance; 50% of population carries in upper respiratory tract at some time

  Increased incidence in blood group A types because pneumococcus has A-like antigens; and in pts after splenectomy because residual RES requires increased antibody coating before phagocytosis can occur (Nejm 1981;304:245)

Pathophys: (Nejm 1995;332:1280) Invasive w pyogenic response; little toxin production; pathogenic via numbers alone; polysaccharide capsule in virulent strains makes phagocytosis hard

Sx:

  Meningitis: Fever, confusion

  Otitis media: Ear pain

  Pneumonia: Fever, chills, sudden onset of pleurisy

Pneumococcal Infections, continued

Si:
  Meningitis: Fever, confusion
  Otitis media: Hot ear
  Pneumonia: Bloody sputum unlike viral or mycoplasma
Crs:
  Pneumonia: Xray clears in 6 wk (Nejm 1970;283:798)
  Meningitis: 50% mortality
Cmplc: Triad w endocarditis, meningitis, and pneumonia often fatal (Am J Med 1963;33:262); empyema
  r/o multiple myeloma if crit low
Lab:
  Bact: Gram-pos diplococci; culture shows optochin-sensitive/bile salt soluble colonies
Rx:
  Prevent w:
  • Adult pneumococcal vaccine (Med Let 1999;41:84), 65% overall effective (Nejm 1991;325:1453; Ann IM 1988;108:653; 1986;104:1–118) at least for elderly (>65) and people at increased risk, eg, splenectomy, COPD, alcoholics, diabetes, chronic renal pts on dialysis, CHF (Ann IM 1984;101:325,348); worth it in all? (Ann IM 1986;104:106 vs Jama 1996;275:194); ineffective in many sick pts who need it the most, eg, VA COPD pts (Nejm 1986; 315:1318). Revaccinate if vaccination in doubt or once 5 yr later at least for high risk pts and those who got 1st dose under age 65 (Mmwr 1997;46:1); local reactions in ~10% of those revaccinated (Jama 1999;281:243)
  • Pediatric conjugated vaccine (Jama 2000;283:1460) @ 2, 4, 6, and 12 mos, or single dose thereafter; decreases pneumococcal otitis media by 20+% (NNT-2 = 5) (Nejm 2001;344:403)
  of disease: since penicillin resistance is now so widespread though regionally variable, 25% nationally (Nejm 2000;343:1917), until know sensitivities, rx w ceftriaxone + vancomycin for life-threatening infections like meningitis; or vancomycin iv w po levofloxacin (Rx Let 2000;7:17) 500 mg po qd × 7–14 d, or 3rd generation fluoroquinolone. Then, if sensitive, switch to penicillin or another β-lactam antibiotic
  Chest PT for pneumonia doesn't speed healing (Nejm 1978;299:624)

SCARLET FEVER

Nejm 1970;282:23; 1970;297:365

Cause: *Streptococcus pyogenes* (rarely *S. aureus,* which causes no sore throat)

Epidem: Respiratory droplets and wound infections. Occurs in children only, since adults usually already immune

Pathophys: Erythrogenic toxin produced by bacteria lysogenized by a specific phage that causes bacterial capsular dilatation, rupture, and toxin release

Sx: Sore throat, fever, rash

Si: Rash, trunkal, especially in creases (Pastia's lines), palpable, viral-like. Spots on soft palate. "Strawberry" tongue. Circumoral pallor

Crs:

Cmplc:

- Acute glomerular nephritis
- Rheumatic fever, in old days 3% in epidemic and 1/2% in endemic type if no rx; now <1/10,000 w/o rx, and <1/100,000 w rx in adults
- Peritonsillar abscess (Quincy abscess), and tonsillar vein phlebitis leading to pulmonary emboli, rx w tonsillectomy (L. Weinstein 3/85)
- Toxic shock syndrome (p 395), which may just be the extreme variant (Nejm 1991;325:783)

r/o other childhood exanthems: roseola, rubeola, rubella, erythema infectiosum (5th disease)

Lab: Sore throat workup protocol (Ann IM 1980;93:244)

Bact: Throat culture, single swab positive in 75%, 2 swabs in 85% β-hemolysis on culture plates. Positive culture may still be just a carrier. Rapid office tests take 10 min–1 hr, cost $2–3 plus lots of time (Med Let 1985;27:49) but may still have to culture if negative (J Peds 1987;111:80)

Hem: Eosinophils increased often

Rx: Penicillin, erythromycin. If sick, treatment speeds healing (Jama 1975;227:1278); but overall often does not (Am J Med 1951;10:300)

STREPTOCOCCAL PHARYNGITIS
Nejm 2001;344:205; 1991;325:783; Ann IM 1989;110:612

Cause: *Streptococcus pyogenes,* group A, β-hemolytic, rarely group C or D

Epidem: Respiratory droplets; occasionally foodborne (Nejm 1969;280: 917); 15% of the population carry in pharynx

Pathophys:

Sx: Sore throat, fever[1] >100°F (>37.8°C), no cough[2]

Si: (Jama 2000 284:2912) Pharyngeal and/or tonsillar exudate[3] (50% sens, 80% specif), anterior cervical tender and/or enlarged nodes[4] (50% sens, 70% specif), T>101° (>38.3°C) often (50% sens and specif).

Notes [1,2,3,4] = crucial si and sx (Ann IM 2001;134:506,509)

Crs: 10 d without rx

Cmplc:

- Acute glomerular nephritis
- Rheumatic fever, in old days 3% in epidemic and 1/2% in endemic type if no rx; now <1/10,000 w/o rx and <1/100,000 w rx in adults
- Peritonsillar abscess (Quincy abscess) and tonsillar vein phlebitis leading to pulmonary emboli, rx w tonsillectomy (L. Weinstein 3/85); occurs w/o strep as well

r/o (A. Komaroff, 1985) chlamydia (21%) especially TWAR, viral (17%) (rhinovirus, coronavirus, adenovirus, parainfluenza virus, respiratory syncytial virus, echo, coxsackie, acute primary HIV infection), mycoplasma (11%), mononucleosis (EBV) (10%), nongroup A strep (9%), legionella (3%), gonorrhea (1–2%), diphtheria; or *Arcanobacterium haemolyticum* (a diphtheroid) pharyingitis and scalatiniform rash, esp common in adults, rx w erythromycin

Lab: Sore throat workup protocol (Ann IM 2001;134:506,509)

Bact: Rapid office throat swab strep tests take 10 min, cost $2–3; are 90+% specific but in practice only 60–70% sensitive (30–50% sens, 95% spec—Jama 1992;267:695) so may need to culture negatives if it is clinically important (Med Let 1991;33:40; J Peds 1987;111:80). New optical immunoassay test 80% sens, 95% specif compared to culture, which is 70+% sens and 99% specif (Jama 1997;277:899). Rarely need full throat culture, single swab positive in 75%, 2 swabs in 85%. β-hemolysis on culture plates. Positive culture may still be just a carrier.

Rx: Penicillin V or erythromycin 250 mg po t-qid, × 10 d at least for rheumatic fever prophylaxis, even bid may be enough (Peds 2000;105:E19; Rx Let 2000;7:25), although 20–40% resistance to erythromycin now being reported in Finland (Nejm 1992;326:292); or azithromycin. Rx immediately (Ann IM 2001;134:506, 509) if h/o fever, adenopathy, no cough, and exudate; or, if 2–3/4 of these criteria met, get rapid strep and rx only if pos

Tonsillectomy and adenoidectomy does decrease recurrence of strep throats in children w 3 or more documented strep throats/yr over several yr (Nejm 1984;310:674, 717)

of hyperendemic outbreak, eg, Marine boot camp (Nejm 1991;325: 92), benzathine penicillin 1 million U q 1 mo or po erythromycin to all group members

STREPTOCOCCAL ERYSIPELAS, CELLULITIS/ WOUND INFECTIONS, NECROTIZING FASCIITIS, AND IMPETIGO

Nejm 1996;334:240

Cause: *S. pyogenes,* group A, β-hemolytic

Epidem: Erysipelas and cellulitis, common; necrotizing fasciitis (NF), rare, 1/yr in big hospital. Invasive strep infections in 1.5/100,000/yr in general population, 3/1000 of household contacts (Nejm 1996;335: 547); but invasive cases are just the tip of the iceberg since same strain will be found causing much more pharyngitis in the community (Jama 1997;277:38)

Pathophys: Erysipelas is mainly in lymphatics

Cellulitis, in subcutaneous tissues

NF, infections dissect along fascial planes, so skin is last to go, and look deceptively benign; 1/3 of the time NF is associated w anaerobic bacteria as well

Impetigo is a superficial skin infection, starts in a break in the skin

Sx: Pain, fever, and rapid spreading in erysipelas, cellulitis, and NF; in impetigo, sx are of a weeping rash usually in a child

Si: Erysipelas has sharp limits, symmetric swelling, usually across bridge of nose

Cellulitis has little edema and indistinct limits

NF has edema, fever, redness, gas crepitation (in 50%), anesthesia (nerve infarction), ecchymosis (thrombosis)

In impetigo, rash has bullae w honey yellow exudate

Crs: In NF, 75% die without surgical debridement within 1–2 d

Cmplc: Toxic shock syndrome (p 395) and acute glomerular nephritis can occur w all

Erysipelas: r/o **erysipeloid** (hands, exposure to raw meat and animals, slower spread; gram-positive rod, culture skin biopsy; rx w penicillin etc.)

Cellulitis: erythema nodosum and endocarditis, r/o acute axillary lymphadenitis (Nejm 1990;323:655)

NF: r/o gas gangrene

Lab:

Bact: In all, culture, and gram-positive cocci in chains on Gram stain

Path: For NF, frozen section biopsy

Serol: ASO titers elevated

Rx: Prevention w bacitracin dressing no better than vaseline (Jama 1996; 276:972)

for all, antibiotics like penicillin, erythromycin although 20–40% resistance now in Finland (Nejm 1992;326:292)

of impetigo, mupirocin (Bactroban) ointment (not cream) (Rx Let 1998;5:11) topically tid as good as po antibiotics; $10/15-gm tube (Med Let 1988;30:55); debated if need to cover for resistant staph, especially nonbullous type (Lancet 1991;338:803)

of NF, extensive surgical debridement first; clindamycin helps decr toxin production

---

9.3 GRAM-NEGATIVE ORGANISMS

WHOOPING COUGH

Nejm 1994;331:16

Cause: *Bordetella pertussis* (similar to *Haemophilus*); occasionally sporadically by adenovirus (Nejm 1970;283:390). From respiratory tract of infected persons especially during catarrhal stage; 90% attack rate

Epidem: Worldwide, worst in developing countries. Highest incidence in children <5 yr. Female morbidity > male. In US, increasing to >2500 cases/yr w many infections in adults

Pathophys: Rapid bacterial multiplication causes decreased tracheal and bronchial ciliary action, which in turn causes infection by strep, staph, etc. Endotoxin produced and released when bacteria die causing cell irritation and occasional death; perhaps neurotoxic effects on CNS

Coughing causes anoxia, which somehow causes hemorrhages

Sx: Catarrhal stage (mild cough) × 2 wk; then paroxysmal coughing. In adults (Ann IM 1998;128:64), nonproductive intermittent chronic cough (>2 wk), 12–21% of those w that sx?! (Jama 1996;275: 1672, 1995;273:1044)

Si: Spasmodic coughing, long drawn out w rapid sharp inhalations (whoops); small petechial hemorrhages throughout body

Crs: Paroxysmal stage lasts 2 weeks

Cmplc: Seizures; secondary pulmonary infection and atelectasis; meningitis; in infants, apnea and death 75% are <1 yr, 40% <3 mo (Ann IM 1972;76:289)

r/o croup (p 656)

Lab:

Bact: Culture sputum or nasal/pharyngeal swab during catarrhal stage; smear shows small gram-neg rods, nonmotile, no spores, encapsulated

Hem: Wbc's increased w high % (usually >50%) lymphocytes, looks like CLL in a child

Serol: Acutely direct fluorescent antibody (DFA) to the antigen; antibody titer increased after 3 wk

Rx: Preventive (CDC rv—Ann IM 1985;103:896):

- Immunize w antigens 1, 2, and 3 in children between age 6 wk and <6 yr; use acellular pertussis as DTaP for immunizations beginning at 2 mo, 70–90% effective compared to placebo while whole cell vaccine is only 40–60% effective and has encephalitic/neurologic cmplc's (Nejm 1996;334:341,349,391, 1995;333:1045; Jama 1996;275:37). No cross-placental transfer
- Hyperimmune globulin
- Antibiotics prophylactically or to sick pts to decrease infectivity, do shorten course: erythromycin 40 mg/kg in children, 1 gm/d in adults; or Tm/S × 10 d, 8 mg/40 mg/kg in children, 320/1600 in adults

CAMPYLOBACTER DIARRHEA
Ann IM 1983;98:360; 1983;99:38; Nejm 1981;305:1444

Cause: *Campylobacter jejuni*

Epidem: Contaminated water, surface water, and municipal water supplies (Ann IM 1982;96:293); similar epidemiology to *Giardia*. Also may be sporadic, foodborne, often by eggs. Cattle, goats, horses, and perhaps wild animals excrete in feces. 3× more frequent than *Giardia;* more common than *Salmonella* and *Shigella* (Harvard Medical School CME lecture 3/85)

Pathophys:

Sx: 1–7 d incubation period
   Diarrhea (100%), cramps (95%), fever (80%), bloody diarrhea (29%)

Si:

Crs: 20% last over 1 wk

Cmplc: Chronic colitis; Guillain-Barré syndrome (Nejm 1995;333:1374; Ann IM 1993;118:847)
   r/o ulcerative colitis relapses

Lab:
   Bact: Culture in 10% CO_2 × 48 h, special media

Rx: Erythromycin if sx >3 d; ciprofloxacin (Arch IM 1990;150:541), or other quinolones though drug resistance appearing because of their use in poultry industry (Nejm 1999;340:1525)

TRAVELER'S DIARRHEA
Nejm 2000;342:1716; 1993;328:1821

Cause: (Jama 1999;281:811) *E. coli* enterotoxigenic type (50⁺%), rarely invasive type (see next p); *Salmonella* spp., *Campylobacter,* rotavirus, et al.

Epidem: In salads, sewer-contaminated water (Crater Lake epidemics—Ann IM 1977;86:714). 30% of all travelers to Mexico get one type or the other, usually within 2 wk of arrival (Nejm 1976;294:1299). Most of acute childhood diarrhea in Brazil (Nejm 1975;293:567)

Pathophys: A toxin is produced while the organisms are attached to gut wall much like *C. perfringens;* heat-labile toxin type is delayed in onset like cholera; heat-stable types cause immediate onset (Nejm

1975;292:933). In the unusual invasive types, colonic wall invasion causes bloody mucus, like *Shigella*

Sx: Toxin-producing types: clear, watery diarrhea may become bloody later; fever (50%)

Invasive types: bloody mucus, fever in most, pain

Si: Toxin-producing types: sometimes low-grade fever; in invasive types, fever

Crs:

Cmplc: r/o other gi infections

Lab:

Bact: Stool smear shows polys in invasive types, none in noninvasive types; if polys present, culture for pathogens on sorbitol-MacConkey agar, O157 antiserum test of cultured *E. coli* (Nejm 1995;333:364)

Rx: (Med Let 1994;36:41)

Prevent in travelers w:

Avoidance of high-risk foods, eg, ice, salads, milk, street foods; of questionable benefit (Jama 1999;281:811)

Antibiotic prophylaxis if willing to risk rx cmplc

- Ciprofloxacin, 1st choice. 500 mg po × 1 dose (Lancet 1994;334:1537) or qd; or ofloxacin (Floxin) 300 mg po qd; or norfloxacin 400 mg po qd
- Doxycycline 100 mg qd × 5 wk (90% effective—Nejm 1978;298:758) but resistance common by 1993; gi excretion means can use in renal or hepatic disease
- Pepto Bismol 60 cc or ii tabs qid (75% effective), has 2 ASA equivalents/60 cc (Med Let 1980;22:63); salicylate probably inhibits prostaglandins, hence effect, or antibiotic effect of bismuth
- Tm/S SS po qd in children, risks allergic reaction

of diarrheal sx when traveling, may be the better approach, with:

- Ciprofloxacin, 1st choice, 500 mg po bid × 3 d (Ann IM 1991;114:731), also gets *Campylobacter, Salmonella,* and *Shigella* as well as the pathogenic *E. coli;* or norfloxacin 400 mg po bid × 3 d; or ofloxacin (Floxin) 300 mg po bid × 3 d; or
- Loperamide HCl (Imodium) 4 mg po then 2 mg after each stool up to 16 mg po qd used w any antibiotic below doesn't hurt, may help (Ann IM 1993;118:377; 1991;114:731); diphenoxylate + atropine (Lomotil) may worsen some types, eg, *Shigella* (Jama 1973;226:1575) and

ID: BACTERIOLOGY

- Azithromycin 500 mg x1, then 250 mg po qd × 4d
- Tm/S (Septra) DS bid × 3–5 d (Ann IM 1987;106:216; Nejm 1982;307:84); resistance more common than w cipro

E. COLI INVASIVE DIARRHEA

Cause: Toxin-producing types like O157:H7 (Nejm 1995;333:364; Ann IM 1988;109:705)

Epidem: O157:H7 type (Ann IM 1995;123:698) in hamburger (Jama 1984;272:1349), sprouts (Ann IM 2001;135:239), drinking water, and swimming lakes (Nejm 1994;331:579). Most common cause of infectious bloody diarrhea in US

Pathophys: Colonic wall invasion and toxin production causes bloody mucus, like *Shigella*

Sx: Incubation period 1–3 d. Bloody mucus, fever in most, pain

Si: Low-grade fever, fecal leukocytes present, initial watery stool becomes bloody

Crs:

Cmplc: Hemolytic/uremic syndrome (in 10%—Jama 1994;272:1349; Nejm 1987;317:1496) or TTP

r/o other gi infections

Lab:

Bact: Stool smear shows polys; if polys, culture for pathogens on sorbitol-MacConkey agar and do O157 antiserum test of cultured *E. coli* (Nejm 1995;333:364); stool toxin titers

Rx: Rehydration and supportive care; at least in children, antibiotic rx increases risk of hemoytic uremic syndrome (Nejm 2000;342:1930), can use ciprofloxacin or Tm/S DS bid × 3 d (Ann IM 1987;106:216)

CHANCROID

Ann IM 1985;102:705; 1983;98:973

Cause: *Haemophilus ducreyi* (Ann IM 1981;95:315)

Epidem: Venereally spread, ie, an STD, associated w syphilis in 15%

Pathophys:

Sx: Painful ulcer after 2–15 d incubation

Si: Adenopathy; tender, "dirty," necrotic ulcer(s); tender bubos (40%)

Crs: Self-limited

Cmplc:

Lab:

Bact: Culture positive in 80%

Rx: (Med Let 1999;41:89)

1st choice for patient and contacts: ceftriaxone 250 mg im once; or azithromycin 1 gm po once

2nd choice, ciprofloxacin 500 mg po bid × 3 d; or erythromycin 500 mg qid × 7 d

in AIDS, azithromycin, cipro, or erythro as above

NONSPECIFIC VAGINITIS (Vaginal Bacteriosis, Bacterial Vaginosis)

Nejm 1997;337:1896, Ann IM 1989;111:551

Cause: (Med Let 1999;41:86) *Gardnerella vaginalis, Mobiluncus,* mycoplasmas, *Ureaplasma,* and other anaerobes that themselves may be primary cause. These are all endogenous flora, not necessarily venereal since occur in 15% of virginal women

Epidem: 3rd most common cause of vaginitis after *Trichomonas* and monilia

Pathophys: Diminished presence of lactobacilli, corresponding increase in pH leading to *G. vaginalis, Mycoplasma hominis* (Nejm 1995;333: 1732,1737), and anaerobe (esp. *Bacteroides*) overgrowth

Sx: Vaginitis w watery discharge, no dyspareunia

Si: Watery discharge evenly coats walls; vinegar-like smell

Crs:

Cmplc: Increased incidence of premature labor (<37 wk) and low birth weight

r/o trichomonal (p 476), monilial (p 143) and other (p 631) vaginitis causes

Lab:

Bact: Vaginal discharge smear shows clue cells (100%—Lancet 1983; 2:1379); pH >4.5–5.0; positive amine ("whiff") test, ie, discharge smells of ammonia (70–80%); few polys. Culture positive in 40% (Obgyn 1984;64:271)

Rx: (Med Let 1994;41:86)

Preventive: Unclear if screening and treating ASX pregnant women decreases prematurity and LBW babies (Am J Prev med 2001; 20(3S):62)

of disease:

Metronidazole (Flagyl) 2 gm qd × 1 →75% cure; or 500 mg bid × 7 d →95% cure (Lancet 1983;2:1379), costs $5; 30% recur in 1 mo, at least if partner not rx'd, although partner rx not clearly helpful (Ann IM 1989;111:551). Or as metronidazole vaginal gel 5 gm bid × 5 d, probably ok in pregnancy, costs $20; or

Clindamycin 300 mg po bid × 7 d; or as 2% vag cream 5 gm q hs × 3–7 d; avoid in pregnancy; costs $27

Sulfa and ampicillin are ineffective (Holmes—Nejm 1980;303:601; 1978;298:1429)

in pregnancy, rx at least women at high risk for preterm labor since rx decreases incidence from 50% to 30% (Nejm 1995;333:1732 vs 2000;342:534,581)

HAEMOPHILUS RESPIRATORY INFECTIONS
Nejm 1990;323:1415; Ann IM 1973;78:259

Cause: *Haemophilus influenzae,* unencapsulated or encapsulated (type B) (Mmwr 1985;34:201)

Epidem: Airborne from respiratory tract of infected person. Worldwide distribution. Infections w unencapsulated types occur in all age groups and are common in people w COPD. Infections with more invasive and malignant encapsulated type now becoming rare with advent of vaccine in children; most now in adults (Ann IM 1992; 116:806). Before Hib vaccine, incidence was 100/100,000 and meningitis in 60/100,000 under age 5.

Pathophys:

Sx:

Si: Otitis media, bronchitis, sinusitis. Encapsulated type can also cause acute epiglottitis (p 173), sore throat w dysphagia, meningitis, pneumonia, but only rarely otitis media (10% of all H. flu otitis media)

Crs: Meningitis has a 5% mortality and a 30% incidence of neurologic sequelae

Cmplc: Encapsulated type causes:
- Sudden death w epiglottitis, especially if sedated or kept supine, or throat stick gags throat, due to cardiac arrest (L. Weinstein 3/85) and airway obstruction
- Retropharyngeal abscess resulting in "quacking" voice, breathe better supine (Weinstein 3/85)

Lab:

Bact: Gram-negative coccobacilli; capsule may be visible in encapsulated type

Xray: Lateral neck soft tissue view to look for epiglottis involvement

Rx: Passive prophylaxis for encapsulated type disease possible w rifampin (Nejm 1987;316:1226) or hyperimmune globulin (Nejm 1987; 317:923)

Active immunization: Hib vaccine conjugated w diphtheria protein to give better immune response in infants (Nejm 1987;317:717); give MSD Pedvax Hib at 2 and 4 mo w DPT and boost at 12 mo (Med Let 1991;33:5), perhaps a 6 mo shot if using one of the other vaccines; all appear interchangeable (Jama 1995;273:849). Vaccinating mother in 3rd trimester may help where risk is high (Jama 1996;275:1182)

of active disease: ampicillin, but 8–20% of all US isolates now resistant; in life-threatening illness, ceftriaxone or rarely used chloramphenicol. Tm/S if mild infection and may be or is resistant to ampicillin

of cmplc's: steroids and tracheotomy for acute airway obstruction; steroids for meningitis, like dexamethasone 0.15 mg/kg iv 20 min before antibiotic, then q 6 h × 4; decreases cmplc's especially deafness (Nejm 1990;319:968)

KLEBSIELLA PNEUMONIA ETC

Cause: *Klebsiella pneumoniae* (enterobacteriaceae)

Epidem: Fecal contamination usually; a normal inhabitant of large bowel and often in upper respiratory tract too

1% of all pneumonias; increased incidence in males >40 yr

Klebsiella *Pneumonia Etc, continued*

Pathophys:
Sx: Brown-red, thick ("currant jelly") sputum; fever, chills; pleurisy
Si: Fever; consolidation si's, often much less impressive than xray
Crs: Rapidly progressive; 25–50% mortality
Cmplc: Empyema; multiple drug resistance acquisition in hospital (Ann IM 1971;74:657)
Lab:
  Bact: Gram stain shows gram-neg rods w capsule
  Hem: Wbc may be low
Xray: Chest consolidations may be convex, "swollen lobar consolidation"
Rx: Gentamicin + cephalosporin, fluoroquinolone, or 3rd generation cephalosporin until know sensitivities

LEGIONNAIRES' DISEASE (Legionellosis)
  Nejm 1997;337:682; J Inf Dis 1992;165:736; Ann IM 1981;94:164, 1979;90:489–699

Cause: *Legionella pneumophilia* etc. (Ann IM 1980;93:366)
Epidem: Airborne or drinking water-borne (Nejm 1992;326:151)
  Epidemic and endemic. Male > female; summer/fall peaks; many unrecognized cases, 5% of all community acquired pneumonias; spread by air conditioner systems (Nejm 1980;302:365). Increased incidence in patients on dialysis, with DM, COPD, over age 50, on chemotherapy
Pathopys:
Sx: 2–10 d incubation. *Diarrhea (2/3); cough w/o sputum, pleurisy, headache, recurrent rigors; r/o mycoplasma and psittacosis
Si: *Pneumonitis, *fever, slow pulse, confusion, wound infections (UVM—Ann IM 1982;96:173)
  *Most important findings to dx
Crs: High fatality rate if immunocompromised
Cmplc: r/o other atypical pneumonia agents, eg, Pittsburgh agent (Ann IM 1980;92:559) and very similar **Pontiac fever** (Ann IM 1984;100:333)
Lab:
  Bact: Sputum Gram stain shows polys without bugs; gram-neg rod when pick culture, won't stain in tissue. Fluorescent antibody stains

of transtracheal aspirate or sputum, pos in 26% (Ann IM 1979;90:1). Culture requires special media, very fastidious

Chem: LFTs increased (1/2); Na <130 (2/3)

Hem: ESR increased (1/3); polys increased (2/3) w left shift

Serol: Titer >1/250 IgG and IgM

Urine: 3^+ protein (20%), rbc's. Urine antigen by RIA or ELISA, 70% sens, 100% specif; is the clinically most useful test

Xray: Chest shows bilat pneumonia, 1/3 w pleural effusion

Rx: (Nejm 1998;129:328)

Azithromycin, clarithromycin, or erythromycin × 10–14 d; ciprofloxacin 400 mg iv q 8 h or 750 mg po bid, or newer fluoroquinolone; doxycycline, but less effective. Add rifampin in severe disease

MORAXELLA INFECTIONS

Cause: *Moraxella (Branhamella, Neisseria) catarrhalis*

Epidem: High carrier rates in the population

Pathophys: Major pathogen in COPD/chronic bronchitis; 3rd most common bacterial pathogen in otitis media after pneumococcus and H. flu

Sx: Increased sputum production, cough

Si: Fever fairly uncommon

Crs:

Cmplc:

Lab:

Bact: Gram neg diplococci

Hem: WBC usually <10,000

Xray:

Rx: Ciprofloxacin, 2nd generation cephalosporins, macrolides, Tm/S, tetracyclines

GONORRHEA (gc)

Cause: *Neisseria gonorrhoeae*

Epidem: Venereal; common; bacteremia associated w deficient complement factors, eg, C_5', C_6', C_7', C_8' (Ann IM 1983;99:35).

Coincident *Chlamydia* infection in 15% male heterosexuals, 25% females (Nejm 1984;310:545)

Pathophys: Infects mucus membranes of gu tract (Nejm 1985;312:1683). IgA protease on surface distinguished infectious *Neisseria* from commensals (Nejm 1978;299:973) as do pili. Septicemia more commonly w strains w fewer gu sx, leading to rash, polyarthralgias w negative joint taps (an immune complex disease, Ann IM 1978; 89:28); later one joint may evolve to a single hot infected joint (Nejm 1968;279:234)

Sx: Male: urethral discharge, but 2/3 asx (Nejm 1974;290:117); anal infections, more often asx (Ann IM 1977;86:340); pharyngitis (Nejm 1973;288:181)

Female: Bartholin cyst (80% acute Bartholin's gland cyst infections are due to gc); vaginal discharge, dysuria, pelvic inflammatory disease, pain typically occurring w menses or pregnancy, abnormal menstrual bleeding due to endometritis

Si: Urethral, anal or pharyngeal discharge; in female, abdominal distension, "chandelier sign" (severe pain w cervical motion), pus in cervix

Crs: 2–7^{+} d latent period

Cmplc:
- Bacteremia w purpuric or vesicular pustule on broad erythematous base or later, hemorrhagic bullae
- Endocarditis, 80% have arthritis too; w monoarticular arthritis, 3% will have endocarditis
- **Fitzhugh-Curtis syndrome,** hepatic capsule inflammation (Nejm 1970;282:1082)
- Polyarthritis and tenosynovitis (rv of all septic arthritis; Nejm 1985;312:764)

r/o *Trichomonas, Candida,* chlamydia (Nejm 1974;291:1175), syphilis, Reiter's, appendicitis in women

Lab:

Bact: Gram stain, in male 1st, culture only if unclear on Gram stain; in female, smear of cleanly wiped cervix to look for >3 polys/hpf w intracellular gram-negative cocci, has a 67% sensitivity, 98% specificity

Culture: in women; in male only if unclear on smear. Reculture all after rx and recheck VDRL if negative first time. Penicillinase producing strains now in US

Serol: Screen for associated complement deficiencies w CH_{50} level (Nejm 1983;308:1138)

Rx: Preventive tetracycline, in neonates, 1% ointment once, or erythromycin; are better than $AgNO_3$ (Nejm 1988;318:657)

of disease (Med Let 1999;41:86), general rules: regimens now must be good vs penicillinase-producing organisms; 1st generation cephalothins and phenoxymethyl penicillin are ineffective; tetracycline inadequate for gc but treat all w azithromlycin 1 gm po × 1, or doxycycline 100 mg bid × 7d to get chlamydia

1st:
- Ceftriaxone 125–250 mg im × 1 ($10); gets syphilis, and both pharyngeal and resistant gc; or
- Cefixime (Suprax) 400 mg po × 1 ($5); or
- Cefpodoxime 200 mg po × 1 ($3) (Med Let 1992;34:107)
- Ciprofloxacin 600 mg po × 1; no good vs syphilis; resistance appearing (Ann IM 1996;125:465)
- Ofloxacin 400 mg po × 1

2nd:
- Spectinomycin 2 gm im × 1; if penicillin allergy and pregnant; no good vs syphilis or vs gc pharyngitis, resistance develops quickly (Nejm 1987;317:272)

of cmplc's (Mmwr 1993;42:STD supplement 1) arthritis and/or septicemia, hospitalize and tap joint, irrigate it if worsens. 10 million U aqueous penicillin until afebrile × 3 d then 7 d cefoxitin 1 gm qid iv, or spectinomycin 2 gm bid im

MENINGOCOCCAL MENINGITIS
(and Adult Meningitis)
Nejm 2001;344:1378

Cause: (Nejm 1997;337:970) of adult meningitis:

Age 20–60: 1st, pneumococcus; 2nd, *Neisseria meningitidis* (Serogroup Y > C > B > A); 3rd, *Listeria;* rarely now, *H. influenzae*

Age 60+: 1st, pneumococcus; 2nd, *Listeria;* 3rd, others

Epidem: Serogroup A in epidemics in developing countries; rare in US, 1/100,000/yr or < 3000 cases/yr; groups B (ET-5 strain—Jama 1999;281:1493) Y, and C are sporadic and in epidemics in US (Jama 1995;273:383, 390)

From respiratory tract of carriers (<3% of general population) or patients w meningococcal pneumonitis (Ann IM 1979;91:7). Increased after influenza infection (Nejm 1972;287:5). Bacteremia recurs in patients w complement deficiencies of C_6', C_7', or C_8'. (40% of all adult meningitis is nosocomial, often gram negatives, although meningococcal never is)

Incr by exposure to tobacco smoke

Pathophys: IgA protease on surface distinguishes infectious from commensal meningococcus (Nejm 1992;327:864). Impaired protein C activation in sepsis (Nejm 2001;345:408)

URI leads to bacteremia 1st, then
- Metastatic infections of meninges, eye, pericardium, joints, and/or cardiac valves
- Shwartzman phenomenon
- Immune complex arthritis w/o permanent damage

Sx: Fever, unusual changed affect/mental status (85%), stiff neck

Si: Fever >100°F (>37.8°C) (95%), stiff neck (88%), petechial rash w central focal necrosis (66%) (purpura fulminans, pictures—Nejm 1996;334:1709), focal neurologic deficits (28%), seizures (23%)

Occasionally meningococcal pneumonia alone (Ann IM 1975;82:493)

Crs: Without rx, death in hrs; w rx, 25% mortality (in pneumococcal meningitis, mortality higher and morbidity >50%)

Cmplc:
- CNS thrombophlebitis w focal seizures and deficits, cranial nerve neuropathies (Nejm 1972;286:882), communicating hydrocephalus
- Myocarditis in 75% at postmortem, 20% have aseptic pericardial effusions (Ann IM 1971;74:212)
- Adrenal hemorrhage and insufficiency (Waterhouse-Friderichsen syndrome)
- Chronic bacteremia without CNS involvement, fever, or rash

In compromised host, r/o *Listeria, Cryptococcus,* toxoplasmosis, and other treatable causes of meningitis

Lab:

Bact: CSF has >10 white cells/mm^3, usually (87%) >200, mostly polys; glucose <40 mg% (50%); protein >45 mg% (96%), usually >100 mg%; Gram stain shows intracellular gram-neg diplococci. Culture best in 10% CO_2. Blood cultures

Xray: CT scan if focal si's before LP (Nejm 2001;345:1727), but START ANTIBIOTICS 1ST

Rx:

Prevent in epidemic or in endemic areas by:

- Decreasing intimate contact;
- Immunize w:

    Quadrivalent polysaccharide antigen (Menomune) (Med Let 2000;42:69) 0.5 cc sc × 1; vs serogroups A, C, Y, and W-135; 67% effective in epidemic but not under age 2 (Jama 2001;285: 177; 1998;279:435); used in epidemics, routinely in Army, and may be indicated in dorm-living college students especially dorm-living freshmen (Jama 2001;286:688); $75/dose;

Oligosaccharide-protein conjugate vaccines (like Hib vaccine for H. flu) vs type C and perhaps A, more effective in infants (Jama 2000;283: 2795, 2842; 1998;280:1685; 1996;275:1499)

- Administering prophylactic antibiotics (Nejm 1982;307:1266) to family, day care companions, and close friends, not school or hospital personnel unless 2 cases occur in a school (Jama 1997; 277:389): 1st, ciprofloxacin 500 mg po z1; 2nd, rifampin 600 mg po qid × 2 d; or ceftriaxone

Of acute unknown adult meningitis (Med Let 1999;41:96): cefotaxime or ceftriaxone pending cultures, w vancomycin up to 4 gm qd to cover resistant pneumococcus. With sensitivities, can truncate to penicillin 24 million U iv qd in q 2 h bolus × 1 d then q 4 h for meningococcal type and covers 64% of pneumococcus as well (Nejm 1997;337:970); doesn't eliminate carrier state; same choices in head trauma since most likely organism is pneumococcus; rarely chloramphenicol if penicillin-allergic, but alarming appearance of chloro resistant meningococcus appearing (Nejm 1998;339:868) in developing countries

Of other gram negatives (Ann IM 1990;112:610): cefotaxime, ceftizoxime, or ceftriaxone for nonpseudomonas types but not *Listeria* (requires 3 wk penicillin). Ceftazidime and gentamicin for *Pseudomonas*. Ampicillin + chloramphenicol or ceftriaxone or cefotaxime for H. flu, and drop the second drug if organism turns out to be ampicillin-sensitive

PEDIATRIC MENINGITIS
Ann IM 1990;112:610

Cause: (Nejm 1997;337:970)
Age <1 mo: 1st, group B strep; 2nd, *Listeria;* 3rd, pneumococcus; 4th, vaginal flora, *Listeria,* and *Staph epidermidis*
Age 2–24 mo: 1st, pneumococcus; 2nd, meningococcus; 3rd, group B strep; 4th, H. flu
Age 2–18: 1st, meningococcus; 2nd, pneumococcus; 3rd, H. flu
Epidem: Overall incidence much reduced now since H. flu vaccines (Nejm 1997;337:970)
Increased incidence in premies
Pathophys: Age 6–24 mo: cranial bruits due to increased intracranial pressure
Sx: Age <6 mo: poor appetite, seizures (30%)
Age 6–24 mo: seizures (30%), petechial rash especially w H. flu and *N. meningitidis*
Si: Age <6 mo: no stiff neck, no fontanelle bulge
Age 6–24 mo; bulging fontanelle, stiff neck, cranial bruits (20% false neg and pos—Nejm 1968;278:1420)
Crs: (Nejm 1997;337:970) Age <6 mo, worse mortality than age 6–24 mo yr
Cmplc: (Nejm 1997;337:970) Age <6 mo significantly worse morbidity than age 6–24 mo
In both, morbidities include cranial nerve palsies especially of VI, VII, and VIII; sensorineural hearing loss 6% w H. flu, 32% w pneumococcus, 10% w *N. meningitidis* (Nejm 1984;311:869); detect w evoked potentials (Pediatrics 1984;73:579); subdural empyemas and effusions, hydrocephalus, retardation, seizures. H. flu morbidity >6 yr later = 20% (Pediatrics 1984;74:198)
Lab: CSF protein increased, glucose decreased, wbc >10/mm^3; Gram stains

Rx:

> Preventive: age 6 mo–6 yr: rifampin to intimate contacts of H. flu as well as meningococcal cases and to pt on hosp discharge to clear nose (Mmwr 12/24/84)
>
> Therapeutic (Med Let 1999;41:96): See individual organism pages
>
> Age <6 mo (Med Let 1999;41:96): ampicillin and ceftriaxone, or cefotaxime plus gentamicin
>
> Age 6 mo–6 yr (Med Let 1999;41:96): ceftriaxone 100 mg/kg iv qd, or cefotaxime w vancomycin to cover resistant pneumococcus pending cultures
>
> In both: dexamethasone 0.15 mg/kg iv 20 min before antibiotic, then q 6 h × 4; decreases cmplc especially deafness in H. flu types (Nejm 1990;319:968) and perhaps other bacterial types as well (Lancet 1993;342:457; Nejm 1991;324:1525) esp pneumococcal (Jama 1997;278:925)

BITE WOUND INFECTIONS

Nejm 1999;340:85,138

Cause: Anaerobes, *Pasteurella multocida* and *canis,* strep, staph, *Moraxella,* and *Neisseria* in animal bites

Epidem: *P. multocida* is the organism in >50% animal bite wound infections especially from cats, which can also induce infections in scratches

Pathophys:

Sx:

Si: Cellulitis

Crs: 70% develop within 1 d, 90% in 2 d, 100% in 3 d

Cmplc:

Lab:

Rx: dT shot if indicated

> Prophylactic antibiotics reasonable if deep punctures (esp from cats), hand wounds, or surgical repair needed, w:
>
> 1st: Augmentin (amoxicillin and clavulinic acid) po, or Unasyn (amp + sulbactam) iv; or
>
> 2nd: Penicillin; or
>
> 3rd: Tetracycline, or ampicillin, or oxacillin 500 qid × 5 d, or erythromycin, or cephalothin

TULAREMIA (Rabbit Fever)

Nejm 2001;345:1637; Vermont epidemic—Nejm 1969;280:1253

Cause: *Francisella (Pasteurella) tularensis*

Epidem: From infected rodents and lagomorphs, by eating or handling, or by being bitten by arthropod (tick) vector (50% of transmissions occur in this way). Worldwide wherever large rabbit/rodent populations, eg, muskrats in Vermont; endemic in Martha's Vineyard, MA, rabbits (Nejm 2001;345:1601)

Pathophys: Endotoxin production and rapid multiplication, transient bacteremias lead to all parenchymous organ involvement

Sx: 5 d incubation

Fever (97%), malaise (60%), headache (23%), nausea and vomiting (8%), pleuritic chest pain (5%)

Si: Ulcerated papule (94%) at site of entry, very infective; regional lymphadenopathy (70%); fever and septicemia

Crs: 2 wk duration on average; 15% relapse later

Cmplc: Tularemic pneumonia, probably need to inhale to get

Lab:

Bact: Gram-negative bacilli; culture of blood, sputum, or local ulcer on special medium

Serol: Available from health departments, agglutinin titers

Rx: 1st choice, streptomycin 15 mg/kg im bid × 14 d, or gentamicin; 2nd, tetracycline or chloramphenicol

YERSINIA GASTROENTERITIS

Nejm 1989;321:16

Cause: *Yersinia* (a pasteurella) *enterocolitica*

Epidem: Fecal/oral; associated w poor sanitation; can live and reproduce at 39°F (4°C), hence can occur in winter too. Animal reservoirs, especially pigs (Nejm 1990;322:984). Contaminated chocolate milk in NY school epidemic (Nejm 1978;298:76); meat and milk products, fecally contaminated water. Person-to-person transmission rare, but can occur especially w blood transfusions

Pathophys: Bowel wall invasion

Sx: Headache, sore throat, fever (FUO occasionally), abdominal pain, chronic and recurrent diarrhea

Si: Exudative pharyngitis especially in adults (Ann IM 1983;99:40), ι erythema nodosum, polyarthritis (Bull Rheum Dis 1979; 29:100)

Crs: 2⁺ wk, even w antibiotic rx

Cmplc: Misdiagnosed as appendicitis and as regional enteritis (Nejm 1990;323:113). Massive gi bleed or perforation; thyrotoxicosis (Ann IM 1976;85:735); bacteremia, especially if iron overloaded, which fuels growth, 50% fatal; postinfectious arthropathy (HLA B27-associated)

r/o other more common forms of gastroenteritis (NV + D) like viral esp from "small round-structured viruses" (Jama 1997;278:563)

Lab:

Bact: Gram-negative rod, an enterobacteriaceae; grows best at 77°F (25°C) in 24–48 h; facultative anaerobe

Serol: Passive hemagglutinin titer >1/512 diagnostic but 30% false negatives

Rx: Questionable that rx helps uncomplicated cases

In patients w focal, extraintestinal infections or bacteremia: 1st choice is gentamicin + doxycycline pending sensitivities; maybe fluoroquinolones, maybe chloramphenicol or tetracyclines alone

PSEUDOMONAS INFECTIONS

Ann IM 1975;82:819

Cause: *Pseudomonas aeruginosa* (rv of rare species—Ann IM 1972;77:211)

Epidem: From respiratory or gi tract droplets; normal skin flora

Very old, very young, and immunocompromised patients most frequently infected. Occasional hospital epidemics from anesthesia bags, hot and cold nebulizers (Nejm 1970;282:531). Hot tub folliculitis epidemics (Arch IM 1985;135:1621)

Pathophys: Exotoxin A production causing some of pathogenesis and antibody to it offers some protection (Nejm 1980;302:1360)

Sx: Pneumonias, septicemia, skin and wound infections

Si: Cutaneous ecthyma gangrenosum (in a very small %) w black necrotic center, indurated, in groin or axilla; r/o mucor and aspergillosis

Crs:
Cmplc: r/o "pseudobacteremia" w *Burkholderia (Pseudomonas) cepacia,*
which grows in povidone/iodine prep solution (Nejm 1981;
305:621) or in albuterol neb bottles (Ann IM 1995;122:762)

r/o **meliodosis,** tropical *Burkholderia (Pseudomonas) mallei* causes
subcutaneous "farcy" infections; recrudesces up to 10 yr later, and
as "glanders" it cavitates in liver, spleen, and lung hence looks like
tbc; skin abscesses. In lab personnel too (Nejm 2001;345:256;
1981;305:1133)

Lab:
Bact: Gram-neg rod
Rx: Preventively avoid hot/cold nebulizers; there is no effective
decontamination
of acute disease: tobramycin (or gentamicin) + piperacillin (or
mezlocillin, ticarcillin, or azlocillin); or ceftazidime + ciprofloxacin
if penicillin allergic
of *P. pseudomallei,* tetracycline or chloramphenicol × 1–6 mo at high
doses

TYPHOID (Enteric) FEVER

Inf Contr Hosp Epidem 1991;12:168; Nejm 1970;283:686,739

Cause: *Salmonella typhae*
Epidem: Fecal/oral, from carriers (2–3% of recovered population),
probably resides in gallbladder
Increased incidence in US foreign travelers, cirrhotics, patients w
tumors especially of CNS, hemolytic anemias especially sickle cell
anemia, aortic aneurysms especially thoracic
Pathophys: Endotoxin production; intracellular organisms; ingestion
results in gi lymph nodes picking up and the nodes' subsequent
necrosis over 2 wk leading to septicemia and further node
involvement plus ulceration
Sx: 6–22 d incubation period
Fever >100°F (38.5°C); constipation, more rarely diarrhea
Si: Fever (100%), bradycardia P < 100 (80%), spleen (75%), hepatomegaly (30%), macular rash (rose spots) over lower chest (5%)

Crs: Fever gradually up, then gradually down over days even with rx

Cmplc: Mortality even w rx especially if septicemia; relapse (10%); metastatic infections to lung, brain, joints, aorta (10%); hemorrhage (7%); perforation (3%); pneumonia and/or multiple pulmonary emboli

Lab:

Bact: Blood culture, 50–80% positive in 1st 2 wk; marrow (26%) positive even when blood negative. Stool culture goes positive in 80% after 1 wk. Gram stain shows gram-negative rods. Stool mucus methylene blue stain shows wbc's, mostly mononuclear unlike polys of salmonellosis, shigellosis, and ulcerative colitis (Ann IM 1972;76:697)

Serol: Widal's test positive after 2 wk, an antibody vs O, H, and Vi antigens

Rx:

Preventively:

Keep carriers away from food, water; chlorinate water; cholecystectomy, or ampicillin 6 gm qd w 2 gm probenecid (Med Let 1968;10:51), or ciprofloxacin (Nejm 1991;324:392) for carriers

Immunize (Med Let 1994;36:41) with:

- Live attenuated Ty21a vaccine (Vivotif) po qod × 4 beginning at least 2 wk before departure, good for 5 yr; or
- Capsular polysaccharide conjugated vaccine (Vi-rEPA) im × 2, 6 wk apart, ~95% effective even in children age 2–5 (Nejm 2001; 344:1263,1322)

of active disease:

- Ciprofloxacin, no resistance yet (Jama 2000;283:2668); or
- Cephalosporins, 3rd generation like ceftriaxone, no resistance yet (Jama 2000;283:2668); or
- Chloramphenicol 4 gm qd × 4 wk; 15 gm/d when acute; or 15 gm qd × 14 d (Nejm 1968;278:171), some resistance (Nejm 1973; 289:463)
- Ampicillin as good as chloro although some resistance too (Nejm 1969;280:147)
- Tm/S (Nejm 1980;303:426)

of delirium leading to coma and/or shock, dexamethasone 3 mg/kg × 1, then 1 mg/kg q 6 h × 48 h, decreases mortality from 55% to 10% (Nejm 1984;310:82)

ID: BACTERIOLOGY

SALMONELLOSIS; PARATYPHOID

Cause: *Salmonella paratyphi* and other nontyphoid species

Epidem: Fecal/oral from carriers, 1/3 carry for 1 yr after infection, some forever; pet reptiles, 90% carry (ME Epigram 3/99); birds, especially poultry from gi tracts and including chicken eggs, eg, ice cream epidemic when pre-mix transported in tank truck that had just carried eggs (Nejm 1996;334:1281); cider (Mmwr 1997;46:4); orange juice (Jama 1998;280:1504); beef/hamburger, (Nejm 1987; 316:565), especially in patients on antibiotics; carmine dye (ground-up insects) in food or as stool marker (Nejm 1967;276: 829); marijuana (Nejm 1982;306:1249); sprouts (Ann IM 2001; 135:239)

Increased incidence in cancer patients (Nejm 1967;276:1045), 1/400 leukemics, lymphomas, and colon cancer patients; 1/2000 patients w other cancers; 1/9000 patients w/o cancer

2nd most common food poisoning after staph and before clostridial

Pathophys: Endotoxin production by intracellular organisms in small and large bowel

Sx: Nausea, vomiting, and diarrhea

Si: Diarrhea, may be as watery as in cholera

Crs: 12–72 h incubation, unlike staph; several day duration; recover spontaneously after 1 wk

Cmplc: Septic arteritis and aneurysms (Nejm 1969;281:310)
r/o staph (less diarrhea) and clostridial food poisoning

Lab:

Bact: Gram-negative rods on stool culture. Stool smear w methylene blue shows polys unlike typhoid fever but like other colitis, eg, ulcerative, *Shigella, E. coli,* etc. (Ann IM 1972;76:697)

Hem: White counts in normal range, no correlation w severity

Rx: Antibiotics contraindicated (ACP J Club 1999;130:15) because if rx, then carry in stool longer (27% vs 11% at 31 d), and in vivo resistance develops in 10% (Nejm 1969;281:636); but ciprofloxacin or Tm/S is used if fecal leukocytes, fever, and other measures of severity are bad (Arch IM 1990;150:546); ciprofloxacin does help, but prolongs convalescent excretion (Ann IM 1991;114:195), and quinolone resistance now appearing, probably due to use in animal feeds (Nejm 1999;341:1420)

Opiates could theoretically worsen due to decreased motility

BACTERIAL DYSENTERY

Cause: *Shigella* spp (*dysenteriae, flexneri, boydii, sonnei*)

Epidem: Fecal/oral especially via water supplies, organisms die fast w drying; or person to person. Increased incidence in Asia (*dysenteriae*), also most malignant; *sonnei* most benign. Infective dose low (~100 organisms) when compared w other bacterial diarrheas

Pathophys: Shiga endotoxins, noninvasive so no bacteremias; superficial mucosal ulcerations, can produce DIC, hemolytic anemia, renal microangiopathy (Nejm 1978;298:926)

Sx: Nausea, vomiting, and severe diarrhea w cramps (75%); fever (75%); 50% of cases have both

Si: Bloody stool, watery like cholera

Crs: Incubation period = 8^+ h, average 2–4 d; duration ~1 wk

Cmplc: Incapacitating w low mortality, except *dysenteriae* often fatal Reiter's syndrome precipitation; perhaps causes ulcerative colitis?

Lab:

Bact: Gram-negative rod; stool culture. Stool smear shows polys (Ann IM 1972;76:697)

Rx: Symptomatic: oral or iv lyte/fluid replacement, opiates to slow diarrhea, although theoretically could worsen by decreasing motility
Antibiotics: ciprofloxacin (Ann IM 1992;117:727) 500 mg po bid × 5 d for *S. dysenteriae*, 1 gm po × 1 ok for other species; or azithromycin 500 mg po day 1, 250 mg qd day 2–5 (Ann IM 1997; 126:697); or Tm/S (Nejm 1980;303:426); ampicillin 500 mg qid, questionably effective

CHOLERA

Nejm 1985;312:343; Ann IM 1981;94:656

Cause: *Vibrio cholerae* or new non O-1 strains

Epidem: Sewage in drinking water. Carriers (in gallbladder) = 3–5% of world population (Ann IM 1970;72:357); primarily in Asia, S America, and N Africa; increasing number of cases/yr in US, (Jama 2000;284:1541). Many asx cases

Pathophys: Na pump inhibition by entero/exotoxin; glucose important to that pump (Nejm 1985;312:28)

Sx: Diarrhea; sometimes fever

Si: "Rice water" diarrhea up to 15 L/d; "dishwater hands" from volume
  depletion

Crs: Benign if replace H_2O and salt iv or via NG tube

Cmplc: Mortality significant in symptomatic disease without rx; increased
  anion gap acidosis (Nejm 1986;315:1591)

Lab:

  Bact: Gram-negative rod, flagellated; culture carriers post Mg^{2+} purge
    (30% false neg—Ann IM 1970;72:357)

  Chem: Stool cyclic AMP increased

Rx: (Mmwr 1991;40:562; Med Let 1991;33:107)

  Vaccination w killed vaccine; 0.5–1 cc × 2 then q 1 mo if heavy
    exposure anticipated (Ann IM 1971;74:412); 50% effective, but not
    for new O-1 strains. New live attenuated oral vaccine more effective
    (Lancet 1990;335:958), but not yet available in US

  of acute disease:

  - Oral rehydration solutions (p 739); catch up, then stool output +
    100 cc q 1 h (Ann IM 1975;82:101) or iv Ringer's lactate
  - Antibiotics: doxycycline 300 mg po × 1 or 100 mg po bid × 3 d;
    or in children, Tm/S 5 mg/25 mg/kg po bid × 3 d; or ciprofloxacin

VIBRIO DIARRHEA AND WOUND INFECTIONS

  Ann IM 1988;109:261,318; 1983;99:464; Nejm 1985;312:343

Cause: *Vibrio vulnificus* and *parahaemolyticus*

Epidem: Southern seawater exposure. Various species live in sea, hence gi
  disease from raw oyster ingestion (MMWR 1996;45:621), shell cut
  wound infections, swimming (Ann IM 1983;99:169)

Pathophys:

Sx: Nausea, vomiting, diarrhea w cramps w/in 4 d of consumption;
  bloody diarrhea in <50%; fever, headache; ear pain; wound pain

Si: Otitis media, cellulitis, gangrene

Crs: 2–4 d (Nejm 1985;312:343)

Cmplc: Septicemia, often fatal, especially in compromised host (Nejm
  1979;300:1) like alcoholics in whom can cross gut barriers

Lab:

  Bact: Culture w special medium (TCBS) broth

Rx: Preventive: immunocompromised avoid eating raw oysters
Tetracyclines (Med Let 1991;33:107)

9.4 ANAEROBES

BOTULISM

Ann IM 1998;129:221; Nejm 1973;289:1005

Cause: *Clostridium botulinum* (types A, B, E are the most common human pathogens)

Epidem: Heat-resistant spores contaminate
- Canned foods or opened cans kept for days unrefrigerated (Ann IM 1996;125:558) leading to bacterial proliferation of exotoxin, which then is ingested w/o further heating, eg, homemade salsa, relish, canned vegetables or meats, garlic in oil, etc.
- Wounds where bacteria proliferate and produce exotoxin (80% type A, 20% type B)

Spores common in dirt and dust

Pathophys: Exotoxin is heat-labile, extremely toxic (<1 lb could kill the world); inhibits transmitter release at all cholinergic endings
In infants and occasionally in adults (Nejm 1986;315:239) w impaired gastric acid, can generate toxin in human gi tract

Sx: Incubation period of 12 h to several days; mild gi sx; descending paralysis of motor and autonomic nerves starting w cranial nerves: double vision, dysphagia, dysarthria; upper respiratory tract paralysis w trouble breathing and swallowing

Si: "Myasthenia gravis that doesn't respond to edrophonium (Tensilon)" though some may a little (Ann IM 1981;95:443); flaccid paralysis

Crs: Pts can survive and recover w respirator and other supportive care for weeks to months

Cmplc: r/o myasthenia, Guillain-Barré, diphtheria, CVA, Eaton-Lambert syndrome; intoxication w organophosphates, CO, paralytic shellfish toxins

Lab:
Bact: Smear of food shows gram-pos bacilli; food and/or stool culture grows obligate anaerobe; extract kills mice
CSF: Normal

ID: BACTERIOLOGY

Botulism, continued

    Noninv: EMG shows low-amplitude response to nerve stimulation increased by 50/s repetitive stimulation (Nejm 1970;282:193); 15–40% false neg

Rx: Preventively heat all canned food prior to serving; immunization impractical on widespread scale

    of disease: passive immunization w polyvalent horse antitoxin helps before severe sx set in, available from CDC; type-specific if possible. Debride wounds. Gastric lavage if food recently ingested. Supportive care, eg, respirator, etc × weeks to months usually successful; guanidine not helpful (Nejm 1971;285:773)

PSEUDOMEMBRANOUS COLITIS
Nejm 1994;330:257; Med Let 1979;21:97

Cause: *Clostridium difficile*

Epidem: Associated w antibiotic rx, usually broad-spectrum types and especially clindamycin (Nejm 1999;341:1645), and/or cancer chemoRx. Also the cause of 20% of all antibiotic-associated diarrhea w/o pseudomembranous colitis

Pathophys: Proliferates when there is suppression of normal bowel flora by various broad-spectrum antibiotics; cytotoxic toxin production. IgG antibody to the toxin develops variably and is protective (Nejm 2000;342:390)

Sx: H/o antibiotic use, esp cephalosporin or clindamycin > 6 d before loose but not watery diarrhea onset; occasionally fever, abdominal pain

Si: Raised plaques (pseudopolyps) on sigmoidoscopy or colonoscopy, "swollen rice grains," bleed when scraped; rectum may be spared often

Crs:

Cmplc: 15–20% relapse rate w rx

Lab:

    Bact: Fecal leukocytes by methylene blue stain or Gram stain of stool

    Chem: Toxin assayable in stool by various methods; by tissue culture assay, 94–100% sens, 99% specif; by latex agglutination assay (poorest test but most often used), 50% sens, 99% specif; by enzyme-linked methods, 75% sens, 99% specif; order if positive fecal leukocytes stain

Hem: Increased polys

Rx: (Med Let 1989;31:94)

Prevent by restricting clindamycin use (Ann IM 1994;120:272)

of colitis, stop antibiotics and give metronidazole (Flagyl) 250 mg po qid × 10–14 d, perhaps iv if ileus; as good as vancomycin and costs a small fraction of what vanco costs (Lancet 1983;2:1043). Or vancomycin 125 mg po qid × 10–14 d, increase to 500 mg qid in resistant cases but do not give iv since is not secreted into bowel where the organism is

GAS GANGRENE
Nejm 1973;289:1129

Cause: *Clostridium perfringens* (*C. welchii*), or *C. novyi;* via wound contamination w dirt

Epidem: (Nejm 1972;286:1026): In most soils; 8% of people carry in stool. Frequent agent in septic abortions.

Pathophys: Exotoxin produced in tissues leading to cell necrosis via lecithinase, which splits cell walls, collagenase, and other enzymatic activity. CO_2 produced in wounds. Obligate anaerobes; need to live in dead tissue

Sx: Severe pain

Si: Fever, severe toxemia, necrotic skin; sweet smell

Crs: Rapid spread, leading to death in hours or days

Cmplc: Shock, rapid hemolysis.

r/o more benign anaerobic crepitant cellulitis (Ann IM 1975;83:375) in diabetics when *E. coli* or *Klebsiella* anaerobically metabolizes glucose; other anaerobes (p 429)

Lab:

Bact: Smear shows large gram-pos sporulating bacilli, which in culture produce lecithinase and CO_2

Chem: Elevated bilirubin (hemolysis)

Xray: Gangrene: tissue gas throughout muscle after 18 h; unlikely to be gas gangrene if occurs earlier and/or without edema and inflammation (Nejm 1968;278:758)

Gas Gangrene, continued

Rx: Gangrene: hyperbaric O_2 inactivates the toxin; antitoxin 75,000 U iv q 6 h may stop the hemolysis? Antibiotics: high-dose penicillin + gentamicin. Surgery to excise dead tissue

CLOSTRIDIAL FOOD POISONING

Nejm 1973;289:1129

Cause: *Clostridium perfringens*. Food (food poisoning) contamination w dirt

Epidem: (Nejm 1972;286:1026) In most soils; 8% of people carry in stool. 3rd most common type of food poisoning after staph and *Salmonella*

Pathophys: Exotoxin produced in food before or rarely after ingestion causing watery diarrhea via Na pump effects. Obligate anaerobes; need to live in dead tissue

Sx: 12 h incubation period, then diarrhea without vomiting; no fever

Si:

Crs: Mild, only 1% call doctor; lasts 12 h

Cmplc: r/o other diarrheal illnesses

Lab:

    Bact: Smear shows large gram-pos sporulating bacilli, which in culture produce lecithinase and CO_2

Xray:

Rx: Fluid replacement oral or iv

TETANUS, LOCKJAW

Nejm 1973;289:1293; 1969;280:569

Cause: *Clostridium tetani,* via wound contamination with dirt

Epidem: Present in most soils; 535 cases in 1965 in US; ~4 cases/100 million, mainly in southern states; Texas had 56% of cases; highest incidence in very young and very old (inadequate immunization); <3% of patients have hx of ever having had tetanus toxoid; increased incidence in "skin popping" drug addicts. Females > males

Pathophys: Exotoxin production and transported both via circulation to CNS (probably most significant in humans), and along motor nerves to CNS (but can't correlate wound distance from CNS w morbidity and mortality in humans)

Sx: Puncture wound or laceration (58%), or postpartum, postsurgery, skin ulcers

1–54 d incubation period, median = 8 d, 88% within 14 d; short incubation period in patients under age 50 is poor prognostic sign

Si: Spastic paralysis; tonic convulsive contractions precipitated by intrinsic or extrinsic muscle movement; no or rarely fever

Crs: 60% mortality

Cmplc: r/o **"stiff man syndrome,"** autoimmune antibodies against GABA neurons (Ann IM 1999;131:522; Nejm 1990;322:1555) induced muscle spasms over years, seen w hypopituitarism, IDDM, Graves, and other endocrinopathies (Nejm 1988;318:1012,1060; 1984;310:1511); occasionally is an autoimmune paraneoplastic syndrome in breast cancer (Nejm 1993;328:546)

r/o malignant neuroleptic syndrome (p 526)

Lab:

Bact: Smears show gram-pos bacilli; culture shows fastidious anaerobe, pos in 32% of proven cases

Rx: Prevent w toxoid vaccine (CDC rv—Ann IM 1985;103:896) im, primary series of 3 over 1 yr, then q 10 yr, more frequently increases risk of reaction w/o increasing protection (Nejm 1969;280:575); some argue that routine dT booster is unnecessary in adults (Lancet 5/11/85, p1089); booster of dT is enough even for dirty wounds if last dT was less than 5 yr ago (Nejm 1983;309:636)

Tetanus human immune globulin 250 U im, for dirty wounds w vaccine if not sure has had primary series; give coincident w vaccine in different im area

of disease: metronidazole 500 mg iv q 6 h (Nejm 1995;332:812); human immune globulin; respirator (Ann IM 1978;88:66)

ANAEROBIC INFECTIONS (Except Clostridial)

Cause: *Bacteroides fragilis* and other species; anaerobic streptococcus; microaerophilic streptococcus

Epidem:

ID: BACTERIOLOGY

Pathophys: Abscess formation very often; almost always 2 or more organisms; perivascular localization causes thrombophlebitis

Sx: Brain abscess extrasubdural empyema; peridontal abscess; lung abscess; appendiceal/diverticular abscesses; hepatic abscess (Lancet 1/16/82 p134); PID/septic abortion; sinus abscess

Si: Putrid pus (fatty acids); palpable gas in tissues, but r/o gas gangrene, or *E. coli* gas formers in diabetic

Crs: Indolent, may be relatively asymptomatic for months

Cmplc: Thrombophlebitis often

r/o clostridial gas gangrene, which has incubation <3 d, marked toxemia, severe pain, lots of swelling, necrotic blistered skin, minimal gas, sweet smell, gas extension and infection into muscle, which is all in contrast to anaerobic infections

Lab:

Bact: Culture anaerobically

Rx: Anticoagulate w low threshold because of DVT predisposition
Antibiotics (Med Let 1999;41:95):

- Clindamycin; w gentamicin if may have aerobes; ampicillin alone ok in PID if not too toxic; better than penicillin in pulmonary abscess (Ann IM 1983;98:466, maybe not 1983;98:546); often used w penicillin for brain abscess
- Metronidazole (Flagyl) po or iv (Med Let 1981;23:13); cidal vs all anaerobes except microaerophilic gram-positives; diffuses well into abscess spaces
- Amoxicillin + clavulanic acid (Augmentin)/ampicillin + sulbactam (Unasyn)/piperacillin + tazobactam (Zosyn)
- Penicillin G, or ampicillin, ~10 million U qd; for brain abscess, perhaps w chloramphenicol
- Chloramphenicol; can be used alone for brain abscesses or w penicillin
- Cefoxitin or cefotetan; are 90% effective vs bacteroides
- Imipenem + cilastatin (Primaxin)

9.5 ACID FAST ORGANISMS

TUBERCULOSIS

Am Rv Respir Crit care Med 2000;161:S221; 1994;149:1359; Ann IM 1993;119:400

Cause: *Mycobacterium tuberculosis* and *bovis*

Epidem: Inhalation of respiratory droplets, of infected persons; but once on drugs probably little infectivity despite positive smears (Nejm 1974;290:459). Reinfection may be as important as reactivation, at least in homeless. Epidemic description at Bath Iron Works (Ann IM 1996;125:114)

Incidence, 25,000 new US cases/yr; these rates were increased in the 1990s from HIV patients, prisons, homeless populations (Nejm 1992;326:703) and the foreign born (Jama 1997;278:304). 3/4 cases from pts w previous positive PPD. 25 million positive PPDs in US, only 5–10% ever result in active disease, whereas HIV pos pts who contract tbc become active cases at 5–10%/yr. In elderly and foreign born, 90% of cases are reactivation, whereas only 60% are in younger pts and the homeless (Jama 1996;275:305), and 1/3 are recent infections (Nejm 1994;330:1692,1703,1750) to 3/4 are now due to exogenous reinfection (Nejm 1999;341:1174)

Incidence higher (Mmwr 5/18/90) in diabetics, institutionalized, household contacts, HIV-infected (Nejm 1992;326:231; 1991;324:289,1644), alcoholics, gastrectomy, silicosis, immunosuppressed including pts on TNF agents (Nejm 2001;345:1098), postpartum (Ann IM 1971;74:764) patients, blacks (Nejm 1990;322:422), and w highly virulent strains (Nejm 1998;338:633)

C. bovis now very rare due to pasteurization of milk

Worldwide 33% prevalence and causes 6% of all deaths (Jama 1995; 273:220, MMWR 1993;42:961)

Pathophys: (Nejm 1967;277:1008)

Primary infection by inhalation to lower lungs leading to local node involvement and asx bacteremia causing gradual hypersensitization via lymphocytic response and eventual calcification and scar = sterile Ghon complex

Secondary disease is a reactivation and hypersensitivity reaction to bacteria spread by asx bacteremia to lung apices and upper kidneys

ID: BACTERIOLOGY

where high O_2 concentrations prevent Ghon complex-type sterilization

Sx: Fever, weight loss, night sweats, cough, sputum production, hemoptysis

Si: Same as sx

Crs: Mortality 6%/yr, 12% at 2 yr but 50% at 2 yr if HIV pos and 80% if have AIDS (Jama 1996;276:1223)

Cmplc: Apical lung abscess; peritonitis (Nejm 1969;281:1091); meningitis; epididymitis; PID; endometritis; splenic and hepatic abscesses; nontender, scarring skin sores/abscesses; arthritis (especially bovis); pericarditis (Nejm 1964;270:327); osteomyelitis, especially of spine **(Pott's disease)**; pleuritis (Am Rev Tbc 1955; 71:616); laryngitis, very infectious (Ann IM 1974;80:708); hypercalcemia (25%) from vitamin D sensitivity (Ann IM 1979; 90:324)

Antibiotic resistance, geographically variable, 25% of cases resistant to INH and/or rifampin (Nejm 1993;328:521,527); multiple drug resistance epidemics in AIDS patients now (Nejm 1992;326:1514) esp in New York City (Jama 1996;276:1229)

Lab:

Bact: Sputum or urine AFB smears; cultures of sputum, gastric aspirate, urine, peritoneal fluid (1 L spun down—Nejm 1969;281: 1091). RIAs now possible in 3 wk

Path: Biopsy of liver pos in high % of miliary, or of peritoneum if ascites protein >2.5 gm % (64% true pos-Nejm 1969;281:1091)

Serol: Interferon γ assay (Jama 2001;286:1740) more specif and sens than skin test

Skin tests: Intermediate strength (IPPD, 5 U), positive if ≥5 mm in HIV pts (Ann IM 1997;126:123) or pts w pulmonary scars or recent contacts, >10 mm in others or perhaps even >15 mm in very low risk; repeat in 2–3 wk to get booster effect, 1/3 more become positive in elderly (Nejm 1985;312:1483) but of questionable significance in the young (Ann IM 1994;120:190). Ignore old BCG immunization in interpreting, esp if > 5–10 yr ago. False negs w overwhelming infection, sarcoid, or other anergy. Delayed reactivity (IPPD neg at 48 h, pos at 6 d in 25% of SE Asians (Ann IM 1996; 124:779)

Urine: Acid, sterile, wbc's and rbc's, protein

Xray: Chest shows apical scarring and/or Ghon complex
IVP characteristically shows beaded ureters

Rx: (Am Rv Respir Crit care Med 2000;161:S221)

Prevent w:

- Hospital preventive policies (Nejm 1995;332:92) respiratory isolation in negative pressure rooms (debatably—Ann IM 2000;133:779) until 3 negative smears of HIV pts w abnormal chest xray, plus regular skin testing programs (Nejm 1995;332:92; Ann IM 1995;122:658)
- BCG vaccination to entire at-risk population (Jama 1994;271:698)
- INH 300 mg po qd × 9 mo for PPD reactors and household contacts under age 35 (Arch IM 1990;150:2517) as well as over 35 if previous neg test or in epidemic (Ann IM 1996;125:114), or perhaps in all since hepatitis risk is small (<1/1000 under age 35, 2/1000 35–65, 3/1000 >65—Jama 1999;281:1014), <1/50,000 die (Ann IM 1997;127:1058); supplement w B_6(pyridoxine) only if alcoholic and/or malnourished (S Sears 12/94), not for asthmatics on steroids (Ann IM 1976;84:261); in HIV-pos pts w pos PPD or anergic, 300 mg po qd w B_6 50 mg po qd forever (Lancet 1993; 342:268) decr incid by 2/3 at 2 yr (Nejm 1997;337:801)
- Rifampin 600 mg alone × 4 mos; or + pyrazinamide 20 mg/kg po qd × 2 mo for pos PPD in HIV pts as effective as 12 mo of INH (Jama 2000;283:1445)
- Other options for latent tbc (Rx Let 2000;7:40): rifampin 600 mg qd × 4 mo; rifabutin alone if on some protease inhibitors; pyrizinamide + ethambutol

of active disease (Nejm 2001;345:189; Med Let 1995;37:67; Ann IM 1990;112:393,397,407): contact local health dept, use 4 drugs initially in all and continuing in AIDS (Nejm 1999;340:367; Ann IM 1987;106:25); use tiw directly observed rx for all cases to prevent further drug resistance (Jama 1995;274:945; Nejm 1994; 330:1179; 1993;328:576) or biw rx after 2 wk of qd rx; prevalence of drug resistance incr from 10% to 36% if take meds for < 1 mo (Nejm 1998;338:1641)

1st line:

- INH 300 mg qd × 6 mo or b-tiw × 9 mo, w pyridoxine only if >300 mg qd to prevent neuropathy. Adverse effect: hepatitis
- Rifampin 600 mg qd or b-tiw × 9 mo, less toxic than streptomycin or INH or longer acting form, rifapentine (Priftin) (Med Let 1999;41:21; Rx Let 1998;5:46) biw × 2 mos then q wk

ID: BACTERIOLOGY

thereafter. Adverse reactions: drug interactions, red body fluids, incr urate. $90/mo

- Pyrazinamide 0.5–40 mg/kg/d or b-tiw × 2 mo, w above allows 6-mo cure courses (Am Rev Respir Dis 1991;143:700,707). Rifamate (INH + rifampin) or "Rifater," a combination pill of all 3 (preferable—Ann IM 1995;122:951). Cure rates ~98% (Am Rev Respir Dis 1982;126:460)
- Ethambutol 15 mg/kg pos qd, use as 4th drug until know sensitivities (Med Let 1995;37–67). Adverse effects: retrobulbar neuritis, check visual acuity regularly, rarely reversible
- Streptomycin 250–1000 mg im qd or 20 mg/kg biw

2nd line drugs:

- Capreomycin
- Ciprofloxacin
- Clofazimine
- Cycloserine
- Ethionamide
- Kanamycin/amikacin
- Levofloxacin
- Ofloxacin
- Aminosalicylic acid
- Rifabutin
- Rifapentine

of antibiotic-resistant tbc: 3 drugs to which organism test susceptible × 12–24 mo; frequent now in AIDS pts (Nejm 1993;328:1137; 1992; 326:1514; Ann IM 1992;117:177,191) and infection can be w previously cured strain so must use 4 drugs (Ann IM 1987;106:25)

ATYPICAL TUBERCULOSIS

Cause: Atypical *Mycobacterium* spp. (MOTT: mycobacterium other than tuberculosis)

Epidem: *M. scrofulaceum* and *kansasii* (MSK) (AnnIM 1998;129:698): Endemic in soil (*kansasii*); little person-to-person spread. In midwest especially

M. avium and *intracellulare* (MAI): Major problem in AIDS where is 3rd most common opportunistic infection after pneumocystis and Kaposi's (Nejm 1996;335:428)

M. fortuitum and other fast growers (FG): (Ann IM 1970;73:971) Normal throat inhabitant?

Pathophys:

Sx:

> *MSK:* Pulmonary, scrofula, skin ulcers. Seen in AIDS pts (Ann IM 1991;114:861)
>
> *MAI:* Pulmonary, especially in COPD, AIDS, and previously damaged lung but not always (Nejm 1989;321:863)
>
> *FG:* Pulmonary; subcutaneous abscess; corneal infection

Si: Pulmonary

Crs:

> *MAI:* Quite virulent in HIV pts
>
> *FG:* Spontaneous resolution w/o rx or w debridement

Cmplc:

> *MSK:* Full gamut like regular tbc; drug resistance common
>
> FG: r/o *M. marinum*, which causes **swimming pool granuloma** (Nejm 1997;336:1065)

Lab:

> *Bact:* All are nicotinic acid nonproducers in contrast to *M. bovis* and *tuberculosis.* All are acid fast; grow at 77°F (25°C); are avirulent to guinea pigs; chromogen characteristics: MSK shows photochromogen; MAI, no chromogen; FG no chromogen and fast growth (2–7 d); r/o scotochromogen types, which are rarely clinically significant
>
> *Skin tests:* MSK and MAI are specific and cause 2nd strength PPD to be positive

Rx:

> for MSK: rifampin etc. (Ann IM 1971;74:758)
>
> for MAI (big problem in AIDS pts)
>
> prophylaxis (Nejm 1996;335:428), routinely in all AIDS pts w CD_4 counts <100–200/cc (Nejm 1993;329:828) or perhaps only if <100, if no disseminated *M. avium* complex disease yet; can d/c prophylaxis when CD_4 >100 again after HIV rx (Nejm 2000; 342:1085)
>
> - Rifabutin, similar to rifampin, retards dissemination in AIDS pts (Med Let 1993;35:36) 300 mg po qd prophylaxis; prevents 55% of expected cases, no resistance develops but can induce rifampin resistance (Nejm 1996;334:1573)
> - Clarithromycin 500 mg po bid (Nejm 1996;335:384) prevents 69%, resistance develops in 45%

- Azithromycin 1200 mg po q wk (Nejm 1996;335:392) prevents 59% of expected cases; or used w rifabutin prevents 85%; resistance develops in 11%

of disease: surgery, if possible, + 3–4 drugs (Nejm 1996;335:377, 1993;329:898; Ann IM 1994;121:905) like clarithromycin or azithromycin + ethambutol + clofazimine or rifabutin or rifampin or cipro or amikacin; interferon γ may also help (Nejm 1994; 330:1348)

LEPROSY

Cause: *Mycobacterium leprae*

Epidem: Unknown mode of transmission, seems to require prolonged (>1 mo) exposure, probably skin and nasal discharge. 3–5 yr incubation. Tuberculoid type is not infectious (Ann IM 1978; 88:538)

15 million in world; especially children and young adults

Pathophys:
- Lepromatous type like sarcoid and Hodgkin's, involves impaired delayed hypersensitivity. Granuloma formation leads to nerve compression? IgG and IgA increased while IgM normal (Ann IM 1969;70:295; Nejm 1968;278:298). T lymphs in lesions are all suppressor cells
- Tuberculoid type, in patients w strong response; all T cells in lesions are helper cells (Nejm 1982;307:1593)

Both types infect colder tissues, hence hands, feet, ears, nose, peripheral nerves

Sx: Years incubation period; eczematous rash; numbness (85%)

Si: Lepromatous to tuberculoid spectrum: nodular accumulations in skin, mucous membranes, and other organs, especially on face, organisms are in these "globi"; to thickened peripheral nerves; to decreased sensation in extremities leading to mutilation and loss, pain and temperature sensation diminished

Absent wheal and flare response; vitiligo

Crs:

Cmplc: Arthritis, septic w bacteria in joint histiocytes (Nejm 1973;289: 1410); secondary amyloid; **erythema nodosum leprosum** w painful skin nodules, fever, wasting, rx'd w thalidomide (Med Let 1996;38:15)

Lab:

Bact: AFB-positive smears of globi as well as blood and buffy coat since bacteria both free and in wbc's in lepromatous type, decrease in numbers correlates w rx over months, average rx duration = 105 mo (Nejm 1972;287:159); and of marrow histiocytes (Nejm 1979;300:834)

Path: Skin bx of globi and/or nerve bx show epithelioid cell collections w/o distinct tubercles; nerves surrounded by microscopic tubercles

Serol: VDRL, cryoglobulin, rheumatoid factor often pos in lepromatous, not tuberculoid types

Rx: Prevent w BCG immunization?, questionable results (Ann IM 1978; 88:538); isolation unnecessary; DDS (Dapsone) effective prophylaxis for household contacts (Ann IM 1978;88:539)

of disease, triple rx w clofazimine (Med Let 1987;29:77) 50–100 mg po qd, +sulfones, eg, DDS (Dapsone = diaminodiphenylsulfone), +rifampin; or combinations of minocycline, clarithromycin, ciprofloxacin, and augmentin. Cmplc of rx: erythema nodosum leprosum, rx w thalidomide (Med Let 1998;40:104)

May become noninfectious in weeks (Ann IM 1976;85:82) to 3 mo; 2$^+$ yr course, longer w lepromatous type

9.6 SPIROCHETES

LYME DISEASE

Nejm 2001;345:115; 1993;329:936; 1989;320:133

Cause: *Borrelia burgdorferi* spread by *Ixodes dammini* tick bite (same tick also spreads babesiosis and pts may get both—Ann IM 1985; 103:374)

Epidem: Deer tick, also infests white-footed deer mice. Northeastern and northwestern US. HLA DR$_4$ and DRw2 B-cell allotypes associated w increased CNS, cardiac, and arthritic involvement (Nejm 1990; 323:219). Most common tickborne spirochetal disease in US; attack rates up to 66% of people living in a highly endemic area over 7 yr

(Nejm 1989;320:133); annual incidence = 20–80/100,000/yr; also common in N. Europe (Nejm 1995;333:1319)

Pathophys: Sometimes an immune complex disease, but organisms now identified in joints most of the time (Nejm 1994;330:229). Clinical syndromes very much like primary, secondary, and tertiary syphilis; but much overlap between stage 1 and 2 sx complexes

Sx: (Nejm 1991;325:159) Tick bite (should remove w tweezers) hx in 80% (Nejm 1995;333:1319); disease rare if tick on <24 h, usually takes 72 hr and most ticks associated w disease have stayed on a week (Nejm 1992;327:543)

Stage 1: Arthralgias (98%), malaise (80%), headache (64%), fever (60%), stiff neck (aseptic meningitis); ringworm-like rash erythema chronicum marginatum (ECM) in 77% (Nejm 1995;333:1319)

Stage 2: Neurologic and cardiac

Stage 3: Arthritis; chronic neurologic changes

Si:

Stage 1: Fever, lymphadenopathy; and erythema chronicum migrans, a warm "ringworm" around bite (ECM), median diam = 15 cm (pictures—Ann IM 1991;114:490; 1983;99:76) present in 60–80%

Stage 2: Neurologic: lymphocytic meningitis (15%) and meningoencephalitis, peripheral motor or sensory neuropathies, facial nerve palsies including Bell's palsy. And/or cardiac: myocarditis (8%), like rheumatic fever w heart block but valve disease rare or never; sometimes heart block is only sx, no fever or even malaise; usually transient, ~6 wk after primary infection

Stage 3: Recurrent polyarthritis at 1st, then 1–2 large joints; onset up to 4–6 mo after skin rash w decreasing recurrences over years (Ann IM 1987;107:725). Late keratitis (Nejm 1991;325:159)

Crs: Stage 1 lasts 3–4 wk. Sx and si of stages 2 and 3 may be chronic and recurrent over mo-yr. Even after rx, especially if given >3 mo after sx, residual arthralgias, fatigue, memory problems may persist (Ann IM 1994;121:560). Very benign crs in children (Nejm 1996;335;1270)

Cmplc: Chronic myocardiopathy (Nejm 1990;322:249). Neurologic (Nejm 1990;323:1438): chronic encephalopathy in 90% of those who have stage 2 neurologic sx; also chronic polyneuropathy and leukoencephalitis

r/o Ehrlichiosis, babesiosis (p 466) as separate or concomitant infection (Nejm 1997;337:27; Jama 1996;275:1657)

Lab:

Hem: ESR >20 mm/h (53%), crit >37% (88%), wbc <10,000 (92%)

Path: Pos silver stain or culture of rash edge for organisms in 86% (Jama 1992;268:1311)

Serol: (Jama 1999;282:62; Ann IM 1997;127:1109) need reliable lab; IgM and IgG ELISA titer increased (Nejm 1983;308:733) and pos Western blot; rare false positives, most in low-prevalence populations, in syphilis, and SBE (Ann IM 1993;119:1079); ≤5% false neg especially in late stages (Ann IM 1987;107:730), seen if early po antibiotic rx or early in crs, or w some labs which run 10–50% false neg and up to 25% false pos (Jama 1992;268:891). Immune complex measurement (Jama 1999;282:1942)

Synovial fluid: Organisms usually present by PCR (Nejm 1994; 330:229)

Rx: (Med Let 2000;42:37; Jama 1995;274:66; Ann IM 1991;111:472)
Prevent w:

- Permethrin (Nix) rx of clothing and DEET at 75$^+$% concentration (Med Let 1989;31:46)
- Remove ticks within 24 h
- Vaccinate w Osp-A antigen (Lymerix) (Rx Let 2000;7:11; 1999; 6:3; Med Let 1999;41:29,46; Nejm 1998;339:209,216,263) 3 shot series at 0, 1, and 2–6 mo w q 1 yr boost, for ages 15–70, not children; ~75% effective after 3 doses, unclear how long immunity lasts and long term safety unclear, could cause autoimmune arthritis (Med Let 1999;41:46)

Prophylactic rx after tick bite perhaps, doxycycline 200 mg po ×1, if engorged and in high-prevalence area (Nejm 2001;345:79 vs. 133)

of stage 1 (Med Let 1989;31:57): to decrease post rash arthritis and illness (Ann IM 1983;99:22)

- 1st: Tetracycline 250 mg qid or doxycycline 100 mg bid × 21 d; or, for children and pregnant women, amoxicillin 250–500 mg po tid × 21 d, but misses concomitant *Ehrlichia* infections; or
- 2nd: Erythromycin 250 mg po qid × 10 d, or penicillin 20 million U qd iv × 10 d, or cefuroxime 500 mg po bid × 21 d (Ann IM 1992;117:273)

of stages 2 and 3: doxycycline 200 mg po bid or amoxicillin as above but for 4–6 wk (Nejm 1994;330:229) or ceftriaxone 2 gm iv/im × 14–21 d especially if bad arthritis or cardiac/neurologic findings, only 1/13 failures (Nejm 1988;319:1661); or penicillin G 20 million U qd iv × 10–21 d for cardiac, or neurologic abnormalities and/or

ID: BACTERIOLOGY

meningitis (Ann IM 1983;99:767), cures 55% of arthritis. Avoid intraarticular steroids (Nejm 1985;312:869)

of acute non-meningitis disseminated disease: doxycycline 100 mg po bid × 21d, equally effective as ceftriaxone 2 gm im qd × 14d (Nejm 1997;337:289)

of heart block: antibiotics and temporary pacer (Ann IM 1989;110: 339) since usually transient

of chronic encephalopathy: 60–85% improve w ceftriaxone rx given even after several years

if pos titers or hx and chronic fatigue/fasciitis syndrome, antibiotic rx not helpful (DBCT—Nejm 2001;343:85; Ann IM 1993;119:503, 518)

SYPHILIS (Lues)

Nejm 1992;326:1060

Cause: *Treponema pallidum*

Epidem: Incidence = 20^+/100,000 in US, increasing since 1985; spread via direct contact (venereal) with primary (1°) or secondary (2°) lesion

Pathophys: In 2°, marked bacteremia. Tertiary (3°) types probably represent hypersensitivity reactions since few organisms are present. Gummas, from endarteritis obliterans, which causes necrosis, eg, in aortic media. Three types of neurosyphilis:

- **Tabes dorsalis**
- Meningovascular
- **General paresis of the insane** (GPI), primary parenchymal involvement

All 3° complications are increased in AIDS (Nejm 1987;316:1600)

Sx:

1°: Painless chancre

2°: Rash, round with pigmented center; fever; headache; alopecia; eye pain from iritis

Si:

1°: Chancre with edema (looks like squamous cell cancer), and nonsuppurative lymphadenitis

2°: Macular/papular/pustular rash w pustules, annular-appearing as ages, on palms and soles; split papules at mouth corners and other moist body areas (condyloma lata); diffuse lymphadenopathy; meningitis

3°:

- Neurosyphilis: Argyle-Robertson pupils (small, unequal, reactive to accommodation not light); general paresis dementia; meningovascular, strokes, meningitis and cranial nerve palsies (Nejm 1994;331:1469,1516) most commonly seen within 3–4 yr of primary infection especially in AIDS pts, tabes dorsalis w motor long tract and sensory losses usually in lower extremities
- Vascular including aortitis w AI and aneurysms in 10%
- Gummas in 15%; 75% are cutaneous

Congenital: onset at age 14^+ weeks even if seronegative at birth; si: rash, fever, hepatosplenomegaly, rhinitis, lymphadenopathy, elevated LFTs, CSF cells, and protein (Nejm 1990;323:1299); notched permanent (Hutchinson's) teeth, in 25%; interstitial keratitis in 50%; saddle nose

Crs:

1°: 9–90 d, 20–30% develop secondary syphilis

2°: Months if no rx

Cmplc:

1°: r/o herpes and chancroid (both tender)

2°: Obstructive pattern hepatitis (Nejm 1971;284:1422); nephrosis from immune complex disease (Nejm 1975;292:449)

3°: Cirrhosis (Med Clin N Am 1964;48:613)

r/o **bejel/pinta** from *T. carateum,* spread by skin-to-skin contact w lesions, as well as by flies in pinta. Bejel in Arabia, pinta in Central and South America. Primary disease consists of a nonulcerating papule; secondary, of pigmented skin lesions later becoming depigmented and hyperkeratotic; tertiary of cardiovascular and nervous system involvement. Rx w penicillin

r/o **yaws** from *T. pertenue* spread skin to skin in many tropical areas, especially affecting children. An ulcerating papule w "strawberry" scar formation. Rx w penicillin

Lab:

Bact: Dark field shows bacteria w 8–14 spirals, ~7 m long; false positives in mouth from normal treponema flora there

CSF: Do LP 1 yr post rx of 1° or 2° types if VDRL or FTA still positive; in meningovascular syphilis elevated protein, and cells are present; VDRL positive in 50% but can be negative even if bacteria present, getting FTA hence better. Probably best to just rx for 3–4 wk without LP if asx (Ann IM 1986;104:86)

Serol: (rv—Ann IM 1986;104:368)

- VDRL or RPR is positive in 76% of 1° cases (if negative, dark field positive still), 100% of 2° cases; and 75% of 3° cases; false pos (>1/16) in mononucleosis, malaria, collagen vascular diseases, sarcoid, leprosy, yaws, pinta
- TPI is positive in 50% of 1°, 98% 2°, and 90% of 3° cases
- FTA (Nejm 1969;280:1086) positive in 90% 1°, 99% 2°, 98% 3° cases; false positives in only 30% VDRL false-positive patients, some w yaws, pinta, or in 10% lupus but is atypical (beaded—Nejm 1970;282:1287); remains positive all life

Xray: Congenital type has lytic areas (bites) in long bones, subperiosteal

Rx: (Med Let 1999;41:89) same even if HIV positive (Nejm 1997;337:307)

Prevent by partner notification, usefulness limited (Ann IM 1990;112:539)

of early disease (1°, 2°, or latent <1 yr): 1st, benzathine penicillin (Bicillin) 2.4 million U im × 1, or azithromycin 1 gm po × 1 (Ann IM 1999;131:434); 2nd, doxycycline 100 mg po bid × 14 d; or 3rd, erythromycin 500 mg po qid × 14 d

of late, short of neurosyphilis: 1st, benzathine penicillin 2.4 million U im weekly × 3 wk; or 2nd, doxycycline 100 mg po bid × 4 wk

of neurosyphilis: penicillin G 2–4 million U iv q 4 h × 10–14 d; or 2nd, procaine penicillin 2.4 million U im qd + probenecid (Benemid) 500 mg po qid × 10–14 d

of congenital: penicillin G 50,000 U/kg im/iv q 8–12 h × 10–14 d, or procaine penicillin 50,000 U/kg im qd × 10–14 d

If penicillin allergy: ceftriaxone im qd × 10 d, or tetracycline 2 gm qd or doxycycline 100 mg po bid × 15 d (12% failure rate) or erythromycin 2 gm qd × 10 d (30 d for tertiary) (12% failure rate). Rx for 28 d if late latent disease

rx crs: <1% relapse; follow VDRL, goes negative in 3–6 mo; w CNS lues, follow CSF cells; Herxheimer reaction (endotoxin sx w fever) within hours after penicillin (Nejm 1976;295:21). Longer rx in AIDS where early neurosyphilis develops (Nejm 1994;331:1469, 1488,1516; Ann IM 1991;114:872; 1988;109:855) and penicillin rx only transiently effective since long-term cure normally depends on immunity

9.7 MYCOPLASMA/CHLAMYDIA

CHLAMYDIAL ATYPICAL PNEUMONIAS AND URIs

Jama 1997;277:1214; Clin Inf Dis 1992;15:757; Ann IM 1987;106:507; Nejm 1986;315:189

Cause: *Chlamydia pneumoniae* (TWAR agent) which was previously thought to be *psittaci* (Nejm 1986;315:161)

Epidem: 100,000 cases/yr in US; nearly half of all adults have a titer

Pathophys: Pneumonia and bronchitis

Sx: 7–14 d incubation period

Sore throat and hoarseness often 1st sx; fever only early in crs; dry cough often late in crs

Si: Minimal findings on chest exam; worse in elderly

Crs: Long (weeks) even w rx

Cmplc: Chronic infections may increase MIs? (Ann IM 1996;125:979, 1992;116:273)

r/o mycoplasma (cold agglutinins)

Xray: Chest, may show atypical pneumonic infiltrate

Lab:

Serol: Paired sera allow dx of nonspecific chlamydial infection retrospectively

Rx: Tetracycline or erythromycin 500 mg qid × 10–14 d

CHLAMYDIAL NONSPECIFIC URETHRITIS (NSU), PROCTITIS, MUCOPURULENT CERVICITIS, PELVIC INFLAMMATORY DISEASE

Nejm 1994;330:115; Ann IM 1988;108;710; 1986;104:524

Cause: *Chlamydia trachomatis;* in NSU in men, also *Ureaplasma* and *Mycoplasma* spp

Epidem: Venereal; over 50% of nonspecific urethritis episodes in males; 11% of proctitis in gay males (Nejm 1981;305:195); 12%

prevalence in Maine women (Maine Epigram 5/87), 7–15% in Army women recruits (Nejm 1998;339:739). Transmission rates males to females and vice versa nearly equal as are the asx infection rates (Jama 1996;276:1737)

Pathophys:

Sx: 1/3 asx in males

Si: Urethral discharge in male; proctitis, mild in gays

Cervical swab shows yellow mucopurulent discharge (14% false pos—Nejm 1984;311:1; Ann IM 1982;97:216)

Pharyngitis, from fellatio (Ann IM 1985;102:757)

Crs:

Cmplc: Epididymitis (the etiology in 1/2 the cases of epididymitis); endometritis, PID, perihepatitis like Fitzhugh-Curtis syndrome of gonorrhea; male sterility (Nejm 1983;308:502,505; Am J Pub Hlth 1993;83:996) and female sterility (worse than gc). r/o gc and mycoplasma PID

Acute conjuctivitis in newborn (ophthalmia neonatorum) (r/o herpes simplex w ulcerations) from gc or chlamydia, latter more common, 5% of all U Wash deliveries; a smaller % have pneumonitis, from 1 to 60 d postpartum, average 15 d, rx w erythromycin × 14 d (Med Let 1995;35:117)

Lab:

Bact: Single swab culture is 100% specif, 75% sens (Ann IM 1987; 107:189); smears: males have >4 polys/hpf by urethral swab even if no discharge; females have 10^+ polys/h0f (at 1000×), 17% false pos, 10% false neg (Holmes—Nejm 1984;311:1)

Path: Pap smear detection unreliable

Serol: Enzyme immunoassay method (ELISA) on secretions or urine (Jama 1993;270:2065) can be done in <30 min; 80% sens, 98% specif (Ann IM 1987;107:189); use to screen. DNA amplification assay of urine very accurate, 89% sens, 99% specif, ? availability (Nejm 1998;339:739,768; Ann IM 1996;124:1)

Rx:

Prevent w:

- In adult, barrier methods or birth control pills
- At birth, povidone iodine 2.5% soln gtts OU is more effective, less toxic, and cheaper (Nejm 1995;332:562) than tetracycline,

erythromycin, or silver nitrate gtts, which still miss some gc, hence have a 10–20% incidence of ophthalmic disease in newborns of infected mothers (Nejm 1989;320:769)

Screen: (p 680)

- All multiple partnered asx men (jama 1996;276:1737), and women to reduce PID sterilization rates from 2% to 1%/yr (Nejm 1996;334:1362), or all women under age 25–30 (Nejm 1998;339: 739, 768; Ann IM 1998;128:277)
- All pregnant women early and at 36 wk w cultures if expected prevalence >7% (Ann IM 1987;107:188), or at least lower socioeconomic groups, and rx positives w erythromycin 500 mg qid × 7 d; this strategy decreases postnatal eye and lung infections, when given asx mothers prepartum, from infections in 50% of infants to 7% (Nejm 1986;314:276)

of active disease (Med Let 1999;41:85) by treating patient and partner (Med Let 1994;36:1; Nejm 1978;298:490) with:

- 1st: Azithromycin (Zithromax) 1 gm po × 1 (Jama 1995;274:545; Nejm 1992;377:921; Med Let 1991;33:119)
- Tetracycline 500 mg qid × 7 d (Ann IM 1982;97:216), 250 qid × 14–21 d, or doxycycline 100 bid × 7 d, or × 2– 3 wk for proctitis
- Ofloxacin 300 mg po bid × 7 d
- Minocycline 100 mg po hs × 7 d (Ann IM 1993;119:16)

2nd (1st choice in pregnancy):

- Erythromycin 500 mg qid × 7 d or × 3 wk after tetracycline failure (Ann IM 1990;113:21) that may be due to tetracycline-resistant *Ureaplasma,* for adults; nonestolated types ok in pregnancy (Med Let 1991;33:119); 12.5 mg/kg/d po or iv × 14 d for neonatal pneumonia or conjunctivitis
- Amoxicillin

PRIMARY ATYPICAL PNEUMONIA

Rev Inf Dis 1990;12:338; Mayo Cl Proc 1986;61:830; Nejm 1981; 304:80; 1971;285:374 (Emory fraternity epidemic)

Cause: *Mycoplasma pneumonia* (pleuropneumonia-like organism [PPLO]; Eaton agent)

Epidem: Probably airborne respiratory droplets. Highest incidence in young adults; 10% of all their respiratory diseases; 49% attack rate in single-exposure epidemic. Intimate and prolonged contact, eg, intrafamilial, usually necessary for spread

Pathophys: Intracellular infection

Sx: Malaise (85%), cough (85%), headache (77%), fever (65%), sore throat (44%), sweats (37%), myalgias (41%), arthralgias

Si: Bronchitis; pneumonia (27%); vesicle on tympanic membrane (bullous myringitis), 12% overall, more common age 5–15 yr; rash

Crs:

Cmplc: Hemolytic anemia w cold agglutinins (Nejm 1977;296:1490); peri- and myocarditis (Ann IM 1977;86:544); Guillain-Barré syndrome (Ann IM 1981;94:15)

Lab:

Serol: Specific comp-fix antibodies increased. Nonspecific cold agglutinins increased (IgM), 35–75% of patients will be positive after 7 d of illness (Ann IM 1977;86:547); r/o collagen vascular disease, lymphoproliferative disease, mononucleosis

Xray: Chest infiltrates; and/or pleural effusions (in 25%—Nejm 1970; 283:790)

Rx: Macrolide drug of choice because effective and also gets pneumococcus, eg erythromycin, azithromycin, or clarithromycin; tetracycline, but 50% after rx still have nonresistant organisms in respiratory tract (Nejm 1967;277:719) although same may also be true for erythromycin

9.8 RICKETTSIA AND RELATED ORGANISMS

ROCKY MOUNTAIN SPOTTED FEVER

Nejm 1993;329:941; Ann IM 1976;84:752

Cause: *Rickettsia rickettsiae*

Epidem: Carried by ticks (large and visible) from wild rodent reservoirs. Endemic in Rocky Mountain rodents; also on Cape Cod and throughout most mid-Atlantic states including Virginia and North Carolina; also seen in lab technicians working w ticks. 700–1000 cases/yr in US

Pathophys: Angiitis due to endothelial infection causing proliferation and thrombosis via activation of kallikrein-kinin system (Ann IM 1978; 88:764). Subclinical DIC changes in platelet and clotting system detectable even before sx (Nejm 1988;318:1021)

Sx: Seasonal; 95% of cases between April and August. Tick bite (most recall) or dog contact. Incubation period, 5–7 d. Severe frontal headache (90%) is usually first sx; myalgias (80%), emesis (60%)

Si: Rash (90%), centripetal progression (extremities to trunk), palm and sole involved (in 2/12); toxic w fever leading to confusion (in 10/13); muscle tenderness, especially calf and thigh; diffuse angiitis; skin necrosis regardless of pressure points

Crs:

Cmplc: Mortality without rx = 25%; w rx, 5%. Carditis, cerebral edema, DIC

r/o Babesiosis; (p 466) rat bite fever; **rickettsial pox** (Nejm 1994;331:1612) from *Rickettsia akari,* seen all over US, initial lesion at mouse mite bite, 1 wk latency then fever, malaise, and chicken pox-like vesicular lesions, not too sick, can rx w tetracycline; other rickettsial pox in other parts of world, eg, **North Asian rickettsiosis, African tick bite fever** (Nejm 2001;344:1504), **Queensland tick typhus, typhus**

Lab:

Hem: Thrombocytopenia (Nejm 1969;280:58) and DIC

Path: Skin bx of rash positive on immunofluorescent stain (available from CDC)

Serol: Antibody increased by immunofluorescence or microagglutination by day 15. Weil-Felix test: in Rocky Mountain spotted fever, OX2 and OX19 positive, OXK negative; in rickettsial pox, all neg

Rx: 1st, tetracycline; or 2nd, chloramphenicol

CAT SCRATCH FEVER

Nejm 1997;337:1876; 1994;330:1509; Ann IM 1993;118:388

Cause: *Bartonella (Rochalimaea) henselae* (Nejm 1994;330:509; Ann IM 1993;118:331). *Afipia felis,* a closely related organism, may be the cause in some cases

Epidem: Young cats, infected for a few weeks; transmit via bites, scratches, and fleas; 80% of cases are in pts under age 21

Cat Scratch Fever, continued

Pathophys:
Sx: Bite or scratch by kitten (90% have had by hx); 7–14 d incubation; then papule at site of scratch. Papule at site of infection; fever (<50%), adenopathy (40% of nodes suppurate)
Si: As above
Crs: All benign including cmplc
Cmplc: Encephalopathy/encephalitis (10%), conjunctivitis, purpura (suppressed platelets), mesenteric adenitis, endocarditis (Ann IM 1996;125:646); hypercalcemia (Jama 1998;279:532)

in AIDS patients (Ann IM 1988;109:449) and otherwise immuno-compromised hosts, disseminated disease; **bacillary angiomatosis** (Nejm 1997;337:1876,1888,1916;1995;332:419,424), which looks somewhat like Kaposi's sarcoma, cutaneous and deep tissue infections as well as osteolytic bone lesions; and **peliosis hepatis** (Nejm 1992;327:1625; 1990;323:1573,1581), occasionally also seen in the immunocompetent (Ann IM 1993;118:363)

Lab:
CSF: Protein increased; occasionally mononuclear cells in 10%
Bact: Small pleomorphic gram-neg
Hem: Elevated ESR and white count w left shift; eosinophils elevated modestly
Path: Biopsy shows organism w Warthin-Starry and silver stains
Serol: Bartonella henselae titers >1/64 (84% sens, 96% specif—Nejm 1993;329:8), from CDC, available commercially as well
Skin test: DHS pos in 30 d, homemade from ground-up nodes; no longer used due to AIDS and other viral risks
Rx: None may be indicated in mild disease except aspiration of fluctuant nodes to decrease sx
of disease:
- Erythromycin 500 mg po qid or other macrolide, especially for disseminated forms
- Doxycycline 100 mg po bid, especially for disseminated forms if can't tolerate erythromycin
- Ciprofloxacin 500 mg po bid (Jama 1991;265:1563)
- Tm/S for children
- Gentamicin iv × 5 d (West J Med 1991;154:330)
- Ceftriaxone, cefotaxime, or amikacin (J Clin Microbiol 1991; 29: 2450)

9.9 MISCELLANEOUS

Bactericidal activity titer (serum) of unproven use even in SBE (Nejm 1985;312:968); others say is useful (in osteo—Am J Med 1988;83:218; in SBE—Am J Med 1985;78:262)

Catheter-induced phlebitis and colonization: tip culture and Gram stain (Nejm 1985;312:1142); plastic Teflon tips no worse than steel (Ann IM 1991;114:845); change over guidewire if no obvious infection, or use new site if obvious infection and culture tip, >15 colonies is significant (Nejm 1992;327:1062)

Fever, false negatives: oral temperature will be $2^{+\circ}$F less than rectal if respiratory rate >20, difference increases w more rapid respirations (Nejm 1983;308:945)

Fever of unknown origin (FUO) (Petersdorf 100 patients—Med 1961;40:1, update—1982;61:269; Ann IM 1969;70:864; MGH—Nejm 1973;289:1407). Definition: fever >101°F (>38.3°C) daily 3^{+} weeks and 1 week hospital or physician workup (p 832) for differential when fever associated w polyarthritis). See Table 9.9.1

Handwashing: Chlorhexidine (Hibiclens) use is better than soap + isopropyl alcohol (Nejm 1992;327:88)

Penicillin allergy (Jama 2001;285:2498; Am J Med 1999;107:166; Arch IM 1992;152:930,1025; Ann IM 1987;107:204; Nejm 1985;312: 1229); 5% have cephalothin cross reactivity (Nejm 2001; 345:804)

Penicylloyl-polylysine (Prepen-major determinant skin test positive in 80% of people allergic to benzyl penicillin G, cephalothin, and benzyl penicillinoic acid) scratch (10 U/cc), then intracutaneous; will detect 96^{+}% of reactors, 100% of anaphylactics; 50% false positive for skin reactions, 75% for anaphylaxis

If tests negative, proceed; if positive, phenoxymethyl penicillin elixir in progressive po 100-U increments, double q 15 min to 1.3 million U total. Beware: penicillin IgE allergy attenuates over years so patients may have anaphylaxis and 5 yr later not be allergic by above tests

ID: BACTERIOLOGY

Table 9.9.1 Fever of Unknown Origin (% per Petersdorf series)

Infections (36%)	Collagen-vascular (13%)	Miscellaneous (30%)	Neoplasms (19%)	No dx (2%)
Tbc (11)	Rheum fever (6)	Regional enteritis	Disseminated or localized of pancreas, liver, kidney (9)	
Liver/biliary (7)	SLE (5)	Pericarditis	Lymphoma/ leukemia (8)	
Abdominal abscess (4)	Unclassified (2)	Allergic hepatitis	No histologic dx (2)	
Pyelonephritis (3)	RA (84% present as FUO in children—Nejm 1967;276:11)	Thyroiditis		
Psittacosis (2)	Polymyalgia rheumatica	Myelofibrosis		
Cirrhosis and bacteremia (1)		Erythema multiforme		
GC arthritis (1)		Panniculitis (Weber-Christian disease)		
Malaria (1)		Neuroleptic malignant syndrome		
Yersinia		Drug fever (protean nature, rv—Ann IM 1987;106:728)		
Fastidious bug, eg, microaerophilic strep		Pulmonary embolus		
SBE		Sarcoid		
Osteomyelitis		FMF		
Cholangitis		Ruptured spleen/ pancreas		
Sinusitis		Factitious (self-induced or faked)		

but on reexposure will resensitize fast. Thus must retest every time want to use in patient w positive hx

Prophylactic antibiotics

- Bacterial endocarditis (SBE) (Med Let 1999;41:80; Jama 1997; 277:1794; Nejm 1995;332:38): Use anytime bacteria-containing mucosa is breached, esp if indication is high risk (h/o SBE, artificial valve, cyanotic heart disease, surgical shunts):

  For dental procedures that cause bleeding (case control study finds no benefit?—Ann IM 1998;129:761,829), T+A, surgery on gi or upper respir mucosa, sclero rx of varices, esophageal dilatation, OB surgery, cystoscopy, urethral dilatation, urethral catheterization if UTI, urinary tract/prostate surgery, I+D of infected tissue, vaginal hysterectomy, infected vag delivery

  Not for sigmoidoscopy (Ann IM 1976;85:77), other endoscopy w bx, cesarian section, normal vaginal delivery (Ann IM 1983;98:509)

  Antibiotic choice:

  For dental and upper respiratory tract give 1 hr po or 1/2 hr iv before procedure, amoxicillin 2 gm; if penicillin-allergic, clindamycin 600 mg iv/po, or cephalexin 2 gm iv, or cefazolin 2 gm iv, or azithromycin 500 mg po

  For procedures below diaphragm, ampicillin 2 gm alone or if high risk w gentamicin 1.5 mg/kg (up to 80 mg) 1/2 hr before + 1 gm amoxicillin/ampicillin po/iv 6 hr later; if penicillin-allergic, substitute vancomycin 1 gm iv for amoxicillin/ampicillin

- Leukemics: ? Norfloxacin (Ann IM 1987;106:1, 7) or ciprofloxacin
- Splenectomy patients: Phenoxymethyl penicillin 250 mg bid (Med Let 1977;19:3), consider especially if not immunized, or use prn fever
- Surgical (Med Let 1999;41:75): Cephazolin (vancomycin if allergic or lots of MRSA around) for all except colorectal/appendectomy where use cefotetan or cefoxitin to help w anaerobes. Single iv dose, half-hour preop or at least <2 h preop (Nejm 1992;326:281) for clean cardiovascular, orthopedic, and cranial surgery; clean or contaminated ENT, gi, and gyn surgery including C/S for PROM and therapeutic abortion. In gyn surgery, antibiotics help most w fast as compared to prolonged surgery, and abdominal more than vaginal hysterectomy (Nejm 1982;307:1661). For dirty wound or ruptured viscus surgery, rx as infected × 7–10 d, ie, not prophylaxis
- Prosthetic joint patients: Erythromycin before dental work (Am J Pub Hlth 1990;79:739)

ID: BACTERIOLOGY

Protective isolation no benefit (Nejm 1981;304:433,448) but at least eliminate salads in granulocytopenics

Sepsis/septic shock, Gram-negative shock Ann IM 1994;121:1, 1994;120:771; 1990;113:227; Nejm 1993; 328:1471

Pathophys: Systemic inflammatory response (SRS) define by P >90, respir >20, T >96.8–100.4°F (>36–38.0°C), pCO_2 <32, WBC >12,000 or <4000; progresses to sepsis, which progresses to septic shock (Jama 1995;273:117). Nitric oxide production may be a mechanism that can be rx'd w inhibitors (Jama 1996;275:1192)

Cmplc: Encephalopathy correllates w severity of sepsis and Glasgow coma scale score (Jama 1996;275:470)

Rx: In shock, steroid bolus no help, may worsen (Crit Care Med 1995; 23:1294; Nejm 1987;317:653,659); rx w iv fluids and antibiotics to cover staph and *Pseudomonas* like 3rd generation cephalosporin + aminoglycoside (Med Let 1999;41:97); NSAIDs help fever but no improvement in survival (Nejm 1997;336:912)

Experimental monoclonal anti-endotoxins of no help (Jama 2000;283: 1723; Ann IM 1994;121:1); nor is tumor necrosis factor receptor rx (Jama 1997;277:1531; Nejm 1996;334:1697)

Activated protein C if shock and end organ failure, improves survival by 6% (NNT = 16) (Nejm 2001;344:699)

Traveler's advice (Nejm 2000;342:1716; Med Let 1999;41:39; CDC web site: www.cdc.gov, or phone information: 888-232-3228); consider, depending on the destination and length of stay:

• Traveler's diarrhea prophylaxis and/or rx prn (p 306)
• Immunizations for hep A and B as combo vaccine Twinrix at 0, 1 and 6 mo, cost $92/dose (Med Let 2001;43:67); Japanese B encephalitis, measles if born after 1956 and haven't had 2 doses of vaccine over age 1, meningococcus, polio, diphtheria/tetanus, typhoid, and yellow fever
• Malaria prophylaxis (CDC phone: (770)488-7788)

Chapter 10
Infectious Disease: Fungal Infections

D. K. Onion and S. Sears

10.1 ANTIFUNGALS

Med Let 1997;39:86

AZOLES
Nejm 1994;330:263

All can cause nausea and vomiting, rashes, and hepatotoxicity; all impair cytochrome 450 enzymes so impair metabolism of many drugs (Med Let 1996;38:72) like erythromycin, non-sedating antihistamines, benzodiazepams, cisapride

- Amphotericin B, 1 mg test dose, 0.3–1 mg/kg iv in D5W over 2 h, or perhaps better over 24k (Bmj 2001;322:579) qd or qod × wk, or as 100 mg/cc oral suspension for AIDS oral candidiasis (Med let 1997; 39:14), or liposomal amphotericin B, which may be less toxic (Nejm 1999;340:764); vs *Candida,* mucor, *Cryptococcus,* histolmosis, blastomycosis, and extracutaneous sporotrichosis. Adverse effects: RTA and renal damage especially >4 gm, chills (rx with meperidine 25 mg iv or prevent w hydrocortisone, ASA, acetaminophen, or antihistamines), hypokalemia, anemia, phlebitis, hypotension, pulmonary toxicity (Nejm 1981;304:1185)

    Lipid complex form (Abelcet) (Ann IM 1996;124:921) has less renal toxicity but costs $300–500/d

- Fluconazole (Diflucan) (Ann IM 1990;113:183); 100–400 mg po/iv qd; vs *Candida, Cryptococcus;* none of H$_2$-blocker interference or

453

testosterone problems of ketoconazole. Adverse effects: alopecia (12–20%) after 2 mo rx (Ann IM 1995;123:354), toxic interactions w non-sedating antihistamines like terfenadine (Jama 1996;275:1339)

- Itraconazole (Sporanox) (Med Let 1993;35:7); 200–400 mg po qd × 6–12 mo; may be less toxic than ketoconazole; used vs histo, blasto, invasive aspergillosis; 80–90% effective, but amphotericin still better if life threatening; $10/d for 200 mg qd. Adverse effects: toxic interactions w non-sedating antihistamines (Jama 1996;275:1339), some benzodiazepines and statins (Rx Let 2000;7:17)

- Ketoconazole (Nizoral) (Ann IM 1983;98:13); 0.2–1 gm po qd; rarely used vs coccidioidomycosis, *Candida, Cryptococcus,* blastomycosis, and histoplasmosis; less toxic than amphotericin but generally a little less effective too. Adverse effects: usual as above, Antabuse-like effect, need gastric acid to absorb, anti-testosterone synthesis causes impotence and gynecomastia (Nejm 1987;317:812), decr levels w rifampin (Nejm 1984; 311:1681) and H_2 blockers

- Miconazole (Monostat); topical, po/iv; vs *Monilia,* tinea; chronic mucocutaneous candidiasis (Med Let 1986;21:31). Adverse effects: incr warfarin and phenytoin (Dilantin) levels, hypoglycemia w oral hypoglycemic agents

ECHINOCANDINS

- Caspofungin (Cancidas) (Med Let 2001;43:58) 50 mg iv qd × 30 + d for invasive aspergillosis if amphotericin B or itraconazole can't be used; $10,000/mo

FLUORINATED PYRIMIDINES

- Flucytosine (5-fluorocytosine; Ancobon); 50–150 mg/kg/d po divided qid; w amphotericin for *Cryptococcus,* blastomycosis, and *Candida;* renal excretion. Adverse effects: enterocolitis, dose-dependent leukopenia resistance development prevents using alone

10.2 SYSTEMIC INFECTIONS

ASPERGILLOSIS

Cause: *Aspergillus*

Epidem: Ubiquitous; environmental, eg, from construction, especially from bird guano; air conditioners; a pathogen primarily in the immunocompromised, esp AIDS (Nejm 1991;324:654)

Pathophys: Fungus ball, allergic (Ann IM 1982;96:286), and invasive types. Invasive type is associated w severe and persistent leukopenias and AIDS (Nejm 1991;324:654). Enters through nose in immunocompromised host if nose first sterilized by antibiotics (Ann IM 1979;90:4), or through skin ulcers or iv sites (Nejm 1987; 317:1105)

Sx: Hemoptysis w fungus ball type; asthma w allergic type

Si:

Crs: Invasive type has a 50% survival if start rx within 4 d of infiltrate appearing; much worse if wait (Ann IM 1977;86:539)

Cmplc:

Lab:

> *Bact:* Gram stain shows mycelia in sputum 1/3 of time; blood culture shows occasionally positive if systemic; nose culture 40% false negative, 10% false positive (Ann IM 1979;90:4)
>
> *Hem:* In allergic type, eosinophilia
>
> *Serol:* In allergic type, RIA-specific IgG and IgE (Ann IM 1983;99:18)
>
> *Skin test:* In allergic type shows immediate wheal and flare (Ann IM 1977;86:405)

Rx: in allergic type: steroids, itraconazole 200 mg po qd-bid × 16 + wk (DBCT—Nejm 2000;342:756), electrostatic dust-free filters help (Ann IM 1989;110:115)

in systemic invasive types:

- 1st: Amphotericin 1 mg/kg qd until improve, then double-dose qod, then q 1–2 wk × 3–12 mo
- 2nd: Itraconazole (Sproanox)
- 3rd: Caspofungin (Cancidas)

BLASTOMYCOSIS

Nejm 1986;314:529,575

Cause: *Blastomyces dermatitidis*
Epidem: Airborne in rotten wood dust. North America especially around the Great Lakes and southeastern US
Pathophys:
Sx: 3–12 wk incubation period. Asx (50%), cough (45%), headache (32%), chest pain (30%), weight loss (28%), fever (25%)
Si:
Crs: Usually self-limited, 3–4 wk (Nejm 1974;290:540)
Cmplc: r/o **South American blastomycosis** caused by paracoccidioidomycosis (*Paracoccidioides brasiliensis*), which is transmitted by thorn pricks and causes skin disease that looks like leprosy; rx'd w sulfonamides
Lab:
Bact: Diphasic but yeast form in tissue; *brasiliensis* has multiple budding in yeast form
Serol: CF antibodies positive in only 10% (Nejm 1974;290:540); immunodiffusion positive in 28% of true positives; enzyme immunoassay positive in 77%
Skin test: Doubtful usefulness, positive in <40% proven cases (Am Rev Respir Dis 1988;138:1081; Nejm 1986;314:529,575)
Xray: Positive chest xray if pulmonic
Rx: Amphotericin, or miconazole, or ketoconazole 400 mg qd po × 6 mo (low dose) results in 80% cure; high dose (800 mg qd) results in 100% cure but 60% side effects (Ann IM 1985;103:861, 872); not for meningitis. Perhaps itraconazole

Alternative for North American blastomycosis, 2-hydroxystilbamidine iv, if confined to skin or noncavitary in lung; amphotericin is just as good (Nejm 1974;290:320)

Alternative for South American blastomycosis, sulfonamides

COCCIDIOIDOMYCOSIS (Valley Fever)

Nejm 1995;332:1077

Cause: *Coccidioides immitis*
Epidem: Airborne spread (inhalation) of mycelial stage infective spores; endospores spread in body (description of storm-scattered epidemic

in California—Nejm 1979;301:358). American southwest, especially Arizona, Texas, and Calif., eg, San Joaquin valley (Stockton to Bakersfield); worst in wet season, especially in patients exposed to dirt in spring and late fall

Increased prevalence (reactivation?) in diabetics and patients on steroid rx, in AIDS and other immunocompromised pts

Sx: Hemoptysis; granulomatous reactions of face and neck; primary cocci picture (Nejm 1972;286:507) of pneumonitis (Nejm 1970;283:325), flu-like syndrome w generalized pruritus macular/papular rash; acute polyarthritis (Nejm 1972;287:1133)

Si: Erythema nodosum, pleural effusion

Crs: Mortality 1% in whites, 20% in Asians and Mexicans with disseminated disease. Recurrent up to 10 yr after amphotericin rx (Nejm 1969;281:950)

Cmplc: Hypercalcemia (Nejm 1977;297:431); extrapulmonary lesions, onset 1+ yr after primary pulmonary infection, eg, bones, joints, skin, meninges

Lab:

Bact: Mycelial form (white, fluffy, distinctive) dangerous to lab personnel. Diphasic but no yeast forms in tissue. Urine culture frequently positive if concentrated by lab, even when don't suspect disseminated disease. Prostate secretions culture also often positive in same circumstances (Ann IM 1976;85:34)

Serol: Comp-fix antibody titer >1/16 suggests disseminated active disease. Positive in 14/15 (Nejm 1970;283:326); decreases w successful rx. Counterimmunoelectrophoresis titer has 8% false-negative rate (Ann IM 1976;85:740)

Skin test: 20–50% false neg but still useful (Am Rev Respir Dis 1988; 138:1081); indicates present or past disease

Xray: Nodular pneumonitis; primary pneumonias; coin lesions; thin-walled cavities, r/o rheumatoid nodules and pneumatoceles

Rx: Beware steroids

Meningitis after acute rx must be rx'd w lifelong suppression (Ann IM 1996;124:305) of acute disease (Nejm 1987;317:334):

- Amphotericin 0.5 mg/kg iv 2x/wk to total of 30 mg/kg if sick, if comp-fix is increased, or if hx of and on steroids; 20% relapse (4/20—Nejm 1970;283:325); intrathecal for meningitis, many complications especially w reservoir (Nejm 1973;288:186).

- Ketoconazole po is at least static in many moderate pulmonary/
  skin infections (Ann IM 1982;96:436,440); vs meningitis (Ann IM
  1983;98:160)
- Fluconazole 400 mg qd po × years effectively suppresses
  meningitis (Ann IM 1993;119:28) and treats >50% of
  non-meningeal infections (Ann IM 2000;133:676)
- Itraconazole 200 mg po bid, cures 63% of non-meningeal
  infections (Ann IM 2000;133:676)

CRYPTOCOCCOSIS
Rev Inf Dis 1991;13:1163; Ann IM 1981;94:611

Cause: *Cryptococcus neoformans*

Epidem: Ubiquitous fungus. Airborne; birds are probable vectors,
especially pigeons, grows well in bird guano. Worldwide. Increased
incidence in patients w lymphomas, and/or on steroids, AIDS

Pathophys:

Sx: Meningitis, pneumonitis (Am Rev Respir Dis 1966;94:236)

Si:

Crs: Without rx, nearly 100% dead in 1 year; with rx, 70% survival, 18%
relapse in 29 mo (Ann IM 1969;71:1079) (rv of good and bad
prognosis test results—Ann IM 1974;80:176)

Cmplc: Renal papillary necrosis (Nejm 1968;279:60); resistant prostatitis
despite rx (Ann IM 1989;111:125)

Lab:

Bact: Smear sputum, CSF, urine; round nucleoli, large nonstaining
capsule, looks like lymphocyte; India ink preparation (drop of ink
to CSF) reveals large clear (large capsules) organisms but 35% can
have CNS crypto and neg India ink prep (NIH—Ann IM 1969;
71:1079)

Culture yeast form on rice/Tween agar at 72°F (22°C) and 98.6°F
(37°C); need large volumes of CSF to find

Serol: Antigen by latex fixation or comp-fix is the only clinically useful
test; antigen in bronchopulmonary lavage fluid 100% sens, 98%
specif (Am Rev Respir Dis 1992;145:226); for antibody, by indirect
fluorescent antibody (IFA); 92% patients positive for one or the
other in CSF and/or serum (Nejm 1977;297:1440); patients w

positive antigen levels do more poorly; false-positive IFA in 2% normals, 6% blastos, 12% histos. No false-positive antigen tests; hence rx a positive antigen but not a positive IFA (Ann IM 1968; 69:1113,1117)

Skin test: False positive in 31%; interferes w serologic testing (Ann IM 1968;69:45)

Xray: CT scan for mass lesions in head that will decrease w medical rx (Ann IM 1981;94:382)

Rx: Isolation (Ann IM 1985;102:593)

- Amphotericin B 2–2.5 gm total course, 0.3–0.7 mg/kg iv qd (Nejm 1997;337:15), can rx q 1 wk in OPD. No proven advantage in intrathecal use (Ann IM 1969;71:1079), lots of complications especially w reservoir for intrathecal use (Nejm 1973;288:186)
- Flucytosine 50–150 mg/kg/d po qid (Ann IM 1977;86:318; Nejm 1974;290:320); hematologic toxicity; use w amphotericin to prevent resistance and vs meningeal disease × 6 wk (Nejm 1979; 301:126) or occasionally 4 wk in otherwise healthy (Nejm 1987;317:334); in AIDS meningitis rx w amphotericin and flucytosine × 2 wk then fluconazole or itraconazole prophylaxis (Nejm 1997;337:15; 1989;321:794)
- Fluconazole or itraconazole as good as and less toxic than amphotericin in AIDS patients w meningitis (Nejm 1992;326:83, 793); maintenance postepisode prevents recurrence in AIDS patients (Nejm 1997;337:15; 1991;324:580)
- Ketoconazole, or miconazole (Ann IM 1983;98:13; 1980;93:569) if above fails (p 454)

HISTOPLASMOSIS

Cause: *Histoplasma capsulatum*

Epidem: Bats and birds vectors via airborne spores. Frequently in rolling green countryside (opposite of cocci), eg, Ohio Valley (Ann IM 1981;94:331—100,000 patient outbreak in Indianapolis)

Pathophys: Intracellular

3 clinical syndromes:
- Acute primary (pulmonary)
- Chronic cavitary (pulmonary)
- Progressive disseminated (Ann IM 1972;76:557)

Sx: Pulmonary, acute immune complex-type polyarthritis
Si: Chorioretinitis, focal, macular choroid inflammation, and hemorrhage without vitreous reaction (present w all other types of chorioretinitis)
Hepatomegaly; erythema nodosa
Crs: Usually benign
Cmplc:

- Fibrosing syndromes of mediastinum and/or retroperitoneum
- Endocarditis
- Adrenal insufficiency in 50% of disseminated form (Ann IM 1971; 75:511)
- Meningitis, chronic, like *Cryptococcus*
- Ulcerative enteritis, especially of distal ileum and colon

Lab:

Bact: Silver stain demonstrates; can't see w H + E or Giemsa. Culture of liver, marrow, nodes; positive in ~20% (Ann IM 1982;97:680). Slow grower, takes >2 wk; filamentous strands of hyphal sporangia; distinctive chlamydospores when grown at room temp

Hem: Anemia, thrombocytopenia; marrow culture and stain positive (all only in disseminated form—MKSAT 1980)

Serol: (Ann IM 1982;97:680): Comp-fix antibody titer positive in 96% of patients w active, disseminated disease. Immunodiffusion antibody titer positive in 87%. RIA for antigen positive in urine (90%) and blood (50%) in disseminated disease (Nejm 1986;314:83) and more accurate than antibody titers (Ann IM 1991;115:936)

Skin test: Many false positives and negatives, interferes w serologic testing (Am Rev Respir Dis 1964;90:927)

Xray: "Buckshot" calcifications in lungs, spleen
Rx: Steroids for choroid infections

1st: Amphotericin 1/2 mg/kg iv × 2/wk to a total of 35–40 mg/kg initial course (Ann IM 1971;75:511); use prophylactically if past hx and starting steroids (Nejm 1969;280:206), or if patient has AIDS and has been rx'd to cure (Ann IM 1989;111:655)

2nd: Ketoconazole, 400 mg qd po × 6 mo cures 85% all types (Ann IM 1985;103:861) even cavitary disease but not meningitis; or itraconazole (Sporanox) 200 mg po bid, prevents relapse in AIDS (Ann IM 1993;118:610)

SYSTEMIC CANDIDIASIS

Ann IM 1984;101:390

Cause: *Candida albicans* (and rarely *tropicalis*—Ann IM 1979;91:539)
Epidem: Associated w immunosuppression, antibiotics, TPN
Pathophys: Normal flora, opportunistic invasion
Sx: Rapid deterioration in a debilitated patient; suppurative peripheral thrombophlebitis (Ann IM 1982;96:431)
Si: Fever, papular/pustular rash like gc
Crs: 36$^+$% mortality (Nejm 1994;331:1325)
Cmplc: Systemic type: myocarditis, endophthalmitis ("a culture of fungus growing on retina") (Nejm 1972;286:675), hepatosplenic abscess (Ann IM 1988;108:88). Purportedly chronic fatigue syndrome, but doubtful (Nejm 1990;323:1717)

Lab:
  Bact: May grow on blood culture but distinction from benign contamination difficult (Ann IM 1974;80:605)
Rx: (Med Let 1990;32:58; 1988;30:30):
  1st: Amphotericin or fluconazole (Nejm 1994;331:1325)
  2nd: Ketoconazole or perhaps high dose flucytosine but resistance develops esp in HIV pts

MUCOR INFECTIONS

Cause: Mucoraceae (*Mucor, Rhizopus,* etc.) (Ann IM 1980;93:93)
Epidem: Skin infections from elastoplast tape (Nejm 1978;299:1115); or sinusitis. Almost exclusively (25/26) in diabetics, usually in DKA; occasionally in patients w hematologic tumors
Pathophys: Pulmonary or CNS; invades vessels causing infarcts without much inflammation
Sx: Pulmonary; CNS; skin and subcutaneous infections, swelling
Si: Vascular infarcts, "black pus"
Crs: Almost always fatal
Cmplc: r/o other opportunistics (p 494)
Lab:
  Path: Must do bx to diagnose
Rx: Amphotericin iv or topical for cutaneous type
  Surgical debridement

Chapter 11

Infectious Disease: Parasitology

D. K. Onion and S. Sears

11.1 MEDICATIONS

ANTIPARASITIC DRUGS
   Med Let 1998;40:1; Nejm 1996;334:1178

- Albendazole (Zentel) perhaps at 400 mg po qd × 5 d to all immigrants (Nejm 1999;340:773); for cutaneous and visceral larval migrans, pinworms, hookworm, hydatid cysts and cysticercosis, whipworm. Adverse effects: reversible alopecia occasionally, LFT elevations, abdominal pain; rarely leukopenia, alopecia, elevated LFTs
- Artemether (Nejm 1996;335:69,76,124) 2–4 mg/kg im qd for cerebral falcip malaria; adverse effects: long QT syndrome
- Atovaquone (Mepron) 750 mg po tid × 21 d for pneumocystosis, possibly malaria. Adverse effects: rash, nausea, diarrhea
- Bithionol (Bitin) 30–50 mg/kg po × 10–15 doses for lung (*Paragonimus westermani*) and liver (*Fasciola hepatica*) flukes; available from CDC only. Adverse effects: photosensitivity, emesis, diarrhea, urticaria; rarely leukopenia, hepatitis
- Chloroquine HCl, chloroquine phosphate (Aralen) 600 mg base (1 gm) or 10 mg/kg, then 300 mg base (500 mg) or 5 mg/kg at 6, 24, and 48 h for malaria; 300 mg or 5 mg/kg base po q 1 wk for prophylaxis; also used occasionally in amebiasis. Adverse effects: emesis, headache/confusion, pruritus, alopecia, weight loss, worse preexisting dermatitis, myalgias; rarely irreversible retinal damage, nail changes,

neuronal deafness, peripheral neuropathy, myopathy, heart block, hematemesis

- Crotamiton (Eurax) 10% soln topically for scabies; adverse effects: rash, conjunctivitis
- Dapsone (DDS, diaminodiphenylsulfone) 100 mg po qd to prevent *Pneumocystis carinii* pneumonia (Ann IM 1995;123:584). Adverse effects: rashes, headache, gi, mono syndrome, etc.
- Dehydroemetine 1–1.5 mg/kg/d im up to 5 d for severe amebiasis. Adverse effects: arrhythmias, muscle weakness; occasional diarrhea, emesis, peripheral neuropathy, CHF, headache
- Diethylcarbamazine (Hetrazan) for filariasis, 50 mg or 1 mg/kg po on day 1; 50 mg or 1 mg/kg po tid day 2; 100 mg or 2 mg/kg po tid day 3; then 9 mg/kg/d divided for 21 d crs. Adverse effects: allergic/febrile reactions w heavy microfilarial load, gi sx; rarely encephalopathy
- Diethyl-m-toluamide (DEET) (Ann IM 1998;128:934) 35% slow release (HourGuard), or 6.5–10% SR formulations; insect repellent, lasts 3–4 hr, better than Skin-So-Soft, citronella, others
- Eflornithine (difluoromethylornithine, DFMO, Ornidyl) for trypanosomiasis. Adverse effects: anemia, leukopenia, diarrhea, thrombocytopenia, seizures; rarely deafness
- Furazolidone (Furonone) 100 mg or 1.5 mg/kg po qid × 7–10 d for giardiasis. Adverse effects: nausea/vomiting, anaphylactoid reactions, hypoglycemia, headache; rarely hemolytic anemia if G6PD-deficient, Antabuse reaction w alcohol, polyneuritis
- Iodoquinol (Yodoxin) 650 mg or 10–12 mg/kg po tid × 20 d for amebiasis and *Dientamoeba fragilis*. Adverse effects: rash, acne, thyroidomegaly, diarrhea, anal itching; rarely optic neuritis; optic atrophy, peripheral neuropathy
- Ivermectin (Mectizan) for refractory scabies, onchocercal filariasis. Adverse effects: malaise/fever w heavy worm load
- Lindane (Kwell) topically for lice and scabies. Adverse effects: rash, headache, conjunctivitis; rarely seizures, aplastic anemia; all incr if skin vasodilated, eg, in warm weather
- Atovaquone/proguanil (Malarone) (Med Let 2000;42:109) 250/100 mg po qd, start 1–2 d before arrive and keep up 1 wk after departure
- Malathion (Ovide) 0.5% topically for lice; adverse effects: local skin irritation
- Mebendazole (Vermox) varying doses for pinworm, filariasis, hookworm, whipworm, visceral larval migrans, ascariasis. Adverse effects: diarrhea, abdominal pain; rarely leukopenia, hypospermia

ID: PARASITOLOGY

- Mefloquine (Lariam) 250 mg or 25 mg/kg × 1. Adverse effects: vertigo, gi sx, nightmares, headache, confusion; rarely psychoses, seizures, shock, coma, paresthesias
- Melarsoprol (Arsobal) 2–3.6 mg/kg/d iv × 3 d 1st week, then 3.6 mg/kg/d × 3 d iv 2nd and 3rd wk for CNS trypanosomiasis/Chagas' disease. Adverse effects: cardiac injury, albuminuria, hypertension, colic, Herxheimer reaction, encephalopathy, emesis, peripheral neuropathy
- Metronidazole (Flagyl) various doses for amebiasis, *Trichomonas, Balantidium coli,* tapeworms, *Giardia,* hookworm, whipworm, visceral larval migrans. Adverse effects: nausea/vomiting, headache, metallic taste, insomnia, stomatitis, rash, dysuria, paresthesias, Antabuse reaction to alcohol; rarely seizures, colitis, encephalopathy, neuropathy, pancreatitis. No increase in cancer risk (Nejm 1979;301:519)
- Niclosamide (Niclocide) 50 mg/kg up to 2 gm × 1 chewed for *Fasciolopsis* fluke and *Hymenolepis nana* (dwarf tapeworm). Adverse effects: nausea, abdominal pain
- Nifurtimox (Lampit) 8–10 mg/kg/d po in qid doses × 120 d, double doses for children × 90 d for *Trypanosoma cruzi* (Chagas' disease). Adverse effects: anorexia, emesis, weight loss, sleep changes, tremor, paresthesias, polyneuritis, memory loss; rarely seizures, fever, pulmonary infiltrates
- Oxamniquine (Vansil) 15 mg/kg × 1, 10 mg/kg bid × 1 d for children, for *Schistosoma mansoni.* Adverse effects: headache, fever, somnolence, diarrhea, rash, insomnia, LFT elevations, orange urine; rarely seizures, psych changes
- Paromomycin (aminosidine, Humatin) 25–30 mg/kg/d in tid dosing × 7 d for amebiasis, *D. fragilis, Cryptosporidium.* Adverse effects: gi sx, VIII nerve damage (hearing), renal injury
- Pentamidine (Pentam) 2–4 mg/kg im/iv qd × 14–21 d for leishmaniasis, *Pneumocystis.* Adverse effects: hypotension, hypoglycemia/diabetes induction, emesis, renal damage, gi sx, local injection pain, hypocalcemia, cardiotoxicity, hepatotoxicity, delirium, rash; rarely anaphylaxis, pancreatitis, hyperkalemia because is similar to triamterene (Ann IM 1995;122:103)
- Permethrin (Nix, Elimite) topically 1% for lice, 5% for scabies; adverse effects: local irritation
- Praziquantel (Biltricide) 25 mg/kg tid × 1 d for flukes, schistosomiasis, tapeworms. Adverse effects: malaise, sedation, fever, eosinophilia, abdominal pain; rarely rash

- Primaquine 15 mg base (6.3 mg)/d or 0.3 mg base/kg/d × 14 d, or 45 mg base/wk × 8 wk for prevention of *Plasmodium vivax* and *ovale* relapse after leave area. Adverse effects: hemolytic anemia in G6PD pts, neutropenia, gi sx; rare CNS sx, hypertension, arrhythmias
- Pyrantel pamoate (Antiminth) 11 mg/kg (max = 1 gm) × 3 d for hookworm, 11 mg/kg × 1 repeat in 2 wk for pinworm. Adverse effects: gi sx, headache, rash, fever
- Pyrethrins + piperonyl butoxide (RID) topically for lice; adverse effects: allergic reaction
- Pyrimethamine (Daraprim) 25–100 mg (1 mg/kg)/d × 3–4 wk w sulfadiazine for toxoplasmosis. Adverse effects: folate deficiency; rarely rash, emesis, seizures
- Pyrimethamine-sulfadoxine (Fansidar), 3 tabs × 1 on last day of quinine for resistant falcip malaria. Adverse effects: folate deficiency; rarely fatal Steven-Johnson syndrome, emesis, seizures
- Quinacrine (Atabrine) 100 mg or 2 mg/kg tid × 5 d for giardiasis; no longer available in US? Adverse effects: headache, emesis, diarrhea, yellow skin, psychoses, insomnia, blue nails, rash like psoriasis
- Sodium stibogluconate (Pentostam) (pentavalent antimony) 20 mg Sb/kg/d iv/im × 21–28 d for leishmaniasis. Adverse effects: myalgias, arthralgias (90%), LFT elevations (25%), T-wave inversions (30%), weakness, colic, bradycardia, leukopenia; rarely diarrhea, rash, MI, hemoytic anemia, renal damage
- Spiramycin (Rovamycine) 50–100 mg/kg up to 3–4 gm/d × 3–4 wk for toxoplasmosis during pregnancy. Adverse effects: gi sx; rarely allergic reactions
- Suramin Na (Germanin) 100-mg test dose then 20 mg/kg up to 1 gm iv days 1, 3, 7, 14, 21 for sleeping sickness (trypanosomal). Adverse effects: emesis, urticaria, paresthesias, neuropathy, renal damage, optic atrophy
- Thiabendazole (Mintezol) various doses for angiostrongylosis, cutaneous larval migrans, *Dracunculus, Strongyloides.* Adverse effects: nausea/vomiting, vertigo, leukopenia, crystalluria, rash, hallucinations, erythema multiforme, smell changes; rarely tinnitus, cholestasis, seizures, angioneurotic edema

ID: PARASITOLOGY

11.2 PROTIST PROTOZOANS

BABESIOSIS
Nejm 1993;329:943; 1977;297:825

Cause: *Babesia microti*

Epidem: Carried by ticks of cattle, deer mice, and deer (same as Lyme disease); or by transfusion of infected blood (Ann IM 1982;96:601)

In southern New England esp. Nantucket; Fire Island NY; Georgia; Mexico; California (Nejm 1995;332:298); Washington state (Ann IM 1993;119:284). Incidence incr in AIDS and splenectomized patients (Nejm 1980;303:1098)

Pathophys:

Sx: Fever, malaise

Si: Fever, lymphoma-like si's (Ann IM 1981;94:327)

Crs: 7d incubation period. Days of fever; asx carriers, persistent long term infection unless treated, and subclinical infections all common too (Nejm 1998;339:160). May be fatal

Cmplc: r/o ehrlichiosis, disease (p 437), or concomitant infection w same

Lab:

Hem: Intra-rbc parasites, look like malaria

Serol: Indirect immunofluorescence antibody ≥1/64

Rx:

- Atovaquone + azithromycin, which has fewer side effects (Nejm 2000;343:1454)
- Quinine 650 mg or 8 mg/kg tid po + clindamycin 600 mg or 10 mg/kg po (or iv) tid × 7 d (Ann IM 1982;96:601) but tinnitus and abdominal distress result in 20% failing to complete crs (Nejm 1998;339:160)

Exchange transfusion cures acute hemolytic crisis (Nejm 1980; 303:1098)

CRYPTOSPORIDIUM DIARRHEA
Nejm 1994;331:161; 1985;312:1278; Ann IM 1985;103:886

Cause: *Cryptosporidium* spp

Epidem: Fecal-oral dissemination from humans or cattle (Am J Pub Hlth 1989;79:1528) or contaminated water supplies (Nejm 1994;

331:161) even those w filtered water treatment systems (Ann IM
1996;124:459)

Common cause of travelers and other self-limited diarrhea; incr under
age 4 yr, especially in day care centers; associated w *Giardia* for that
reason

Pathophys:

Sx: Usually watery, nonbloody diarrhea (86–93%) × 12 d average;
occasional abdominal cramps (84%); vomiting (48%); anorexia
(20%); fever (12–57%); weight loss (20%); nausea (12%)

Si:

Crs: 7d incubation period, 6–12 d course; all recover in immunocompetent
host (Nejm 1986;315:1643)

Cmplc: Chronic cholecystitis/cholangitis as well as dissemination in AIDS
and other immunocompromised pts

r/o similar intestinal spore-forming protozoa (Ann IM 1996;124:429):

Cyclospora cayetanensis, coccidia-like organism (Nejm
1993;328:1308); causes fatigue and malabsorption w chronic
infection (Ann IM 1995;123:409; 1993;119:377) waterborne
epidemics (Central American imported raspberries—Nejm 1997;
336:1548) and especially in AIDS pts; prophylaxis and rx w Tm/S
(Ann IM 1994;121:654) or cipro as 2nd choice (Ann IM 2000;
132:885)

Enterocytozoon bienensis, intracellular microsporidial protozoan
(Nejm 1992;326:161); causes diarrhea and cholangitis (Nejm
1993;328:95; Ann IM 1993;119:895)

Isospora belli, rx with Tm/S, pyrimethamine (Ann IM 1988;109:474;
Nejm 1986;315:87), or cipro (Ann IM 2000;132:885)

Lab:

Bact: Ziehl-Neelsen acid-fast stain of stool for O + P; 10% false neg;
75% still have present in stool after sx subside (Nejm
1986;315:1643)

Rx: Supportive; and, if necessary as in AIDS, parmomycin 500 mg po
tid × 2 wk, 500 mg bid Maintenance; spiramycin, azithromycin, or
furazolidone

AMEBIC DYSENTERY
Nejm 1984;310:298; 1978;298:262; Ann IM 1978;88:89

Cause: *Entamoeba histolytica,* rarely *D. fragilis*

Epidem: Encysted organisms excreted in feces, contaminate water or food; human carriers disseminate. Degree of infestation correlates inversely with sanitation. Increased prevalence in mental hospitals and gay males

Pathophys: Trophozoite (amebic form) invades wall of colon, secretes autolyzing enzymes, and lives on necrotic tissue in abscess; multiplies by binary fission

Sx: Fever, bloody stool, alternating diarrhea and constipation

Si:

Crs:

Cmplc: Abscess metastases to liver, lung, brain, pericardium, spleen, skin (ulcers)

r/o the much more benign, **ciliate dysentery** caused by *Balantidium coli,* and nonpathogenic strains of *E. histolytica* that are commensals in gay males (Nejm 1986;315:353, 390)

Lab:
Serol: Elevated antibody titers, <10% false neg (Ann IM 1969;71:983); 95% pos after 7 + d of sx in colitis or liver abscess (Gut 1994;35:1018)

Stool: O + P positive in 90% with severe colonic disease; cysts with 4 nuclei, central nucleolus; often overdiagnosed by lab technicians thinking wbc's are amebae (Ann IM 1978;88:89); antigen tests coming

Xray: BE shows deformed cecum, narrowed; rarely megacolon

Rx: Prevent w tetraglycine hydroperiodate, kills cysts in 30 min; water chlorination doesn't kill cysts

of asx disease: iodoquinol 650 mg or 10 mg/kg po tid × 20 d; or paromomycin 8–10 mg/kg po tid × 7 d

of intestinal disease: metronidazole 10–12 mg/kg or 750 mg po tid × 10 d; or tinidazole 50 mg/kg up to 2 gm/d × 3–5 d

of hepatic abscess: metronidazole as above; or tinidazole 800 mg tid × 5 d

AMEBIC MENINGOENCEPHALITIS
Ann IM 1978;88:468

Cause: *Naegleria gruberi,* and *Acanthamoeba* spp

Epidem: Worldwide; natural inhabitant of freshwater; in pts who have been swimming in past week; very rare

Pathophys: Meningoencephalitis with predilection for olfactory, cerebellar, and temporofrontal areas; later develop hematogenous spread and often fatal myocarditis. May invade via nose through cribriform plate and into olfactory bulb

Sx: Headache, swam within past week, fever (*Acanthamoeba* can also cause ocular keratitis in contact lens wearers)

Si: Parosmia (funny smells), cerebellar ataxia, meningoencephalitis without incr CNS pressure

Crs: Almost universally fatal in 4–5 d

Cmplc: Death

Lab:

CSF: Purulent meningitis with "bubbly" amebae on high-power wet mount

Path: Organisms in all organs but gi tract

Rx: A few survivors now (Nejm 1982;306:346; Ann IM 1971;74:923)

Amphotericin B iv and perhaps intracisternally; perhaps ketoconazole, or flucytosine (p 453)

of keratitis: topical 0.1% propamidine + neosporin; or itraconazole po + topical miconazole

MALARIA
Clin Inf Dis 1993;16:449; Nejm 1983;308:875–934

Cause: *Plasmodium vivax, ovale, malariae, falciparum*

Epidem: Sporozoites (in mosquito salivary gland) enter via puncture wound of bite, undergo exoerythrocytic schizogony into merozoites, which evolve to trophozoites (ring forms), then into erythrocyte schizonts or into macro- and microgametocytes, which are then ingested by mosquitoes

Distribution: *vivax* in Southeast Asia, South America; *ovale* in W. Africa; *malariae* in Africa; *falciparum* in Africa, Asia, Oceania, South America

Malaria, continued

Vector: anopheles *Aedes culex* mosquito. Patients heterozygous for
Hgb S, C, E, or G6PD may be more resistant. Duffy blood group
FyFy completely protected vs *vivax* (Nejm 1976;295:302)
Incr susceptibility during pregnancy and 1st 2 postpartum mos (Nejm
2000;343:598) probably due to immunosuppression of pregnancy
Pathophys: 3–4 h fevers, as endotoxins, including tumor necrosis factor
(Nejm 1990;320:1586), are released when schizonts rupture into
merozoites synchronously in blood. *Vivax* infects young (retics)
rbc's only; *malariae,* old rbc's only. *Falciparum* infects all rbc's and
causes "sticky" rbc's, which infarct brain, kidney, lung (Nejm
1968;279:732); no exoerythrocytic phase, hence no late recurrences
Sx:
Vivax: 6–15 d incubation, tertian (qod) fever but 2 crops can cause qd
fevers.
Malariae: 20–25 d incubation, quartan (q 3 d) fevers.
Ovale: quotidian (qd) fevers.
Falcip: <30 d incubation, tertian (qod) fevers but variable
Si: Splenomegaly (*vivax* = 25%, *falcip* = 80%). Black water fever is
hemoglobinuria from massive hemolysis (*falcip*)
Crs: 3.5% mortality for *falcip* in children, usually within 24 h, especially
if change in consciousness, jaundice, repiratory distress, or
hypoglycemia (Nejm 1995;332:1399)
Cmplc:
Vivax: Tropical splenomegaly syndrome (Nejm 1984;310:337)
Malariae: Recurrence possible decades later (Nejm 1998;338:367)
Falcip: DIC (Ann IM 1969;70:134); CVA, coma (steroids no
help—Nejm 1982;306:313); hypoglycemia correlates with severe
falcip disease and diminished hepatic gluconeogenesis, associated
with severe morbidity and mortality in 50% (Nejm 1988;319:1040)
r/o babesiosis in US (p 466)
Lab:
Hem: Vivax, single infections of only young (big) rbc's; circulating
older ameboid trophozoites and schizonts; 16 merozoites/schizont;
Schüffner's dots (small, eosinophilic) in rbc. *Ovale,* oval rbc often
fringed at one end. *Ovale* and *malariae,* "band like" trophs;
8 merozoites/schizont. *Falcip,* multiple infections of each rbc; all
ages and sizes of rbc's; only young, small ring trophozoites (older

trophs and schizonts in RES); 24 merozoites/schizont; Mauer's dots
in rbc (eosinophilic, larger)

Rx: (Nejm 1996;335:800) (CDC phone number: (770) 488-7788)

Prevent w DEET (<35%) insect repellant, screening, long sleeves;
vaccine vs sporozoite, becoming practical (Nejm 1997;336:86)

Prophylaxis (Jama 1997;278:1767; Med Let 2000;42:8)

for all including resistant *falcip* (Ann IM 1997;126:963) (all areas
except Central America, Carribean, and parts of Middle East):
1st:
* Mefloquine (Lariam) 250 mg po 1 wk before arrival and q 1 wk
  until 4 wk after departure, $8/pill, but variants of fatigue and
  malaise limit use (ACP J Club 2001;135:68); or
* Doxycycline 100 mg qd; or
* Atovaquone/proguanil (Malarone) (Med Let 2000;42:109)
  250/100 mg po qd, start 1–2 d before arrive and keep up 1 wk
  after departure; costs $1.5 \times$ mefloquine price
2nd:
* Chloroquine and primaquine 30 mg po qd through the week after
  departure from area (Ann IM 1998;129:241) + Fansidar
  (pyrimethamine + sulfadiazine) q 1 wk + proguanil 200 mg
  po qd; or
* Fansidar tabs to take prn fever (avoids severe allergic
  reactions—Ann IM 1987;106:714)
for all except resistant *falcip:*
* Choroquine PO_4 300 mg base (500 mg) q wk, 1 wk prior and
  6 wk after leave +
* Primaquine PO_4 15 mg base (26 mg) with last 2 wk of above to
  radically cure exoerythrocytic phases
of active disease (Call CDC, phone above)
for all except resistant *falcip:*
* Chloroquine 600 mg base (1 gm), then 300 mg at 12, 24, and
  36 hr; or in severely ill, 10 mg base/kg iv over 8 hr then 15 mg/kg
  over 24 hr, or 35 mg/kg im/sc q 6 hr or via NG +
* Primaquine as above
of resistant *falcip:*
* Quinine sulfate 650 mg po tid $\times$ 3–7 d, followed by Fansidar (see
  above) 3 tab $\times$ 1, or
* Tetracycline 250 mg qid $\times$ 7 d, or
* Clindamycin 900 mg po tid $\times$ 3 d, or
* Mefloquine 15 mg base/kg po then 10 mg/kg 8–24 hr later, or

- Quinidine gluconate 10 mg/kg over 1–2 h iv then 0.02 mg/kg/min constant infusion until can take po + exchange transfusion if >10% rbc's infected (Nejm 1989;321:65)
- Artesunate 4mg/kg qd × 3 w Fansidar (Lancet 2000;355:352) of cerebral and severe *falcip* malaria:
- Quinine 10 mg/kg iv/im q 8 hr after 20 mg initial dose, or
- Artemether 2 mg/kg im q 8 hr after 4 mg/kg load (Nejm 1996;335:69,76,124)
- Deferoxamine iron chelation speeds recovery in *falcip* pediatric cerebral malaria by denying organism its vitamins! (Nejm 1992;327:1473)

PNEUMOCYSTIS PNEUMONIA

Cause: *Pneumocystis carinii*

Epidem: Opportunistic, from other people harboring (epidemics in tumor clinic—Ann IM 1975;82:772)

In pts w depressed immunologic responses, eg, hypogammaglobulinemia, premies, hematopoietic malignancy, immunosuppression, AIDS (vast majority of patients with *Pneumocystis* have AIDS), elderly (Nejm 1991;324:246)

Pathophys: Diffuse interstitial pneumonitis

Sx: Dyspnea, nonproductive cough

Si: Normal chest exam or rales; thrush often concomitantly

Crs: Die in weeks without rx (50%), with rx mortality ~3%; those requiring ventilator have a 25% survival to hospital d/c (Jama 1995;273:230)

Cmplc: Osteomyelitis rarely (Nejm 1992;326:999)

r/o other opportunistics (p 494)

Lab:

Bact: Saline-induced sputum (Ann IM 1988;109:7), stain with Giemsa (72% sens), toluidine blue (80% sens), or with indirect immunofluorescence (92% sens) (Nejm 1988;318:589)

Path: Fiberoptic bronchoscopic bx, lavage, brushings

Xray: Chest shows diffuse interstitial infiltrate, starts perihilar, 98% bilateral. Gallium scan shows hot lungs even with neg plain films, but 50% false positives including sarcoid patients (Nejm 1988;318:1439)

Rx: (Med Let 1995;37:87; Nejm 1992;327:1853; Ann IM 1988;109:280)

Preventive (Nejm 1995;332:693; Ann IM 1995;122:755): isolation of infected from other susceptible patients?; under CD4 of 100, Tm/S better than dapsone, which is better than pentamidine.

- Tm/S DS (Arch IM 1996;156:177, Nejm 1987;316:1627) tiw, qd or bid or SS qd, cheaper but tolerated less well than the other 2 (Nejm 1992;327:1836,1842)
- Atovaquone (Nejm 1998;339:1890) 1500 mg po qd, better tolerated than dapsone as backup for Tm/S intolerant pts
- Dapsone 50 mg po bid or qd or biw w pyrimethamine, or perhaps 100 mg po biw (Am J Med 1993;95:573), when Tm/S intolerant, also helps prevent toxoplasmosis
- Pentamidine aerosol neb 300 mg q 4 wk (Med Let 1989;31:91) iv q 2–4 wk, or supine (Ann IM 1990;113:677)
- Pyrimethamine + sulfadiazine (Fansidar) perhaps

Treatment:

- Tm/S 2–15 tab po qd as good as pentamidine (Ann IM 1986;105:37); iv works too (Med Let 1981;23:102) 10–20 mg/kg/d; watch rash and marrow. In AIDS patients with severe disease, give with 40 mg methylprednisolone iv or po q 6 h × 7 d, which markedly improves survival from 20 to 75% (Nejm 1990;323:1445,1451)
- Pentamidine 4 mg/kg/d × 12–14 d (Nejm 1972;287:495), better, less toxic in AIDS patients; watch creatinine
- Tm/Dapsone equi-effective and only 30% become intolerant of it unlike 60% with Tm/S (Nejm 1990;323:776)
- Trimetrexate with leucovorin rescue equi-effective (Med Let 1989;31:5; Nejm 1987;317:978)
- Atovaquone (Meprone) (Ann IM 1994;121:174; Med Let 1993;35:28; Nejm 1991;325:1534), a hydroxynaphthoquinone, 250 mg po tid, which also treats toxo, may be reasonable backup to Tm/S

TOXOPLASMOSIS

Nejm 1985;313:957; 1978;298:550; Ann IM 1976;84:193

Cause: *Toxoplasma gondii*

Epidem: Cats are primary hosts, usually transmitted via cat feces? contaminated water (Nejm 1982;307:666) or dust (Nejm 1979;300: 695); also from poorly cooked meat

15–30% of US population have had; especially in wet hot areas

Immunosuppression can induce. Fetus very susceptible; 40% contract disease when mother gets primary infection between 2 and 6 mo gestation (Nejm 1974;290:110). Increased in AIDS as an opportunistic infection

Pathophys: Inflammation and scarring in brain, liver, spleen, heart, eye. Cysts are inert. Eye lesions probably are due to delayed hypersensitivity reactions. Congenital form somewhat different clinical pattern than acquired

Sx:

Acquired (Nejm 1979;300:695) (90%): Fever, headache (85%), myalgia (60%), rash (20%)

Congenital: Rash

Si:

Acquired: Lymphadenopathy (85%), rash (20%), chorioretinitis

Congenital: Chorioretinitis (100%), icterus, rash, hepatosplenomegaly, hydrops, hydrocephalus

Crs:

Cmplc:

Acquired: Meningoencephalitis (50%), r/o lymphoma (Ann IM 1969;70:514); myocarditis

Lab:

CSF: Congenital: organisms on Wright's stain and grow in mice

Path: Intracellular blue with red cytoplasm; can look like intracellular "grapes" when multiplying in cell. Do brain bx in AIDS patients w meningoencephalitis if don't respond to pyrimethamine + clindamycin within 2 wk (Nejm 1993;329:995)

Serol: Indirect fluorescent antibody positive if >1 : 1000; comp-fix antibody and Sabin-Feldman dye test (interpretation of various mother/child combinations—Nejm 1978;298:550). IgM titers now available

Xray:

Acquired: CT of head shows focal encephalitis with enhancing rings (Nejm 1988;318:1439)

Congenital: In utero, cerebral calcifications and bony "white puffs"

Rx:

Preventive: avoidance of cat litter, sand boxes

Congenital: Prevent w screening titer at 1st ob visit, then q 1 mo toxo titers (if elevated but stable, no problem), and in exposed seroneg pregnant women; abort if convert and fetal infection documented, eg, by amniocentesis PCR methods (Nejm 1994;331:695); or rx with spiramycin; or pyrimethamine + sulfa, which results in 13/15 healthy newborns, other 2 had only retinitis (France—Nejm 1988; 318:271). Or screen newborns for IgM toxo titers; this detects 1 case/6000 infants in New England and subsequent rx allows prevention of future eye disease (Njem 1994;330:1858)

Acquired: 1st choice, pyrimethamine 25–100 mg/d or 2 mg/kg/d × 3 d then 1 mg/kg/d up to 25 mg + sulfadiazine 1–2 gm or 25–50 mg/kg qid × 3–4 wk; or pyrimethamine + clindamycin 1200 mg qid (Nejm 1993;329:995; Ann IM 1992;116:33), which is preferable in AIDS because 40% of such pts can't tolerate sulfa. 2nd choice is spiramycin 3–4 gm/kg or 50–100 mg/kg/d × 3–4 wk of eye involvement: steroids

ID: PARASITOLOGY

11.3 FLAGELLATE PROTOZOANS

GIARDIA DIARRHEA AND MALABSORPTION

Nejm 1978;298:319

Cause: *Giardia lamblia*

Epidem: Encysted form excreted in feces, ingested by new host, resides in duodenum. Animal reservoirs: beaver, dog, muskrat, perhaps deer

Occurs in areas of poor sanitation with raw rural surface (not ground) water; gay males; Southeast Asian refugees, hikers/backpackers including in wilderness areas. Associated with globulin deficiencies, especially of IgA; achlorhydria, nodular lymphoid hyperplasia

Pathophys: Malabsorption due to mechanical obstruction of duodenum, hence fat absorption is especially hard hit

Sx: Loose, watery stools (93%), malaise (80%), bloating and cramps (75%), fatigue, weight loss (73%); true diarrhea in only 30%

"Traveler's diarrhea," which often doesn't start until return from a
    trip, ie, delayed onset

Si:

Crs: 10d incubation period, 10^+ wk duration

Cmplc: Malabsorption, upper gi bleed rarely

Lab:
    Bact: Stool O + P, 70% false neg; 2 "eyed" (nuclei) flagellated
        trophozoite, or 4 nucleated cyst. Examination of duodenal aspirate
        or small bowel bx (<10% false neg)
    Serol: Giardia antigen in stool

Rx: Prevent by: avoiding sewage contamination of water supplies;
    filtration; iodine as 2% solution, 0.4 cc/L of water; or heating to
    158°F (70°C) × 10 min (Am J Pub Hlth 1989;79:1633)
    Chlorination probably inadequate even at 8 mg Cl^-/L × 10 min
of active disease:
- Metronidazole (Flagyl), 1st, 250 mg or 5 mg/kg tid × 5–7 d; or
  alternatively
- Furazolidone 100 mg or 1.25 mg/kg qid × 5 d; no carcinogenicity

TRICHOMONAS URETHRITIS/VAGINITIS
Nejm 1997;337:1896

Cause: *Trichomonas vaginalis*

Epidem: Venereal; 10–25% US adult female population carries
    asymptomatically; present in 30–40% of male partners of infected
    women

Pathophys:

Sx: Profuse, watery vaginal discharge in women, or urethritis in males
    (rarer, many asx—Ann IM 1993;119:844); dyspareunia

Si: Erythematous cervicitis

Crs:

Cmplc: PROM and postpartum endometritis
    r/o bacterial vaginosis (p 407), and candidal vaginitis (p 143)

Lab:
    Bact: Wet prep shows motile, 20-μ flagellate with axostyle undulating
        membrane, 50–70% sens, 100% specif (Am J Med 2000:108:301);

culture possible; rapid DNA and monoclonal antibody tests 90%
sens and 99.8% specif (Am J Med 2000:108:301)

Path: Pap smear presence 60% sens, 97% specif (Am J Med
2000:108:301)

Vag discharge pH = 5–6, w amine smell on "whiff test"

Rx: (Med Let 1999;41:86; 1997;37:117)

Metronidazole 2 gm × 1 po to pt and partner, 90% cure; or
375–500 mg po bid × 7 d, 85–90% cure; local rx no good; ok in
pregnancy but does not decr prematurity complc (Nejm 2001;
345:487)

Tinidazole 2 gm po × 1, 2nd choice

in pregnancy: can use metronidazole; Betadine douche to control sx
suppresses fetal thyroid

11.4   CESTODE HELMINTHS

TAPEWORMS

Nejm 1992;327:692,696,727; 1984;310:298

Cause: *Taenia saginata* (beef), *T. solium* (pork); *Diphyllobothrium latum*
(fish); *Hymenolepis nana* (dwarf tapeworm)

Epidem: Adult worms in "definitive" carnivore hosts (dog, bears, etc),
eggs in feces eaten by human or herbivorous animal ("intermediate
hosts") and then encyst in muscle, etc. In *T. solium* and *H. nana,*
humans can be a definitive host or an intermediate host (muscle
encystment) via autoinoculation or fecal-oral transmission, eg, in
food handlers or in families; humans are only definitive hosts, ie,
worm is in gi tract

Seen especially in children and mentally retarded. Dwarf tapeworm is
most common in US. *T. solium* is endemic in Mexico and in many
immigrants, eg, in California

Pathophys:

Sx: *Taenia* and *D. latum:* rarely cause sx besides complaints of passage in
stool

Dwarf: diarrhea and occasionally obstructive gi sx

Si:

Crs:

Cmplc: *D. latum:* B$_{12}$ and folate deficiencies

    T. solium: cysticercosis in brain (seizures), muscle, and skin (50%); sx
    may take 4–5 yr to develop when larvae die (Nejm 1984;311:1492)

Lab:

    Bact: Stool O + P shows characteristic ova and gravid segments in all
    but echinococcus

    Serol: IHA titers incr with *T. solium* cysticercosis

Xray: In cysticercosis: skull films and CT of head (Nejm 2000;343:420)
    show calcifications

Rx: for adult forms, in gi tract, of *Taenia, D. latum,* and *H. nana:*

    • Praziquantel 5–10 mg/kg × 1; 99% effective (Ann IM 1989;110:
      290); or

    • Niclosamide 2 gm (500 mg under age 2, 1 gm age 2–12 yr) once
      (89% cure), then 1 gm (500 mg age 2–12 yr) po qd × 5 d

    for *T. solium* cysticercosis: surgical excision; albendazole as above or
    praziquantel + dexamethasone (Nejm 1984;311:1492; Ann IM
    1983;99:179)

ECHINOCOCCAL (Hydatid) CYST DISEASE

Cause: *Echinococcus granulosus* and *multilocularis* (hydatid cyst);
    sometimes *T. solium* (see above)

Epidem: Humans are only intermediate host, ie, do not spread eggs in
    stool, rather only have encysted organisms

Pathophys: Like a neoplasm, echinococcal cysts grow over years with
    appearance of secondary cysts

Sx:

Si: Mass effects anywhere

Crs:

Cmplc:

Lab:

    CSF: in cysticercosis: aseptic picture with low sugar; eosinophils

    Serol: IHA titers incr (from CDC) are pos in 90% with liver, 75% with
    lung involvement

Rx: Albendazole 5 mg/kg po tid × 28–56 d + either surgical or percutaneous drainage (Nejm 1997;337:881)

for *T. solium* cysticercosis: surgical excision; albendazole as above or praziquantel + dexamethasone (Nejm 1984;311:1492; Ann IM 1983;99:179)

11.5   TREMATODE HELMINTHS

SCHISTOSOMIASIS

Nejm 1984;310:298; 1980;303:203; Ann IM 1982;97:740

Cause: *Schistosoma mansoni, japonicum,* and *haematobium;* swimmer's itch from *S. dermatidis* (Maine Epigram 8/87)

Epidem: Free-swimming cercariae penetrate skin or ingested, become schistosomulae in host blood, and mature into adults in blood vessels. They then deposit in body tissues selectively (*S. mansoni* and *S. japonicum* about gi tract, *S. haematobium* about bladder); there they mate and lay eggs that work out to feces or urine, are excreted into water where become miracidia, which invade certain snail species and reproduce again, and eventually are released as cercariae. Can live 30–40 yr in human

In *S. dermatidis* swimmer's itch, only cercarial penetration of skin by nonhuman schistosomes occurs; cycle stopped there

S. mansoni in Caribbean, Africa, Middle East; *S. haematobium* in Africa, Far and Middle East; *S. japonicum in* Far East (Nejm 1983;309:1533). *S. dermatidis* in marine or fresh water, incl USA

Pathophys: Focal granulomas, fibrosis, vasculitis

Swimmer's itch due to allergic reaction to worms on 2nd exposure

Sx: Chills, diarrhea, abdominal pain, weight loss, bloody urine/stool

S. dermatidis: swimmer's itch

Si: Hepatosplenomegaly (70%), fever (60%), diarrhea (60%)

S. dermatidis: skin welts or swelling

Crs:

Cmplc: Granulomatous response to eggs anywhere including brain, skin, liver with cirrhosis and varices, gu tract with obstruction and secondary infections (Ann IM 1971;75:49) and immune complex nephritis (Ann IM 1975;83:148)

In swimmer's itch: r/o sea bather's eruptions from anemone medusae
(Nejm 1993;329:542)

Lab:

Bact: Stool/urine show typical eggs: *S. japonicum,* rounded oval with
lateral "knob"; *S. haematobium,* elongated with terminal spine;
S. mansoni, oval with lateral spine

Hem: Eosinophils incr

Path: Biopsy of rectum, liver, bladder may show eggs

Serol: Immunofluorescent antibody titers; skin test pos after 20 wk
(10/10)

Rx: Praziquantel 20 mg/kg bid × 1 d; good vs all types; 70% cure (Nejm
1984;310:298)

Swimmer's itch, no rx

11.6 NEMATODE HELMINTHS

HOOKWORM

Nejm 1984;310:298

Cause: *Ancylostoma duodenale* and *Necator americanus*

Epidem: Larvae penetrate skin in filariform stage (5 d older than
rhabditiform stage), or larvae ingested in feces

Africa, Far East, southern Europe; US, especially in south with
barefoot children and poor sewage

Pathophys: Skin penetration, into circulation, thence to lung, into trachea,
to pharynx where swallowed and then attach to small intestine
where they result in chronic blood loss

Sx: Apathy

Si: Anemia, 150–200 cc/d with *Ancylostoma* when severe infestations;
Necator 1/5 as much, ~0.03 cc/d/worm

Crs:

Cmplc: CHF

r/o *Ancylostoma caninum,* dog hookworm, which can infect humans
and cause abdominal pain (Ann IM 1994;120:369)

Lab:
    Bact: Stool O + P shows eggs same size as *Ascaris,* w thin delicate shell; hatch in 24 h into rhabditiform larvae, which molt into filariform larvae. Can quantify eggs and estimate number of worms
    Hem: Hgb as low as 1–3 gm; Fe deficiency anemia
Rx: Mebendazole (Vermox) 100 mg bid × 3 d; or pamoate, or pyrantel, or albendazole
    $FeSO_4$ for the anemia

LARVA MIGRANS

Nejm 1985;313:986

Cause: *Cutaneous,* "creeping eruption": *Ancylostoma braziliense* and *caninum*
    Visceral: Toxocara canis and *Baylisascaris procyonis* (raccoon ascaris)
Epidem:
    Cutaneous: Dog and cat hookworm larvae penetrate skin but never get into circulation; children get when crawl under buildings
    Visceral: Ingestion of dog feces w eggs; 20% of US dogs have it. Eggs survive several winters. 10% of adults in US have serologic evidence of it
Pathophys:
    Cutaneous: Larvae in skin cause local inflammation; can't penetrate dermal/epidermal junction
    Visceral: Worms invade viscera where permanent granulomas form
Sx:
    Cutaneous: Raised itchy areas of skin up to 2 wk after exposure
    Visceral: Age 1–4 yr usually; often asx or erratic fever, anorexia, rash, seizures, wheezing, cough
Si:
    Cutaneous: Rash
    Visceral: Hepatosplenomegaly, tumor-like growths in eye in older children
Crs:
    Cutaneous: Self-limited, × several wk
    Visceral: Self-limited
Cmplc:
    Visceral: Eosinophilic meningoencephalitis (Nejm 1985;312:1619)

ID: PARASITOLOGY

Larva Migrans, continued

Lab:

  Hem: Eosinophilia in both types

  Path:
  - *Visceral:* Bx (usually not justified since benign crs) of liver, lungs, CNS, muscle show eosinophilic granulomas

  Serol:
  - *Visceral:* Titer ≥1/32 (98% sens, 92% spec); get kit from CDC

  Stool: No eggs in either type

Rx:

  Cutaneous: Thiobendazole topically or 25 mg/kg bid up to 3 gm/d max × 2–5 d; or albendazole

  Visceral: Diethylcarbamazine 2 mg/kg tid × 7–10 d; or albendazole; or mebendazole. Steroids for eye disease

ROUNDWORMS

ASCARIASIS AND TRICHURIASIS (Whipworm)

Nejm 1984;310:298

Cause:

  Ascariasis: Ascaris lumbricoides, pig roundworm

  Trichuriasis: Trichuris trichiura

Epidem: Highest incidence of both is in tropics, where eggs survive more easily, and in children who do more fecal-oral transmission

  Ascariasis: Fecal-oral, 2 wk incubation of eggs necessary outside body before infective

  Trichuriasis: Fecal-oral

Pathophys:

Sx:

  Ascariasis: Only if abnormal site or so many that they block gi tract. After ingestion, migrate to lungs, then coughed up, reingested

  Trichuriasis: Embed in superficial intestinal mucosa, mainly colon; no tissue reaction, hence occasionally diarrhea

Si:

Crs:
Cmplc:

Ascariasis: Small bowel obstruction; perforated bowel; asphyxia due to aspiration; biliary obstruction; hepatic abscess

Trichuriasis: Anemia, malnutrition; rectal prolapse; allergic pneumonitis (in 10%) (rx w steroids—Weinstein, 1987)

Lab:

Bact:

- *Ascariasis:* Stool shows eggs, and adults
- *Trichuriasis:* Stool shows barrel-shaped eggs w mucus plug at both ends; adults, whip is head end, handle is tail end

Rx: (Nejm 1996;334:1178)

- Mebendazole (Vermox) 100 mg bid × 3 d, or
- Pyrantel pamoate (Antiminth) 11 mg/kg (1 tsp/25 kg), or
- Piperazine 75 mg/kg up to 3.5 g qd × 2, or
- Albendazole, or
- Ivermectin

Avoid reinfection; worms live <2 yr

ENTEROBIASIS (Pinworms)

Cause: *Enterobius vermicularis*

Epidem: Females live in colon and lay eggs in perianal region; there reinfected to same host or others by scratching; no tissue penetration 30% of US population under age 20 gets it, all social classes

Pathophys:

Sx: Anal pruritus, vaginitis

Si: Vaginitis

Crs:

Cmplc: Vaginitis can lead to migration into peritoneal cavity where granulomas form; rarely appendicitis

Lab:

Bact: Scotch tape to perianal area early in AM, then paste on slide to examine under microscope to see characteristic eggs, flat on one side

Rx: Mebendazole (Vermox) 100 mg × 1, repeat in 2 wk (Nejm 1977;297: 1437); or pyrantel 11 mg/kg (1 gm max) × 1, repeat in 2 wk; or albendazole; rx all family members at same time, even if asx since probably all have

STRONGYLOIDES INFECTIONS

Arch IM 1987;147:1257

Cause: *Strongyloides stercoralis*

Epidem: Skin penetration by filariform larvae that migrate to blood vessels, thence to lung, from there up to pharynx where are ingested back down the gi tract where embed and produce live young that are released into feces. Can mature in gi tract and autoreinfect, or mature on the ground

Increased prevalence in institutions for retarded; southern areas

Pathophys: Much tissue damage in gi tract; perhaps exotoxin release. As noted above, may in severe cases develop internal autoreinfection

Sx: Abdominal pain, midepigastric; nausea, vomiting, and bloody diarrhea (60–100%); perineal pruritus

Si:

Crs: May persist >30 yr in active stage

Cmplc: Superinfections w secondary gram-neg bacteremias, bowel obstruction and malabsorption in pts w diminished resistance, eg, on steroids (can cause death if already infected—Nejm 1966;275:1093), Hodgkin's, leukemia, SLE, leprosy (Ann IM 1970;72:199)

Acute pneumonitis due to sensitivity reaction w tissue migration; rx with steroids (L. Weinstein, 1987)

r/o *Angiostrongylus,* rat worm; get in Pacific and Southeast Asia from raw undercooked mollusks and crustaceans; causes transient benign eosinophilic meningitis

Lab:

Bact: Stool shows rhabditiform larvae in feces sporadically; must use fresh stool, neg in 25%; duodenal aspirate best and most reliable

Hem: Eosinophilia (50%)

Rx: Prevent by wearing shoes, digging latrines
    of disease
- Thiabendazole 25 mg/kg (3 gm max) bid × 2 d; both tissue and intestinal phases hit; cure in 65%; or
- Ivermectin

TRICHINOSIS

Jama 1983;249:23; Nejm 1978;298:1178

Cause: *Trichinella spiralis*

Epidem: Life cycle: infection from ingestion of meat w cysts, hatch and reproduce for 6 wk in gi mucosa, live young born and many get into skeletal muscle where grow and encyst, some calcify and others remain viable for years

From pigs fed uncooked garbage; polar and other bears

Pathophys: Invasion of skeletal (not heart) muscle by worms, degeneration of invaded fiber causing inflammatory reaction, and finally encysted larvae (in all other tissues this reaction kills larvae)

Sx: Fever, myalgias all over including tongue, diaphragm, etc.; gastroenteritis 24–72 h after ingestion from worms in gi tract

Si: Eye swelling, conjunctivitis, small conjunctival hemorrhages; splinter hemorrhages in nail beds; skin rashes both urticarial and petechial

Crs: GI sx in 24–72 h; other sx peak 1–6 wk after ingestion

Cmplc: Myocarditis, CNS inflammation

Lab:

Chem: CPK, AST (SGOT) markely elevated

Hem: Elevated eosinophils; may be as high as 50%

Path: Muscle bx shows 10–100 larvae/gm tissue; ≤1/gm should not produce sx

Serol: Charcoal flocculation test (Ann IM 1972;76:951)

Rx: Prevent by cooking garbage fed to pigs; cook or freeze pork well
    of disease (Med Let 1990;32:23):
- Mebendazole 200–400 mg po tid × 3 d, then 400–500 mg po tid × 10 d
- ASA for mild disease or
- Steroids to decrease inflammation if becomes life threatening but they also increase life of adult worms

ID: PARASITOLOGY

11.7 ARTHROPODS

LICE

Cause: *Phthirus pubis* (crabs—Nejm 1968;278:950); *Pediculus corporis* (body lice), *P. capitis* (head lice)

Epidem: *P. pubis,* venereal; *P. corporis* and *P. capitis,* via bedding, clothing, and other fomites

Life cycle: 25 d egg-to-egg. Live exclusively on human blood, can't live >24 h without it. Only ~10 adults/pt

Pathophys: Attach to hair; itch and rash due to bites and allergies to louse and its feces

Sx: Pruritus with all; *P. pubis* localized to axillary, perianal, pubic areas, and occasionally in eyelashes (blepharitis)

Si: Lice and nits (egg sacs on hairs) evident w magnifying glass or careful inspection; bites

Crs:

Cmplc: r/o bird lice (eg, from pigeons on air conditioner)

Lab:

Rx: (Med Let 1997;38:6)

Launder clothes, bedding; hang them outside × 24 h will also kill since can't survive >24 h away from body

Meds: rx as below (Rx Let 1999;6:59), perhaps repeat × 1 at 7d

1st:
- Permethrin 1% (Nix); $9/2 oz; 95% cure with one rx at 14 d (Am J Pub Hlth 1988;78:978), but resistance appearing

2nd:
- Permethrine 5% (Elimite) over night, 1st choice for pubic lice (Med Let 1999;41:89), avoid for head lice in children; or
- Malathion 0.5% (Ovide) (Med Let 1999;41:73) lotion × 8–12 hr, then repeat in 1 wk
- Pyrethrins + piperonyl butoxide (Rid, Vonce, A-200, Pronto); 65% cure after 1 rx at 14 d (Am J Pub Hlth 1988;78:978); $5/2 oz

3rd:
- Lindane shampoos (1% gamma benzene hexachloride, Kwell), × 1 usually enough; may need × 3 q 4 d; $5/2 oz, or
- Ivermectin (Mectizan) 200 μgm/kg po × 1

4th:
- Tm/S po bid × 10 d w permethrin topically (Peds 2001;107:E30)

of eye cmplc: 1/4% eserine ophthalmic ointment to lids with cotton tip applicator

of school outbreaks, full guidelines (Maine Epigram 10/86); "nit free policies unrealistic"

SCABIES, COMMON AND NORWEGIAN

Ann IM 1983;98:498; Nejm 1978;298:496; 1968;278:1099

Cause: *Sarcoptes scabiei* var. *hominis,* an arthropod mite

Epidem: Norwegian rare in US except in AIDS pts and alcoholics

Pathophys:

Common: Burrows in skin, leading to allergic reaction

Norwegian: No burrowing, but hides beneath skin scales

Sx:

Common: Itching, worst at night

Norwegian: No itching

Si:

Common: Red papules in intertriginous areas

Norwegian: Hyperkeratotic skin hiding mites

Crs:

Common: Even w rx takes 2 wk for sx to subside

Cmplc:

Lab:

Bact:

Mineral oil scraping of burrow shows mite or eggs under low power

Rx: (Med Let 1993;35:111)

Launder clothes, bedding; hang them outside × 24 h will also kill since can't survive >24 h away from body

Meds:

1st: Permethrin 5% (Elimite) cream (Med Let 1999;41:89) × 8–12 h; 30 gm enough to rx adult; 91% cure; safer than lindane

2nd: Lindane 1% (Kwell) (Med Let 1997;39:6) once though often need repeat; 86% cure; crotamiton 10% (Eurax) if above fails; 60% cure

Experimental: ivermectin 200 μgm/kg po × 1, ii 6mg tabs for avg adult; very effective, esp. w crusting type and/or in immunosuppressed (Nejm 1995;333:26)

ID: PARASITOLOGY

Chapter 12
Infectious Disease: Virology

D. K. Onion and S. Sears

12.1 ANTIVIRAL ANTIBIOTICS

Med Let 2000;42:1 (HIV drugs w interactions lists), 1997;39:69
  (non-HIV drugs))
Most iv courses cost $1000–$4000; rapidly changing field, should check
  most recent Med Let and other journal issues

REVERSE TRANSCRIPTASE INHIBITORS

All inhibit reverse transcriptase, which converts viral RNA to DNA so it
  can be incorporated into nuclear DNA; none touch viral DNA already
  incorporated

Nucleoside analogs (nRTIs): All cause few drug interactions; all can rarely
  cause fatty liver and lactic acidosis
  • Abacavir (Ziagen) (Med Let 1998;40:114) 300 mg po bid.
    Adverse effects: drug fever (3%); available when other regimens
    fail (expanded access protocol: (800) 501-4672)
  • Didanosine (Videx, dideoxyinosine [ddI]) (Nejm 1991;324:137)
    200 mg po qd-bid; vs AIDS, less toxic than AZT and perhaps as
    good; interacts w zalcitabine; avoid taking w food. Adverse
    effects: pancreatitis, peripheral neuropathy. $200/mo
  • Lamivudine (Epivir; 3TC) (Jama 1996;276:111; Ann IM 1996;
    125:161; Nejm 1995;333:1657,1662) 150 mg po bid; for chronic
    active hep B, and w AZT for HIV (Jama 1996;276:111,118).
    $230/mo

- Stavudine (d4T) (Ann IM 1997;126:355) 40 mg po bid; alternative retroviral drug for AZT and ddI failures. Adverse effects: peripheral neuropathy, asx hepatitis, rarely lactic acidosis w incr LFTs (Ann IM 2000;133:192). $250/mo
- Zalcitabine (dideoxycytidine [ddC]) 0.75 mg po tid, vs AIDS often alternating w AZT (Ann IM 1993;118:321). Adverse effects: diarrhea, abdominal pain. $207/mo
- Zidovudine (Retrovir, azidothymidine [AZT]) (Ann IM 1992;117: 487) 200 mg po tid (Nejm 1995;333:1662) or combined w 3TC (Combivir) (Rx Let 1997;4:62) (300 mg AZT + 150 mg 3TC) bid; ok in pregnancy (Jama 1999;281:151; Nejm 1992;326:857). Adverse effects: macrocytic anemia, helped by iv erythropoietin weekly (Nejm 1990;322:1488) and granulocytopenia (Nejm 1989;321:726), both about 1% at 500–600 mg/d; can rx the thrombocytopenia w interferon α and continue rx (Ann IM 1994; 121:423); acetaminophen (Tylenol) worsens toxicity (Nejm 1987; 317:192); myopathy in 5–10% (Nejm 1990;322:1098). $287/mo

Nucleotide analogs
- Adefovir (Preveon) (Jama 1999;282:2305,2355; Med Let 1998; 40:114) 120 mg po qd; used when other triple drug combinations fail (expanded access protocol: (800) 445-3235)

Non-nucleoside analogs (nnRTIs)
- Delavirdine (Rescriptor) 400 mg po tid. $222/mo
- Efavirenz (Sustiva) (Med Let 1998;40:114) 600 mg po hs. Better than the protease inhibitor indinavir when used w 2 nRTIs in triple rx (Nejm 1999;341:1865,1874,1925). Adverse effects: drowsiness, HA, insomnia, rash, nightmares, drug interactions decr protease inhibitor and clarithromycin levels
- Nevirapine (Viramune) (Med Let 1997;39:14) 200 mg po qd × 2 wk, then bid; possibly useful in drug combinations (Ann IM 1996;125:1019); adverse effect: rash. $250/mo

PROTEASE INHIBITORS
(Nejm 1998;338:1281; Jama 1997;277:145): all cost $4000–8000/yr

- Amprenavir (Agenerase) (Med Let 1999;41:64) 1200 mg (8 pills) po bid; adv effects: NVD, peranal paresthesias, rash occasionally severe, many drug interactions
- Indinavir (Crixivan) (Med Let 1996;38:35) 800 mg po tid. Adverse effects: renal stones, incr indirect bilirubin, Cushingoid changes (Nejm 1998;339:1296), incr DVT and PEs (Am J med 1999;107:624). $360/mo

- Nelfinavir (Med Let 1997;39:14) 750 mg po tid; adverse effect: diarrhea
- Lopinavir/ritonavir (Kaletra) combo (Med Let 2001;43:1) 133/33 mg pill or 80/20 liquid, iii tab or i tsp po bid w food. Adverse effects: NV + D, fatigue, headache, hepatocellular enzyme increases, rare pancreatitis, lots of drug interactions
- Ritonavir (Norvir) (Med Let 1996;38:35; Nejm 1995;333:1528) 300–600 mg po b-tid. Adverse effects: NV + D, incr LFTs, paresthesias. $670/mo
- Saquinavir (Fortovase, Invirase) (Nejm 1996;334:1011; Ann IM 1996;125:1039) 600–1200 mg po tid. Adverse effect: drug interactions w non-sedating antihistamines. $570/mo

ANTI-INFLUENZA DRUGS
(Nejm 2000;343:1778)

Neuraminidase inhibitors
- Zanamivir (Relenza) (Jama 1999;282:31; J Infect Dis 1999;180: 254; Med Let 1999;41:91) 10 mg pwdr inhalation qd for prophylaxis eg × 10 d in family members (NNT = 7—Nejm 2000;343;1282, 1331), bid × 5 d for rx of both influenza A and B; no resistance, but avoid in asthmatics and COPD where may precipitate bronchospasm (Rx Let 2000;7:43); $50/5d
- Oseltamivir (Tamiflu) (Jama 2000;283;1016; 282:1240; Nejm 1999;341:1336,1387) 75 mg po qd to prophylact × 7 d, or rx × 5 d decr severity and duration if start w/i 36 hr of sx for influenza A or B. Adverse effects: mild nausea and other gi sx, headache (15%); $50/5d

Other
- Amantadine; 100–200 mg qd (Nejm 1990;322:443), 100 mg qd over age 65, during first 48 h of sx or prophylactically × 10 d after single exposure or × 3 wk in epidemic (Med Let 1978;20:25; Nejm 1973;288:725); helps vs A strains only; may use in elderly nursing home pts even if have used flu shot; renal excretion; works as aerosol too. Adverse effects: CNS (don't drive) especially if renal insufficiency is present (Nejm 1990;322:447). $0.10/pill
- Rimantadine (Med Let 1993;35:109) 200 mg qd or 100 mg po bid × 5 d vs influenza; works similarly to amantadine but w much less CNS side effect (Nejm 1982;307:580); but rapid resistance develops during course of rx (Nejm 1989;321:1696); hepatic metabolism. $1/100 mg
- Ribavirin aerosol, works vs A and B; not available in US

OTHER
(Med Let 1999;41:113; Nejm 1999;340:1255)

- Acyclovir (Zovirax) (Med Let 1994;36:97; Nejm 1992;327:782); renally cleared, increase dose interval when creatinine clearance <50 cc/min. Adverse effects: gi sx; renal damage; resistance now appearing in AIDS patients (Nejm 1989;320:313). $125 for 800 mg 5 × /d× 7 d
    - of herpes simplex virus I and II
      of first episode, 200 mg po 5 × /d× 10 d
      of recurrences, × 5 d, or 400 mg po bid × 1 yr for frequent recurrence prophylaxis
    - of disseminated forms, 5–10 mg/kg q 8 h iv
    - of zoster, 800 mg po 5 ×/d or ×7–10 d may decrease duration of post herpetic neuralgia from 120 d to 60 d
    - of varicella (chicken pox), 20 mg/kg up to 800 mg po qid × 5 d
- Cidofovir (Med Let 1997;39:14; Ann IM 1997;126:257,264) for CMV retinitis; adv effect: renal toxicity
- Famciclovir (Famvir) (Med Let 1994;36:87) 500 mg po tid × 7 d for acute (<72 h) zoster vs 125 mg po bid × 5d (Rx Let 1997;4:62); 250 mg po bid preventivly for chronic hep B and recurrent h. simplex; renal excretion; $130/wk
- Foscarnet (Foscavir), vs CMV retinitis in AIDS (Med Let 1992;34:3; Nejm 1992;326:213)
- Ganciclovir (Cytovene) (Nejm 1996;335:720) iv, or 3000 mg po qd for maintenance (Nejm 1995;333:615); vs CMV in AIDS (Nejm 1986;314: 801; Ann IM 1985;103:377) and in marrow transplant pts (Ann IM 1993;118:173,179). Adverse effects: neutropenia w more frequent bacterial infections (Ann IM 1993;118:173,179), resistance now appearing in AIDS patients (Nejm 1989;320:313)
- Interferon α-2a, 2b, con-1 (Infergen) (Rx Let 1997;4:62), and n3, used in AIDS (Ann IM 1990;112:805) and hep B and C (p 276). Adverse effects: psych disinhibitions and depression, flu sx, marrow suppression
- Penciclovir (Danavir) 1% cream q 2 hr × 4 d for local herpes
- Ribavirin po/iv/aerosol; vs hep C w interferon, lassa fever, influenza, and perhaps RSV. Adverse effects: hemolysis (10%), reversible when stop drug; teratogenesis
- Valacyclovir (Valtrex) 500 mg po bid ×5 d (Rx Let 1997;4:62) vs 1 gm po tid × 7–14 d (Med Let 1996;38:3) for acute zoster and genital herpes simplex; for suppression, 250 mg bid (Rx Let 1997;4:62) vs 500–1000 mg po qd (Med Let 1996;38:3). $100/wk for 1 gm tid

ID: VIROLOGY

12.2 VIRAL INFECTIONS

ACQUIRED IMMUNE DEFICIENCY SYNDROME (AIDS)

Note: Rapidly changing field; identify local consultants and resources

Cause: Human immunodeficiency virus (HIV) type 1 (Nejm 1991;324: 308); rarely in US but commonly in Africa, HIV-2 (Ann IM 1993; 118:211); a retrovirus

Epidem: Spread via sex (3% infection rate w HIV pos semen—Jama 1995; 273:854), but no heterosexual transmission when viral loads <1500/cc (Nejm 2000;342:921); contaminated needles; blood products, eg, screened blood transfusion 1996 risk = 1/500,000 (Nejm 1996;334:1685), factor VIII concentrates (Nejm 1993;329: 1835; 1984;310:69); breast milk (Jama 2000;283:1167; 1999;282: 744; Nejm 1991;325:593); rarely by casual or nonsexual familial contact (Nejm 1987;317:1125), percutaneous inoculation in health care workers, 0.3%/incident, incr w incr volume and probably HIV titer (Nejm 1997;337:1485)

12% prevalence in wives of infected hemophiliacs (Ann IM 1991;115: 764); 0.2% of Massachusetts women positive at delivery (Nejm 1988;318:525) and NY state but NY city rate = 14% (Am J Pub Hlth 1991; 81:May suppl); 5% Baltimore ER patients (Nejm 1988; 318:1645)

Transmission enhanced by the presence of chancroid or other genital ulcers (Ann IM 1993;119:1150)

Prevalence incr in gay males (67% in San Francisco 1984—Ann IM 1985;103:210), intravenous drug abusers, hemophiliacs (Nejm 1983;308:79), female partners of infected males (Nejm 1983;308: 1181)

90% of persons transfused w HIV-positive blood convert to positive themselves (Ann IM 1990;113:733); but only 0.3% become positive after a needle stick from an HIV-positive patient; <0.5% of exposed health care workers convert over 1 yr (Nejm 1988;319: 1118); 30% untreated babies of HIV-pos mothers are pos at 16 mo age (Nejm 1992;327:1192; Am J Pub Hlth 1989;79:1662)

Incidence in 1990s decr in US as are AIDS deaths, probably from preventive maneuvers, drug rx of HIV infection, and prophylaxis and rx of opportunistic infections (Mmwr 1997;46:861)

Pathophys: AIDS defined by HIV infection and T4 count <200
  Increased suppressor T8 and decr helper T4 cells (CD4) (Nejm 1985;
    313:79); deficient production of interferon γ (Nejm 1985;
    313:1504)
  Billions of virions produced daily from infection, w high viral RNA
    mutation rate that allows rapid selection of resistant organisms in
    face of rx (Ann IM 1996;124:984)

Sx: Primary HIV infection (Nejm 1998;339:33; Ann IM 1996;125:259)
  consists of a mono-like syndrome 5–30 d after exposure lasting
  ~2 wk, rarely seek care; w fever (95%), sore throat (70%), wgt loss
  (70%), myalgias (60%), headache (60%), cervical adenopathy
  (50%), maculopapular or other rash involving trunk (40–80%); test
  for w HIV RNA assay (100% sens, 97% specif) (Ann IM 2001;
  134:25)
  AIDS: diarrhea (60%—Nejm 1993;329:14), malaise, weight loss, fever,
    adenopathy, dyspnea (PCP)

Si:
  Early: lymphadenopathy; oral monilia/thrush (exudative, cheilosis, or
    erythematous diffuse rash types) precedes overt disease often (Nejm
    1984;311:354), and multiple other oral manifestations (Ann IM
    1996;125:487); dermatoses including warts and shingles; chronic
    fatigue syndrome
  Later: wasting syndromes, chronic diarrhea, dementias/seizures, FUO,
    thrombocytopenia, cervical dysplasia, KS, hairy leukoplakia
    corrugations on sides of tongue due to reactivation of EB virus
    (Nejm 1985;313:1564)

Crs: See Fig. 12.2.1
  Of HIV infection: variable RNA viral loads in first 4 mos but
    worse/faster crs predicted by levels at 5–18 mos from infection and
    by severity of primary infection sx (Ann IM 1998;128:613; Jama
    1996;276:105); evolution to AIDS 10 yr post-seroconversion varies
    from 0–72%
  Of AIDS: 1997 mortality figures markedly improving w aggressive
    multi-drug rx based on viral loads (Jama 1998;279:450), eg, from
    29 to 9/100 person-years in pts w CD4 counts <100 (Nejm 1998;
    338:853); older data were 50% 1-yr, 15% 5-yr survival (Nejm
    1987;317:1297), 5% 10$^+$ yr survival because of some viral
    attenuated pathogenicity (Nejm 1995;332:201,217); in pts w AIDS
    on AZT, 50% 1-yr survival after CD4 count <50/mm^3

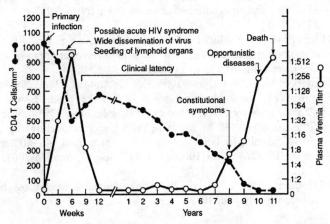

Figure 12.2.1 Typical course of HIV infection. (Reprinted with permission from Pantaleo G, Graziosi C, Fauci AS. New concepts in the immunopathogenesis of human immunodeficiency virus infection. Nejm 1993;328:329.)

Survival worse w increasing age of pt and some HLA MHC types (Nejm 2001;344;1668), but not associated w gender, iv drug use, race, or socioeconomic status (Nejm 1995;333:751)

Cmplc:

- Infections w common bacterial pathogens (Nejm 1995;333:845) as well as opportunistic organisms esp when CD4 <50 (Ann IM 1996;124:333) including:
- *Pneumocystis* (in 1980s was presenting sx in 75%, now much rarer w prophylaxis—Nejm 1993;329:1822)
- Atypical tbc (Ann IM 1986;105:184), especially *M. avium/intracellulare,* rarely *M. haemophilum* (Ann IM 1994;120:118)
- Herpes infections including tongue fissures (Nejm 1993;329:1859); CMV; *Candida;* aspergillosis; *Strongyloides*
- Nocardia
- *Mucor*
- Cryptococcosis, esp meningitis
- *Toxoplasma*
- *Legionella*
- Chlamydia

- *Monilia*
- Torulopsosis
- *Penicillium marneffei,* an SE Asian dimorphic fungus (Nejm 1998; 339:1739)
- Cryptosporidiosis (p 466), *Isospora belli* (p 467)
- *Listeria* (Nejm 1985;312:404)
- Cat scratch *Bartonella (Rochalimaea) henselae* or *quintana* causing bacillary angiomatosis (r/o Kaposi's by bx) and peliosis hepatitis (p 447)
- Syphilis w rapid (<4 yr) appearance of neurosyphilis manifest by strokes, meningitis, and cranial nerve palsies, only transiently suppressed by penicillin regimens (Nejm 1994;331:1469,1488, 1516)
- Tumors including:
- Kaposi's sarcoma (p 515)
- Non-Hodgkin's lymphoma, in 15% after 3 yr of AZT rx (Ann IM 1990;113:276)
- Burkitt's (Nejm 1986;314:874), EB virus associated, in adults
- Leiomyosarcomas (Nejm 1986;314:874), EB virus associated, in children (Nejm 1995;332:12)
- Cervical cancer due to higher prevalence of HPV infection (Nejm 1997;337:1343); get q 1 yr after 2 q 6 mo Paps (Ann IM 1999; 130:97)
- Hematologic including ITP (Nejm 1985;313:1375) and aplastic anemias from parvovirus infections (Ann IM 1990;113:926); and from diminished half-life and megakaryocyte infection (Nejm 1992;327:1779)
- Myocardiopathy, dilated type (Nejm 1998;339:1093; 1992;327:1260)
- Neurologic (Ann IM 1994;121:769) including early subtle CNS degeneration (Nejm 1990;323:864) leading to dementia (Nejm 1995;332:934; Ann IM 1987;107:383); progressive multifocal leukoencephalopathy (Ann IM 1987;107:78) associated w papova/polyoma virus, seen in transplant pts as well, cytarabine rx no help (Nejm 1998;338:1345); cord lesions; aseptic meningitis; peripheral neuropathy (Nejm 1985;313:1538); cerebral toxoplasmosis; cerebral lymphomas
- Nephropathy (Nejm 1989;321:625)

Acquired Immune Deficiency Syndrome, continued

- Rheumatologic including Reiter's without conjunctivitis; and psoriasis w arthritis (Bull Rheum Dis 1990;39:5)
- Suicide (Jama 1996;276:1743)

r/o HTLV I and II infections, former associated w paraparesis, latter w no disease (Ann IM 1993;118:448); rare idiopathic CD4 cell lymphopenia syndrome (Nejm 1993;328:429)

Lab:

Immunol: (Med Let 1997;39:81)

- Viral load, most important test, positive at >50,000/cc in acute primary disease (Nejm 1998;339:33); RNA by PCR, peripheral mononuclear cell viral mRNA levels predict prognosis (Ann IM 1995;123:641) and treatment success (Nejm 1996;335:1091, 1996;334:426; Ann IM 1996;124:984); indicates rapidity of disease progression (Jama 1997;278:983); <10,000/cc good, 10,000–100,000/cc moderately ok, >100,000/cc bad
- T4 helper cells (CD4) <200/cc defines AIDS now (Mmwr 1992; 41(RR-17):1) and predicts opportunistic pneumonias (Ann IM 1989; 111:223); 200–500 = intermediate risk (Nejm 1989; 321:1141)
- ELISA w Western blot test, only 1.5% false positive in low risk military population (Nejm 1988;319:961); if indeterminant, repeat in 1 mo and should become pos if really HIV; if persistently equivocal, get viral load and culture (R. Smith 4/95). Tests negative for 4+ mo incubation period (Nejm 1989;321:941)
- Ora-Sure HIV-1 test from 2 min swab btwn cheek and gum, as specif as serum by ELISA/Western Blot (Jama 1997;277:254)
- P24 nuclear antigen detection either of free antigen or dissociated from IgG antibody-antigen complex (Nejm 1993;328:297); pos usually in early disease including the primary disease syndrome when ELISA still neg in 50% (Nejm 1998;339:33)

Path: Bronchoscopic brushings and lavage are 85% specif and sens for specific infections (Ann IM 1985;102:747)

Urine: Proteinuria >0.5 gm/d in 50%, nephrotic syndrome in 10% (Ann IM 1984;101:429)

Rx: (Nejm 1995;333:450; 1993;328:1686)

Preventive maneuvers

Hospital isolation (guidelines—Ann IM 1986;105:730); risk is very low even w needle sticks (Nejm 1985;312:1)

Screen blood donors w ELISA test (Nejm 1989;321:917,941,947, 966), perhaps others, eg, high-risk spreaders like dialysis staff, psych patients (no—Ann IM 1995;122:641,653; yes—Nejm 1986;315:1562), or maybe all patients and clinicians now (no—Ann IM 1995;122:641,653; yes—Nejm 1991;324: 1498–1508), or perhaps all pts age 15–54 in hospitals w one case of AIDS/1000 discharges (Nejm 1992;327:445)

Consistent condom use prevents disease; 0/124 conversions in HIV neg partners over 2 yr, otherwise 5/100 pt/yr convert (Nejm 1994; 331:341).

In pregnancy (Nejm 1995;333:298), peripartum scalp electrodes, rupture of membranes >4 hr (Nejm 1996;334:1617), and episiotomies. Pre- and peripartum AZT no matter what the maternal viral load or CD4 count (Nejm 1996;335:1621) reduces maternal-fetal transmission from 25% to 8% (Jama 1995;273:977; Nejm 1994;331:1173) and decr to a lesser extent w peri or postpartum rx w/i 1st 6 mo of age (Nejm 1998;339:1409); so rx mother beginning at 28 wk gestation through delivery and infant for 1st 6 wk of life (Nejm 2000;343:982). Rx of prepartum mother viral load to <20,000 (Jama 1996;275:599) or <1000 (Nejm 1999;341:394) or <500 (Nejm 1999;341:385) yields infant infection rate = 0, and is safe for infant (Jama 1999;281:151). Elective C/S reduces infant infection to <190 (Jama 1998;280:55) and w postpartum antibiotics reduces infant infection to 2% (Nejm 1999;340:977). Avoid breast feeding, which has a 6–10+% transmission rate over 1–1.5 yr (Jama 2001;285:2413; 2000;283: 1167; 1999;282:744). All these efforts have decr neonatal AIDS in US by 67% (Jama 1999;282:531)

Vaccines development? (Nejm 1995;333:1331; Ann IM 1996;125:270)

Prophylaxis immediately (<24–48 hr) (CDC prophylaxis/exposure guideline—Mmwr 1998;47[#RR-7]:1) post exposure × 1 mo w AZT (Nejm 1997;337:1485) 300 mg bid + lamivudine (3TC) (Ann IM 1998;128:306; Jama 1998;280:1769) 150 mg bid; may add indinavir 800 mg q 8h or nelfinavir 750 mg tid if exposure substantial

of pregnant women, nevirapine po

Prevention of AIDS-associated infections (Nejm 2000;342:1416; Jama 1998;279:130; and USPHS comprehensive and tabular guidelines—Ann IM 1999;131:873):
- *Pneumocystis* prophylaxis (Nejm 1995;332:693) w CD4 counts <200. Can stop after rx persistently raises CD4 counts >200 (Nejm 2001;344:159,168,222; 1999;340:1301)
  1st: Tm/S SS qd (Arch IM 1996;156:177) or DS tiw, qd-bid; also helps toxoplasmosis
  2nd: Pentamidine aerosol 150–300 mg monthly if CD4 <200 (Nejm 1991;324:1079; 1990;323:769; Ann IM 1989;111:223), least toxic; or
  Atovaquone (Nejm 1998;339:1895) 1500 mg po qd
  3rd: Dapsone 50 mg po bid or qd w pyrimethamine, also helps prevent toxoplasmosis
- *M. avium* (MAI) prophylaxis (p 435) (Rx Let 1999;6:35) if CD4 counts <50 w clarithromycin, azithromycin 1200 mg po q 1 wk, or rifabutin; Can stop after rx persistently raises CD4 counts >100–200 (Nejm 2000;342:1085; 1999;340:1301)
- Pneumovax immunization
- Chickenpox: Vaccination + VZIG if exposed
- Tuberculosis prophylaxis if ppd pos w INH, or rifampin + pyrazinamide, or rifabutin + pyrazinamide (Nejm 1999;340:371)
- Toxoplasmosis after encephalitis, w sulfadiazine + pyrimethamine folate po qd (Ann IM 1995;123:175); or if pos IgG titer and CD4 <200, w Tm/S DS qd or dapsone + pyrimethamine
- HPV w pap smears
of questionable benefit:
- CMV infections w ganciciclovir 1 gm po tid, if CD4 <50–100 decr rates by 1/2 (Nejm 1996;334:1491)
- *Cryptococcus,* histo and cocci w chronic fluconazole, but no prolongation of survival (Nejm 1995;332:700)
- Candidal local mucosal and systemic infections w fluconazole 200 mg po q 1 wk (Ann IM 1997;126:689) but no prolongation of survival (Nejm 1995;332:700) and resistance a problem
- Cryptosproidiosis w careful exposure prevention (see list—Ann IM 1999;131:879)
- Human herpes virus-8 (Kaposi virus) perhaps (Ann IM 1999; 131:891)

- Influenza w vaccine (Ann IM 1999;131:430 vs 1988; 109:383)

of acute primary infection: Triple drug rx (Nejm 1998;339:33):

of disease (Jama 2000;283:381; Ann IM 1998;128(2):1057; CDC guidelines—Jama 1997;278:1962; Nejm 1997;337:725,734, 1996; 335:1081,1091; Ann IM 1997;126:929,939,946); rapidly changing field, should check most recent Med Let and other journal issues

Drug therapy (p 488) triple + for adults and children (Nejm 2001;345: 1522) w HIV viral load RNA levels <5000–10,000/cc no matter the CD4 count (?) at doses incr to get RNA load levels <500; both survival and other measures of disease severity are improved (Jama 2001;286: 2560,2568; 1998;280:1497). Women run lower viral loads but prognosis same so may be use CD4 <500 even if viral loads higher (Nejm 2001;344:720). Simultaneous initiation of triple rx results in >80% still adequately suppressed whereas w sequential initiation <40% suppressed at 2^+ yr (Jama 1998;280:35); tapering to 1–2 drugs after 3–6 mos not as good as cont'd 3 drug rx (Nejm 1998;339: 1261,1269,1319; Lancet 1998;352:185). Multiple drug resistant organisms appearing (Jama 1999;282:1135,1142,1177; Nejm 1998; 339:307) esp in Thailand, prevalent subtype E (Ann IM 1999;131: 502). Avoid combinations of d4T + AZT; or ddC w ddI, d4T, or 3TC

Triple drug rx w:
- 2 nRTIs + a PI or a nnRTI; or
- 2 nRTIs + ritonavir + another PI

Most common triple rx combo: zidovudine (AZT) + lamivudine (3TC) + indinavir; or abacavir w AZT + 3TC as good (Jama 2001;285:1155)

Experimental: interleukin 2 × 5d q 8 wk (Jama 2000;284:183) boosts CD4 counts but at least other immunogen stimulation of CD4 counts have no effect on survival (Jama 2000;284:2193)

Treatment of AIDs-associated conditions:
- of aphthous stomatitis (p 181)
- of wasting syndrome (p 328)
- of diarrhea: rx primary cause if can be found; octreotide 50 mg sc q 8 h (Ann IM 1991;115:705), opiates, loperamide (Imodium), or diphenoxylate-atropine (Lomotil)

OVERALL AIDS PRIMARY CARE STRATEGIES

General: Discuss meaning, definitions, prognosis; risk reduction, avoidance of cofactors; safer sex, birth control; substance abuse issues; community resources, support network, counseling; facilitate dialogue w partner, friends, family; complete and directed physical; build referral network

Asx HIV-positive (usually >500 T4 cells): Viral load, T cells, CBC, chemistries q 6–12 mo, q 6 mo cervical pap smears × 2 then q 1 yr (Ann IM 1999;130:97); PPD and controls; pneumovax, H. flu vaccine, yearly flu shots; hep B status, consider vaccine if still at risk; syphilis serology; baseline toxo and CMV titers; dual or triple drug rx to decr viral load if recent (6 mo) infection but not if asx and >6 mo infected (Rx Let 2001;8:17)

Symptomatic HIV-positive (usually 200–500 T4 cells): Triple rx; CBC, chemistries q 2–4 wk until stable on AZT, then q 4–8 wk; T cells, viral load q 3–6 mo; appropriate evaluation of sx; consider experimental rx's

AIDS and serious HIV infection (usually <200 T4 cells, occasionally only <300): Triple rx although advantage/benefit less clear than when CD4 = 200–500 (Nejm 1996;335:1099); opportunistic organism prophylaxis esp for *Pneumocystis,* MAI, toxo if baseline titer positive, CMV; mental status exams; ophthalmologic evaluation q 6 mo; aggressive evaluation of sx; appropriate rx of opportunistic infections and malignancies; consider experimental rx's, consultation/referral; AIDS-defining dx's and reporting

ARBO VIRAL ENCEPHALITIS

Cause: Several types of arboviruses: St. Louis (Ann IM 1969;71:681), eastern equine, West Nile (Nejm 2001;344:1807), western equine, and La Cross encephalitis

Epidem: *Culex* mosquitoes and ticks from birds and invertebrates. Incidence highest in small children and adults age >50 yr; many inapparent cases, up to 99%; incidence up after rainy winter; equine types kill horses by 1000s and children age <10

Pathophys: Humans and horses don't develop enough viremia to transmit these diseases

Sx: Fever (90%), Guillain-Barré type muscle weakness (56% w W. Nile type unlike others), severe headache (47%), nausea, and vomiting (52%)

Si: Altered mental status (46–86%); frontal lobe si's (78%); stiff neck (71%); cranial nerve palsies, especially of #III, IV, VI, VII (22%); Babinski (30%); seizures (10%)

Crs: 10–21 d; 10–36% mortality, higher if seize; 35–60% of survivors w neurologic morbidity; both predicted by CSF WBC counts and serum hyponatremia (e. equine type—Nejm 1997;336:1867)

Cmplc: SIADH

r/o tick-borne Powassan encephalitis, which has similar clinical presentation (Mmwr 2001;50:761)

Lab:

Serol: ELISA for IgM antibodies; reverse transcriptase PCR identification of viral RNA in CSF

CSF: 1–500 WBCs, 50% lymphs; protein 40–500$^+$ mg%

Xray: MRI shows basal ganglia and thalamic focal lesions (Nejm 1997; 336:1867)

Rx:

Prevention: spray to eliminate mosquito population; kill pigeons and other birds or use them as sentinels and test for antibody titer changes (Nejm 1967;277:12)

of disease: supportive

CHICKENPOX (Cpox) AND HERPES ZOSTER (Shingles)

Nejm 2000;342:635 (zoster); Ann IM 1999;130:922

Cause: Varicella, a herpesvirus

Epidem:

Cpox: <10% repeat infections, probably quite rare (Jama 1997; 278:1520)

Zoster: More common in the elderly and pts w HIV and cancer but not a si of occult malignancy; 10–20% of all persons will have in lifetime

Pathophys: Same organism causes first Cpox, and later shingles (Nejm 1984;311:1362)

Sx:

Cpox: 14 d incubation period; fever, centrifugal rash (on face and trunk 1st, then extremities)

Zoster: Shingles rash; pain often, may precede and sometimes rash never appears

Si:

Cpox: Fever <102°F (<38.8°C); herpetic rash various ages, trunk first and worst. New lesions appear for 4 d

Zoster: Classic herpetic lesions in dermatome distribution w hyperesthesia and pain; cranial and other neuropathies

Crs: Cpox worse w incr age, so adolescents and adults suffer more than children

Cmplc:

Cpox:

- Anterior horn cell myelitis
- Encephalitis leading to cerebellar ataxia
- Pneumonia especially in adults
- Group A β strep cellulitis and toxic shock
- Reye's syndrome
- Rare congenital abnormalities if infected in first trimester, 1/11 (Nejm 1986;314:1542)
- Embryopathy, rate is 2% if infected between weeks 8 and 20 (Nejm 1994;330:901); in pregnancy, 85% of women are immune even if don't recall having had the disease

Zoster:

- Secondary bacterial infections
- Dissemination
- Chronic post-herpetic neuralgias and neuropathies (Nejm 1996;335:32); incidence incr w age, 27% at age 55, 47% at 60, 73% at 70; as is duration, so over age 70 yr lasts >1 yr in 50%; British study found over age 69 3 mo prevalence = 20%, 12 mo preval = 10%, while under age 60 3 mo preval = 2% and 12 mo <1% (Bmj 2000;321:794)
- Guillain-Barré
- Encephalitis/myelitis
- Keratitis, heals well unlike simplex

Lab:

Path: Skin bx or Tzanck prep show intranuclear inclusions and giant cells

Serol: Antibody level to determine past immunity

Rx:

Preventive:

Cpox: Vaccine, live attenuated (Varivax-MSD) (Med Let 1995;37:55) 0.5 cc sc × 1 for age 1–12, × 2 1–2 mo apart if age >13 yr (Mmwr 1995;44:264), must keep frozen until reconstituted, then used w/i 30 min; 100% effective, 86% in field use (Nejm 2001;344:955), more failures if RAD (Jama 1997;278:1495), safe (Jama 2000;284: 1271); duration >20 yr and may decr later zoster incidence (Jama 1997;278:1529; Nejm 1989;320:892; 1988;318:573). Avoid in immunocompromised and pregnant pts
Isolation, children may return to day care or school as soon as lesions are crusted (Nejm 1991;325:1577)

Zoster: V-ZIG (varicella-zoster immune globulin) 125 U/10 kg im; expensive; use if immunosuppressed and exposed, perhaps useful in exposed healthy adult? (Ann IM 1984;100:859)

of disease:

Cpox:

- Acyclovir (Zovirax) 20 mg/kg po qid × 5 d ameliorates course modestly (Ann IM 1992;117:358; Nejm 1991;325:1539) if started in first 24 h but costs $32/d; or 800 mg 5×/d × 7 d (Med Let 1994;36:87) speeds healing × 2 d, costs $125
- Famciclovir (Famvir) (Med Let 1994;36:87) 500 mg po tid × 7 d, similar in all respects including cost of $130/wk
- Valcyclovir (p 491)
- Foscarnet iv q 8 h for disseminated disease in AIDS patients (Ann IM 1991;115:19)

Zoster: Wet soaks when wet, then topical steroids when dry; antivirals may prevent postherpetic neuralgia? (no—Br Med J 1989;289:431; vs do over age 50—J Fam Pract 2000;49:255; or over age 60—Bmj 2000;321:794); but dual rx w steroids and acyclovir × 3 wk does speed healing and comfort (AnnIM 1996;125:376; Nejm 1994; 330:896);

- Famciclovir 500 mg po tid × 7d within 3 d of rash onset speeds healing and decreases neuralgia duration (Ann IM 1995;123:89), use over age 50 or if severe or immunocompromised; or
- Valacyclovir (Valtrex) 1 gm po tid × 7–14 d (Med Let 1996;38:3); similar to famciclovir
- Acyclovir (Ann IM 1987;107:859) iv or po 10 mg/kg q 8 h for severe local, eg, eye, or disseminated, or at onset in immunocompromised host. 800 mg 5 ×/d × 7–10 d speeds

ID: VIROLOGY

healing and decreases acute neuralgia and neuritis (Am J Med 1988;85[2a]:84)

- Prednisone 60 mg tapered to 0 over days/weeks, if over 50, especially if involves head, to decrease postherpetic neuralgia (Nejm 1996;335:40)
- Amitriptyline 10–25 mg po qd × 3 mo decr postherpetic neuralgia (Rx Let 1999;6:26)

of zoster neuralgia (Nejm 1996;335:32) (see also p 579):

- Gabapentin (Neurontin) (Jama 1998;280:1837) 300–1200 mg po tid
- Lidocaine patch 5% (Lidoderm) (Rx Let 1999;6:26,50) × 12 hr qd; or gel or cream topically
- Steroid injections (Arch Neurol 1986;143:836; Ann IM 1980; 93:588)
- Dilantin and/or carbamazepine
- Amitriptyline 12–25 mg po hs, incr q 1 wk; or nortriptyline, or other tricyclic
- TENS
- Phenothiazines
- Nerve block, intrathecal steroid injections (Nejm 2000;343:1514) q 1 wk up to 4 in persistent debilitating disease dramatically helps >80%
- Capsaicin topical cream OTC qid 0.075% (Arch IM 1991;151: 2225 describes use in diabetic neuropathy), questionable benefit (Med Let 1992;34:61), OTC costs $27/oz

COMMON COLD

Cause: Rhinovirus, coronavirus, adenovirus, parainfluenza virus, in order of frequency in adults; other rarer causes include: respiratory syncytial virus (p 662), echo, coxsackie, reovirus, and mycoplasmas

Epidem: Respiratory droplets, most frequently 1–2 d after inoculation, fomites w dried viruses (Nejm 1973;288:1361); hand-to-hand contact (Ann IM 1978;88:463); iatrogenic (adeno 8 conjunctivitis—Nejm 1973;289:1341)

Colds occur q 2–4 mo in average adult American; incr attack rates correlate w increasing individual stress levels (Nejm 1991;325:606)

Pathophys: Infection denudes and alters respiratory epithelial cells, especially the cilia (Nejm 1985;312:463) of nasal pharyngeal mucosa. Sinuses are extensively involved as well (Nejm 1994; 330:25)

Sx: Upper respiratory tract sx in all

Of adenovirus: acute hemorrhagic cystitis, especially in young men (Nejm 1973;289:344, 373); and conjunctivitis

Of reovirus: exanthematous rash

Si:

Crs: Adenovirus conjunctivitis lasts about 21 d

Cmplc: Severe viral interstitial pneumonia possible with all (Nejm 1972; 286:1289)

Of adeno: pertussis syndrome; unilateral deafness due to organ of Corti capillary occlusion rarely (Nejm 1967;276:1406)

Lab:

Rx: (CDC educational materials to decr antibiotic use: (404) 639-2215)

Hot steam 110°F (43°C) nasal inhalation speeds recovery (Proc Natl Acad Sci 1982;79:4766); no, new studies disprove (Jama 1994; 271:1109,1112)

Ipratropium nasal anticholinergic spray helps nasal sx a little (Ann IM 1996;125:89)

Zinc 13 mg lozenges q 2 hr while awake shortens crs by 1/2 (Ann IM 2000;133:245; 1996;125:81); but many studies on both sides of use (ACP J Club 1999;131:69), and causes premature and still births in pregnant women (Jama 1998;279:1962; Med Let 1997;39:9)

Herbal: echinacea OTC preparations may help (ACP J Club 1999; 131:19)

Vitamin C no help (Nejm 1976;295:973)

of rhino: postexposure interferon α-2a nasal inhalation works (Nejm 1986;314:65,71)

COXSACKIE DISEASES

Cause: Coxsackievirus A and B, enteroviruses, eg, enterovirus 71 (Nejm 1999;341:929, 936)

Epidem: Fecal-oral spread. Worldwide; summer predominance; very infectious, epidemics

Pathophys:

Sx: Herpangina causing very sore throat, dysphagia, anorexia, abdominal pain. Hand-foot-mouth disease (HFMD) with URI sx. Acute infectious lymphocytosis (AIL) w diarrhea, weakness, and URI sx. Pleurodynia (Bornholm's disease), a pleural pericarditis causing pleuritic thoracic and abdominal pain. Headache; aseptic meningitis

Si: Herpangina w red, vesicular lesions in pharynx. HFMD has red macules w vesicles on hands, feet, and stomatitis. AIL has documentable muscular weakness. Pleurodynia has fever, and pericardial or pleural rub. Meningitis si

Crs: Herpangina = 1–4 d; HFMD = 4–5 d; pleurodynia = 2–14 d

Cmplc: Polio-like syndromes, pulmonary edema, Guillain-Barré syndrome, encephalitis, chronic myocarditis

Lab:

   Serol: Culture and PCR

Rx: Supportive only

CMV INFECTIONS

   Nejm 1985;313:1270; Ann IM 1983;99:326

Cause: Cytomegalovirus, a herpesvirus

Epidem: Congenital via transplacental transmission; newborn via vaginal infection at birth (Nejm 1973;289:1); blood products and organ transplantation

   Congenitally infected children spread for years (Nejm 1973;288:1370); so too do many others w asx recrudescence (Nejm 1980;303:958); semen and vaginal carriers (Nejm 1974;291:121). Pregnant mothers w children in day care at high risk (Nejm 1986;314:1414). Most fetal damage occurs due to primary infections during pregnancy leading to 10% damaged offspring; but can occur in immune mother too from infection w different strains (Nejm 2001;344:1366), although damage is minimal (Nejm 1992;326:663)

   No incr incidence in female health workers (Nejm 1983;309:950)

Increased in gay men (90% positive by serology—Ann IM 1983;99:326)

Pathophys:

Sx:

Adults: Mononucleosis-like syndrome; rarely sore throat, unlike mono

Si:

Adults: fever, splenomegaly, mild hepatitis in 100%, cervical adenopathy is rare unlike mono

Congenital/newborn: jaundice, hepatosplenomegaly, hemolytic anemia, ITP

Crs:

Adult: 2–4 wk

Cmplc:

Congenital: deafness and mental retardation (Nejm 1976;295:469), now ahead of rubella

Adult: AGN in transplant patients (Nejm 1981;305:57); Guillain-Barré (Ann IM 1973;79:153); retinitis (Nejm 1982;307:94; Ann IM 1980;93:655,664); if immunocompromised, pneumonitis (Ann IM 1975;82:181) and encephalitis (Ann IM 1996;125:489)

Lab:

Hem: Atypical lymphs (Nejm 1969;280:1311); anemia (50%) w positive Coombs' in 20% (Ann IM 1970;73:553)

Serol: Rapid urine DNA hybridization detection method, accurate and fast, is possible (Nejm 1983;308:921). Specific antibody by neutralization, comp-fix, and indirect fluorescent antibody

Xray: Congenital, skull xrays show periventricular calcifications

Rx: Preventively screen women before pregnancy and perhaps in future immunize them? (Nejm 1992;326:663); screen blood products (Nejm 1986;314:1006); and isolate immunosuppressed patients from susceptibles who spread it for weeks

Prophylact immunocompromised with

- Acyclovir (Nejm 1990;320:1381)
- Interferon × 14 wk (Nejm 1983;308:1489)
- CMV immune globulin iv (Nejm 1987;317:1049)

of disease in immunocompromised host:

- Ganciclovir (Nejm 1999;340:1063; 1991;325:1601; Med Let 1989;31:79), which kills CMV but patients still die and resistance to it now developing (Ann IM 1990;112:505; Nejm 1989;320:289); helps retinitis (Ann IM 1985;103:377) if cont'd in suppressive doses, 3000 mg po qd after iv rx (Nejm 1995;333:

ID: VIROLOGY

615) or given prophylactically if CD4 < 50 (Nejm 1996;334: 1491); can stop if CD4 count up and 0 RNA loads after rx (Jama 1999;282:1633). Also available as intraocular implant (Nejm 1997;337:83); but neutropenia a problem (Ann IM 1993;118: 173,179)

- Foscarnet × 2–3 wk, the qd iv maintenance gives better survivals than ganciclovir but costs more ($24,000 vs $7500) (Med Let 1992;34:3; Nejm 1992;326:213)
- Cidofovir iv (Med Let 1997;39:14; Ann IM 1997;126:257,264); adv effects: renal toxicity
- Valacyclovir prevents CMV in renal transplant (Nejm 1999; 340:1462)

ERYTHEMA INFECTIOSUM (Fifth Disease)
Nejm 1989;321:485,536

Cause: Parvovirus B19

Epidem: Endemic and epidemic; spread primarily by respiratory secretions esp in infected young children (Jama 1999;281:1099). Nosocomial epidemics in nursing staffs caring for children in aplastic crisis (Nejm 1989;321:485). In adults, 50^+% are seropositive indicating past infection

Pathophys: P antigen on rbc is prime cellular receptor for the virus; hence the rare pt who is pp (homozygously P antigen-negative) is immune from infection (Nejm 1994;330:1192). Anemias and CHF occur because infection of erythroid progenitor cells results in their lysis acutely, and these conditions then develop if there is already chronic hemolysis for some other reason, or if no antibodies are formed at all as in AIDS (Ann IM 1990;113:926)

Sx: 7–10 d incubation period. 20% of adults and children may be asymptomatic. In children it presents as a rash; in adults it presents as a polyarthritis and malaise

Si: In children, "slapped cheek" may then develop into a diffuse exanthematous, pruritic rash lasting 5–7 d (picture in Nejm 1994;331:1062). In adults, an acute arthritis; and a rash on neck, extremities, trunk but not face

Crs: Arthritis is usually self-limited although it can be chronic and recurrent; rash may recur over weeks or months

r/o other childhood exanthems: chickenpox, rubeola, scarlet fever, rubella, and roseola

Cmplc: Aplastic crisis in patients w underlying chronic hemolysis and occasionally chronic marrow failure (Nejm 1987;317:287)

In pregnant women, spontaneous abortion in 1–3% exposed in first 20 weeks of pregnancy (Nejm 1986;315:77); other fetal anomalies (Nejm 1987;316:183; 1985;313:74) including hydrops fetalis from anemia and CHF (Ann IM 1990;113:926)

Lab:

Hem: Marrow has giant pronormoblasts and/or multiple nucleoli in pronormoblasts

Serol: IgM, IgG antibody titers by ELISA (Jama 1999;281:1099); or, in immunosuppressed, by DNA dot-blot hybridization studies of serum (Ann IM 1990;113:926)

Rx: Isolation may be unnecessary. In cases of persistent infection and marrow aplasia, IgG im qd (Nejm 1989;321:519), or iv (Ann IM 1990;113:926)

GERMAN MEASLES

Cause: Rubella virus

Epidem: Carrier is newborn infant, excretes for >1 yr postpartum. Maternal infection in first 7 wk causes 50% fetal death, 25% malformation rate at birth, premature delivery in 25%, and no problem in 20%; infection at 20 wk gestation and beyond results in no teratology and <10% prematurity rate

Pathophys:

Sx: Malaise; rash

Si: Exanthematous rash, usually; face first, spreads in 3 d; macular-papular; in infant w congenital syndrome as well; r/o other childhood exanthems: roseola, rubeola, scarlet fever, erythema infectiosum (5th disease)

Lymphadenopathy, posterior cervical, 98%; postauricular, 90%; suboccipital, 90%; preauricular, 50%

Conjunctivitis; splenomegaly (25%); fever <102°F; sore gums

Crs: 12–21 d incubation period

Cmplc: Encephalitis (0.01%), myelitis; thrombocytopenia; RA-like syndrome (Nejm 1985;313:1117)

Congenital syndrome: rash, low birthweight, platelets <140,000 (91%), hepatosplenomegaly (75%), congenital heart disease (70%) especially PDA and VSD, cataracts (50%), mental retardation (100%), deafness (55%—Nejm 1968;278:809)

Lab:
Bact: Culture possible but not clinically practical
Serol: Latex, fluorescent antibody, ELISA

Rx: (rv of hospital epidemic control—Nejm 1980;303:541)

Vaccine, live attenuated 1 cc sc; rarely spreads to other family members; although spreads to fetus (25%) if patient pregnant, no fetal damage reported in 683 documented CDC cases (Mmwr 1989;38:289). Give to all childbearing women unless h/o previous immunization beyond age 1 yr or titer pos; may cause transient but not chronic polyarthropathy (Jama 1997;278:551)

HERPES, TYPES I AND II
Nejm 1986;314:686,749; Ann IM 1985;103:404

Cause: Herpes simplex

Epidem: Both types may be venereally spread, 2/3 of the time when active lesions are present but even when no active lesion (Nejm 1986;314:1561) 1/3 of the time (Nejm 1995;333:770)

Type I: at age 14, 25% of whites and 70% of blacks are seropositive (Nejm 1989;321:7). 2/3 new cases are symptomatic; 50% are oral and 50% genital (Nejm 1999;341:1432). Associated w tic douloureux, and appears in those patients when operated on (Nejm 1979;301:225). Epidemics (herpes gladiatorum) among wrestlers (Nejm 1991;325:906)

Type II: about a 20% seropositive prevalence in US adults (Nejm 1997;337:1105); higher in women and blacks (Nejm 1989;321:7). 2/3 new cases are asx (Nejm 1999;341:1432) and shed virus as much (83%) as symptomatic pts (Nejm 2000;342:844)

Pathophys: Type I tends to be orolabial and have complications of encephalitis, while type II tends to be genital and neonatal w complications of meningeal involvement; but clinically full overlap. The two types are distinguishable bacteriologically by serotyping and genotyping (50% different)

Sx + Si: Primary infections are sicker, have fever, tender adenopathy, gingivostomatitis (looks like aphthous stomatitis), pharyngitis, cervicitis, external genital lesions, paronychia (herpetic whitlow, primary and recurrent infection w lymphangitis)

Zoster-like syndrome in newborn (Nejm 1971;284:24)

Recurrent type manifest by classic cold sore, or genital sores

Crs:

Type I recurs less frequently than type II (Nejm 1987;316:144)

Type II primary infection lasts 10 d, recurs 1–2 ×/yr lasting 4 d (Nejm 1978;299:237)

Cmplc: Ocular keratitis by self-inoculation; colitis; aseptic meningitis especially w vulvovaginitis, or recurrently as **Mollaret's meningitis** proven by PCR CSF studies (Ann IM 1994;121:334; Nejm 1991; 325:1082); urinary hesitancy and sacral paresthesias especially w colitis (Nejm 1983;308:868) or vulvovaginitis; disseminated, systemic forms and encephalitis (p 513); neonatal HSV infection w 50% mortality if infection occurs <6 wk prior to delivery (Nejm 1997;337:509)

r/o erythema multiforme, hand-foot-mouth disease (base is not erythematous), and monkey herpes in monkey handlers (Ann IM 1990;112:833)

Lab:

Bact: Culture, can read in 2–3 d; 77% sens in primary herpes (Nejm 1992;326:1533)

Path: Skin biopsy shows inclusions and giant cells; scraped Tzanck prep of skin lesion very sens/specif

Serol: Diagnostic in 97% of secondary infections (Nejm 1992;326: 1533) but does not separate type I from II; commercial kits have false-neg rates >25–50% (Ann IM 1991;115:520); do by Western blot or glycoprotein G immunodot methods; use PCR for CSF

Rx: Prevent by keeping people w cold sores away from newborns and the immunosuppressed; good handwashing technique, condom use (Jama 2001;285:3100); in pregnancy, asx shedding is common so unclear how to handle (Ann IM 1993;118:414), C-section only if clinical lesions when goes into labor because risk of infection in infant is <8% if recurrent disease, ~50% if primary (Nejm 1986; 315:796; 1986;316:240), but <10% of mothers who cultured

ID: VIROLOGY

herpes at delivery have a h/o herpes lesion (Nejm 1988;318:887). Vaccines being developed but so far are ineffective (Jama 1999;282: 331,379)

of disease (Med Let 1999;41:90):

Oral:

- Acyclovir (Zovirax) (Med Let 1994;36:1) 400 mg po tid × 7–10 d for primary; or × 5 d for recurrent episode, then 400 mg po bid prophylaxis reduces recurrences by >50% long term (Nejm 1993; 118:268) (topical is useless—Can Fam Physician 1991;37:92; Med Let 1990;32:5); for all neonatal (iv), whitlow, primary, or frequently recurrent herpes progenitalis, or oropharyngeal stomatitis; renal excretion, dialyzable; resistance appearing in immunocompetent and -incompetent now (Nejm 1993;329:1777); $0.50/pill
- Famcyclovir (Famvir) 125 mg po bid × 5 d at 1st sx of recurrence decr shedding and duration/severity of sx (Jama 1996;276:44); or 500 mg po tid × 7 d for primary or severe infection; 250 mg po bid long term prophylaxis decr recurrence at 6 mo from 75% to 25% and safe (Jama 1998;280:887); 500 mg po bid preventively in AIDS pts w pos serology perhaps (Ann IM 1998;128:21)
- Valacyclovir (Valtrex) 1 gm po tid × 7 d or bid × 5 d (Arch IM 1996;156:1729); 500 mg po qd for long term suppression, cheapest regimen (Med Let 1999;41:90)

Topical:

- Ducosanol (Abreva) (Med Let 2000;42:108) OTC 10% cream 5×/d shortens duration × 1–2 d, works by blocking cell entry not viral synthesis like others so may help if used w first si of recurrence
- Penciclovir 1% cream q 2 hr × 4 d; speeds healing and end of shedding × 1 d (Jama 1997;277:1374; Med Let 1997;39:57) vs no help at least in genital herpes (Med Let 1999;41:90)
- Acyclovir 5% ointment 6×/d not very effective

Herbal: avoid Herp-Eaze (chaparral shrub), which is hepatorenal toxic (Arch IM 1997;157:913)

HERPES: DISSEMINATED, SYSTEMIC, OR ENCEPHALITIS

Nejm 1986;314:686,749; Ann IM 1985;103:404

Cause: Herpes simplex types I and II

Epidem: Occurs in babies under age 3 mo born of mothers w active disease (Nejm 1991;324:450; 1985;313:1327) or to asymptomatic but virus-shedding mothers (56/15,000) (Nejm 1991;324:1247); immunosuppressed; atopics (eczema)

Asx shedding when no lesions in 10–20% w type I or II genital herpes in 1st year after primary infection (Ann IM 1992;116:433)

Pathophys:

Sx + Si:

Encephalopathy: olfactory sensations, focal seizures and si's, low-grade fever, often no skin lesions at all

Disseminated type has classic herpes vesicular rash all over body

Systemic type has fever, malaise, etc.

Crs:

Encephalopathy: rapid course early rx helps, otherwise 70% mortality

Cmplc: Myelitis, hepatitis, pneumonitis, meningitis (Nejm 1982;307: 1060); encephalitis may look like temporal lobe mass lesion, r/o similar **lacrosse viral encephalitis** (Nejm 2001;344:801) for which no approved rx available, mostly in children, 15% have permanent residual defects.

Lab:

Bact: Culture eye, blood, pharynx

CSF: Tzanck prep has a 50% false-negative rate

Path: Brain bx is abnormal

Serol: Diagnostic in 57% (Ann IM 1983;98:958, 977—K. Holmes); most helpful in primary infections, not recurrences

Rx: Prevent by keeping people w cold sores away from newborns and the immunosuppressed; good handwashing technique; in pregnancy culture weekly, C section only if clinical lesions when goes into labor because risk of infection in child is <8% if recurrent disease, ~50% if primary (Nejm 1986;315:796; 1986;316:240), but <10% of mothers who cultured herpes at delivery have a h/o herpes lesion (Nejm 1988;318:887). In sexually active pts about 10%/yr transmit to their partners even when being careful (Ann IM 1992;116:197). Vaccine eventually?

ID: VIROLOGY

of disease:
- Acyclovir for all (Med Let 1994;36:1; Ann IM 1987;107:859) including neonates (Nejm 1991;324:444) 5 mg/kg q 8 h iv × 5–7 d; renal excretion, dialyzable, resistance now appearing (Nejm 1989;320:313) in 5% of cases (Ann IM 1990;112:416); or, if acyclovir-resistant,
- Foscarnet (Ann IM 1989;110:1710), which is better than
- Vidarabine (Nejm 1991;325:551) although often recurrence within 6 wk of rx completion

INFLUENZA

Cause: Influenza virus, types A (most common), B (very young and very old), and C (rare); a myxovirus

Epidem: Worldwide; spread by respiratory droplets. Incidence higher in patients w elevated pulmonary artery pressures, eg, mitral stenosis, pregnancy. School absenteeism increases from 6% to 20% within 2 d of epidemic, best way to monitor. Frequency and severity of A > B > C. 2 types of external antigens; hemagglutinin and neuraminidase; both can undergo antigen shifts; they occur infrequently; there may be a finite and predictable nature to shifts, eg, 1978 A2 variant was similar to 1889–1890 type (Nejm 1978; 298:587)

Pathophys: Ulceration of tracheobronchial tree can cause secondary bacterial infections

Sx: Cough invariably, fever, malaise

Si: Cough, usually nonproductive at first

Crs: 1–2 d incubation period; sx last 5–6 d, malaise may last 2 wk

Cmplc: Secondary bacterial pulmonary infections acutely or during convalescent stage; fulminant viral infection leading to death in 1st 48 h, myocarditis, parotitis (Nejm 1977;296:1391)

Lab:
  Serol: Rapid diagnostic tests 73% sens 95% specif, cost $20 (Med Let 1999;41:121). Comp-fix, FA, or hemagglutination antibodies to types A, B, or C

Rx: (Med Let, yearly update in September; Nejm 2000;343:1778)

Vaccine, 1 cc im, trivalent usually, annually in October if over age 50 or chronically ill; new combination each year based on best guess from previous year's new organisms; usually two A strains and one B strain; 50% effective (reduction in incidence) in the elderly (Jama 1994;272:1661); 25–50% reductions in pneumonia and CHF (Nejm 1994;331:778), in young healthy adults vaccination reduces illness incidence by 25% and work day losses by 40% (Nejm 1995;333:889), and in health care workers caring for elderly mortality of their pts is decr (J Infect Dis 1997;175:1). Adverse effects: generally no different from placebo except sore arm (Nejm 1995;333:889), hepatic metabolism of many drugs decr × 50% for 1 wk, eg, theophylline, warfarin, etc (Nejm 1981;305:1262; questionable—Med Let 1985;27:81). Can give at same time as pneumovax at different site. In children, split virus has fewer side effects; 2 doses 1 mo apart (Nejm 1977;296:567); debatble value in elderly (Jama 1990;264:1139). In cancer patients, diminished response so try to give between chemotherapy courses (Ann IM 1977;87:552); diminished response in nursing home patients too. Not protective in HIV-positive patients (Ann IM 1988;109:383).

Live attenuated intranasal A vaccines give added protection (Ann IM 1992;117:625) and are effective in children as well (Nejm 1998; 338:1405)

Drug prophylaxis and rx of disease (p 490) w zanamivir, oseltamivir, amantadine, or rimantadine

KAPOSI'S SARCOMA

(Nejm 2000;342:1027)

Cause: Human herpes 8 virus (HHV-8) coinfection w HIV (Nejm 1999; 340:1863; 1998;338:948; 1997;336:163; 1996;334:1168,1292, Jama 1997;277:478)

Epidem: HHV-8 is spread venereally and perhaps more importantly orally in saliva (Jama 2002;287:221; Nejm 2000;343:1369), and by needle sharing (Nejm 2001;344:637) at least among gay men and immunosuppressed pts, some endemic pockets in Africa and Near East; also transmitted by transplants (Nejm 2000;343:1378)

Kaposi's Sarcoma, continued

Pathophys:
Sx + Si: Violaceous skin eruptions, ulcers on legs, r/o angiomatosis (see above)
Crs: 80% mortality if immunosuppressed, not bad if not
Cmplc: r/o bacillary angiomatosis by bx
Lab:
Path: Spindle-shaped tumor cells
Rx: Intralesional hCG (Nejm 1996;335:1261); interferon α helps 50% (Nejm 1983;308:1071; debatable—Ann IM 1990;112:582) given w anti-viral rx; vinblastine 4–8 mg iv q 1 wk (Ann IM 1985;103:335); topical alitretinoin (Panretin) (Rx Let 1999;6:22) $2000/60 gm
Radiation helpful for localized disease

MEASLES

Cause: Rubeola, a paramyxovirus
Epidem: Spread by direct contact w patient in day 2 or more of incubation period. Worldwide, common. Mortality up to 50% in developing countries, highest (0.1%) in rural infants over age 1 (Am J Pub Hlth 1980;70:1166); higher in vitamin A-deficient patients (Nejm 1990; 323:160)
Pathophys: Respiratory tract involved, nose to bronchial tree.
Viremia within 2 d of contact. Koplik's spots and skin lesions are areas of local intracellular viral replication (Nejm 1970;283:1139).
Encephalitis is hypersensitivity damage, not infectious (Nejm 1984; 310:137)
Sx: Fever of infection, w rash, on day 2 after exposure, is rare.
4–6 d prodrome of gradually increasing fever to 104°F (40°C), brassy cough, nasal discharge (coryza), photophobia, and then rash
Si:
• Koplik's spots on buccal mucosa, white on red base, opposite molars
• Conjunctivitis, palpebral only
• Vascular spiders on soft palate
• Rash, "brown paint spilled over head and neck," starts around ears, macular/papular, can be on palms and soles when severe

- Fever increasing to 105–106°F (40.5–41.1°C) w rash appearance, then decreasing to normal in 24 h

Atypical measles in previously vaccinated = lymphadenopathy, pulmonary infiltrates, distal rash including palms and soles, high fever (Ann IM 1979;90:873–887)

Crs: 12–14 d incubation period. 2–10% mortality in developing countries (Nejm 1985;313:544)

Cmplc:

Early: Hecht's giant cell pneumonia in adults; secondary bacterial infections of lung, ear; thrombocytopenia (rare); encephalitis in 0.1%, 65% of these will have neurologic residua, subclinical in 15–20% (L. Weinstein, 1986)

Late: subacute sclerosing panencephalitis 10–20 yr later (Nejm 1975; 292:990), a slow virus effect, associated w diminished DHS and IgA levels (Nejm 1985;313:910), cf progressive multifocal leukoencephalopathy from papovavirus (Nejm 1973;289:1278), or AIDS (p 492)

r/o other childhood exanthems: roseola, rubella, scarlet fever, erythema infectiosum (5th disease)

Lab:

Hem: Wbc decr, if increased look for bacterial infection, encephalitis, or viral pneumonia; platelets depressed usually

Path: Skin bx of rash shows intranuclear inclusion bodies

Serol: Antibody by neutralizing, hemagglutination, or comp-fix

Rx: Passive prophylaxis w IgG

Active immunization w live attenuated virus vaccine, after age 15 mo, still ~15% won't take, these patients later sustain outbreaks as adults (Nejm 1987;316:771); give after only 9 mo age in developing countries (Nejm 1985;313:544); under 2 mo <2/3 respond (Jama 1998;280:527). Continued outbreaks in US preschoolers w low vaccination rates and in school children because of vaccine failures; revaccinate at age 5 (Nejm 1989;320:75) or 10 (Med Let 1989;31: 69); 2 shot series 98% effective (Jama 1997;277:1156). Safe even if allergic to eggs (Nejm 1995;332:1262)

Vitamin A 200,000 IU × 2 increases survival in developing countries (Nejm 1990;323:160)

of depressed platelets, if bad enough: steroids

ID: VIROLOGY

MONONUCLEOSIS
Ann IM 1993;118:45

Cause: Epstein-Barr virus (Nejm 2000;343:481), a herpesvirus

Epidem: Spread by intimate contact w carrier. 18% of adults are asx, oral excreters (Nejm 1973;289:1325). Especially in college age adults; only in previously EBV antibody-negative; at Yale freshmen class = 75% antibody-negative, but only 35% negative after 4 yr; apparent to inapparent infections = 2:1 (Yale—Nejm 1970;282:361)

Pathophys: Lives in only B lymphocytes (Nejm 1979;301:1133) and mouth epithelial cells; replicates only in latter (Nejm 1979;301: 1255). IgM antibody response (heterophile) decr rapidly (Nejm 1966;274:61). EBV antibody (IgG, anti-early antigen) persists for years and correlates w cancer risk (Ann IM 1986;104:331; Nejm 1985;312:750). Diminished DHS transiently (Nejm 1974;291:1149)

Sx: Macular rash; sore throat; fever, low grade w malaise; pain behind eyes helps tell from strep throat, r/o rubella, flu; alcohol worsens malaise

Si: Pharyngitis, purulent sterile tonsillitis; splenomegaly (50% males; 25% females); hepatitis, low grade, especially if age >40 yr (Nejm 1975;293:1273); eyelid edema; *palatal petechial rash, *lymphadenopathy (40%), especially postauricular and posterior cervical (r/o secondary syphilis and CMV). Genital ulcers lasting 30 d (Nejm 1984;311:966)

Crs: Usually benign

Cmplc: Rare encephalitis w residual impairment (L. Weinstein 3/85); Guillain-Barré and Bell's palsy, often EBV-positive without clinical mono (Nejm 1975;292:392); ruptured spleen; hemolytic anemia; pharyngeal obstruction; rash in 100% if give ampicillin; nasopharyngeal cancers; B-cell lymphoma (Nejm 1983;309:745) and AIDS associated or post-transplant lymphoproliferative disease (Nejm 1993;327:1710,1750); leiomyosarcomas (Nejm 1995;332: 19); thymic cancer (Nejm 1985;312:1298); Hodgkin's (Nejm 1989; 320:689); hairy leukoplakia in AIDS (S. Sears, 8/97); perhaps multiple sclerosis (Jama 2001;286:3083)

r/o mono-like syndrome caused by CMV (p 506) and human herpesvirus 6 (Nejm 1993;329:168)

---

*If neither present, no point getting monospot (Ann IM 1982;96:505).

Lab:

Chem: Amylase elevated even without pancreatitis due to salivary source

Hem: Wbc shows >50% monos and lymphs w >10% atypical lymphs (serrated where touch rbc, clear cytoplasm, often vacuolated) (Nejm 1969;280:836), r/o hep A, rubella, toxoplasma, phenytoin (Dilantin) (Nejm 1981;305:722), Graves' disease, CMV especially postpump, PAS

Serol: EBV immunofluorescent antibody >1/80

Heterophile by rapid slide (monospot), will be positive if titer >1/40 but if too high must be diluted 1st; false positive w serum sickness; or by sheep rbc agglutination by patient serum, w which serum sickness is distinguished by absorbing sera 1st w guinea pig kidney cells, while mono still agglutinates, and 2nd by beef cells, after which serum sickness still agglutinates. Heterophile goes negative over 6–12 mo

Rx: Symptomatic, steroids for pharyngeal obstruction, hemolytic anemia, or severe neurologic sx

Acyclovir no help in chronic fatigue syndrome (Nejm 1988;319:1692) or acute mono

MUMPS

Nejm 1968;279:1357

Cause: Mumps virus, a paramyxovirus

Epidem: Common; all susceptible exposed patients get neutralizing antibody, 60% get sx

Pathophys: A parotitis

Sx: Nausea and vomiting, fever, pain, and swelling in front of ear and at jaw angle

Si: Parotid enlarged (9/13), unilateral in 15%; ear pushed out, jaw angle obliterated; r/o influenza et al., which can also cause parotitis (Nejm 1977;296:1391). Opsoclonus (dancing nystagmus) and small pupils; fever; aseptic meningitis, 25% have CSF cells, usually benign, can have without parotitis

Crs:

Cmplc: Pancreatitis, often; meningoencephalitis; orchitis in adult; arthritis, large joint, asymmetric; pneumonia; diabetes induction

Lab:

Chem: Amylase elevated

CSF: Cells in 25%; glucose diminished, protein incr for a long time, often (Nejm 1969;280:855)

Serol: Antibody titers elevated, reliable index of immunity; skin test not helpful

Rx: Isolation of patients of little value since spreads before sx. Passive immunization w hyperimmune IgG not effective (Med Let 1968;10: 14). Active immunization w live virus gives lifelong immunity (Ann IM 1983;98:192)

POLIO

Cause: Polio virus, an enterovirus

Epidem: Fecal-oral spread; peak incidence in summer and fall. Paradoxically occurs in countries w good sewage systems; correlates inversely w infant mortality, when <70/1000, many persons not infected in infancy when protected w maternal antibody and hence are susceptible when older when the disease is much more damaging. Most cases now acquired outside of US in persons immunized as children or as vaccine-associated (see below). But global eradication now nearly 90% complete

Only 0.1–1% cases show clinical si's, ie, most are subclinical. Increased clinical incidence in pregnant or ovulating females; after T + A bulbar polio is increased, even if T + A was years ago (L. Weinstein 6/67)

Pathophys: Hits anterior horn cells and sympathetic ganglia; starts in gi reticuloendothelial system; inhibits RNA polymerase

Sx: Fever, malaise, drowsy, headache, nausea, diarrhea or constipation, sore throat; may have stiff neck, low-back pain

Si: An aseptic meningitis; meningismus for 2–10 d; flaccid paralysis, maximum in a few days, maximum recovery in 6 mo. Spinal type may be in muscles of lumbar, dorsal, or cervical areas; bulbar type in upper (cranial nerves III–VIII), lower (CN IX–XII), or medullary (immediate threat to life)

Crs: 6–18 d incubation period. Death in 15% if patient >15 yr old; in 2.5% if patient <15 yr

Cmplc: Encephalitis; viral pneumonia

Late post-polio muscular atrophy due to reactivated CNS infection (Nejm 1991;325:749) w partial motor neuron dysfunction and dropout but not total dropout (Nejm 1987;317:7; 1986;314:959) including dysphagia from bulbar involvement (Nejm 1991; 324:1162)

r/o other causes of "viral" meningitis: coxsackie, echo, viral hepatitis, leptospirosis, et al. (p 576)

Lab:

CSF: Aseptic meningitis picture

Serol: Comp-fix, and neutralizing antibody titers

Rx: (Ann IM 1982;96:630)

Gamma globulin for passive, short-lived protection

Vaccine:

IPV (Salk); killed virus, primary 3 shot series then boost × 1 in 4–5 yr and on foreign travel; lasts 6^+ yr; 70% effective; preferred to OPV in US to avoid spread to immunocompromised

OPV (Sabin) (Nejm 1977;297:249), live attenuated, 90% effective, spreads to other intimate contacts, elicits gi RES secretory IgA immunity as well as systemic unlike Salk (Nejm 1968;279:893); used now in developing countries where benefit of spreading it seen as offsetting risk to immunocompromised

RABIES (Hydrophobia)

Ann IM 1998;128:922; Nejm 1993;329:1632

Cause: Rabies virus, a rhabdovirus

Epidem: From saliva of infected animal, inhaling infected guano in bat caves, or corneal transplants (Nejm 1979;300:603). Bats may be reservoir since not killed by it. Cats are now most commonly affected domestic animal. Most common wild animals affected: bats, foxes, skunks, raccoons; and prey species like rabbits, woodchucks and goats (Me Epigram 12/95)

Cyclic prevalence q 100 yr, peaked in 1965. 20 cases in US 1960–1980 (Ann IM 1984;100:728); incr again in US so that 22 cases

1990–1996. Over 20 cases in animals annually in Maine alone (ME Epigram 12/95)

Pathophys: Spreads along nerves to CNS

Sx: H/o animal bite except in bat rabies where often no h/o bite or even bat contact (Mmwr 1995;44:625)

Pain/paresthesias at exposure site in 50%; difficulty swallowing in 65%; fever; priapism; nausea and vomiting; Guillain-Barré-like syndrome

Si: Encephalitis w tonic contractions of muscles, especially throat on minimal stimulation (hence hydrophobia)

Crs: 15–60 d incubation (depends on nerve length), rarely up to 6 yr later (Nejm 1991;324:205)

Fatal unless rx'd before sx, usually, although some severe cases now recovering w supportive care, ie, respirator, etc. (Ann IM 1976; 85:44). 2/38 survived 1960–1980

Cmplc: May be misdiagnosed as Guillain-Barré

Lab:

CSF: Elevated protein after 1 wk; cells are a mix of lymphs and polys, 6–300/mm^3

Path: Negri bodies in brain at post

Serol: Half positive after 1 week of sx, 2/3 after 1–1/2 wk, all positive by 2 wk of sx

Rx: Vaccinate (Med Let 1998;40:64) w human diploid cell vaccine (HDCV) (Imovax); rabies vaccine absorbed, or purified chick embryo cell (PCEC) (RabAvert); all ~$700/5 shot series; chloroquine malaria prophylaxis may prevent adequate immunization (Nejm 1986;314:280)

• Primary series postexposure = HDCV im on day 1, 3, 7, 14, 28
• Preexposure = day 1, 7, and 28 im, or 1/10 im dose intradermal day 1, 7, 21, or 28
• Booster
- Post repeat exposure after previous primary series w shots day 0 and 3
- Every 2 yr to veterinarians and other high-risk people

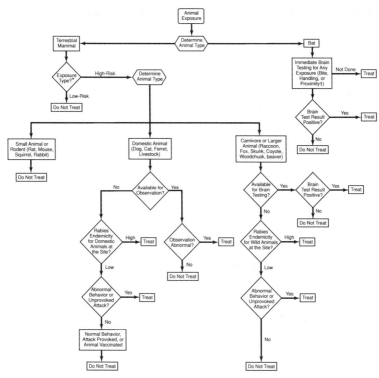

Figure 12.2.2 Algorithm for Determining Appropriateness of Animal Exposure Treatments. Asterisk indicates that high-risk exposure includes bite or body fluid exposure (saliva, cerebrospinal fluid, brain); low-risk exposure includes handling or scratch only, with no body fluid or low-risk body fluid (blood, urine, stool) only. Some sites considered a scratch by a wild carnivore or larger animal as a significant body fluid exposure. Dagger indicates for explanation of proximity bat exposures, see the Advisory Committee on Immunization Practices guidelines. (Reprinted with permission, Journal of the American Medical Association, 2000;284:1003. Copyrighted 2000, American Medical Association.)

For acute single exposure: vaccinate as above + HRIG (immune globulin) 20 IU/kg, 1/2 in wound, 1/2 im in deltoid in adult, thigh in child, not gluteal area (Nejm 1987;316:1256,1270); use liberally even if no bite in bat exposures (Mmwr 1995;44:625)

of disease: supportive care, like respirator, etc. See Fig. 12.2.2

ROSEOLA (Exanthem Subitum, 6th Disease)

Cause: Human herpesvirus 6

Epidem: 14% of febrile children under age 2 in ER have it, cause of 1/3 of febrile seizures under age 2 yr (Nejm 1994;331:432; 1992;326:1145)

Pathophys:

Sx: High fever to 105°F (40.5°C) × 3–4 d, defervesce, then rash in 10%

Si: Viral exanthem, fever

Lab:

Rx: Symptomatic

Chapter 13
Neurology

D. K. Onion

13.1 HYPERTHERMIA

MALIGNANT HYPERTHERMIA
Nejm 1993;329:484; 1983;309:416

Cause: Genetic plus anesthesia or other stress; autosomal dominant

Epidem: Prevalence = 1/14,000 people can develop if stressed; a history of one safe anesthesia is no guarantee next will be ok

Pathophys: Abnormal calcium channel in muscles causes Ca^{2+} release into muscles and intense contractions

Sx: None

Si: Intraoperatively tachycardia and tachypnea precede muscle rigidity and then high fever

Crs: High mortality

Cmplc: r/o neuroleptic malignant syndrome (p 526); and simple **heat stroke,** in the elderly with impaired thermoregulation and anhydrosis, 10% mortality, or in healthy adults exercising in the heat (Nejm 1993;329:484)

Lab:

Chem: Platelet ATP studies distinguish? (Letter—Nejm 1980;303:642)

Path: Muscle bx of relatives shows abnormal in vitro responses to drug stimulation if they too are susceptible

Rx: Prevent by avoiding halogenated gases and muscle paralyzers; may try to prevent with dantrolene (Dantrium) 1 mg/kg po × 2 d prior to elective surgery; avoid calcium channel blockers

of acute attack: stop anesthesia; dantrolene (Dantrium) 1 mg/kg push, repeat up to response or 10 mg/kg

NEUROLEPTIC MALIGNANT SYNDROME
Med Clin N Am 1993;77(1):185; Nejm 1993;329:485; 1985;313:163

Cause: Neuroleptic drugs (major tranquilizers) including phenothiazines, butyrophenones, thioxanthenes, loxapine, and rarely clozapine (Nejm 1991;324:746)

Epidem: ~0.2–0.5% of pts given these drugs will develop; unrelated to dose; 96% of cases occur within 30 d of starting the drug; 30% of those who have had before will get again if reexposed. Incidence is incr with exhaustion, dehydration, organic brain syndrome, and depot phenothiazines

Pathophys: Diminished CNS dopamine

Sx: 1–3 d onset, up to 5–10 d after drug stopped, or 10–30 d after im depot types

Si: Fever >100.4°F (>38°C) in 87%, rigidity and hypertonia ("lead pipe") (97%), changes in mental status (97%), autonomic instability (pallor, diaphoresis, BP changes, tachycardia, arrhythmias), akinesia, involuntary movements, tremor

Precipitated by dopamine agonists like metaclopramide (Reglan), or amoxapine (Asendin) sometimes

Crs: 10% mortality in 3–30 d; before 1984 and aggressive rx, mortality was ~25%

Cmplc: Respiratory failure, myoglobinuric renal failure, cardiovascular collapse, arrhythmias, pulmonary embolus

r/o **heat stroke** (Ann IM 1998;129:173): fever >105°F (>40.6°C), altered mental status (100%), anhidrosis; associated w exertion or infection in elderly in presence of hot humid weather; cmplc include DIC (50%) and renal insufficiency, 20% in-hospital mortality; rx w cooling

Also malignant hyperthermia (p 525); idiopathic **acute lethal catatonia** drug interactions with MAO inhibitors; central anticholinergic crisis, which responds to iv physostigmine; tetanus; stiff-man syndrome (p 429); myotonia; meningitis or encephalitis; thyroid storm

Lab:

Chem: CPK elevated, may be >16,000 IU; aldolase elevated; elevated LFTs (due to pyrexia-induced fatty changes?)

Hem: Wbc 15,000–30,000 with L shift

Urine: Myoglobinuria (67%)

Rx: Stop neuroleptics then give
- Dantrolene (Dantrium) 1–2 mg/kg iv initial dose, then up to 10 mg/kg/d iv or po divided in q 6 h doses; beware of concomitant calcium channel blocker use, +
- Bromocriptine 2.5–10 mg po tid, or amantadine 100 mg po bid, or perhaps L-dopa

Nitroprusside iv/minoxidil po worked in 1 patient when dantrolene failed, controlled fever and BP (Ann IM 1986;104:56)

Prevent myoglobinuric ATN by iv fluids, mannitol infusion, and NaHCO$_3$ iv to alkalinize the urine

13.2 VASCULAR DISEASE

TRANSIENT ISCHEMIC ATTACK

Cause: Carotid or aortic arch (Nejm 1992;326:221) plaque and/or platelet emboli, cardiac emboli, vascular spasm, hypercoagulable states, and idiopathic

Epidem:

Pathophys: Plaque ulceration correlates poorly with TIA and it is hard to accurately make that dx (Curr Concepts Cerebro Dis 1987;22:19); occasionally is vasospastic and can rx w calcium channel blocker (Nejm 1993;329:396)

Sx: Lateralized neurologic sx, usually lasting <5–10 min but by definition always <24 h

Anterior circulation sx: amaurosis fugax (Stroke 1990;21:201), weakness of arm > face > leg paresis (middle cerebral artery pattern), leg > arm > face paresis (anterior cerebral artery pattern)

Posterior circulation sx: bilateral blindness, diplopia, numbness in face and mouth, slurred speech, quadriplegia

Si: Carotid bruit, but correlates poorly with symptomatic disease (Ann IM 1994;120:633); in elderly, asx bruit present in 10% and does not correlate with CVA rate in or out of affected carotid distribution; 60% disappear over 3 yr (Ann IM 1990;112:340)

Flow reversal through supraorbital artery (feel, then occlude preauricular artery, if lose pulse then flow is reversed) indicates significant carotid stenosis or occlusion

NEUROLOGY

Crs: Subsequent stroke, 5% w/i 2 d (Jama 2000;284:2901), 8% in first
   month, 5%/yr for 3 yr, 3%/yr thereafter; 41% will die of MI

Cmplc: r/o tumor, can mimic exactly (Arch Neurol 1983;40:633); r/o
   carotid or vertebral dissections (see below)

Lab:

Noninv: (All about 85% sens and 90% specif—Ann IM
   1995;122:360; 1988;109:805,835) Not substitutable for
   angiography unless local comparisons made (Nejm 1998;339:1415,
   1468; Stroke 1995;26:1747) but still is often done
   • Carotid doppler or duplex ultrasound
   • Magnetic resonance angiography

Xray: CT/MRI to r/o tumor, bleed; carotid angiography, if ready to
   operate; % stenosis denominator is normal carotid, not bulb or post
   stenotic dilated area, Europeans calculate differently (Nejm
   1998;339:1415)

Rx:

of asx carotid bruit: (see below)

Meds:
   • Aspirin 30 mg qd after 300 mg load as good as higher doses and
     has fewer side effects (Nejm 1991;325:1261); or as Aggrenox
     (Med Let 2000;42:11; Rx Let 2000;7:6; 1999;6:62) 25 mg ASA +
     200 mg dipyridamole po bid; not clearly better than ASA alone;
     $90/mo
   • Ticlopidine (Med Let 1992;34:65) 250 mg po qd may be as good
     as ASA (Nejm 1989;321:501) but causes gi side effects often and
     agranulocytosis in 1%, $80/mo
   • Warfarin for people age >60 yr w Afib and intrinsic heart disease,
     hypertension, LVH, or previous TIA (Ann IM 1994;121:41,54)
     (see below); or ASA or ticlopidine if bleeding risk w warfarin
     judged too high (Ann IM 1994;121:45)

Surgical endarterectomy (Jama 1992;268:3120) of stenosis >70%
   (Nejm 1995;332:238), in patients with TIA or mild CVA reduces
   strokes by 17% (NNT = 6) (Nejm 1991;325:445); stenosis of
   50–70% in symptomatic pts equivocally helped (Nejm
   1998;339:1415). If asx carotid stenosis >60–70%, NNT-5 = 16
   (Nejm 2000;342:1743; Jama 1995;273:1421,1459 vs Nejm
   2000;342:1693), and clearly if >80% (Ann IM 1995;123:720 vs
   723; ACP J Club 1995;123(1):2; Lancet 1995;345:209); but still

debatable if asx (S. Kolkin 5/97) since NNT-3 = 36 (ACP J Club 1999;130:59), and cost per stroke avoided = $500,000 (Ann IM 1997;126:338). No help if stenosis is <50% (Lancet 1996; 347:1591);

Presumes a combined cmplc rate of angiography and surgery of <4%; often much higher morbidity in community hospitals, but only 1⁺% in big centers (M. Samuels 3/85; Jama 1998;279;1278, 1282).

Temporal artery graft, not indicated except in rare intracranial stenosis (Nejm 1987;316:809; 1985;313:1191). Aspirin + dipyridamole no help postendarterectomy to prevent recurrence (Ann IM 1992; 116:731)

CAROTID OR VERTEBRAL ARTERY DISSECTION

Nejm 2001;344:898; Neurol 1995;45:1517

Cause: Spontaneous, or trauma that is often trivial ("hairdresser's stroke")

Epidem: 1/100,000/yr for vertebral and 2.5/100,000/yr for carotid; 2% of all ischemic CVAs but 10–25% of those age <50; peak in 40s. Increased in Ehler-Danlos, Marfan's, osteogenesis imperfecta, polycystic kidney disease, and with positive family hx

Pathophys: Intimal tear in extracranial portions of the vessels

Sx: Age 35–55 yr

Carotid: sometimes h/o minor neck twist or trauma; facial pain (50%), unilateral headache (66%) often hemicrania, cerebellar ischemic sx (63%), retinal ischemia w amaurosis fugax, cranial nerve palsies (10%), dysgeusias, tinnitus (35%) often pulsatile

Vertebral: posterior neck pain (50%)/headache (66%); cerebral, cerebellar, brain stem ishcemic sx (90%), eg, lateral medullary plate syndrome (p 532)

Si: Horner's syndrome (46%) (p 575); bruit (24%) (Nejm 1994;330:393; Arch Neurol 1986;43:1234; Neurol Clin 1983;1:155)

Crs: Contralateral dissection in 2%, usually w/i 1 mo; rarely in same artery

Cmplc: Raeder's neuropathic pain (p 575); CVA; blindness

Lab:

Xray: MRI/MRA (Nejm 1996;335:1368) usually diagnostic; or angiography

NEUROLOGY

Rx: Heparin followed by warfarin × 3 mo; surgery sometimes if
   progresses

EMBOLIC STROKE

   Nejm 1992;326:1672; Med Aud Dig 1985;32:13

Cause: Atherosclerotic plaque, esp carotid, and protruding atheromatous
   plaque >4 mm in thoracic aorta (Nejm 1996;334:1216); mitral
   stenosis; SBE and atrial myxoma; cardiac valve prostheses; from
   silent DVTs (Ann IM 1993;119:461) paradoxical through ASD,
   may be silent (Ann IM 1986;105:695) 40% of patients age <55 yr
   with CVA have patent foramen ovale (Ann IM 1992;117:461; Nejm
   1988;318:1148); post-MI mural thrombus, 5% of patients with big
   anterior MI develop a mural thrombus, most in first 10 d (Nejm
   1989;320:392); chronic Afib (Arch Neurol 1984;41:708); billowing
   mitral valve (Nejm 1980;302:138)
   Also from fat emboli (p 728), and air emboli esp in divers (Ann IM
   2001;134:21)
Epidem: 31% of all strokes; incidence incr ×5 in atherosclerotic Afib, ×
   17 in rheumatic Afib (Neurol 1978;28:973); 35% lifetime incidence
   of stroke in Afib, 3/4 are embolic (Curr Concepts Cerebro Dis
   1986;21:5). Associated with homocystinuria (p 241), hypertension,
   and smoking (Nejm 1986;315:717)
Pathophys:
Sx: Very abrupt onset; seizures with onset occasionally, unlike thrombotic
   CVA
Si: Occlusion patterns like thrombotic stroke
Crs: 15% 30-d mortality
Cmplc: Like thrombotic strokes
Lab:
   CSF: Protein may be slightly elevated and may have some (<1000)
      rbc's
   Noninv: Echo cardiogram, 2D with contrast to find ASD at least in
      young pts without obvious cause (Ann IM 1992;117:922;
      1986;105:695) or LV thrombus (80+% sens); or TEE, 100% sens,
      99% specif for LA thrombus (Ann IM 1995;123:817)

Rx: (Nejm 1994;121:41)
Prevent by:
ASA prophylaxis po qd (Am J Med 2000;108:205)
Modifying risk factors like HT and smoking (Nejm 1995;333:1392)
Surgical endarterectomy (see above)
By anticoagulating all chronic or intermittent atrial fibrillators with
warfarin (Nejm 1992;327:1451), at least those over age 60; or, if
bleeding risk of warfarin seems too high, perhaps ASA (Nejm
1990;322:863) although some studies suggest no help (Ann IM
1995;123:649 but counted angina and MIs as well?), or if that fails,
ticlopidine; doing so decreases CVA rate × 2.5% on average, but at
2 yr, rate with rx is 1% compared to 7% on placebo, ie, number
needed to rx (NNT-2 yr = 16) (Nejm 1990;323:1505); PT of
1.2–1.5× control adequate (Nejm 1992;327:1406); no need to
anticoagulate if age <60 yr, no h/o TIA, no valve disease, normal
echo, and no hypertension (Ann IM 1994;121:41, 54); annual
bleeding risk ~2.5% (Ann IM 1992;116:6). Anticoagulate anterior
MIs with therapeutic heparin doses in first 10 d (Nejm
1989;320:352, 392)

THROMBOTIC STROKE
Nejm 1992;326:1672

Cause: Atherosclerosis; hypotension; migraine; high dose (≥100 μgm)
(Ann IM 1978;89:58), but maybe not low-dose estrogen (Nejm
1996;335:8 vs Jama 2000;284:72 meta-analysis) bcps; arteritis
caused by radiation, collagen vascular diseases, drug use (Ann IM
1972;76:823); infection leading to venous thrombosis or carotid
occlusion especially in children with tonsillitis; trauma to carotid or
head that may cause spasm most often seen in patients with
migraine hx; hematologic causes like polycythemia, sickle disease,
TTP, DIC, dysproteinemias; inherited clotting factor abnormalities,
like factor V (Leiden) and prothrombin gene position 20210
mutation, which cause venous thrombosis incidence incr especially
w BCP use (Nejm 1998;338:1793)

Epidem: Large vessel (half are carotid) type = 34% of all strokes;
lacunar = 19% of all strokes. 3% are in pts age <40 yr (Curr
Concepts Cerebro Dis 1982;17:15)

Incidence decr by 1$^+$ drinks/wk (Nejm 1999;341:1557) or <2 drinks qd (Jama 1999;281:53)

Associated with "crack" cocaine use (Nejm 1990;323:699), homocystinuria (p 241), hypertension, and smoking (Nejm 1986; 315:717; 1988;318:937), immediate postpartum period (Nejm 1996;335:768)

Pathophys: Carotid type usually a watershed distribution in anterior circulation; vertebral basilar syndromes (Curr Concepts Cerebro Dis 1980;15:11)

Sx: TIA hx (80%); nocturnal onset (60%)

Si: Specific occlusion patterns:

Middle cerebral: face and arm motor; expressive aphasia (Broca's)

Carotid watershed: parietal aphasias, weakness arm > face > leg

Posterior cerebral: homonymous hemianopsia, hemisensory loss, memory loss (Curr Concepts Cerebro Dis 1986;21:25)

Lateral medullary plate syndrome (posterior inferior cerebellar artery—Curr Concepts Cerebro Dis 1981;16:17): ipsilateral pain and temperature loss on face, contralateral for rest of body, hoarseness, swallowing dysfunction, Horner's, hiccoughs, ipsilateral cerebellar si's

Supraorbital/preauricular artery test (see TIA) positive if carotid occlusion.

Crs: 15% 30-d mortality; <15% return to work (Nejm 1975;293:955); survival (as well as incidence) correlates inversely with systolic BP prior to stroke (Ann IM 1978;89:15)

Cmplc: Pulmonary emboli, pneumonias, UTIs, poststroke depression (probably physiologic not psyche phenomenon) (Stroke 1994;25:1099), swallowing dysfunction in 45% (Stroke 1999;30:744)

Lab:

CSF: Normal

Xray: CT scan normal first 2–4 d, positive later; MRI abnormal within hours (rv—Curr Concepts Cerebro Dis 1989;24:13)

Rx:

Prevent (Nejm 1995;333:1392) by same maneuvers mentioned above for embolic stroke; plus by hypertension control; incr K$^+$ intake (Nejm 1987;316:235); smoking cessation; i ASA qd (Arch IM 1999;159:1248; Lancet 1999;353:2179; Ann IM 1991;115:885), better than warfarin (Nejm 2001;345:1444); perhaps HMG-CoA statin rx of elevated cholesterol (Nejm 2000;343:317; Ann IM 1998;128:89), or low HDL w fibrates (Circ 2001;103:2828)

Supportive care (Curr Concepts Cerebro Dis 1989;24:1): keep pCO_2 at 25–30 mm Hg if on respirator; monitor; give 100–125 cc/h of Ringer's or D5S; rx diastolic BP >140 or systolic >230 acutely with iv nitroprusside, if dias persists >105 or sys >180 for hours then rx with labetalol iv or po and/or nifedipine sl or po; mannitol 25–50 gm as 20% soln over 30 min q 3–12 h and/or furosemide iv; ASA po qd improves outcome (Lancet 1997;349:1569,1641). Acute care in designated stroke units in England dramatically improves mortality/morbidity (BMJ 1997;314:1151)

Rehab helps 80% and can keep out of nursing home (Curr Concepts Cerebro Dis 1980;15:21). Speech rx of aphasia of questionable help (Lancet 1984;1:1197 vs Arch Neurol 1986;43:653). Heparin sc if hemiparesis acutely to prevent DVT, which occurs in 70% (Ann IM 1992;117:353)

Experimental treatments:
- Acute thrombolysis (Nejm 2000;343:710; Med Let 1996;38:99, hotly debated—Nejm 1997;337:1309) within 3 hr of onset (Jama 1999;282:2019) if BP <185/110 and no ASA or heparin for at least 24 hr afterward, but not clearly beneficial (Jama 2000;283:1145; ACP J Club 1999;130(2):34; 1998;129(2):52; Lancet 1998;352:1245)
  - TPA 0.9 mg/kg up to 90 mg max, given 10% as bolus, 90% over next 60 min; better results in 20% (NNT = 5) evident at 3 and 12 mo, not acutely, ~2–10% bleed into CVA (Nejm 1999;340:1781; 1995;333:1581 vs Jama 2000;283:1151; 1995;274:1017)
  - streptokinase; ? no benefit w harmful CNS bleeding (European SK trial—Nejm 1996;335:145) vs borderline helpful if given in tertiary care stroke center w 3^+% risk of fatal CNS bleed and 12% better outcome at 3 mo (Jama 1996;276:961,995)
  - Urokinase intra-arterial (Jama 1999;282:2003) possibly up to 6 hr post onset
  - Ancrod (Jama 2000;283:2395, 2440) iv × 72 hr adjusted to fibrinogen level may be as good as TPA w same 5% bleed risk; available in Canada
- Heparin, low molecular wgt, sc qd-bid × 10 d improves 6 mo function and survival (NNT = 5) (Nejm 1995;333:1588) vs no

help long-term (Jama 1998;279:1265). IV heparin for "stroke in progress" no help (Ann IM 1986;105:825) although ASA may be worth trying
- ASA alone may be as good as thrombolysis (ACP J Club 1996;124:58; Lancet 1995;346:1509)
- Unsuccessful experimental treatments: nimodipine, a calcium channel blocker (ACP J Club 2000;133:20; Lancet 1990;336:1205); acute hemodilution (Curr Concepts Cerebro Dis 1988;23:31). Surgical extraintracranial bypass no help (Nejm 1985;313:1191)

of poststroke depression: SSRIs (Stroke 1994;25:1099), or nortriptyline (Lancet 1984;1:297)

HEMORRHAGIC STROKE

Nejm 2000;342:29(SAB); 1997;336:28; 1992;326:1672

Cause:
Subarachnoid: aneurysm or AV malformation (Nejm 1983;309:269)
   Hemorrhage into brain substance (Nejm 2001;344:1450): cerebrum, cerebellum, or brain stem

Epidem: Risk incr by use of α agonists for nasal congestion or wgt loss (Nejm 2000 343:1826,1886; Med Let 2000;42:113)
Subarachnoid: 7% of all strokes; 1% of all adults have an aneurysm. 2% of all w subarachnoid hemorrhage and aneurysm have polycystic kidneys. Associated w iv (not "crack") cocaine use (Nejm 1990;323:699); sometimes familial; also w Ehlers-Danlos and Marfan's syndromes, and type I neurofibromatosis
Brain: 9% of all strokes. Increased in smokers (Nejm 1986;315:717) and "crack" cocaine users (Nejm 1990;323:699). 50% are due to hypertension, 17% from amyloid angiopathy, 10% from anticoagulation rx, 5–10% from brain tumors, 5% from smoking, 5% from "crack," etc.

Sx:
Subarachnoid: Headache, severe often "worst in life," thunderclap-like (Nejm 2000;342:29), usually w emesis (r/o colloid cyst of 3rd

ventricle—Nejm 1995;332:1267); may have loss of consciousness; low back pain

Brain: With cerebellar: severe vertigo (unable to walk or stand), headache, and vomiting. With cerebral: decr level of consciousness, sudden onset, headache, and vomiting

Si:

Subarachnoid: Hypertension, stiff neck, **Parinaud's si** (upward gaze paralysis), subhyaloid retinal hemorrhages. Specific patterns: pons = Horner's si, cranial nerve nuclei, pyramidal tract

Brain: With cerebellar: awake, alert even w ophthalmoplegias; acute hypotonia; conjugate gaze paresis, skew deviation.

With cerebral: motor and always sensory deficits; seizure (13%) w onset or w/i 48 h

With brainstem: early loss of consciousness, brainstem si's, quadriplegia

Crs:

Cmplc:

Subarachnoid: Secondary cerebral vessel thrombosis; r/o "hereditary" cerebral hemorrhage w amyloidosis (Nejm 1984;311:1547)

Lab:

CSF: Some intracerebral bleeds and all subarachnoid bleeds show bloody tap (protein >1 g %; rbc's (100% sens, 80% spec); xanthochromia present in immediately spun CSF in 90% but also in 30% traumatic taps; w traumatic tap, rbc's decrease ≥10-fold from 1st to 3rd tube (80% sens, 60% specif—Ann IM 1986;104:880)

Noninv: EKG shows abnormal anterior MI patterns w SA bleeds (Nejm 1974;291:1122; J Neurosurg 1969;30:521)

Xray: CT before LP to r/o mass lesion; overall, 25% of subarachnoid bleeds won't show blood on CT so must LP after CT neg. False negativity by CT varies over time (Nejm 2000;342:29): 2% 1st 12 hr, 8% next 12 hr, 14% day 2, 25% day 3, 42% day 5.

MRI or MRA to find AVMs, r/o cerebral cavernous malformation, inherited in Hispanics and present w seizures in 3rd–4th decades (Nejm 1996;334:946)

Rx: Prevent SAH by hypertension control; aneurysm surgery if transient or mild sx, or asx aneurysm >10 mm (Nejm 1998;339:1725); screening 1° relatives w MRA and operating on even <5 mm aneurysms causes more harm than good, 11/18 had residual neurol damage (Nejm 1999;341:1344). Bucrylate embolization of av malformations, can cause late bleeding (Nejm 1986;314:477)

of acute SAH, calcium channel blockers (Neurol 1998;50:876) like
nimodipine 60 mg po q 4 h × 21 d (Med Let 1989;31:47; Curr
Concepts Cerebro Dis 1989;24:31), or rarely nicadipine iv;
hemodilution to hematocrit of 32% with colloid after phlebotomy
helps limit damage in spasm (Curr Concepts Cerebro Dis
1988;23:31). Surgery or other ablation of aneurysms before rebleed,
20% will w/i 2 wk

of intracerebral bleed: dexamethasone for cerebral edema no help
(Nejm 1987;316:1229)

of intracerebellar bleed: aspiration surgery if >3 cm diameter (Nejm
2001;344:1455)

13.3 HEADACHE

TENSION-TYPE (Muscle Contraction) HEADACHE

Cause: Vascular spasm?

Epidem: Very common; 40–50% of the population have each year (Jama
1998;279:381)

Pathophys: Intra- and extracranial vessels somehow cause pain; perhaps
other end of migraine spectrum? (Med Aud Dig 1979;26:16);
"doesn't exist," all psychogenic (M. Samuels 8/88); all due to
posterior cervical muscle spasms?

Sx: Never completely headache-free; worse late in day; cap distribution;
"band around the head"; stiff neck; no relief in pregnancy; ergot no
help

Si: Tender scalp vessels superficially; tender occipital muscles

Crs:

Cmplc: May "mix" with migraine type

r/o trigeminal neuralgia (limited to 5th cranial nerve distribution),
angioma (headache, preceding scotomata), tumor, trauma, sinusitis
(get xray), Fiorinal- or ergotamine-induced headache (put on
steroids × 2–3 wk to get off—M. Samuels 8/88), whiplash headache
from muscle spasm or arthritis in cervical zygapophyseal joints
(Nejm 1994;33:1047)

Lab:

Rx: ASA and sedation; other NSAIDs

TCAs help with or without depression, started low and gradually incr to tolerance, eg nortriptyline 10–75 mg or amitriptyline 10–100 mg po hs, alone or combined w stress management counseling (Jama 2001;285:2208)

Chiropractic manipulation no help (Jama 1998;280:1576)

MIGRAINE HEADACHE

Nejm 1992;326:1611; Ann Neurol 1984;16:157; Curr Concepts Cerebro Dis 1983;18:21

Cause: Genetic?

Epidem: Perhaps autosomal dominant with incomplete penetrance; 80% have pos family hx. Higher incidence in obsessive/compulsive, patients with family hx of epilepsy, after psychological trauma, and patients who had motion sickness as children

Common and classic: female:male ratio = 3–4:1; in women on bcps incidence incr × 9, 10% have each year, 15% have in lifetime. Cluster: male:female ratio = 10:1

Pathophys: (Nejm 1994;331:1713) Angiographically documented cerebrovascular constriction, shunting; perhaps from 5-HT induced vascular and neurogenic (Nejm 1991;325:353) changes, perhaps sludging leads to brain ischemia, which causes vasodilatation and pain especially in external carotid distribution. Or all neurologic deficits due to "the spreading depression of Leao"

Sx: (Nejm 1982;307:1029)

Common (80%): Slow onset over 4 h, no scotomata or other aura; prodrome of yawning, euphoria, depression; usually bilateral; lasts 4–72 h

Classic (10%): Precipitated by bright light, sound, or idiopathic; usually unilateral headache follows 20–30 min scotomata, which spread then recede, or other sensory, speech, or motor aura. Headache lasts 4–72 h; associated with NV + D, polyuria, and hemiplegias, all on opposite side of headache and scotomata. Consistently on one side 90% of time

Cluster (10%): "A migraine packed into 1 h." Clusters of several/week for ~1 mo; precipitated by vasodilators like alcohol, nitroglycerin during cluster period only; sweating, tearing, flush, salivation, runny nose; nocturnal; severe, may precipitate suicide

Si: Ergotamine trials help most but not all

Common: Eye tearing, face and neck muscle stiffness

Classic: On affected side, small pupil, external carotid pain; carotid sinus pressure temporarily relieves headache

Cluster: Horner's syndrome

Crs:

Classic: Relief with illness, steroids; after attack, ~1 week immunity from recurrence

Cmplc: CVA

r/o glaucoma (distinguished by cupped discs), epilepsy (scotomata last longer with migraine), trauma/tumor (in migraine no permanent scotomata except in very old, varies to opposite side 10% of time, headache not worse with Valsalva)

Lab:

Noninv: EEG shows spike patterns (46%—Nejm 1967;276:23)

Xray: CT/MRI unnecessary if classic sx (Neurol 1994;44:1191,1353)

Rx: (Med Let 1995;37:17; Nejm 1993;329:1476)

Prevention:

Common and classic: Stop birth control pills; i ASA po qod (Jama 1990;264:1711); then,

1st: • β blockers like propranolol, works in 70+%, 80–240 mg in bid doses or long-acting forms qd, or timolol (Blocadren) 10 mg po bid or 20 mg po qd

2nd: • Methysergide with 2 wk holiday q 3 mo to prevent fibrosis syndrome

3rd: • Calcium channel blockers like verapamil and nimodipine (Ann IM 1985;102:395; Headache 1983;23:106)

4th: • Valproate (Arch Neurol 1995;52:281) as Depakote ER 500–1000 mg po qd (Rx Let 2001;8:16); high dose riboflavin 400 mg po qd (Neurol 1998;50:466)

• ACE inhibitors (Rx Let 2001;8:12)

• Gabapentin 300–2400 mg po qd divided (Rx Let 2001;8:34)

Cluster: Avoid vasodilators; lithium 300+ mg qd (Med Let 1979;21:78); verapamil 120 mg po tid (Neurol 2000;54:1382)

Rx of acute attack

Common or classic (Med Let 1998;40:97): Stepped care (Jama 2000; 284:2599) based on severity or during attack w re-evaluation q 2 hr

- 1st: ASA/acetaminophen/caffeine (Excedrin) i–ii tab po × 1; much better than placebo by RCT, NNT = 4 (Arch Neurol 1998;55: 210), or
- ASA 900 mg + metoclopramide 10–20 mg po, as effective as po sumatriptan (Lancet 1995;346:923)
- 2nd: Triptans; beware drug interactions w MAO inhibitors, ergots, bcp's, cimetidine, and SSRIs, which could produce an excessive serotonergic response but rarely do (Rx Let 1999;6:68)
  - Zolmitriptan (Zomig) (Med Let 1998;40:27) 2.5–5 mg po, can repeat in 1–2 hr, $13/dose
  - Sumatriptan (Imitrex) (serotonin [5-HT] analog) 6 mg sc × 1 helps 90% within 2 h; or 100 mg po × 1 helps 50% within 2 h; or as nasal spray 20 mg/dose helps w/i 15 min like sc, but expensive ($20/dose) (Arch Fam Med 1998;7:234; Rx Let 1997;4:49; Med Let 1992;34:91; Nejm 1991;325:316,322) and may precipitate coronary artery disease
  - Rizatriptan (Maxalt) (Rx Let 1998;5:47) 5–10 mg po/sl q 2 hr up to 30 mg/24 h
  - naratriptan (Amerge) (Rx Let 1998;5:16) 1–2.5 mg, may repeat × 1 4 hr later, takes 4 h to work

Cluster: Prednisone 40–60 mg po qd × 7 d (Nejm 1980;302:449); chlorpromazine 100–700 mg qd (Nejm 1980;302:449); indomethacin; sumatriptan (see above)

Other options:

- Caffeine/ergotamine 1 mg po or 2 mg pr <6 mg/24 h, <10 mg/wk; overdose can cause vascular occlusion (Nejm 1970;283:518) especially when on β blockers or erythromycin
- Dihydroergotamine 0.5–1 mg iv/im/sc repeat q 1 hr; nasal spray (Migranal) (Med Let 1998;40:27; Neurol 1986;36:995) i inh each nostril repeat in 15 min; max on all + 3 mg/24 h; fewer side effects than ergotamine; $15/dose
- Ergotamine 2 mg sl q 30 min × 2 prn
- Butorphanol (Stadol) i nasal spray, may repeat × 1 in 1–2 h
- Lidocaine 4% intranasally, decr headache by 50% in 50% w/i 15 min (Jama 1996;276:319)
- Valproate 300–500 mg iv over 15–30 min (Rx Let 2001;8:12)

TIC DOULOUREUX; TRIGEMINAL NEURALGIA

Nejm 1986;315:174

Cause: Idiopathic

Epidem: Most age >50 yr old; may occur as a cmplc of multiple sclerosis

Pathophys: Unknown

Sx: Paroxysms of neuralgic, unilateral pain in trigeminal nerve distribution, many patients may identify specific actions that trigger the sx; maxillary and mandibular branches more frequently involved than ophthalmic; precipitated by touch. Occasional painless sensory neuropathy precedes (Nejm 1969;281:873)

Si: Pain on rotation of tongue blade inside cheek with teeth lightly clenched is diagnostic of syndrome, absence is diagnostic of remission (Trans Am Neurol Assoc 1966;91:163)

Corneal reflex preserved

ENT consult to look at posterior nasal space?

Recheck si's q 2 mo since frequent remissions

Crs: Frequent spontaneous remissions in 50%

Cmplc: r/o cluster headache, postherpetic neuralgia, 5th cranial nerve pressure by tumor, arteritis, syphilis

Lab: (Nejm 1969;281:873)

Hem: ESR to r/o arteritis

Serol: VDRL

Xray: MRI

Rx: (Nejm 1996;334:1123)

Meds:

- 1st: Carbamazepine (Tegretol) 100 mg po bid × 24 h, increase by 100 mg q 12 h until pain controlled up to 1200 mg/d; 70% effective long term. Adverse effects: agranulocytosis and aplastic anemia, thus get CBC q 1 week × 3 mo, then q 1 mo × 3 yr (Med Let 1975;17:76) or more recently weekly × 6 then q 6 mo is acceptable; nausea and vomiting; vertigo; urinary retention; multiple CNS reactions (Ann IM 1971;74:449)
- 2nd: Phenytoin (Dilantin)
- Others: Baclofen (Lioresal) 10–20 mg po t-qid; a muscle relaxant, effective in 70%, less toxic (Ann IM 1984;100:906), used alone or with above, don't stop abruptly (seizures), taper by 5–10 mg qd q 1 wk (Ann Neurol 1984;15:240)
- Gabapentin (Neurontin) 300–1200 mg po tid

Surgical microvascular decompression helps >75% immediately and long term (Nejm 1996;334:1077). Radiofrequency probe destruction of nerve results in 90% success (3% have anesthesia, 10% recur—Nejm 1973;288:680). Other surgical procedures sometimes include nerve section, or alcohol or phenol injection; both cause permanent numbness.

13.4 SEIZURE DISORDERS

Nejm 2001;344:1145; 1999;340:1565

EPILEPSY: PARTIAL COMPLEX AND ABSENCE (Petit Mal) TYPES

Nejm 1992;326:1671; 1983;309:536

Cause: Petit mal (PM): genetic autosomal dominant, 10% penetrance
Epidem:
Pathophys:
   Partial complex (PC): Seizure stays unilateral; in temporal lobe and inferior optic radiation
   PM: Slow waves in basal ganglia
Sx: Stereotypic, similar w each attack
   PC: Auras, déjà vu, visceral (nausea)
   PM: Classically short (seconds) lapses with facial (eye blinking, etc.) or extremity movement
Si: Stereotypic, similar w each attack
   PC: Lip smacking and automatic limb movements; change in consciousness, unlike simple partial seizures; last > 1 min
   PM: Patient unaware of lapse, no postictal confusion, no lateralizing si's; last <15 sec, hyperventilation induction
Crs:
   PC: Onset in adolescence to adulthood
   PM: Onset at age 3–4 yr usually, always by age 11; 50% outgrow in 10 yr especially if IQ >90, male, and otherwise normal (Neurol 1983;33:559)

Cmplc:
PM: In pregnancy, congenital malformations, infant drug withdrawal (Nejm 1985;312:559); 50% go on to have grand mal seizures as adults

Lab:
Noninv: EEG in PM shows 3/sec slow waves during and even often between attacks; may be precipitated by a respiratory alkalosis (hyperventilation); less often conclusive in PC

Rx:
PC: (Nejm 1996;334:165; Med Let 1995;37:37; Ann IM 1994;120:411):

1st,
- Carbamazepine (Tegretol) 400–1200 mg qd po (therapeutic level = 6–8 μgm/cc ≥2 h after last dose and ≥3 d after last dose change (Jama 1995;274:1622); drug/food interactions: grapefruit increases levels (Rx Let 1998;5:68), INH potentiates and is potentiated (Nejm 1982;307:1325). Adverse effects: nystagmus, drowsiness, ataxia, nausea, teratogenic, spina bifida in 1% (Nejm 1991;324:674), agranulocytosis, and aplastic anemia, so get CBC q 1 wk × 6
- Oxcarbazepine (Trileptal) (Med Let 2000;42:33) 300–1200 mg po bid; as effective as carbamazepine and better tolerated, no hematologic, hepatic, or dermatologic toxicity; does cause ataxia, incr phenytoin levels, interferes w bcps, phenobarb and phenytoin can decr levels, not effected by by erythromycin or cimetidine; $180/mo
- Phenytoin (Dilantin) (p 545) and/or
- Valproate 1–3 gm po qd divided (see below)

2nd,
- Phenobarbital 150–250 mg po qd or 0.6 mg/kg at 25–50 mg/min (therapeutic level = 15–30 μgm/cc ≥3 h after last dose and ≥20 d after last dose change (Jama 1995;274:1622)). Adverse effects: sedation; drug interactions, valproic acid toxicity, in utero intelligence impairment of fetus esp. in 3rd trimester (Jama 1995;274:1518); or
- Primidone (Mysoline) 750–1500 mg po qd (therapeutic level = 6–12 μgm/cc); works like and is partly broken down to phenobarbital; or

- Felbamate (Felbatol) (see below)
- Gabapentin (Neurontin) (Nejm 1996;334:1583; Med Let 1994;36:39) 900–1800 mg po qd divided; renal excretion; no interactions with other meds. Adverse effects: few, fatigue, ataxia, gi. $81/mo. Or
- Lamotrigine (Lamictal) (Nejm 1996;334:1583; Med Let 1995; 37:21) 50 mg po qd gradually incr to 300–500 mg po qd in bid doses; hepatic metabolism; levels decr by most other seizure meds but incr by valproate. Adverse effects: headache, N + V, ataxia, diplopia, rash esp w valproate concomitant use. $50/mo. Or
- Levetiracetum (Keppra) (Med Let 2000;42:33) 500–1500 mg po bid; adjunctive to other rx; no drug interactions. Adverse effects: anxiety, somnolence. $100/mo
- Topiramate (Topamax) (Med Let 1997;39:52) 200–400 mg po qd; adv effect: mental slowing; or
- Tiagabine (Gabitril) (Med Let 1998;40:45; Rx Let 1997;4:65) 4mg qd - 16 mg tid po, GABA reuptake inhibitor; used as adjunct w others; levels decr by phenytoin, carbamazepine, and phenobarb but their levels unaffected
- Zonisamide (Zonegram) (Med Let 2000;42:94) 100–600 mg po qd, a sulfa; adv effects: rashes, renal stones

Surgical resection for refractory and special cases, pursue if 1st line meds don't work (Jama 1996;276:470; 1996;334:647)

PM:
1st,

- Valproic acid (Nejm 1980;302:661) 1–3 gm po qd eg as Depakote DR b-tid (Rx Let 2001;8:16) (therapeutic level 50–100 μgm/cc, ≥2 h after last dose and ≥3 d after last dose change (Jama 1995; 274:1622)); also helps **myoclonic seizures.** Adverse effects: spina bifida in fetus (Sci Am Text Med 1984), depressed platelet stickiness, hair loss, essential tremor (Neurol 1983;33:1380), pancreatitis (Rx Let 20007:53); polycystic ovaries in ~50% of women because blocks testosterone to estradiol conversion (Nejm 1993;329:1383); or
- Ethosuximide (Zarontin) 750–1000 mg po qd (therapeutic level = 40–100 μgm/cc). Adverse effects: gi sx, dyskinesias and psychiatric changes after stopped, fatigue, headache

2nd,
- Clonazepam 0.5–5 mg po tid (also helpful for myoclonic seizures); or
- Lamotrigine (Lamictal) (see above); or
- Felbamate (Felbatol) (Med Let 1997;39:51) 300–900 mg po qid; increases levels of other seizure meds (Med Let 1993;35:107) and has high incidence of aplastic anemia (Jama 1994;272:995) and hepatic failure
- Tiagabine as above

GRAND MAL EPILEPSY
Nejm 1992;326:1671; 1990;323:1468

Cause: 20% idiopathic; 80% due to organic disease; trauma (subdural, scar), infection, neoplasia, vascular (AV malformation, CVA), degenerative disease (MS, Alzheimer's), metabolic (intoxications, anoxia, hypoglycemia, fever, hypo-Na, alkalosis, hypo-Mg, hypo-Ca)

Epidem:

Pathophys: Crosses midline; functional brain transection at midbrain (decerebrate)

Sx: Auras, Jacksonian progression, and postictal Todd's paralysis all indicate focal onset/origin; precipitated by menses

Si: Tonic decerebrate posturing evolving to clonic phase after 1–2 min. Postictal amnesia, confusion, often Todd's paralysis

Crs: Can stop meds (taper over 6 wk—Nejm 1994;330:1407) in children after 2 yr, especially if EEG has no slowing with or without spikes, 60–75% won't recur (Nejm 1998;338:1715). No decrease in IQ due to seizures (Nejm 1986;314:1085) unless complicated by status epilepticus

Cmplc: Status epilepticus (Nejm 1998;338:970), seizures >5 min or failure to awaken between tonic-clonic seizures, causes brain damage after 1 h even with normal vital si's (Nejm 1982;306:1337). In pregnancy, congenital malformations and infant drug withdrawal (Nejm 1985;312:559). Not a significant cause of car accidents (Nejm 1991;324:22)

r/o:

In adults: migraine, syncope, TIA, Meniere's; **Hysterical/Pseudo seizures** which have longer, less precise onset and end, "more pelvis," ie, pelvic thrusting, side-to-side head movements, eyes tightly shut, and alternating movements of limbs

In children: breath holding, long QT, night terrors, sleep walking, febrile seizures (p 665) (Nejm 1992;327:1122); **Lennox-Gastaut syndrome,** rx'd w lamotrigine (Nejm 1997;337:1807) or felbamate

Lab:

Chem/urine: Drug screen to r/o illicit drug ingestion

Noninv: EEG abnormal in 30–50%; 60–90% with repeated studies

Xray: MRI to r/o organic damage

Rx: (Nejm 1996;334:168; Med Let 1995;37:37; Ann IM 1994;120:411)

Withdrawal successful in 2/3 if sx-free after 2 yr (Nejm 1988;318:942) unless focal neurol si's, focal type seizure, or abnormal EEG; prophylactic rx beyond 1 week after head surgery/trauma no use (Nejm 1990;323:497); consider surgical rx if 1st-line drugs not enough (Nejm 1996;334:647)

1st,

- Phenytoin (Dilantin) 300–400 mg qd or fosphenytoin (Cerebyx) 10 mg/kg iv load then 5 mg/kg qd (therapeutic level = 10–20 μgm/cc, $\geq$2 h after last dose and $\geq$6 d after last dose change (Jama 1995;274:1622) for psychomotor (PC), not petit mal. Adverse effects: displaces T_3 and T_4 from TBG, hence lowers levels but TSH ok (Jama 1996;275:1495); rare idiosyncratic mono syndrome with hepatotoxicity due to inherited sensitivity to metabolites (Nejm 1981;305:722); many drug interactions causing elevated levels, eg, with warfarin, disulfiram (Antabuse), INH, chloramphenicol, chlordiazepoxide (Librium), Thorazine, phenylbutazone, methylphenidate (Ritalin), estrogens; interactions lowering levels occur with phenobarbital, primidone, carbamazepine; phenytoin also decreases folate (hence fetal toxicity) and vit D levels, and increases theophylline levels (Nejm 1982;307:1189); drug intoxication leads to a drunken state, cerebellar si's, gingival hyperplasia, rashes, hirsutism. Or
- Carbamazepine (p 540), or
- Valproic acid (p 543)

NEUROLOGY

2nd,
  - Phenobarbital (p 542), or
  - Primidone (Mysoline) (p 542), or
  - Felbamate (Felbatol) (p 543), or
  - Lamotrigine (p 543)
of status epilepticus (p 6)

13.5   SLEEP DISORDERS

OBSTRUCTIVE SLEEP APNEA
Nejm 1996;334:99; Ann IM 1987;106:434

Cause: Obesity; genetic component since often familial (Ann IM 1995;122:174)

Epidem: Associated with alcohol use, which worsens apnea, and with hypertension in obese older males; are they cause or effect (Ann IM 1985;103:190)?; congestive heart failure (Ann IM 1995;122:487); testosterone rx worsens (Nejm 1983;308:508). 1–5% of men age >60 yr; 4% of men age 30–60; 2% of women (Nejm 1993;328:1230)

Pathophys: Anatomically smaller pharynx predisposes (Nejm 1986;315:1327)

Sx: Daytime somnolence (in 80%) due to disturbed sleep; history of deep snoring and apneic episodes from roommate; but such hx is only ~65% sens/specif for sleep apnea (Ann IM 1991;115:356); and HT and/or obesity; if 2 of 3 present, sleep apnea will be documented (>5, 10^+ sec apneas/hr sleep) w 86% sens, 77% specif in general adult primary care population (Ann IM 1999;131:485)

Si: Hypertension (90%) (Jama 2000;283;1829; Nejm 2000;342:1378; Ann IM 1994;120:382)

Crs:

Cmplc: Cor pulmonale; car accident incidence incr × 6 (Nejm 1999;340:847, 881), ASHD and CVAs (Am J Med 2000;108:396)
  r/o
  - Narcolepsy (p 548)
  - Restless leg syndrome (see below)

- Normal elderly sleep patterns (Nejm 1990;323:520)
- **Central sleep apnea,** rare, rx with protriptyline 10–25 mg po hs or other tricyclic to suppress REM sleep especially if apnea occurring during REM, or progesterone as a central stimulant, or theophylline in CHF (Nejm 1996;335:562)

Lab:
    Noninv: Polysomnography (sleep) studies are definitive and probably best first test (Ann IM 1999;130:496), positive if >5, 10^+ sec apneas/hr sleep

Rx: Avoid sleep meds and alcohol
    Weight loss, even modest (eg, 20 lb) helps (Ann IM 1985;103:850)
    Nasal CPAP (Ann IM 2001;134:1015,1065; Lancet 1999;353:2100) helps daytime drowsiness and function if impaired, but not if pt has no complaints even w 30^+ apneic spells/hr of sleep
    Rarely tracheostomy or uvulopalatopharyngoplasty (Ann IM 1985;103:190), and/or maxillofacial surgery

RESTLESS LEG SYNDROME

ACP J Club 2000;132:24; NIH Mar 2000 publ #00-3788; Ann IM 1996;125:576; Neurol 1996;46:92

Cause: Primary cause: probably genetic autosomal dominant
    Secondary causes: iron deficiency, diabetes, drug-induced (TCAs, lithium, SSRIs), uremia, cord and peripheral nerve diseases, transiently in pregnancy (20%)
Epidem: Common; $2–5^+$% prevalence; incr w age, but 35% of adults w severe disease have onset in childhood; strong familial association
Pathophys: CNS disorder
Sx: Creepy crawly leg (usually) paresthesias relieved by movement. Positive fam hx. Sleep interference
Si: Normal neurologic exam; involuntary periodic jerking limb movements, esp when asleep (nocturnal myoclonus)
Crs:
Cmplc: r/o nocturnal muscle cramps
Lab:
    Chem: r/o secondary causes w iron and TIBC, ferritin, BUN/creat, FBS

NEUROLOGY

Rx: (Rx Let 1999;6:39)
- Dopaminergics like Sinemet and Sinemet CR, pergolide 0.10–0.75 mg po hs (Neurol 1999;52:944), bromocriptine, pramipexole (Mirapex), ropinirole (Requip)
- Anticonvulsants: valproate, gabapentin (Neurontin)
- Opiates: propoxyphene, Tylenol #3 hs
- Other: clonidine, baclofen, or clonazepam (Klonopin)

NARCOLEPSY

Nejm 1990;323:389; Ann IM 1987;106:434

Cause: Genetic in 15%; autosomal dominant; associated with HLA-DR2 in 100%

Epidem: Males and females equally affected; prevalence = 1–10/10,000 population; incidence incr by 60× in other family members; associated with SIDS families (Nejm 1978;299:969)

Pathophys: Drop directly into REM sleep, which causes paralysis, dreams, and loss of postural tone, all of which can also occur inappropriately when awake

Sx: Positive family history; onset usually in teens, 80% by age 30 yr, all <40 yr

Periodic inappropriate drowsiness 30 s–15 min, awake refreshed

Cataplexy: REM-type episodic loss of postural tone precipitated by excitement, laughter, surprise, nostalgia; lasts usually <1 min; 30% have when 1st present, 50% have eventually

Hypnagogic hallucinations: vivid dreams at onset of, or coming out of sleep

Sleep paralysis (60%): can't move as going into sleep or coming out but latter not diagnostic; lasts up to 10 min

Si:

Crs: Onset usually between ages 15 and 35; benign usually, doesn't progress after first 3–4 yr

Cmplc: Accidents, especially with cars; secondary psych problems, especially depression

r/o familial sleep paralysis on awakening (benign), sleep apnea hypersomnolence

Lab:

Noninv: EEG shows immediate REM sleep or at least slow wave sleep very abbreviated (1–2 min); not true in all narcoleptics, and amphetamines can mask

Rx: Nap 15–20 min at least 1–3/day

1st
- Methylphenidate (Ritalin) up to 200 mg qd; must give drug holidays 1×/12 mo or increase doses to levels that cause severe dependence; worse during these holidays

2nd
- Amphetamines like methamphetamine 10–60 mg qd, or dextroamphetamine 5–50 mg qd

Others:
- Modafinil (Provigil) (Med Let 1999;41:30) 200–400 mg po qd in am; many drug interactons; comparable to 2 cups of coffee?; $150/mo
- Imipramine or desipramine 25 mg tid for cataplexy (decreases REM) but beware incr BP when used with amphetamines

13.6 MOVEMENT DISORDERS

HUNTINGTON'S CHOREA

Nejm 1986;315:1267

Cause: Genetic, autosomal dominant, on chromosome #4; senile type rarely genetic

Epidem: Origin in England; brought here by colonists; may have been the etiologies of several Salem witches; "Woody Guthrie disease"
Equal racial incidence

Pathophys: CAG triplet repeats (36–121) on chromosome #4 (Nejm 1994;330:1401) somehow cause degeneration of caudate and lenticular nuclei, as well as frontal lobe; γ-aminobutyric acid (GABA) deficient in these areas (Nejm 1973;288:337)

Sx: Onset usually around age 35 yr
Chorea of arms, legs, face; pediatric onset often has no chorea and looks like Parkinson's

Si: Chorea and dementia with preservation of memory longer than problem solving skills

Crs: Live about 15 yr after diagnosis of the disease

Cmplc: Suicide common (~7%)

 r/o inherited cerebellar ataxia, myoclonus in Alzheimer's, Creutzfeldt-Jakob disease, Wilson's disease abetalipoproteinemia/ acanthocytosis, tardive dyskinesia, and infarction of basal ganglia

Lab: L-dopa evocation trial: gradually increase from 250 mg to 1 gm qd, usually increases chorea (reversibly) at least in patient with barely perceptible, questionable si's (Nejm 1972;286:1332; Lancet 1970;2:1185)

 DNA restriction fragment length methods can detect in asx patients in at least 1/2 of cases (Nejm 1988;318:535); and this information provided with counseling decreases anxiety in the high- as well as the low-risk groups (Nejm 1992;327:1401)

Xray: CT and MRI characteristically show caudate atrophy

 PET scans in asx show decrease in glucose metabolism in caudate nucleus (Nejm 1987;316:357)

Rx: Prevent by genetic counseling

 of disease: phenothiazines like haloperidol (Haldol) or other ancillary drugs like reserpine to decrease chorea

PARKINSON'S DISEASE (Paralysis Agitans)

 Nejm 1998;339:1044,1130; 1992;326:1613

Cause: Idiopathic, vascular, or postencephalitis lethargica (1918 flu); some genetic component, occasionally autosom dom (Jama 1999;281:341)

Epidem: Present in high % of US elderly: 15% by age 65–75, 30% by 75–85, 50% over 85 (Nejm 1996;334:71). Early onset type assoc w genetic mutations (Nejm 2000;342:1560).

 Increased incidence in Guam of a variant with more dementia, where is associated with ALS (O. Sacks, Island of the Color Blind, A. Knopf, 1996; Nejm 1970;282:947)

 Decr incidence in coffee and other caffeine users (Jama 2000;283:2674)

Pathophys: Relative dopamine deficiency in basal ganglia with concomitant incr inhibitory GABA activity

Sx: Tremor, akinesia, drool, characteristic stooping posture

Si: 4 major sx; dx if at least 2/4 present:
- Tremor, 3–4/sec, "pill rolling"
- Bradykinesia, with masked facies; a paucity of movement; slow finger tapping; can still respond to true danger easily though
- Rigidity, cogwheeling muscle type
- Gait disturbance: forward falling, shuffling; diminished arm swing, prolonged turning

Also seborrhea; low-volume voice

Crs: Progressive; risk of death (Nejm 1996;334:71) 2× that of pts w/o, worse if gait disturbance

Cmplc: Inanition, dementia (probably intrinsic, not due to L-dopa—Med Aud Dig 9/79), upper airway obstruction due to tremor and stiffness of upper airway muscles (Nejm 1984;311:438); postural hypotension (p 562) from sympathetic denervation (Ann IM 2000;133:338)

r/o (Bmj 1995;310:447) parkinsonism induced by phenothiazines, metoclopramide (Reglan) (Jama 1995;274:1780), Wilson's disease, reserpine (Nejm 1976;295:816), manganese toxicity (Nejm 1970; 282:5), CO_2 toxicity, drug impurity in heroin addicts (Nejm 1985; 312:1418), **progressive supranuclear palsy** w paresis of downward gaze, and multisystem atrophy subtypes (**olivopontine cerebellar atrophy, striatonigral degeneration, Shy-Drager syndrome,** and **cortical basal ganglionic degeneration** (Nejm 1993;324:1560)

Lab:

Noninv: Evoked potentials (Nejm 1982;306:1140,1205)

Path: Substantia nigra and locus coeruleus have lost melanin-containing neurons; remaining neurons have lacy bodies with eosinophilic inclusion bodies in cytoplasm

Rx: (Med Let 1993;35:31; Nejm 1993;329:1021; BMJ 1993;307:469)

Avoid metoclopramide (Reglan), a CNS dopa antagonist

to slow progression? but used less now because may incr mortality (Bmj 1995;311:1602; ACP J Club 1996;124:57):
- MAO B inhibitors,
- Selegiline (L-deprenyl, Eldepryl) (Nejm 1993;328:176; Neurol 1992;42:339). Adverse effects: interactions with meperidine (Demerol) (Can J Psych 1990;35:571) causing sedation, and w tricyclics and SSRI antidepressants causing severe agitation; insomnia; depression

of major sx:

1st, unless over age 70 or demented (Rx Let 1999;6:57):

- L-dopa with carbidopa, a decarboxylase inhibitor, = Sinemet 25/100 or 250 (not 10/100); up to 100 mg carbidopa qd and as little L-dopa as can get away with (2–8 gm qd); Sinemet CL 50/200 mg sustained release may be preferable and save money, but it takes 30% more than other forms since less bioavailable, start 1/2 po bid, may need plain Sinemet to jump start in morning (Med Let 1991;33:92). Adverse effects (drug holidays no help):
  - Postural hypotension, due to diuretic effect (Nejm 1971;284:865), nausea, and vomiting (Ann IM 1970;72:29) most frequently
  - Mental changes, especially hallucinations in older patients (Neurology 1983;33:1518)
  - On-off phenomena partly due to meal-induced absorption changes (Nejm 1984;310:483) most commonly in patients age <60 yr
  - Wearing off too soon, and start hesitation, especially after 5 yr of use
  - Dyskinesias, dystonias, and athetosis always within 5 yr (rx with lowering dose and adding bromocriptine, antihistamine, amantadine, or baclofen); the major reason for waiting to add L-dopa (Nejm 2000;342:1484)
  - Peripheral adrenergic effects, which lead to loss of weight and appetite (use the higher doses of carbidopa to prevent, and pretreat 2–3 d before start L-dopa)
  - Overall decr effectiveness after 3–5 yr

2nd, dopamine agonists (Med Let 2001;43:59), although unclear if their fewer side effects but lesser motor improvements than L-dopa make them preferable (Jama 2000;284:1971):

- Pergolide (Permax) 0.25–1.5 mg po bid up to 8 mg tid; dopamine agonist like L-dopa and bromocriptine. >$60/mo
- Ropinirole (Requip) (Rx Let 1998;5:29) 3–5 mg po tid, slowly incr dose; hepatic metabolism. Adverse effects: nausea, syncope, drowsiness, headache; incr levels w cipro, decr w antipsychotics and metoclopramide
- Pramipexole (Mivapex) (Jama 2000;284:1931) 0.125–1.5 mg po tid; renal clearance. Adverse effects: hallucinations, nausea,

somnolence including sudden deep sleep w/o warning (Rx Let 1999;6:57), incr levels w cimetidine. >$160/mo

- Bromocriptine (Parlodel) 5–10 mg po tid alone or with L-dopa, or if L-dopa fails. Adverse effects: orthostatic BP changes, sweating, mental status changes. >$240/mo

Ancillary meds:

- Amphetamines like dexedrine 5 mg po b-tid help akinesia and psych depression
- Anticholinergics (inhibit the dopamine-uninhibited acetylcholine neurons), like antihistamines, eg, diphenhydramine (Benadryl) 50 mg tid po, or bentropine (Cogentin), or trihexyphenidyl (Artane) (Nejm 1971;284:413), help tremors
- Amantadine 100 mg po bid, effect diminishes in 6 mo, helps 64% (Jama 1972;222:792), helps rigidity and bradykinesia
- Estrogen replacement therapy

COMT (catechol-O methyl transferase) inhibitors:

- Tolcapone (Tasmar) (Med Let 1998;40:60; Rx Let 1998;5:16) 100–200 mg po tid; works as a L-dopa booster; helps w early "wearing-off" phenomenon; use when other drugs fail. Adverse effect: signif hepatotoxicity (Rx Let 1998;5:71), pulled off Canadian mkt; $162/mo for 100 mg tid
- Entazapone (Comtan) (Med Let 2000;42:7) 200 mg po w each L-dopa dose; less hepatotoxicity; $1.75/pill

Surgical:

- Pallidotomy ? (Nejm 2000;342:1708; 1997;337:1036, 1996;334:114, Med Let 1996;38:107) for bradykinesia and tremor; unilateral thalamotomy, or continuous uni- or bilateral thalamic electrical stimulation (Nejm 2000;342:461) for severe tremor unresponsive to meds; or
- Electrical stimlulation of subthalamic nucleus (Nejm 1998;339:1105), occasionally causes severe acute depression w left substantia nigra placement (Nejm 1999;340:1476); or
- Fetal dopa-producing brain cell implants to caudate nucleus or putamen perhaps (Nejm 2001;344:710; 1995;332:1118)

13.7 MUSCLE WEAKNESS

GUILLAIN-BARRÉ SYNDROME (Acute Infectious Polyneuritis)

Nejm 1992;326:1130; Ann Neurol 1990;27:s21

Cause: Often viral, probably several types including Epstein-Barr virus (7/24 children—Nejm 1975;292:392); and *Campylobacter jejuni* (Nejm 1995;333:1374), 1/3 cases have a h/o such as a precedent. Occasionally/rarely follows flu shots (Nejm 1998;339:1997; 1981;304:557), CMV, and HIV

Epidem: All ages, both sexes equally. 1–2 cases/100,000/yr

Pathophys: Allergic polyneuropathy leads to demyelination and decr conduction velocity especially at root exit on cord dorsum (hence areflexia); must get ventral root too, though pathologically unimpressive. Can experimentally mimic by sensitizing animals with injections of dorsal root homogenates and Freund's adjuvant

Sx: URI, mild, precedes by 1–3 wk. Vague sensory losses, including, often early on, paresthesias of toes and fingers, which then extend proximally; deep aching at onset is very characteristic; proximal muscle weakness evolves over 24 h

Si: No sensory losses; afebrile; diminished reflexes always; proximal weakness >> distal involvement; always symmetric; no mental changes; facial nerve palsies (60%): cranial nerves X, XI, XII often; V occasionally; II, III, IV, VI rarely

Crs: Deteriorate after admission; start improving within 3 wk; back to normal in 16 mo, though slight decrease in reflexes and foot drop may persist; no relapses. *Campylobacter* type has worse outcome w 60% at 1 yr still w moderate to severe disability, compared to only 25% for other causes (Nejm 1995;333:1374)

Cmplc: Insidious respiratory paralysis, monitor by having count to 20 in 1 breath; glomerular nephritis (Ann IM 1973;78:391)

r/o cord compression, especially if CSF protein ≥2.5 gm %; collagen vascular disease; diabetic neuropathy; multiple sclerosis; polio; diphtheria; myasthenia; heavy metal toxicity; infectious mono; amyloid; rabies (Nejm 1979;300:603); botulism; red tide disease; Lyme disease; HIV; CNS neoplasia; sarcoid meningitis; chronic, HLA-associated; tick paralysis (Nejm 2000;342:90), rapidly ascending paralysis, rx'd by finding and removing tick

Lab:

CSF: Increased protein to 120–300 mg % by end of first week; wbc's <5000–6000

Noninv: Nerve conduction velocities profoundly decreased; if normal several days into course, find another dx

Rx: 1st: Supportive care including respirator; iv steroids no help (Lancet 1993;341:586)

2nd: Immune globulin iv high dose, eg, 0.4 gm/kg/d × 5 d if can't walk and <2 wk of sx; will help 1/2 in 1 mo (Nejm 1992;326:1130); or plasmapheresis/exchange at a tertiary care center for patients who can't walk or are progressing rapidly; both equi-effective though combination use not (Lancet 1997;349:225)

MYASTHENIA GRAVIS

Nejm 1994;330:1797

Cause: Autoimmune

Epidem: Especially in young females, and in males age 65–75 yr; female:male = 3:1 overall. Associated with:
- Thymomas, especially in older males; 30% have; 30% of patients with thymomas have myasthenia
- Thyrotoxicosis, especially Hashimoto's
- Collagen vascular disease, especially SLE
- HLA B8
- Penicillamine (BMJ 1975;1:600)

Pathophys: Antibodies to neuromuscular junction acetylcholine receptors (Nejm 1977;296:125); measured antibody doesn't correlate with disease severity; but some patients have more lethal antibody function than others (Nejm 1982;307:769)

Sx: Precipitated by thyrotoxicosis, muscle-paralyzing anesthesia, antibiotics like streptomycin etc., quinine (including gin and tonic), quinidine, perhaps Dilantin, procainamide, propranolol (Ann IM 1975;83:834)

Diplopia, muscle fatigue with repetitive use

Si: Increased weakness with repeated use, often in extra-ocular muscles first, or pharynx; reflexes intact

Crs: Prognosis much poorer if thymoma present (Neuro 1966;16:431); remissions during times of stress often, eg, pregnancy

NEUROLOGY

Cmplc: Respiratory failure; transmission to fetus, normalizes within 6 mo as maternal IgG decreases

r/o botulism; Guillain-Barré; polio; ALS; Graves disease; curare poisoning; **snake bite,** acetylcholine receptor blockade, rx with edrophonium (Tensilon), etc. (Nejm 1986;315:1444) or anti-venom Fab fragments iv w/i 6 hr (Med Let 2001;43:55); **Eaton-Lambert syndrome,** a similar disease associated with cancer especially of lung and pancreas (Nejm 1989;321:1267) and caused by antibodies to calcium channels responsible for neurotransmitter acetylcholine release (Nejm 1995;332:467)

Lab:

Noninv: EMG shows fatigue with >2/sec stimulation; posttetanic facilitation present; edrophonium test can be diagnostic, do double blind with saline, 2 mg then 8 mg iv causes no side effects (tearing, incr sputum, cramps) if myasthenia rather than cholinergic crisis

Serol: Antithymus and antinuclear antibodies in ~60% (Ann NY Acad Sci 1966;135:557,644)

Rx: (Nejm 1973;288:27) Avoid neomycin-like drugs; maintain K$^+$

1st, anticholinergics:
- Pyridostigmine (Mestinon) 30–60 mg po qid; or
- Neostigmine (Prostigmin) 0.5–1.5 mg im q 1–6 h or 15+ mg po qid long-release type

2nd, immunotherapy:
- Prednisone ~100 mg po qod alone, magically good results at NIH (Ann IM 1974;81:225; Nejm 1972;286:17); start low, work up to avoid crisis (Nejm 1974;290:81)
- Azathioprine (Imuran)
- Cyclosporine 6 mg/kg/d po helps (Nejm 1987;316:719); short-term options
- Plasmapheresis (Nejm 1984;310:762), with prednisone and/or azathioprine if thymectomy and anticholinergics not enough (Med Let 1979;21:64; Nejm 1977;297:1134); or
- Immunoglobulin high dose 400 mg/kg/d × 5 d (Nejm 1992;326:107; Acta Neurol Scand 1991;84:81)
- Surgical: thymectomy, for severe disease in all groups, but especially for pts with onset between puberty and age 60 yr; 2% operative mortality

13.8 DEGENERATIVE CNS DISEASES

MULTIPLE SCLEROSIS
Nejm 2000;343:938; 1997;337:1604

Cause: Perhaps autoimmune, perhaps ppt'd by EBV infection (Jama 2002;286:3083). Genetic component indicated by 25% concordance with monozygotic twins but only 2% with dizygotic twins and siblings (Nejm 1986;315:1638)

Epidem: Transmissible somehow (Faroe Island epidemic after WW II troop occupation); incr incidence with birth and/or childhood distance from equator; equal sex ratios, although females get at younger age; onset at age 10–50 yr, bell-shaped curve; 1/1000 of population have disease (probably tip of carriers)

Pathophys: Autoimmune attack of myelin basic protein by T cells (Nejm 1987;317:408) or by tumor necrosis factor-α, which is measurable in CSF (Nejm 1991;325:467); or of neuronal glia (Nejm 1977; 297:1207); decr suppressor T cells (Nejm 1987;316:67). Axonal demyelination and ultimately transection (Nejm 1998;338:278)

Sx: Motor (most often ataxia) nearly always hyperreflexia and positive Babinski's; and sensory tract (most often visual) sx, confusion, depression

Si: Diagnose by 2 or more attacks of neurologic deficits in different parts of CNS, which last >24 h, not by CSF or MRI lesions (Nejm 1993;329:1764,1808)

Loss of abdominal reflexes early, in contrast to ALS

Lhermitte's si: electric shock sensation to extremities with neck flexion (posterior column stretch), r/o any disease involving cervical or thoracic cord

Crs: Worse with hot climate, late onset; slightly fewer relapses in pregnancy and slightly more relapses postpartum (Nejm 1998;339: 285); 25% are benign with 1–2 episodes and minimal disability

Types:
- Acute attack
- Initially remitting/relapsing (80–90%), but many evolve to progressive; M:F = 1:2
- Initially progressive (10–20%); M = F; superimposed subsequent relapse/remit cycles don't improve prognosis (Nejm 343:1430, 1486)
- Stable (Nejm 1987;317:442)

Multiple Sclerosis, continued

Cmplc: Pain, neuralgia including trigeminal (Nejm 1969;280:1395)
 Optic neuritis; 40% of MS pts will have it sometime; up to 75% of
  women and 34% of men with isolated optic neuritis will develop
  MS up to 15 yr later (Neurol 1988;38:185; Nejm 1973;289:1103,
  1140); r/o Sjögren's syndrome, which can mimic (Ann IM
  1986;104:323)

Lab:

 CSF: Oligoclonal bands (90%), present throughout disease; elevated
  myelin basic protein (90%) (Nejm 1982;307:1183); IgG/albumin
  ratio elevated (70%)

 Noninv: Brainstem evoked potentials, no false positives except for
  other similar diseases like Friedreich's ataxia; ~10% false negatives
  in early MS

Xray: MRI, 25% false negatives (Neurol 1993;43:905; Jama
 1993;269:3146), and many false positives

Rx: Avoid flu shots in pts w definite MS
 of remitting/relapsing (not chronic progressive):
  • Interferon β-1b (Betaseron) sc qod or β-1a (Avonex, Rebif)
   3 million IU tiw im q wk × years, decreases relapse rate and
   severity by 50%; $1000/mo (Lancet 1998;352:1491,1498; Ann
   Neurol 1996;39:285; Neurol 1995;43:641; 1993;43:641,655,
   662; Med Let 1996;38:63; 1993;35:61). Weekly im Avonex × yrs
   w 3 d of iv then 11 d of po steroids, given on 1st demyelinating
   si/sx and UBOs on MRI , decr MS × 1/3 (Nejm 2000;343:898)
  • Glatiramer (Copaxone) (copolymer I) (Med Let 1997;38:61;
   Neurol 1995;45:1268) 20 mg sc qd, reduces recurrences from
   85% to 60%/yr; $1000/mo
 of progressive MS: mtx, cyclophosphamide, cyclosporine
 of acute attack: (hyperbaric and plasmapheresis rx no longer thought
  useful)
  • Cyclophosphamide (Cytoxan) 400–500 mg iv qd × 7–10 d; alone,
   best 1st choice now, but many still disagree with its use, eg,
   Canadian multicenter study (Lancet 1991;337:441); with ACTH,
   decreases morbidity (Nejm 1983;308:173,215)
  • ACTH 25 U tapering to 5 U iv qd × 2 wk, then 40 U tapering to
   20 U im × 1 wk, then stop; or short course of steroids, eg, methylprednisolone 1000 mg iv in 3 h qd × 3, then taper in 7–14 d

of incontinence (p 325)

of neuralgias, with carbamazepine, phenytoin (Nejm 1969;280:1395)

of muscle spasms (Med Let 1997;39:62; Nejm 1981;304:29,95), in order of efficacy:
- Baclofen, a GABA agonist, 5–20 mg po tid, or even chronically intrathecally via pump (Nejm 1989;320:1517); or
- Tizanidine (Zanaflex) (Med Let 1997;39:62) 4mg hs to 6$^+$mg tid. Adverse effects: dry mouth, sedation, dizziness, hypotension, rare visual hallucinations and hepatitis; or
- Diazepam (Valium), but makes sleepy; or
- Dantrolene 300 mg qd, but causes weakness

of fatigue (Rx Let 2000;7:41): amantadine, methylpenidate (Ritalin), modafinil (Provigil)

AMYOTROPHIC LATERAL SCLEROSIS
Nejm 2001;344:1688

Cause: Genetic in 10%, autosomal dominant, on chromosome #21 at least half the time (Nejm 1991;324:1381)

Epidem: 1/25,000 persons in US will die of it; 50× incr prevalence in Guam (Nejm 1970;282:947) along with a unique dementing variant of Parkinson's; both associated with a specific HLA genotype and decr delayed hypersensitivity (Nejm 1978;299:680)

Pathophys: Degeneration of anterior horn cells and motor Betz's cells of cerebrum progressively up from caudad portion of body. Can start anywhere in cord. Circulating antibody inhibits protein stimulation of axonal sprouting secreted by denervated muscle, primary or secondary effect? (Nejm 1984;311:933). Perhaps defective glutamate transport systems permit neurotoxic levels to build up (Nejm 1992;326:1464) or autoimmune IgG against calcium channels (Nejm 1992;327:1721)

Sx: Paresis and leg weakness

Si: Marked muscle atrophy, usually upper extremity, accompanied by asymmetric fasciculations and hyperreflexia of the atrophic muscles; fasciculations of tongue; paraplegia; and no sensory abnormality or sx, which distinguishes it from cervical disc disease

Crs: Fatal over 3–5 years

Cmplc: Dysphagia, respiratory paralysis, dysphonia, and dysarthria
 With paraplegia, r/o mass lesion, syphilis, B_{12} deficiency, parasagittal
  meningioma, Shy-Drager syndrome (p 551, 561), postpolio
  muscular atrophy (Nejm 1986;314:959)

Lab:
 Path: Muscle biopsy shows neuronal degenerative changes; cord shows
  atrophy with decr anterior horn cells and lipofuscin in degenerated
  corticospinal tracts

Rx: Riluzole (an antiglutamate) 50–200 mg po qd slows progression
  minimally (Lancet 1996;347:1425), perhaps in pts w bulbar onset
  but not with limb onset disease (Med Let 1995;37:113; Nejm
  1994;330:585,636)

13.9 NEUROPATHIES

BELL'S PALSY

 Nejm 1982;307:348

Cause: Herpes simplex (majority) (Ann IM 1996;124:27); ? EBV (Nejm
  1975;292:392); sarcoid, usually bilateral; Lyme disease (Nejm
  1985;312:869)
 Other causes of facial nerve paralysis: h. zoster (10%; called the
  Ramsay-Hunt syndrome), basilar skull fracture (5%), otitis media
  (2%), birth (2%), other including syphilis (1%)

Epidem: Increased incidence in diabetics (Nejm 1982;307:348), or are
  those diabetic nerve infarcts?

Pathophys:

Sx: Facial weakness, acute onset, may also be painful; incr noise
  sensitivity from diminished stapedial reflex

Si: Cranial nerve VII weakness; decr taste on anterior tongue (helpful if
  absent taste because it distinguishes from primary motor disease, eg,
  polio); only true occasionally, since often the process is more distal
  and chorda tympani is spared

Crs: 90% recover completely, only 50% if Ramsay-Hunt syndrome. If
  there is some residual motion on affected side, patient always
  recovers (Nejm 1975;292:748)

Cmplc: Corneal ulceration, prevent by taping lid, especially hs. Misregeneration of the nerve, causing "jaw winking" of orbicularis ori with orbicularis oculi and vice versa; parasympathetics regenerate incorrectly sometimes leading to eye tearing when taste good food ("crocodile tears")

Lab:

Noninv: EMG at 2 weeks if still fibrillation; consider decompression of nerve then

Rx: Protect eyes w Lacrilube gtts and hs taping

Steroids, as prednisone 60 mg po qd tapered over 10 d to 5 mg (Nejm 1972;287:1268,1298), double-blind study shows results in less denervation (Laryngoscope 1993;103:1326); consider especially if no motor function at all

Acyclovir (p 491) w steroids (Ann IM 1996;124:63)

Surgery no help (Nejm 1975;292:748)?, perhaps decompression if flat EMG at 2 wk; physical therapy program no help (Nejm 1982;307:348)

DYSAUTONOMIAS

Mccvd 1985;54:7

Cause: Primary degeneration of autonomic system, alone in Bradbury-Eggleston syndrome (BES), or combined w multisystem atrophy in Parkinson's disease (Ann IM 2000;133:382), olivopontocerebellar atrophy (prominent Parkinsonian si), striatonigral degeneration (prominent cerebellar si's), Shy-Drager syndrome (SDS) (acquired), and Riley-Day Syndrome (RDS) (congenital).

Secondary causes: CNS injury from spinal cord injury esp above T6, amyloid neuropathy, Guillain-Barré syndrome, diabetic neuropathy, cancer, HIV infection, porphyria, pernicious anemia, tabes dorsalis from syphilis, drug toxicity like alcoholic neuropathy

Epidem: RDS in Eastern European Jews

Pathophys: RDS from decr dopamine → norepinephrine conversion; BES and SDS from autoimmune antibodies to ganglionic Ach receptors (Nejm 2000;343:847) causing multineurosystem degeneration; diminished or no sympathetic CNS stimulation on standing

NEUROLOGY

Dysautonomias, continued

Sx:

Postural hypotension: Heat intolerance; constipation (occasional diarrhea), dysphagia; nocturia, frequency, urgency, incontinence, urinary retention; erectile and ejaculatory failure; stridor, apnea; parkinsonism, ataxias

RDS: Absent taste; intermittent skin blotching

SDS: A mix of autonomic failure, Parkinson's type sx, and sometimes cerebellar sx

Si:

Postural hypotension: Anhidrosis; anisocoria, Horner's syndrome; stridor, apnea; parkinsonism, cerebellar si's

RDS: Loss of anterior tongue papillae; poor coordination; absent deep tendon reflexes; paroxysmal hypertension; defective temperature control and sweating; absent corneal reflexes

SDS: Dementia, tremor

Crs:

Cmplc: Autonomic dysreflexia = hypertensive crisis precipitated in quadriplegics by distended viscus (NE Rehab Hosp lecture 10/89)

r/o vasovagal syncope; carotid hypersensitivity; postural tachycardia syndrome (Nejm 2000;343:1008), incr pulse w/o decr BP in young women w partial sympathetic denervation of legs

Lab: In RDS and SDS, methacholine sc causes eye tearing, transiently improved taste; in eye, i gtt methacholine causes potentiated miosis (denervation supersensitivity). Histamine intradermally causes no flare

Noninv: Measure with expiratory-inspiratory respiratory variation in sinus rates, if <10, suspect neuropathy present (BMJ 1982;285:559)

Rx:

of postural hypotension: Avoid diuretics, vasodilators and tricyclics, increase salt intake; atrial pacing at 100/min (Nejm 1980; 302:1456); try

- Dihydroergotamine 6.5–13 μgm/kg sc in AM (Ann IM 1986;105:168), w
- Caffeine 250 mg po half-hour ac (Ann IM 1986;105:168; Nejm 1985;313:549)
- Fludrocortisone (Florinef) 0.1+ mg po qd (Nejm 1989;321:952)
- β blockers

- Anticholinergics like disopyramide (Norpace) (Jama 1995; 274:961)
- Midodrine 10 mg po tid (an α agonist) (Med Let 1997;39:59; Jama 1997;277:1046)
- Ibuprofen (Motrin) ir indomethacin (Indocin) (Sci Am Text Med, 1986);

of SDS: L-dopa + above

If anemic (hct <40%), old or young, rx w erythropoietin (Ann IM 1994;121:181; Nejm 1993;329:611)

LIPIDOSES (Niemann-Pick (NPD), Gaucher's (GD), Tay-Sachs (TSD), and Wolman's Disease (WD))

Nejm 1991;325:1354 (GD); Ann IM 1975;82:257 (all)

Cause: Genetic, autosomal recessive

GD on chromosome #21

Epidem:

NPD: Children age 2–5 yr

GD: Children and adults, especially in Jews (1/850)

TSD: Jews only, gene prevalence 1/30 Ashkenazi Jews

Pathophys: Neurologic disorder due to distension of neuron with lipid, displacement of nucleus toward axon hillock. All cause enlargement of RES organs, bone involvement, etc. General increase in brain size. All have a defective catabolic enzyme

NPD has cholesterol and sphingomyelin foam cells

GD has an enzyme defect at glucosylceramide (a glucocerebroside) → sphingosine + folic acid (Nejm 1971;284:739)

TSD has ganglioside foam cells due to hexosamidase A deficiency (Nejm 1970;282:15)

WD has cholesterol foam cells exclusively in RES

Sx: Bone pain, fractures, failure to thrive, and seizures

Si: Pathologic fractures; neurologic si's, large head, seizures, amaurosis; cherry red macular spot; splenomegaly, anemia, bleeding; pingueculae

Crs:

NPD and *GD:* Most die before age 5 yr

TSD die before age 5 yr, although one gene type presents in adolescence

WD present and die by age 3 mo

Cmplc: GD, pulmonary hypertension (Ann IM 1996;125:901)
r/o carnitine deficiency, presents as Reye's syndrome (Nejm 1980;303:1389)

Lab:
Chem: GD, elevated acid phosphatase, nonprostatic portion, incr B_{12} binding proteins (Nejm 1976;295:1046)

TSD, incr AST (SGOT), hexosaminidase A absent in homozygote, intermediate levels in heterozygote (Nejm 1970;283:15)

Hem: GD, low platelets (hypersplenism)

Path: NPD, nerve bx shows foam cells

GD, marrow shows foam cells, spindle-shaped with eccentric nuclei

WD, RES biopsy shows foam cells

Urine: 24-h collection analyzed for glycoceramide (Nejm 1971;284:739)

Xray: Erlenmeyer flask-like lesion, lucent, often in lower femur

Rx: *NPD,* genetic counseling by detecting heterozygote (Nejm 1974;291:989)

GD, genetic counseling; splenectomy helps CBC but may speed course; marrow transplant (Nejm 1993;328:745; 1984;311:84,1606); or iv enzyme, alglucerase (Ceredase) (Ann IM 1994;121:196; Nejm 1992;327:1632; 1991;324:1464), which costs $250,000–500,000/yr, or recombinant type (Cerezyme) (Ann IM 1995;122:33)

TSD, screen serum or tears with hexosaminidase-based test (Nejm 1973;289:1072), confirm with DNA-based test (Nejm 1990;323:6)

13.10 MYOPATHIES

PSEUDOHYPERTROPHIC MUSCULAR DYSTROPHY (Duchenne's Muscular Dystrophy)

rv of all muscular dystrophies—Am J Med 1963;35:632

Cause: Genetic, sex-linked; occasionally autosomal recessive

Epidem: Mostly males; most common of all muscular dystrophies

Pathophys: Decreased calcium uptake, but normal muscle efficiency early in course of disease affecting both fast and slow fiber bundles (Nejm

1969;280:184); deficient dystrophin, a muscle protein (Nejm 1988;318:1363)

Sx: Aggressive: onset age 1–5 yr. Calf hypertrophy early, later may decrease; symmetric pelvic involvement, w waddle gait and Gowers' si

Benign: onset usually age 6–18 yr, but can range 2–35. Calf, deltoid, infraspinatus hypertrophy; pelvic 1st, then shoulder in pts age 5–10 yr

Si: As above

Crs: Aggressive: relentless, often rapid progression, in bed by age 10 yr

Benign: able to walk 25–30 yr after onset; life expectancy into 4th–5th decades

Cmplc: Progressive skeletal deformities; death due to wasting, inanition, infection; pseudo-gi obstruction and gastric dilatation due to smooth muscle involvement (Nejm 1988;319:15); myocardiopathy in both patients and female carriers (83%), gradually progressive (Jama 1996;275:1335)

r/o metabolic myopathies: acid maltase deficiency; carnitine deficiency (Nejm 1985;312:370); other sex-linked muscular dystrophies: Becker's dystrophy, and Emery-Dreifuss muscular dystrophy (Ann IM 1993;119:900)

Lab:

Chem: Elevated CPK (in carrier females too), aldolase, and AST (SGOT); all elevated early before clinical sx and si, decrease later with burnout

Path: Muscle bx shows dystrophy before clinical sx and si's, ie, random-sized fibers; lipomatosis; incr connective tissue in interstitium; degenerative changes like hyalinization, vacuolization, etc.; nuclear shrinkage; basophilic staining of some fibers

Rx: Prevent by prenatal dx at age 18–20 wk in utero via amniotic CPK (Nejm 1977;297:968); or DNA probe techniques via amniocentesis sample of early pregnancy (Nejm 1987;316:985) or by activation of myogenesis (Nejm 1993;329:915)

Prednisone 0.75 mg/kg qd × 6 mo increases strength (Nejm 1989;320:1592)

MYOTONIC DYSTROPHY

Cause: Genetic, autosomal dominant on chromosome #19

Epidem: 1/8000

Pathophys: Abnormal insulin fasting levels and incr response to stimulation (Nejm 1967;277:837). In vitro the sarcoplasmic reticulum shows incr rapidity of calcium uptake initially and normal total uptake, suggesting fast but not slow fibers most affected (Nejm 1969;280:184) and may thus explain some of the myotonia

Sx: Onset age 20–25 yr

Si: Weak jaw, weak sternocleidomastoids, ptosis; early frontal balding; myotonia (unable to release grasp); cataracts; gonadal atrophy. Muscle percussion (thenar eminence) with reflex hammer causes localized myotonic contraction

Crs:

Cmplc: Diabetes mellitus; flaccid esophagus with secondary reflux and strictures; billowing mitral valve (Ann IM 1976;85:18), Vtach and heart block (Jama 1995;274:813) contribute to 15–30% incidence of sudden death (Ann IM 1991;115:607)

r/o other myotonic syndromes (Nejm 1993;328:482) including: cold myotonia (autosomal dominant), excitement myotonia (autosomal dominant), both of which respond to quinidine; "stiff-man syndrome" (p 429); hyperkalemic periodic paralysis

Lab:

Chem: Flat glucose tolerance test with normal FBS; decr urinary ketosteroids

Noninv: EMG has a diagnostic pattern

Serol: IgG low (incr catabolism), without other globulin changes. Southern blot analysis w DNA probe detects the abnormal gene 90$^+$% of the time (Nejm 1993;328:471)

Rx: Acetazolamide rx helps sx but causes severe muscle weakness of quads (Ann IM 1977;86:169)

REFLEX SYMPATHETIC DYSTROPHY SYNDROME (Complex Regional Pain Syndrome, Causalgia, Shoulder-Hand Syndrome)

Bull Rheum Dis 1986;36:#3

Cause: Previous injury/arm pain

Epidem: Up to 25% of patients with locally painful organic disease

Pathophys: Diminished sympathetic tone leads to incr vascular responsiveness to adrenergic stimulation (Ann IM 1993;118:619)

Sx: H/o painful organic injury, eg, MI, trauma, CVA, or cervical disc disease. Burning pain with tenderness in an extremity usually; swelling; dystrophic skin changes; vasomotor dysfunctions; bilateral in 40%; hot/cold sensations

Si: Tenderness, dystrophic skin changes, vasomotor instability, edema

Crs: Progressive leading to atrophy over 1+ yr

Cmplc: r/o rheumatoid arthritis, septic joint, SLE, Reiter's, peripheral neuropathy

Lab:

Xray: Local osteoporosis; bone scan positive over affected joints

Rx: Prevent w early mobilization

of sx (Nejm 2000;343:654): local hot/cold; prednisone 15 d tapering rx po 60 mg to 0 mg qd divided; intensive PT; sympathetic ganglion blocks, eg, stellate; surgical sympathectomy; TENS (transcutaneous electrical nerve stimulator) unit; implanted spinal cord stimulator (Nejm 2000;343:618); chronic intrathecal baclofen infusion (Nejm 2000;343:625)

13.11 TUMORS

SUBDURAL HEMATOMA, Chronic

Cause: Head trauma, in older patients, may be mild (eg, sitting down hard) if also volume-depleted

Epidem: Predominantly in patients age <1 yr and >50 yr

Pathophys: Vein wall tear; no sx's until >50 cc; forms semipermeable membrane that absorbs fluid and thus becomes a tumor; ipsilateral upper motor neuron si's from contralateral cerebral peduncle being pressed against the tentorium, and ipsilateral 3rd cranial nerve deficit from herniating temporal lobe tip pressure especially dilated

NEUROLOGY

nonreactive or poorly reactive pupil before abnormalities of extraocular movements, but later as expands opposite pyramidal tract also becomes compressed

Sx: Headache and confusion (essential, to consider dx)

Si: Progression over days to weeks, from confusion and equivocal contralateral hyperreflexia, to severe headache and ipsilateral hyperreflexia and pupillary dilatation, to varying contralateral pupillary changes (Neurol 1990;40:1707), and finally to bradycardia, hypertension, coma, and fixed dilated pupils

Crs: Chronic >15 d–6 mo (7.5% mortality)

Cmplc: Chronics are bilateral 20% of time, hence no lateralization r/o much more obvious acute <3 d (55% mortality); and subacute 3–15 d (15% mortality);

Lab: LP dangerous to do without CT first, but often will show incr pressure and xanthochromia

Xray: CT scan, rarely need arteriogram. Skull films to look for fracture

Rx: of acute: rapid craniotomy and decompression within 4 h helps prognosis (Nejm 1981;304:1511); plus steroids and osmotic agents of subacute and chronic: craniotomy and decompression

PSEUDOTUMOR CEREBRI

Nejm 1983;308:1077

Cause: Idiopathic

Epidem: Associated with anemia; vitamin deficiencies and intoxications, especially vitamin A toxicity, eg, acne rx with isotretinoin and tetracyclines (Neurol 1984;34:1509; FDA Bull 1983;13:21); chronic hypoxia; post-head trauma; post-otitis media; hypoparathyroidism; start of thyroid replacement in myxedematous patients; steroid administration and withdrawal (Addison's); lateral sinus thrombosis. Mostly in young, overweight women

Pathophys:

Sx: Headache, visual field losses; no impairment of consciousness

Si: Enlarged blind spot, central vision losses; later, inferior quadrantic defects/visual field constrictions. Papilledema without hemorrhages or exudates

Crs:
Cmplc: Visual loss, monitor rx w quantitative visual perimetry
Lab:
  CSF: High pressures (>200 mm), normal CSF
Xray: CT shows small or normal ventricles
Rx: Repeated LPs; 2–6 weeks of steroids
  Surgical shunt rarely needed

MENINGIOMA

Nejm 2001;344:114

Cause: Neoplasia; chromosome #22q deletions and thereby assoc w
  neurofibromatosis type 2
Epidem: Peak incidence between age 50–70 yr; rare <20; 20% of all brain
  tumors, 25% of all cord tumors. Increased in irradiated children
  (Nejm 1988;319:1033), and patients with breast cancer.
  Female:male = 2:1
Pathophys: Most commonly over hemisphere convexities; also deep in
  cleft (parasagittal), over sphenoid ridge, olfactory groove, spinal
  cord. Slow growing with few si's of brain damage. Often have
  estrogen and progesterone receptors. 2% are malignant
Sx: Headache, seizures (often first sx)
Si: Of subtle mass lesion
Crs: Very slowly progressive. After resections, 10–20% recurrence at 10 yr
  if thought to have been completely resected, 80% if obviously could
  not get all
Cmplc:
Lab:
  Path: Uniform size cell whorls; these may calcify to form psammoma
  bodies
Xray: Skulls show hyperostosis or radiolucency of underlying bone, large
  feeding vessel impression, foramen spinosum enlarged due to middle
  meningeal enlargement, 33% are calcified (Fraser, Edinburgh 1968)
  CT scan usually is diagnostic; often do not show up on MRI unless
  gadolinium-enhanced
Rx: Surgery
  Radiation as adjunctive rx if unresectable or only partially resectable
  Perhaps hormone rx in future

MEDULLOBLASTOMA

Nejm 1994;331:1505; 1991;324:464

Cause: Neoplasia

Epidem: Usually in children; 20% of all pediatric brain tumors; usually cerebellar (70% of all childhood tumors are in posterior fossa)

Pathophys: Often starts in vermis of cerebellum; incr pressure due to hemorrhage, gliosis, and both local and diffuse edema due to incr venous pressure from incr intracranial pressure

Sx: Truncal ataxia, sx of incr intracranial pressure like headache, vomiting, etc., over weeks

Si: Papilledema

Crs: Highly malignant 30–70% 5 yr remissions, 92% 5 yr survival; and perhaps 50% cure, 60% in girls vs 25% in boys (Jama 1998; 279:1474)

Cmplc: Metastases down spinal cord; hydrocephalus from aqueductal stenosis; uncal and cerebellar foramen magnum herniations (p 567, 576)

Lab:

Path: High nuclear/cytoplasmic ratio, round oval nuclei, scant stroma, many mitoses, small cells, pseudorosettes

Xray: CT/MRI useful to initially dx but not much help as surveillance for recurrence; hx and PE picks up 83% of recurrences (Nejm 1994; 3330:892)

Rx: Combinations of surgery, craniospinal irradiation, and chemotherapy

ASTROCYTOMA

Grade I (astrocytoma); grades 2 (glioma) and 3 (astroblastoma) = anaplastic astrocytoma; grade 4 (glioblastoma) (Nejm 2001;344:114; 1991;324:1471,1555)

Cause: Neoplasia; chromosome #10 deletion, etc.

Epidem: 50% of all brain tumors (pediatric—Nejm 1991;324:463). Occasionally associated w both types of neurofibromatosis and Turcot's syndrome

Pathophys: In children, in cerebellum and pons; in adults, in spinal cord (most common spinal cord tumor), cerebrum and cerebellum

Sx: Seizures, CNS mass lesion sx's including headache

Si: Depends on location

Crs: Without rx, <6 mo for grade 4 glioblastoma, 5% 2-yr survival; but others are low-grade tumors compatible with survival for many years, eg, 50% 2-yr survival for anaplastic astrocytoma

Cmplc:

Lab:

Path: Biopsy to be sure is not lymphoma, abscess, etc.

Xray: MRI

Rx: Radiation; chemotherapy first in very young children, allows brain maturation (Nejm 1991;324:463), in adults w temozolomide (Temodar) (Med Let 1999;41:123); surgical resection

CRANIOPHARYNGIOMA
Nejm 1994;331:1506; 1991;324:1555

Cause: Neoplasia

Epidem: Mainly in children

Pathophys: Suprasellar tumor arising from pharyngeal epithelium

Sx: Adults: headache; bitemporal hemianopsia; hypothalamic dysfunction including personality changes, obesity, diabetes insipidus, sleep changes

Children: growth failure

Si:

Crs: Slow growing, with rx live at least 15 yr

Cmplc: Panhypopituitarism postop (80–90%)

Lab:

Xray: MRI or CT shows calcification in 95%

Rx: Surgery difficult in floor of 3rd ventricle, 70% able to be completely resected, 90% cures w postop radiation

Radiation: quite sensitive, gives 5–10 yr of asx life; often used postsurgery

13.12 MISCELLANEOUS

Aphasias (N. Geschwind; Curr Concepts Cerebro Dis 1981;16:1; Nejm 1971;284:654); definition: unable to name an object
- Nonfluent; Broca's area; associated with hemiplegia, arm > face > leg
- Fluent:

Wernicke's; posterior superior temporal; can't comprehend or repeat
Conduction; parietal lobe above Sylvian fissure; comprehends but can't repeat
Anomic; angular gyrus; comprehends and repeats
Isolation of speech area; above and below Sylvian fissure; can't comprehend but repeats

Caloric stimulations (calorics): With ear canal irrigation, normally fast nystagmus component to same side as warm stimulation and opposite side of cold stimulation. No fast component if cortex out (coma); good way to distinguish feigned coma. Patterns (measure seconds duration and/or inverse of onset lag): right ear end-organ damage = Warm L + Cold L > WR + CR; central (brainstem) = WL + CR > WR + CL

Coma prognosis: 0% if 3 days out fewer than 2/3 eye si's (corneal, pupillary, doll's eyes) in medical, nonoverdose, nontraumatic coma (Ann IM 1981;94:293); predictors after cardiac arrest (Curr Concepts Cerebro Dis 1987;22:1; Jama 1985;253:1420). Persistent vegetative state prognosis: ~50% become conscious after 6–12 mo if traumatic, only ~10% in nontraumatic types (Nejm 1994;3330:1572)
Glasgow coma scale (best efforts) (Nejm 1991;324:1477); ≤8, needs ICU and intubation; scoring:
Opens eyes: spontaneously (4); to speech (3); to pain (2); none (1)
Verbal: oriented (5); confused (4); inappropriate (3); incomprehensible (2); none (1)
Motor: spontaneous/obeys (6); localizes pain (5); withdrawal (4); flexion to pain (3); extension to pain (2); none (1)
Rx: Hypothermia to 91.4°F (33°C) × 24 hr may help in traumatic coma (Nejm 1997;336:541); postarrest thiopental (Nejm 1986;314:397) or calcium channel blockers (Nejm 1991;324:1225) no help

CSF eosinophilia: Helminths or lymphoma (Ann IM 1979;91:70)

CSF, increased protein: Usually <100 mg %, medical causes: (1) diabetes, (2) hyperparathyroidism, (3) myxedema, (4) rheumatoid arthritis (Ann IM 1979;90:786)

Delirium (organic brain syndrome) (Ann IM 1990;113:941; Nejm 1989;320:578)

Cause: Drugs, long list (Med Let 1993;35:65); primary intracranial diseases; systemic diseases secondarily affecting the brain; withdrawal from alcohol/sedatives; metabolic like hypo/hyper-Na, hypoglycemia, and UTI in patient with atonic bladder leading to elevated NH_3 levels (Nejm 1981;304:766); infectious, eg, syphilis, crypto; brain mets; status epilepticus, petit mal or partial complex seizures (Neurol 1983;33:1545)

Epidem: High incidence in elderly; eg, 50% of patients with hip fracture develop it; 15% of elderly develop it after general surgery; higher rates in those with dementia

Sx: Hallucinations, often visual as well as auditory

Si: Acute onset and fluctuating course; transient (days-weeks; unlike permanent dementia) global (unlike acute psychosis) disorder of cognition and attention. Inattention, loss of attention span is most prominent deficit; test by serial 7's; serial digits up to 7, eg, phone numbers; spell "world" backward. Disorganized thinking and/or altered level of consciousness; typically "sundown," ie, worsen at night

Rx: Prevent in hospitalized elderly (Nejm 1999;340:669) by programs directed at cognition, sleep, immobility, hearing, vision, and dehydration; reduces incidence from 15% to 10%

Find and rx the primary cause

Dermatomes and cutaneous nerves: See Fig. 13.12.1

Electrodiagnostic methods (Ann IM 1981;95:599): EMG, NCV, evoked potentials (Nejm 1982;306:1140,1205)

Fragile X syndrome (Nejm 1991;325:1673,1720)

Epidem: 1/1000 males, 1/2000 females; X-linked, 80% penetrance in males, 65% in heterozygote females due to triplet repeats (Nejm 1996;335:1222); most common inherited form of mental retardation after Down's syndrome

Sx: Mental retardation

NEUROLOGY

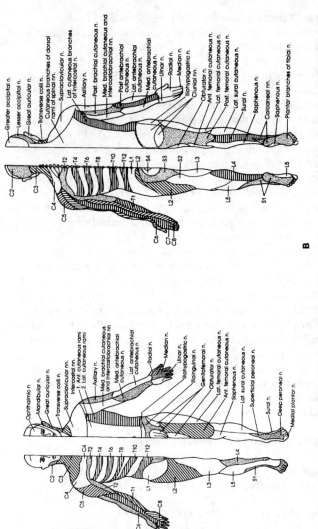

Figure 13.12.1   Dermatomes and cutaneous nerve distribution. (A) Anterior view of dermatomes (*left*) and cutaneous areas supplied by individual peripheral nerves (*right*). (B) Posterior view of dermatomes (*left*) and cutaneous areas supplied by individual peripheral nerves (*right*). (Reproduced with permission from Carpenter, Sutin, eds. Human neuroanatomy. Baltimore: Williams & Wilkins, 1983:179.)

A

Ophthalmic n.
Mandibular n.
Great auricular n.
Transverse colli n.
Supraclavicular nn.
Intercostal nn.
1. Ant. cutaneous rami
2. Lat. cutaneous rami
Med. brachial cutaneous and intercostobrachial nn
Med. antebrachial cutaneous n.
Lat. antebrachial cutaneous n.
Axillary n.
Radial n.
Ulnar n.
Median n.
Iliohypogastic n.
Ilioinguinal n.
Genitofemoral n.
Obturator n.
Lat. femoral cutaneous n.
Ant. femoral cutaneous n.
Saphenous n.
Lat. sural cutaneous n.
Superficial peroneal n.
Sural n.
Deep peroneal n.
Medial plantar n.

C2
C4
C3
C2
C3
T4
T2
T6
T8
T10
C5
T12
C6
L1
C7
C8
T1
L2
L3
L4
L5
S1

B

Greater occipital n.
Lesser occipital n.
Great auricular n.
Transverse colli n.
Cutaneous branches of dorsal rami of spinal nn.
Supraclavicular n.
Lat. cutaneous branches of intercostal n.
Axillary n.
Post. brachial cutaneous n.
Med. brachial cutaneous and intercostobrachial nn.
Post. antebrachial cutaneous n.
Lat. antebrachial cutaneous n.
Med. antebrachial cutaneous n.
Ulnar n.
Radial n.
Median n.
Iliohypogastic n.
Clunial nn.
Obturator n.
Ant. femoral cutaneous n.
Lat. femoral cutaneous n.
Post. femoral cutaneous n.
Lat. sural cutaneous n.
Sural n.
Saphenous n.
Calcaneal nn.
Saphenous n.
Plantar branches of tibial n.

C2
C3
C4
C5
C6
C7
C8
T2
T4
T6
T8
T10
T12
L1
L2
T1
S4
S3
S2
L3
L4
L5
S1
L5

Si: Long face, large testicles, big ears, big chin
Rx: Prenatal dx

Frontal lobe si's: Gegenhalten (paratonia), snout, suck, palmomental, grasp, pathologic laughing and weeping; rx latter with low dose (25–75 mg) amitriptyline (Nejm 1985;313:1480)

Head injuries In sports (Jama 1997;277:1190; 1991;266:2867)
    Grade 1
Dx: Confusion <15 min without amnesia
Rx: q 5 min exams; return to game ok if no amnesia or sx after 20 min
    Grade 2
Dx: Confusion >15 min without amnesia; or any amnesia
Rx: q 5 min exams; no return to game; recheck next day; no practice ×
    1–2 wk
    Grade 3
Dx: Loss of consciousness
Rx: Neck collar; hospitalize; observe × 24 h; no practice × 2 wk
    In ER: CT if LOC or amnesia for even and any of the following sx/si: headache, vomiting, >60 yr old, drug or alcohol intoxication, short term memory deficit, trauma evidence on physical exam above clavicles, seizures. Otherwise CT not necessary, no false negs (Nejm 2000;343:100:138); hypothermic rx no help (Nejm 2001;344:556)

Horner's syndrome (oculosympathetic paresis): Ipsilateral ptosis of eyelid, decr facial sweating, and miosis of pupil unresponsive to cocaine 10% gtts because is denervated (Nejm 1997;337:1359); all due to interruption of sympathetics either at apex of chest (eg, Pancoast syndrome), or w carotid diseases like aneurysm or dissection; r/o Raeder's paratrigeminal syndrome (Acad Emerg Med 1996;3:864), which manifests as a Horner's w/o loss of sweating and w neuralgic pain, seen w carotid dissection

Immune globulin iv rx (Ann IM 1997;126:721) may help several autoimmune neurologic diseases, very expensive, $6000–12,000/mo

NEUROLOGY

Innervations: See Table 13.12.1

Table 13.12.1

Reflex	Innervation
Biceps	C_{5-6}
Supinator	C_{5-6}
Triceps	C_{6-7}
Abdominal	T_{8-12}
Cremasteric	L_1
Quadriceps	L_{3-4}
Ankle	L_5-S_1

Intracranial mass effect treatment: 1st, hyperventilation; if that fails, mannitol 0.5 gm/kg iv or furosemide 1 mg/kg. Brain masses, tumors, subdurals, hemorrhage, CVA all produce diminished mental status due to lateral brain shifts (Nejm 1986;314:953)

Meningismus si's: Kernig's = hamstring spasm with straight leg raising; Brudzinski's = neck flexion causes hip flexion

Meningitis, definitions and causes
• Aseptic meningitis (predominant lymphocytes in CSF; if polys in first LP, re-do in 6–12 h to look for change to lymphs—Nejm 1973;289:571); * indicates normal CSF glucose

Treatable: tuberculosis, SBE,* fungal (crypto), tumor, Listeria, h. simplex, NSAIDs (Ann IM 1983;99:343), syphilis, subdural* or epidural* abscess (eg, in spine due to a disc abscess), cysticercosis (*Taenia solium*—Nejm 1984;311:1492), leptospirosis, partially rx'd bacterial, RA (Ann IM 1979;90:786), rickettsial, Lyme disease, HIV, cat scratch fever, *Borrelia* (relapsing fever), high dose immunoglobulin rx (Ann IM 1994;121:254)

Untreatable: sarcoid, viral including enteroviruses* (polio, coxsackie, echo), mumps,* mono,* rabies, lymphocytic choriomeningitis* in lab person, arbovirus,* rarely CMV (infants)

• Septic meningitis: CSF sens/specif numbers (Ann IM 1986;104:880): glucose <40 mg % (40% false neg), <1/3 of blood glucose (30% false neg), antigen studies (10–40% false neg)

Movement disorders:
Chorea (irregular joint movement):
• Rheumatic Sydenham's chorea (distal)

- Hemiballismus, from vascular damage from ASCVD or in SLE (if proximal, rx with Haldol (Nejm 1976;295:1348))
- Huntington's chorea

Athetosis (writhing):

- Huntington's chorea, can't keep tongue extended
- Tardive dyskinesia after phenothiazine rx (Ann IM 1981;94:788); lip smacking, tongue and perioral and periorbital tics; rx with perhaps clozapine (which has cmplc of seizure and agranulocytosis—Nejm 1991;324:746) (p 691), or vit E 1600$^+$ U/d (Rx Let 1999;6:3)

Asterixis (failure of postural tone) in hepatic or other (eg, CO_2 retention) metabolic encephalopathy

Torticollis: basal ganglia disease; inherited (Nejm 1973;288:284); rx with botulinum toxin (Med Let 2001;43:63) q 3 mo; expensive

Myoclonus: (muscle contractions of CNS origin); all movement but palatal type (central tegmental tract lesion) disappear with sleep; rx with barbiturates or L5-HT + carbidopa (Nejm 1980;303:782), r/o myoclonic epilepsy (Nejm 1986;315:296)

Tics:

- Simple benign
- **Tourette's syndrome** (Nejm 2001;345:1184; Jama 1995;273:498)

Cause: Genetic, autosomal dominant (Nejm 1986;315:993) but incomplete penetrance so M:F = 4:1

Epidem: 3–5/10,000; associated w ADHD (p 654)

Sx: Motor tics, vocal tics usually sniffs or grunts but may be swearing or echoes of own or others' speech; obsessive touching of hazardous things, eg, stove burners

Si: Above plus often obsessive compulsive counting, checking rituals, etc.

Crs: Onset around age 7 yr, progressive into adulthood

Cmplc: ADHD in 60% (Jama 1998;279:1100)

Rx: 1st, haloperidol (Haldol) augmented w nicotine gum (Am J Psychiatry 1991;148:793), or pimozide (ORAP) 1–16 mg qd (Med Let 1985;27:3); 2nd, w clonidine (Lancet 1979;(2):551); 3rd w benzodiazepines

Tremor ("involuntary motion back and forth about a point") (Ann IM 1980;93:460, M. Samuels 3/85)

- Parkinsonism tremor (at repose, better with action/intention, 3/sec)

NEUROLOGY

- Constant tremor (at repose, increases with action/intention, 9/sec, all "soluble in alcohol"):
  - Exaggerated physiologic tremor from hyperthyroidism, coffee, tea, theophyllines, adrenergic stimulation, lithium, drug withdrawal; rx with propranolol 10–40 mg or others, β blockers (Nejm 1975;293:950), peripheral effect within minutes
  - **"Essential" tremor,** idiopathic and familial; can co-exist with parkinsonism or other degenerative neurologic disease; rx (Rx Let 2000;7:3) with propranolol (best of β blockers), which helps 50%, weeks to work (probably CNS effect), primidone 50–250 mg bid, gabapentin (Neurontin), rarely clozapine
  - Wilson's disease (Nejm 1978;298:1347)
- Coarse intention (cerebellar) tremor, peripheral and/or truncal ataxia; rx with limb weights, INH 600–1200 mg qd helps perhaps via GABA; causes:
  - Multiple sclerosis
  - Tumor, primary or metastatic; or paraneoplastic syndromes seen with breast or gyn tumors (Nejm 1990;322:1844)
  - Alcoholic degeneration, only in legs
  - Vascular diseases of cerebellum: cerebellar hemorrhage or thrombotic medullary plate syndromes
  - Foramen magnum syndrome from short neck or Paget's disease by compression of vertebral artery
  - Genetic ataxias: Friedreich's ataxia, hereditary, ataxia telangiectasia, diminished pyruvate oxidation (Nejm 1976; 295:62), olivopontocerebellar ataxia, vit E deficiency (Nejm 1995; 333:1313)

Vocal tremor; stuttering/cluttering; worsened by tricyclics and other anticholinergics; helped by bethanechol 5 mg po tid (Nejm 1993;329:813)

Muscle weakness
- Motor neuronal disorder, eg, ALS
- Polyneuropathy
- Neuromuscular transmission: myasthenia, Eaton-Lambert, lithium or β blockers; curare, snake bite (Nejm 1986;315:1444)
- Myopathy:

Electrolyte abnormalities, eg, low K or PO_4

Endocrine: hyper or hypothyroid, Cushing's, acromegaly, vit D deficiency, hyperparathyroid

Infections: toxo, trichinosis, cysticercosis
Immune: poly/dermatomyositis, sarcoid, amyloid
Drug/toxin: alcoholic, steroids, colchicine, rifampin, chloroquine, clofibrate, emetine, β blockers, diuretics

Neuropathy, peripheral (Nejm 1979;300:546) Diabetic, uremic, myxedemic, alcoholic, idiopathic, familial, amyloid (diminished pain and temperature; associated with autonomic neuropathy too), leprosy (diminished pain and temperature especially in vitiligo patches), toxic (N-hexane—Nejm 1971;285:82)

Pain, chronic, rx (Ann IM 1980;93:588)
Medications:
NSAIDs
Narcotics
Psychoactive agents:
- Carbamazepine (for tic douloureux) 400–800 mg po qd;
- Phenytoin (for tic or peripheral neuropathy) 300–400 po qd;
- Gabapentin (Neurontin) (Rx Let 1999;6:53; Jama 1998;280:1831,1837,1863) 300–1200 mg po tid, incr slowly. Adverse effects: somnolence, dizziness, confusion
- Imipramine, desipramine, amitriptyline (not helpful in HIV neuropathy—Jama 1998;280:1590), haloperidol, fluphenazine, chlorpromazine, SSRIs (J Gen Int Med 1997;12:384)

Mexiletine (Mexitil) 200 mg po qd to tid, last resort, related to lidocaine; adverse effect: arrhythmias
Electrical stimulation (TENS)
Acupuncture (not helpful in HIV neuropathy—Jama 1998;280:1590)
Neurosurg ablation
Injections
Biofeedback
Hypnosis
Behavioral modification

Paraplegia, causes:
Treatable:
- B_{12} deficiency (subacute combined degeneration)
- Syphilis (general paresis of the insane)
- Mass lesion including disc, cervical spondylosis and metastatic cancer (Nejm 1992;327:614)

NEUROLOGY

- Parasagittal meningioma
- Shy-Drager syndrome (p 551, 561)

Untreatable:
- Multiple sclerosis
- ALS
- Syringomyelia
- Chronic progressive myelopathy due to HIV infection (Nejm 1988;318:1195)

Pupillary abnormalities
- Argyll-Robertson pupils: react to accommodation, not to light; caused by syphilis or diabetes
- Adies pupils: dilated unilaterally (80%), slow (5 min) reaction to light and accommodation; idiopathic cause
- Horner's syndrome (p 575)
- Uncal herniation (p 567)
- Cranial nerve #III palsy from aneurysm of internal carotid

Sleep: Circadian sleep cycles and work (Nejm 1983;309:534; Sci 1982; 217:460); bright lights at beginning of work and dark rooms to sleep in, very effective (Nejm 1990;322:1253)

Insomnia, review of causes and rx (Nejm 1990;322:239); medications (p 688) used 50–90% of time in hospital and probably no help (Ann IM 1984;100:441); in elderly, aerobic exercise 3–4×/wk helps (Jama 1997;277:32)

Third cranial nerve palsies (p 640 for innervations of eye movements): Eye deviates laterally; diabetic type spares pupil; aneurysm of internal carotid does not

Transient global amnesia (Curr Concepts Cerebro Dis 1983;18:13): Perhaps bilateral temporal lobe ischemia; lasts minutes to hours (<24 h): usually in pts age >50 yr, no associated neurologic deficits, no permanent damage, rarely recurs

Vertigo/dizziness: Past pointing with finger-to-nose testing with closed eyes, a vestibular not cerebellar sign

- Causes of dizziness in:
  Primary care practice (Ann IM 1992;117:898):
  - Vestibular (54%) ("an illusion of motion"), of which 1/3 are benign positional vertigo
  - Psychiatric (16%)
  - Presyncope (6%)
  - Dysequilibrium (2%), imbalance when moving, sense of falling; usually from musculoskeletal and/or sensory deficit
  - Hyperventilation (1%)
  - Multiple other causes (13%)
  - No cause found (8%)

  Elderly; present in 25% over age 72; may be a syndrome (Tinetti—Ann IM 2000;132:337) like delirium or falls in which elements of several of these causes contribute: anxiety, depression w or w/o medications, impaired balance (test by turning circle in <4 sec), post MI, postural BP drop (mean BP decr by >20%), 5$^+$ meds, hearing impairment

- Causes of acute vestibular syndrome (Nejm 1998;339:680; 1984;310:1740):

1. **Labyrinthitis**
   Cause: Perhaps viral
   Crs: Better in 2–3 d, residual mild sx for up to 2 yr
   Rx: With small doses iv diazepam (Valium), or dimenhydrinate (Dramamine) po, or scopalomine as Transderm (Ann IM 1984; 101:211), steroid taper × 3 d, especially if see within 1st 24 h

2. **Benign positional vertigo** (Nejm 1999;341:1590): Move patient from sitting to supine with first one, then other ear down (Hall-Pike head-hanging test), appears after a 5–20 sec delay and will pass in 1–2 min; rarely lasts >1 yr. Caused by canalithiasis; best rx'd (80% successful) w canalith repositoning w Epley maneuvers (Otolaryng Clin NA 1996;29(2):323; Otolaryngol Head Neck Surg 1995;112:154). Meclizine (Antivert) 25 mg po q 12 h or prn of modest help; surgery also possible

3. **Cerebellar hemorrhage** (p 534) or stroke; sudden onset, severe, assoc w other brainstem findings, lasts weeks, needs acute CT/MRI to r/o neurosurgically reversible cerebellar bleed and/or brainstem swelling

4. Cerebellar-pontine angle tumor (p 170)

NEUROLOGY

5. Temporal bone fracture, usually with severe hearing loss though not always (Nejm 1982;306:1029)
6. Floccular-nodular or insular seizures
7. Meniere's disease with tinnitus and diminished hearing though both may not start at once
8. Inner ear hemorrhage, acute, w hearing loss; See Fig. 13.12.2

$\longrightarrow$

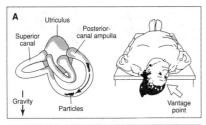

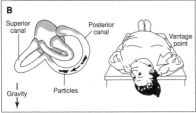

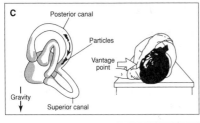

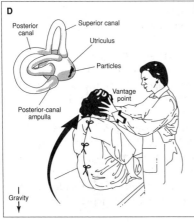

Figure 13.12.2 Bedside Maneuver for the Treatment of a Patient with Benign Paroxysmal Positional Vertigo Affecting the Right Ear. The presumed position of the debris within the labyrinth during the maneuver is shown in each panel. The maneuver is a three-step procedure. First, a Dix–Hallpike test is performed with the patient's head rotated 45 degrees toward the right ear and the neck slightly extended with the chin pointed slightly upward. This position results in the patient's head hanging to the right (Panel A). Once the vertigo and nystagmus provoked by the Dix–Hallpike test cease, the patient's head is rotated about the rostral–caudal body axis until the left ear is down (Panel B). Then the head and body are further rotated until the head is face down (Panel C). The vertex of the head is kept tilted downward throughout the rotation. The maneuver usually provokes brief vertigo. The patient should be kept in the final, facedown position for about 10 to 15 seconds. With the head kept turned toward the left shoulder, the patient is brought into the seated position (Panal D). Once the patient is upright, the head is tilted so that the chin is pointed slightly downward. Reproduced with permission from Furman JM, Cass SP. Benign paroxysmal positional vertigo. Nejm 1999;341:1594. Copyright 1999, Mass. Medical Society. All rights reserved.

NEUROLOGY

Chapter 14
Obstetrics/Gynecology

D. K. Onion and R. DeJong

14.1 BREAST DISEASE

BREAST CANCER

Nejm 1998;339:974; 1992;327:319,390,473

Cause: Neoplasia; genetic component in some (esp Ashkenazi Jews) w BRCA-1 or -2 gene, mutations of p 53 area of chromosome #17; BRCA-1 present in 10% of women w cancer onset before age 35 (Nejm 1996;334:137,143), women w gene have 85% lifetime risk for breast and 60% risk for ovarian Ca while BRCA-2 women have same breast cancer risk but less ovarian Ca risk, but environmental factors may ameliorate (Nejm 1997;336:1448)

Epidem: Incidence = 100/100,000 women, 37/1000 women die of it; 45,000 die/yr in US; 12% of women will get in their lifetime; 0.5% of all male cancers (Ann IM 1992;117:771)

Increased incidence with: obesity; infertility; smoking in postmenopausal women who are slow acetylators (Jama 1996;276:1494); late motherhood (age >30 yr); uterine cancer; h/o breast cancer in 1st degree relatives (×3–10); postirradiation, eg, Hiroshima, fluoroscopy, even thymus radiation in childhood (Nejm 1989;321:1281), and mammography over age 40 causes 40/million women after a 20-yr lag (Nejm 1989;321:1285); moderate alcohol use (Nejm 1987;316:121), linear incr w incr use (Jama 1998;279:535); hereditary ataxia telangiectasia heterozygotes who may represent 9% of all US breast cancer (Nejm 1986;316:1289), and in whom radiation from mammograms etc. may increase incidence a lot (Nejm 1991;325:1831); generally in women exposed to more estrogen, eg, those w high bone densities (Nejm 1997;336:611), in high risk women who have used BCPs (Jama 2000;284:1791), and debatably in perimenopausal users of estrogen and/or progesterone where relative risk incr × 1.7 (Jama 1999;281:2091 vs 2141; Nejm 1995;332:1589; 1989;321:293) vs no incr risk (Ann IM 1997;127: 973); low dietary vit A intake (Nejm 1993;329:234); fibroadenomas of breast before age 24 yr (Nejm 1994;331:10); in males w gynecomastia

No increase with: abortions (Nejm 1997;336:81); birth control pill use (Nejm 1986;315:405 vs Lancet 1996;347:1713); high dietary fat consumption (Nejm 1996;334:356; 1987;316:22); low fiber intake (Jama 1992;268:2037); thyroid hormone rx (Ann IM 1977;86:502); silicone breast implants (Nejm 1995;332:1535; exposure to PCBs or DDT (Nejm 1997;337:1253); "fibrocystic disease" except in the 1/3 w proliferative or atypical pathology who are at incr risk (Nejm 1985;312:146)

Lowered incidence in: women w first pregnancy before age 30–35, 1/3 fewer if first pregnancy before age 23, although pregnancy transiently increases risk for ~15 yr or until 2nd pregnancy, especially if over 35 w 1st pregnancy, but protects long term (Nejm 1994;331:5); nursing (more is better) protects against premenopausal type only (Nejm 1994;330:81; 1987;316:229 vs Lancet 1996;347:431); women who regularly exercise

Sx: Breast mass, usually nontender; nipple discharge or bleeding sometimes. Self-exam helps when combined w regular clinical exams? (Nejm 1979;301:315; 1978;299:265,271 vs Jama 1987;257:2197); silicone model practice helps (Ann IM 1990; 112:772)

Si: Breast mass, nontender, single, firm, in upper outer quadrant in 60%. Sometimes bloody breast discharge. **Paget's disease of breast,** an areolar dermatitis, if present is strongly correlated w cancer.

Crs: 55% 5-yr survival; w adjuvant CMF, 95% 2-yr survival w positive nodes compared w 70% without CMF (Nejm 1976;294:405); survival worse w increasing age (Nejm 1986;315:559)

Cmplc: Metastases, to skeleton have prognosis better than those to viscera. Cancer in opposite breast in 7–12%

r/o **"Fibrocystic disease"** (Nejm 1985;312:146; 1982;307:1010) present clinically in 50% of women, histologically in 90%

Ductal carcinoma in situ (Nejm 1999;340:1499; Ann IM 1997;127: 1013, 1023), 5–10% prevalence in autopsy series, half progress to invasive cancer over 5–8 yr, represent 50% of mammographically detected cancers because often cause microcalcifications, rx'd w lumpectomy and, if resection margins <10 mm, radiation (Nejm 1999;340:1455)

Lab:

Chem: Screen pts in high risk families for breast and ovarian Ca w BRCA-1 and -2 testing (Jama 1996;275:1885); cost = $2000; beware of over-enthusiastic application (Nejm 1997;336:1448)

Path: Aspiration cytology for invasive cancer w experienced pathologists, 95% sens, 98% specif. Breast bx; in situ ductal and lobular Ca's are relatively benign but need local resection and irradiation (Jama 1996;275:913,948; Nejm 1993;328:1581); estrogen receptors (ER) crucial to f/u rx; must freeze tissue within 30 min to −70°F (−57°C); progesterone receptors (PR) now also used

Xray: Mammograms (p 675)

Rx: (Nejm 1998;339:974; Jama 1995;273:142) Classified by TNM (lesion size, nodes, mets) system

Prevent by various screening strategies including self-exam, clinical exam, mammography (p 675), aspiration of lesions (Ann IM 1985;103:79,143):

for BRCA-1 and -2 mutations: see table (Jama 1997;277:999); prophylactic mastectomy (Nejm 1999;340:77,141; 1997;336:1472) reduces risk by 90%, NNT = 33.

for high risk women:

• Estrogen receptor blockers, which suppresses ER$^+$ tumors effectively (Jama 1999;281:2189) but not ER$^-$ ones (Jama 2001;286:2251) like

- Tamoxifen 20 mg po qd × 5yr (Med Let 1999;41:1; Nejm 1998;339:1609); also helps lipids and osteoporosis although incr risk of thromboembolic disease and endometrial Ca

- Raloxifene (Evista)

• Surgical prophylactic mastectomy, eg, w BRCA 1 or 2 mutations (Nejm 2001;345:159; Jama 2000;284:319)

Surgery, if <4–5 cm, lumpectomy, axillary node vs sentinel node (Nejm 1998;339:941 vs 990) dissection, and radiation (Nejm 1995;332:

907); if <2.5 cm, quadrectomy, axillary node dissection, and, especially if age <55 yr, radiation (Nejm 1993;328:1587)

Postop prophylaxis:

- Tamoxifen, if age >50 yr, ER positive, and positive nodes, 10 mg po bid × 1–2+ yr doubles survival and disease free time (Ann IM 1985;103:324) as well as helping lipids (Ann IM 1991;115:860) and bone density (Nejm 1992;326:852). Adverse effects: endometrial cancer and thromboembolic risks incr, hot flashes helped a little by clonidine (Ann IM 2000;132:788)
- CMF (cytoxan, methotrexate, 5-FU), if axillary nodes positive and especially if premenopausal, 21–28-d cycles, at full strength to toxicity (Nejm 1995;332:901), less not helpful (Nejm 1994;330: 1253; 1981;304:45) × 4–6 mo; or 4 cycles of doxorubicin then 8 cycles of CMF (Jama 1995;273:542); or CDF (cytoxan, doxorubicin, 5-FU); or mtx, cytoxan, 5-FU, prednisone × 6–7 mo (Ann IM 1991;114:621). All decrease 5-yr mortality × 20–25% (Nejm 1988;319:1681), but all also have significant adverse effects (Nejm 2001;344:1997), like wgt gain, ovarian failure, fatigue, cognitive dysfunction, and cardiac toxicity in doxorubicin regimens.

These regimens may also help in patients w negative nodes but lesions >1 cm^3 (NIH consensus conf 6/18/90;8:#6; FDA Drug Bull 1990;20(2):5), but significant benefit still questionable (Nejm 1994;330:805; 1992;326:1756; 1991;324:160; Ann IM 1989;111:1,703). Modest (1/1000) long-term leukemia risk w radiation and/or chemotherapy especially w melphalan (Alkeran) (Nejm 1992;326:1745)

- Radiation along w CMF improves survival (Nejm 1997;337:949, 956)

Postop f/u for metastatic disease: routine PEs and annual mammograms enough, no survival benefit in annual bone scans, labs, chest xrays, or liver imaging done on asx pts (Jama 1995;273:142; 1994;271:1587,1593)

of metastatic disease:

- Radiation good for local recurrences and bone pain
- Chemotherapy first if ER neg w CMF or adriamycin + vincristine, paclitaxel (Taxol) (Nejm 1995;332:1004); trastuzumab (monoclonal antibody) or capecitabine (Med Let 1998;40:106)
- Endocrine rx first if ER positive or over age 50, w tamoxifen 20 mg po qd; or just as good or better w pure antiestrogen

aromatase inhibitors, which prevent peripheral adrenal androgen conversion to estrogens but w/o endometrial or thrombo-embolic cmplcs, like anastrozole (Arimidex) (Med Let 1996;38:61), exemestane (Aromasin) (Med Let 2000;42:35), and letrozole (Femara) (Med Let 1998;40:43). In premenopausal women, surgical oophorectomy, or medically w leuprolide, an FSH inhibitor; adrenalectomy, surgically or medically w aminoglutethimide + dexamethasone (as good as surgical—Nejm 1981;305:545); androgens; pituitary ablation

- Autologous hematopoietic stem cell transplantation + high dose ChemoRx ? (Nejm 2000;342:1069,1119 vs Jama 1999;282:1335)
- Bisphosphonates if bone mets to prevent sx: pamidronate (Nejm 1996;335:1785) iv q mo, or clodronate (Nejm 1998;339:357) po qd
- Megestrol 400–800 mg po qd to stimulate appetite (Ann IM 1994;121:393)

14.2   VAGINAL/UTERINE/TUBE DISORDERS

VAGINAL CARCINOMA
Nejm 1987;316:514

Cause: Clear cell and squamous cell types; latter from human papilloma virus infection chronically (Nejm 1986;315:1052)

Epidem: Clear cell type incr by maternal estrogen (especially DES) use during first trimester 1/1000 in utero-exposed females get clear cell type; DES exposure does not incr any other cancers (Jama 1998;280:630). 30–50% of squamous type occur in women who have had a hysterectomy for human papillomavirus disease

Pathophys: In clear cell type, adenosis (uterine cervical columnar cells) is present in vagina, then a 2nd carcinogen hits this susceptible tissue and the cells undergo malignant degeneration? May also start in cervix

Sx: Irregular menses or spotting in young female in clear cell type; peak onset age 19, 91% are age 15–27 yr; h/o maternal estrog use in 72%
Squamous type, occurs usually in postmenopausal female

Si: Carcinomatous mass in both types

In clear cell type, poor I_2 staining of vaginal mucosa = adenosis

Crs: Clear cell type is very malignant, survivals to date only in lesions <1 cm²; recurrences can be late

Cmplc: Clear cell, distant mets; squamous cell, local invasive disease

Lab:

Path: Pap smear in clear cell type shows adenosis present in 11% of cervical, 27% of vaginal pool specimens. In squamous type, 20% false-negative paps; debate whether paps are indicated posthysterectomy (Obgyn 1984;64:699; Am J Obgyn 1980;148:695), probably should be done when h/o HPV even posthysterectomy but otherwise useless (Nejm 1996;335:1559, 1599)

Biopsy areas that stain poorly w I_2, bleed, or feel funny

Rx: Preventive (description of New York State clear cell screening program—Nejm 1981;304:47)

Surgery for both types as primary rx; radiation is equally effective and used for advanced invasive disease

CERVICAL CARCINOMA

Nejm 1996;334:1030; Ann IM 1990;113:214

Cause: Human papilloma (venereal wart) virus (HPV) (p 147), esp types 16, 18, 31, 33, 35 (Nejm 1989;320:1437; 1986;315:1052; Obgyn 1984;64:16)

Epidem: Sexual intercourse transmits the virus, hence also associated w genital herpes of cervix and vulva (Nejm 1981;305:517,483). HPV incidence in college women high (>40%), resolution and recurrence common (Nejm 1998;338:423)

Most common cancer in women after breast and lung. 65% of all female genital cancers; 95% are over age 30 yr. Incidence = 20/100,000, 16,000/yr in US women; CIS = 120/100,000; 5000 deaths/yr in US

Increased incidence w early onset of sexual activity, number of sexual partners, h/o other STDs esp HIV (Jama 2000;283:1031; Nejm 1997;337:1343) and chlamydia (Jama 2001;285:47), smoking, birth control pill use (slight), and w asymptomatic macular and raised warty lesions on male partners (Nejm 1987;317:916)

Pathophys: HPV genome becomes integrated into cellular DNA and causes malignant transformation. Squamous dysplasia may resolve, or untreated, may evolve to invasive carcinoma

Sx: Usually none; may have vaginal bleeding, especially postcoital; vaginal discharge; pelvic pain, when invasive

Si: Cervical erosion and mass

Stage 0: Carcinoma in situ

Stage I: Confined to cervix only

Stage II: Not to pelvic wall and not in lower third of vagina

Stage III: To pelvic wall

Stage IV: Rectum or bladder involvement

Crs: 5-yr survival 50% overall (old data); 100% w CIS; 25% in stage IV w surgery

Cmplc: Ureteral obstruction; lymphatic mets, usually local; pregnancy worsens; postop sexual dysfunction in 25% (Nejm 1999;340:1383)

Lab:

Path: Pap smear q 1 yr if <35 and/or multiple partners; q 5 yr if >35 and <8 lifetime partners (Canadian Walton Rept—Can Med Assoc J 1982;127:581) and no h/o abnormal paps or STDs in pt or partner; alternatively at least q 3 yr at age 20–65 (Ann IM 1990;113:214); and in elderly >65, get 2–3 paps 3 yr apart if not previously done then stop (Ann IM 1992;117:520). Unnecessary if s/p hysterectomy for benign disease (Nejm 1996;335;1559,1599, Jama 1996;275:940). 5–10% false neg rate in best labs. Atypical squamous cells uncertain significance (ASCUS), should be <5% of paps; about 25% will turn out to be serious higher grade lesions; either check for HPV DNA (Jama 1999;281:1605,1645) or follow pap q 6 mo × 2–3 yr after rx of any infection and colpo if + DNA or repeat ASCUS pap. Papnet, Autonet, and Thin Prep improved sensitivity technologies are expensive but may eventualy be useful if move to q 4 yr screening (Jama 1999;281:347) their use for rescreening of 10% unnecessary (Jama 1998;279:235, 240) and much more expensive than manual rescreening (Jama 1998;279:235,240)

Colposcopy w bx if pap shows dysplasia, recurrent atypia 3 or more times in a row (J Reprod Med 1989;34:634; Am J Obgyn 1987;156:628), papillomavirus, or if see warts or condyloma. Looking for (Jama 2001;285:1506): cervical intraepithelial

neoplasia (CIN) I (mild dysplasia, or low-grade squamous intraepithelial lesion), CIN II (moderate dysplasia), CIN III (severe dysplasia) and carcinoma in situ (CIS); high-grade squamous intraepithelial lesion (HSIL) includes CIN II and III, and CIS
HPV DNA screening may eventually replace PAP (Jama 2000;283:81, 87,108; Nejm 1999;341:1633,1687)

Rx:

of low grade SILs: f/u paps since most regress and resolve, especially in young women (Nejm 1998;338:423)

of dysplasia: local colposcopic destruction by cryo rx, laser, or loop excision all equieffective for 90% of dysplasia

of high-grade lesions or difficult dx situations: usually loop excision, or occasionally cone bx

of carcinoma stage I and early II: radiation and surgery equieffective w 80% stage I and 50% cures of advanced stage II, as well as stages III and IV: radiation; w advanced local disease even I B, cisplatin chemoRx w radiation improves survival (Nejm 1999;340:1137, 1144,1154,1198)

ENDOMETRIAL CARCINOMA
Nejm 1996;335:640

Cause: Prolonged, unopposed (by progesterone) estrogen (estradiol especially) exposure from many possible sources including:
- Estrogens given for menopausal sx (Nejm 1979;300:9,218), risk persists 10^+ yr after cessation (Nejm 1985;313:969)
- Stein-Leventhal syndrome
- Granulosa/theca cell tumors ($100 \times$ incidence)
- Anovulation, especially perimenopausal
- Turner's syndrome
- Tamoxifen use

Genetic syndromes w breast and right sided colon cancers

Epidem: 20% of all female genital cancers; 4th most frequent cancer in women; 34,000 cases/yr, 6000 deaths/yr in US; rare before age 40 unless ovarian pathology, median age at dx = 63, only 25% occur in premenopausal women. Lower incidence in smokers, because of smoking's antiestrogen effect (Nejm 1986;315:1305)

Endometrial Carcinoma, continued

Incidence in US is decreasing since the early 1980s, perhaps due to the
incr use of progesterone (Am J Pub Hlth 1990;80:935) in ERT

Pathophys: Continuous estrogen stimulation causes hyperplasia and
eventually can convert to carcinoma; rarely metastasizes distantly

Sx: Postmenopausal vaginal bleeding, r/o atrophic uterine mucosa,
bacterial endometritis, polyp; or premenopausal metrorrhagia; or
intermenstrual bleeding

h/o infertility, irregular menses, late menopause, obesity, estrogen
replacement, hypertension, diabetes

Si: Pelvic/uterine mass

Stage I: Confined to fundus

Stage II: In cervix and fundus

Stage III: Extension beyond uterus

Stage IV: Extension to pelvis

Crs: With rx, 70+% overall 5-yr survival; 75% stage I, 60% stage II, 30%
stage III, and 10% stage IV; estrogen supplementation-induced type
is less malignant? (Ann IM 1978;88:410)

Cmplc: Metastases, usually local. Incr risk of subsequent colorectal Ca
(Ann IM 1999;131:189)

Lab:

Noninv: Transvaginal ultrasound, endometrial thickness >5 mm 90%
sens, 48% specif (Nejm 1997;337:1792) vs 96% sens and 92%
specif if not on HRT; and 77% specif if on HRT (Jama 1998;280:
1510), perhaps do before bx and skip bx if neg?

Path: Pap smear positive in only 18% (Nejm 1974;291:191);
endometrial aspiration bx in office or D + C w tumor grading 1–3

Rx: Prevent by always withdrawing at least q 3 mo w progesterone, eg,
medroxyprogesterone (Provera) 10 mg qd × 10 d when using
estrogen for menopause or osteoporosis, or if obese and having
irregular menses, or other chronic estrogen stimulation situation
(Obgyn 1984;63:759)

Surgery for stages I and II, w or w/o pre-/postirradiation; for stages III
and IV, individualized rx including radiation, surgery, as well as
hormonal w progesterone (as Megace), and chemotherapy w
cyclophosphamide, 5-FU, adriamycin

ENDOMETRIOSIS
Nejm 1993;328:1759

Cause: Ectopic uterine mucosa, unclear why; various theories include embryonic residua, transtubal transport of endometrial fragments and implantation, coelomic metaplasia, "retrograde menstruation," and lymphatic, surgical, or vascular metastases?

Epidem: 10% prevalence in menstruating women

Pathophys: Ectopic foci of functioning endometrium cause pain when bleed into confined, nonuterine areas. Commonly on ovaries but also beneath peritoneum of bladder, tubes, bowel, pelvic scars postop. Can result in tubal or ovarian sterility. Sx severity correlate poorly w anatomic findings

Sx: Acquired premenstrual or menstrual pain, dyspareunia, pain on defecation; sterility; but often asx

Si: Tenderness on pelvic exam; retroverted fixed uterus; pelvic mass

Crs: Progressively worse until menopause or pregnancy

Cmplc: Infertility

r/o pelvic inflammatory disease, adenomyosis, ovarian tumor

Lab:

Endo: Laparoscopy, usually diagnostic, shows hemorrhagic spots or cysts, often scarred

Xray: Ultrasound may show irregular pelvic mass; but is a poor test except to r/o other causes of pelvic pain; frequent false negatives

MRI is 90% sens/specif for endometriosis in women w pelvic pain

Rx: (Nejm 2001;345:266):

NSAIDs for pain

Birth control pills, typically high progesterone content ones; either cyclic or continuous

Danazol 200–800 mg po qd, a weak androgen; 200-mg pill costs $1 (Ann IM 1982;96:625). Adverse effects: androgenic side effects

GnRH (gonadotropin-releasing hormone) analog, nafarelin 400 μgm nasal spray qd (Med Let 1990;32:81; Nejm 1988;318:485) or leuprolide (Lupron) 3.75 mg im depot q 1 mo for up to 6-mo course. Adverse effects: cost ($300+/mo), estrogen deficiency sx including bone loss, which can be prevented w qd sc PTH (Nejm 1994;331:1618)

Progesterone: medroxyprogresterone 20–100 mg po constantly × 6–12 mo or cyclic 20 d rx; depo-provera 150 mg im q 3 mo; levonorgestrel implant (Norplant) q 5 yr (Med Let 1991;33:17)

Surgical: laparoscopic electro- or laser cautery helps fertility in mild to moderate cases improve from 18% to 30% and is better than hormonal manipulation (Nejm 1997;337:217); TAH + BSOO is 90% successful in relieving pain

UTERINE LEIOMYOMA (Fibroids)

Cause: Mechanical stress?; estrogen stimulation?, eg, from birth control pills

Epidem: Premenopausal women primarily affected, usually appear age 30–50 yr; fibroids shrink in postmenopausal women and rarely cause sx. Increased prevalence and incidence in blacks

Pathophys: Intramyometrial stress causes localized smooth muscle proliferation? Estrogens increase rate of formation. Bleeding is from overlying endometrium stretched? and/or poor uterine contractions during menses hence spiral arteries bleed. Pain due to contractions against mass during menses

Sx: Menorrhagia; pain; sense of fullness; urinary frequency; obstipation; but often asx

Si: Anemia, pelvic mass

Crs: Benign

Cmplc: Infertility; anemia from menorrhagia; ureteral compression and blockage; sudden bleed into fibroid w pain and enlargement; necrosis and calcification (10%); benign metastasizing type (Nejm 1981;305:204); leiomyosarcomas (<1%)

Lab:

Hem: Iron deficiency anemia

Path: Intramural, 90% in fundus, 8% in cx, rarely in round or broad ligaments

Xray: Incidental finding on KUB, calcified in 10%, especially in older women

Ultrasound usually diagnostic, though can't r/o cancer

Rx: Wait for sx; cyclic BCPs low in estradiol to decrease bleeding, though still may stimulate growth; gonadotropin-releasing hormone agonists (Nejm 1991;324:97) (p 774) decrease estradiol by feedback inhibition, shrink fibroids and cause medical menopause, may be used presurgically

Surgical hysteroscopic resection of submucous types; or myomectomy ("shelling out") may allow future pregnancies; hysterectomy

ECTOPIC PREGNANCY

Nejm 1993;329:1174

Cause: Implanted conceptus outside uterine cavity; intraabdominal fertilization

Epidem: 2^+% of all pregnancies; 89,000/yr in US, increasing incidence (Mmwr 1995;44:46), mutiple reasons including antibiotic rx of PID before sterility results. 95% are tubal; but also can be ovarian, cervical, or abdominal (0.5%)

Post tubal ligation rate is 1/1000 over 10 yr, higher (30/1000) after electocoag tubals (Nejm 1997;336:762)

Pathophys: Scarred tubes (rarely uterus) slow transfer and as a result the blastocyst implants wherever it is on day 6. Chorionic villous trophoblasts perforate basement membrane and muscle layers of tubes. If death of embryo occurs first, endometrium is shed and this results in brownish, modest vaginal bleeding; if trophoblast erodes first, this results in massive intraperitoneal bleeding

Sx: Nearly all in 1st trimester; missed period, although withdrawal bleed may mask; most occur at about 8 wk gestation, earlier for isthmus, later for cornual

Abdominal/pelvic pain similar to menstrual/uterine pains; vaginal bleeding; shoulder pain from diaphragmatic irritation by blood

"Funny period, funny pain, funny pregnancy," followed by "syncope in the bathroom"

Si: Abdominal/pelvic mass (present in <50%) and tenderness; cervical tenderness if blood in pelvis; shock

Crs: Without surgery, death in 186/102,000 population (Obgyn 1984;64:386)

Cmplc: Shock, surgical sterility

r/o PID, ruptured ovarian corpus luteum or follicle cyst, endometriosis cyst, appendicitis

Lab:

Chem: Serum HCG positive in all, repeat in 48 h, should double in normal pregnancy, decrease if abortion, rise slowly if ectopic. Progesterone level <25 ngm/cc

Paracentesis or culdocentesis: May show blood in peritoneum

Urine: Pregnancy test positive in all w β-HCG >50 U and 90+% are therefore positive at first missed period

Xray: Ultrasound of pelvis w vaginal probe, if see intrauterine pregnancy, then dx is essentially ruled out, although the very rare circumstance of twins w one ectopic does occur

Rx: (Nejm 2000;343:1325):

Methotrexate 50 mg/M^2 im × 1 (Nejm 1999;341:1974), 91% successful overall, best if HCG <15,000 mIU/cc, follow w HCG levels post rx on days 4, 7, and q 1 wk until <15mIU, usually takes 35 d; or

Laparoscopic salpingostomy

Laparotomy for rupture w hemoperitoneum

PELVIC INFLAMMATORY DISEASE

Nejm 1994;330:115

Cause: (Med Let 1999;41:86) Chlamydia causes over half of mild cases (Ann IM 1981;95:685; Nejm 1980;302:1063) (p 443), maybe most; *Neisseria gonococcus* (15%), anaerobes, mycoplasma. All via sexual intercourse, especially w multiple partners; IUD use previously thought to incr risk (Nejm 1985;312:937,941,984; Med Let 1980;22:87) now felt to have minimal effect

Epidem:

Pathophys: Lower genital tract infections ascend cervical canal usually just before or during menses, to tubes and ovaries

Sx: Pain in lower abdomen, constant or colicky; dyspareunia; dysuria; tenesmus; dysmenorrhea; nausea and vomiting; anorexia

Si: Adnexal mass (20%) and tenderness or pain on cervical motion ("Chandelier si"); fever; cervical discharge

Crs:

Cmplc: Infertility (15^+% w each episode); ectopic pregnancy; pelvic abscess; septic thrombophlebitis; surgical excision of reproductive organs

r/o endometriosis, adenomyosis, ectopic pregnancy

Lab:

Bact: GC culture, chlamydia screens

Hem: WBC elevated; ESR elevated in 1/3; the higher the ESR, the more likely sterility

Noninv: Laparoscopy if dx unclear or improvement slow

Xray: Pelvic ultrasound; CT scan for possible abscess

Rx: Prevent w condom use (Am J Pub Hlth 1990;80:964); birth control pills help (Jama 1984;251:2553)

Screen asx women for chlamydia if expected prevalence is >7%, reduces PID by 1/2 (Nejm 1996;334:1362); or perhaps all women and maybe men under age 25 w PCR techniques (p 680) (Nejm 1998;339:739,768)

of disease (Med Let1999;41:86); pain and tenderness is adequate indication to initiate rx (Mmwr 1993;42:76)

Outpatients:

1st: Cefoxitin 2 gm im + probenecid 1 gm po, or ceftriaxone 250 mg im × 1 then doxycycline 100 mg bid × 14 d

2nd: Ofloxacin 400 mg po bid + metronidazole 500 mg po bid × 2 wk

Inpatients: hospitalize if

• Dx is unclear,

• Mass is present,

• Unable to keep po meds down,

• Peritoneal si's present,

• Outpt rx failure, or

• If expect poor compliance

• Rx w:

1st: Doxycycline 100 mg q 12 hr iv + cefoxitin 2 gm iv q 6 h ("FoxyDoxy") or cefotetan 2 gm iv q 12 h until better, then doxycycline 100 mg po bid × 14 d

2nd: Gentamicin 2 mg/kg iv × 1 then 1.5 mg/kg iv q 8 hr + clindamycin 900 mg iv q 8 hr until better, then f/u w po doxycycline × 14 d

3rd: Ofloxacin + metronidazole; amp/sulbactam + doxycycline; ciprofloxacin + doxy + metronidazole; all followed by doxy × 14 d

Rx of partners for gc if culture is positive, otherwise just for chlamydia

14.3 OVARIAN DISORDERS

POLYCYSTIC OVARY SYNDROME (Stein-Levinthal Syndrome)

Ann IM 2000;132:989; Nejm 1995;333:853; 1994;330:460; 1988;318:558

Cause: Probable genetic autosomal dominant

Epidem: Present in 1.5% of infertile patients, 75% of anovulatory women, 87% w hirsutism; only 2.8% of patients w polycystic ovaries by laparoscopy have the syndrome. Increased prevalence in seizure pts, especially those on valproic acid, 50% of whom have it (Nejm 1993;329:1383); and in IDDM often w insulin resistance

Pathophys: Hyperandrogenism + anovulation

Two theories (Nejm 1992;327:157)

1. Obesity induces by incr conversion of androstenedione to estrone in fatty tissues, which causes pituitary FSH suppression and incr LH; this leads to ovarian LH-stimulated androgen production, which in turn causes follicle atrophy and further stimulation of peripheral fat conversion to more estrone. More common in insulin-dependent diabetes because insulin resistance stimulates ovarian conversion of steroids to androgens (Nejm 1998;338:1876; 1996;325:617,657; Ann IM 1982;97:851); or IDDM may cause the syndrome by deficiency of a D-chiro-inositol-containing phosphoglycan that mediates insulin action (Nejm 1999;340:1314)

2. Onset in teens of abnormal LH surge (Nejm 1983;309:1206) induced or intrinsic ovarian increase in 17-hydroxylase and C-17,20-lyase (see Fig p 189) causing increases in 17-OH progesterone, estrone, and androstenedione, which in turn cause further LH surges and masculinization (Nejm 1992;327:157; 1989;320:559)

Sx: Syndrome onset age 20–40 yr. Oligo- or amenorrhea (80%); infertility (35–75%); obesity (37%); hirsutism (65%); acne (25%); visual acuity sx

Si: Withdrawal bleeding w progesterone; large ovaries, palpable if not too obese; hirsutism usually without masculinization. Astigmatism, myopia, hyperopia? Obesity

Crs:

Cmplc: Endometrial cancer; possibly higher incidence of coronary artery disease (Ann IM 1997;126:32) and ASCVD in general; HT; diabetes; infertility

Lab: Usually unnecessary; diagnose clinically

Chem: Androstenedione, testosterone (>2 SD above mean), and LH elevated, or high normal; glucose intolerance, incr lipids

Path: Ovaries 2–3× normal size, cystic follicles; microscopically show variable theca cell hyperplasia and luteinization

Xray: Pelvic ultrasound may show polycystic ovaries

Rx: Weight reduction if obese

Medroxyprogesterone 10 mg qd or other progesterone × 10 d q 1–3 mo to prevent endometrial cancer

of hirsutism (p 627)

of infertility (p 628): clomiphene; insulin secretion inhibition w metformin 500 mg po tid (Nejm 1998;338:1876); human menopausal gonadotropin/menotropins (Pergonal); rarely wedge resections or laser drill holes of ovary done

if insulin resistant diabetes present, as it often is:

- Metformin 500–850 mg po tid (Rx Let 2000;7:16; Nejm 1996;335:617,657), often w glitazones, which lower insulin levels that drive peripheral estrogen to androgen conversion; or
- Perhaps D-chiro-inositol 1200 mg po qd (Nejm 1999;340:1314)

OVARIAN CARCINOMA

Jama 1995;273:491; Nejm 1993;329:1550; 1992;327:197; 1985;312:415,474

Cause: Neoplasia; 5–10% familial association w breast cancer chromosome #17 BRCA-1 gene deletion (Nejm 1997;336:1125; 1996;335:1413)

Ovarian Carcinoma, continued

Epidem: 5th ranking fatal female cancer in US, ahead of cervical and
uterine; 1/70 lifetime risk is 1/20 if a 1st degree relative has had
ovarian cancer; 13,300 deaths/yr in US; 22,000/yr incidence in US

Increased w low parity, mumps, perineal talc use, infertility drug use
especially clomiphene >1 yr (11 × increase in incidence—Nejm
1994;331:771), ERT users × 2 esp after 10 yr (Jama 2001;285:
1460)

Decreased incidence (40%) w bcp use, even 3 mo of rx protects for
15$^+$ yr (Nejm 1987;316:650); w high FSH levels post menopausally
and w low androgen levels (Jama 1996;274:1926)

Usually postmenopausal women age 50–60 yr; 5% of cases are familial

Pathophys: Epithelial type cancer, 35–50% serous, 6–10% mucinous

Sx: Often asx until widespread; pelvic or lower abdominal mass, pelvic
discomfort, urinary or bowel dysfunction; increasing abdominal
girth

Si: Abdominal or pelvic mass, often (50%) bilateral; may be huge
(largest = 148 kg); ascites. Occasionally unique polyarthritis,
palmar fasciitis syndrome (Ann IM 1982;96:424)

Cmplc: r/o common, benign ovarian corpus luteum cyst by rechecking
pelvic during a different part of menstrual cycle, getting ultrasound
if increasing in size, doing surgery if >5 cm; germ cell or sex cord
struma types, 13–20% of ovarian cancers, very treatable; mets from
elsewhere (Krukenberg's tumors); Meig's syndrome

Lab:

Chem: Ca-125 monoclonal antibodies elevated in 80% but not useful
as screening test (Nejm 1992;327:197) unless two 1st degree
relatives w same type of ovarian cancer (Jama 1995;273:491);
serum inhibin levels elevated in many, especially mucinous
cystadenocarcinomas, like Ca-125, not useful screen but helpful
postop tumor marker (Nejm 1993;329:1539)

Path: "Borderline malignant" cell types of both serous and mucinous
have much better prognosis than numbers shown above, eg,
85–95% 5-yr survival

Xray: Pelvic ultrasound; screen w vaginal probe if pos fam hx as above

Rx: Prevent in BRCA-1 and -2 w BCPs, which decr incidence by 50$^+$%?
(Nejm 1998;339:424 vs not helpful 2001;345:235)

Preventive screening w tumor markers ineffective primarily due to low
prevalence (Ann IM 1994;121:124; 1993;119:901), and w pelvic

exams because fast growing and usually already spread when palpable

Staging laparoscopy/otomy to fully judge extent of metastases, eg, often on diaphragm

Debulking surgery after initial chemotherapy (Nejm 1995;332:629)

Chemotherapy for most except good histology stage Ia, especially for stages III and IV with (Med Let 1996;38:96):

1st: Cisplatin (Nejm 1996;335:1950) iv or intraperitoneal, or carboplatin (Med Let 1993;35:39) + paclitaxel (Taxol) (Med Let 1993;35:39; Nejm 1996;334:1; 1995;332:1004; 1992;327:197) or cyclophosphamide

2nd: Topotecan (Hycamtin) combinations

Possibly: Altretamine (Hexalen) (Med Let 1992;3:76); marrow stem cell transplant after high dose chemoRx (Ann IM 2000;133:504)

Leukemia risk w melphalan (Alkeran) may not warrant its use (Nejm 1990;322:52)

14.4 PREGNANCY-RELATED CONDITIONS

SPONTANEOUS ABORTION (Miscarriage)

Cause: Idiopathic usually; sometimes "lupus anticoagulant," antiphospholipid (cardiolipin) antibodies (p 112)? (Nejm 1997;337: 154, 1991;325:1063; Nejm 1985;313:1322 vs Bull Rheum Dis 1992;40(6):3); or structural (eg, uterine septum, fibroids)

Epidem: 15–20% of all pregnancies. Most at 10 weeks (Nejm 1988;319: 189). 1/3 have chromosome abnormalities, 1/2 are blighted ova, 1/10 due to bad placenta (A. Hertig 1968). Late (>20 wk) assoc w Leiden factor V and prothrombin gene mutations (Nejm 2000; 343:1015)

Incr (× 1.4–1.8) by smoking and cocaine use (Nejm 1999;340:333); w coffee use (Nejm 2000;343:1839; 1999;341:1688), or w video display terminals (Nejm 1991;324:727), or w NSAIDs esp in 3rd trimester (Rx Let 2001;8:14)

Pathophys:

Sx: Crampy pain, spontaneous vaginal bleeding, passage of tissue means fetal death

Si: Open cervical os and/or tissue means inevitably will abort

Crs: When threatened (bleed), 50% will eventually lose pregnancy

Cmplc: Sepsis, uterine necrosis leading to myoglobinuria and ATN, DIC; significant depression (Jama 1997;277:383), onset within 1 mo, esp if childless (20$^+$% incidence) or past h/o depression (50%) incidence

r/o ectopic, molar pregnancy, self-induced abortion

Lab: If ≥3 spontaneous abortions, chromosomal studies looking for balanced translocation

Rx: Emotional support

D + C if

- Heavy bleeding;
- >8 wk gestation, since will bleed longer and more heavily;
- Is 2nd SAB, to r/o intrauterine anatomic abnormalities; or if
- Infected

in Lupus anticoagulant pts, ASA + prednisone prophylaxis no help (Nejm 1997;337:149)

INDUCED ("Therapeutic") ABORTION

Cause:

Epidem: No, or minimal, incr risk of spontaneous abortion in future pregnancies after an abortion (Nejm 1979;301:677)

Pathophys:

Sx:

Si:

Crs:

Cmplc: Septic abortion if not done medically (Nejm 1994;331:310), but even then infection occurs in 1% (prophylactic tetracycline 500 mg po qid × 5 d decreases to 0.25%); uterine perforation; retained products of conception; **postabortal syndrome:** bleeding, in absence of retained tissue, which spontaneously resolves or is rx'd w methergine

No incr in breast cancer risk (Nejm 1997;336:81; Jama 1996;275:283, 321)

Lab:

Path: Confirm gestational tissue and r/o mole

Rx:

of 1st trimester pregnancy (Nejm 2000;342:946):

- Mifepristone (Mefeprex, RU-486) (Med Let 2000;42:101; Nejm 1993;329:404), an antiprogesterone, in 1st 2 mo of pregnancy, 200–600 mg po followed in 1.5–2 d w misoprostol (Cytotec) 400 μgm po (Nejm 1998;338:1241) or 800 μgm vaginally (Jama 2000;284:1948; Nejm 1995;332:983); causes 95[+]% to abort completely (Nejm 1998;338:1241; 1993;328:1509; 1990;322:645; Med Let 1990;32:112). Adverse effects: Möbius syndrome (facial paralysis and limb defects) if fail to abort (Nejm 1998;338:1881); cost: $100/200 mg
- Suction evacuation, or
- Misoprostol (Cytotec) (Nejm 2001;344:38, 59) 200 μgm vag q 12 h; a prostaglandin that causes 90% to abort within 2 d; 55% need subsequent D + E. Adverse effects: fever (11%), abdominal pain (57%), emesis (4%), diarrhea (4%). Cost $1; or
- Methotrexate 50 mg/m^2 im, followed in 3–7 d by misoprostol 800 μgm vag × 1 and repeated in 1–7 d if no abortion; 90[+]% complete abortions, 4–9% require vacuum extraction w or w/o dilatation (Med Let 1996;38:39; Nejm 1995;333:537; Jama 1994; 272:1190)
- Epostane (prevents progesterone synthesis) 200 mg qid × 7 d at 5–8 wk causes 84% to abort within 2 wk, usually at 5 d (Nejm 1988;319:813)

of 2nd trimester pregnancy:

- Prostaglandin E$_2$ (Nejm 1994;331:290) 20 μgm vaginally q 3 h; aborts 80% within 2 d, 70% will need a D + C as well. Adverse effects: fever (63%), pain (67%) and abdominal cramping, emesis (33%), diarrhea (30%). Cost $300
- D + E up to 18[+] wk

PREGNANCY

Cause: Unprotected intercourse

Epidem: 20% abort before clinically apparent, another 10% abort later (Nejm 1988;319:189)

Pathophys: (Ann IM 1984;101:683)

Sx: Early: nausea and vomiting (50%); breast engorgement; missed period. Quickening at 20 wk, 1–2 wk earlier in experienced multiparous women

Si: Soft uterine neck, blue cervix by 6 wk. Fetal heart by doppler at 9–12 wk; by feto- or stethoscope at 18–20 weeks.

Crs: 39–42 wk for maximal perinatal survival in singleton births, 37–38 wk for twins (Jama 1996;275:1432)

Cmplc: Adverse outcomes are not incr by long hours or stress (residents—Nejm 1990;323:1040)

- Asthma management is nearly the same as in the nonpregnant, but be aware that β agonists like terbutaline inhibit labor (Nejm 1985; 312:897), iodides induce fetal goiter (Lancet 1990;1:1241); tetracyclines stain fetal teeth
- Bleeding and/or contractions (pain):
  - 1st trimester: ectopic or threatened abortion, mole, septic abortion
  - 2nd trimester: mole, pyelonephritis, placenta praevia, incompetent cervix, or bicornuate uterus
  - 3rd trimester: premature labor, previa, or abruption, which can be caused by trauma (Nejm 1990;323:1609)
- Cardiac disease rx (Nejm 1993;329:250) generally stenotic lesions (AS, MS) a greater problem than insufficiency lesions (MR, AI) because of incr cardiac output during pregnancy (J. Love 12/94); rare (1/10,000) MI (Ann IM 1996;125:751)
- Diabetes: incr C-section rates because of incr rates of toxemia, macrosomia, and congenital malformations (Nejm 1986;315:989)
- GI: (Ann IM 1993;118:366) esophageal reflux, nausea and vomiting, bloating/constipation from diminished LES pressure and motility; gallstones (2%) and sludge (present by ultrasound in 31% of pregnancies) occur but often revert to normal postpartum (Ann IM 1993;119:116)
- Hyperemesis gravidarum, usually in 1st trimester; for rx see below
- Liver disease, various types including acute fatty liver of pregnancy, intrahepatic cholestasis, et al. (Nejm 1996;335:570)
- Low birth weight (p 661)
- Premature rupture of membranes, if before 32 wk gestation, rx for group B strep w ampicillin/amoxicillin 250 mg + perhaps erythromycin for chlamydia (Jama 1997;278:989)

- Rheumatologic disorders: safe medications (Bull Rheum Dis 1992;41(2):1)
- Stroke risk not incr during but is incr for 1st 6 wk post partum (Nejm 1996;335:768)
- Thyrotoxicosis (Nejm 1985;313:562) more common when high HCG levels from gestational trophoblastic disease since HCG structurally close to TSH (Nejm 1998;339:1823); more common postpartum in IDDM pts (10%) (Ann IM 1993;118:419)
- Toxemia of pregnancy (p 613)
- Urologic: pyelonephritis from physiologic dilatation or ureters and/or decr motility and/or compression; proteinuria associated w toxemia; nephrogenic diabetes insipidus in 3rd trimester (Nejm 1984;310:442); chronic renal failure (Nejm 1985;312:836)

Lab: Routine initial prenatal package: UA and culture, hgb/hct in 1st and 3rd trimesters, ABO and Rh type, VDRL, chlamydia antigen, gc culture, pap smear; rubella titer (if neg, advise on avoiding exposure during pregnancy and offer postpartum immunization—Nejm 1992;326:663,702); HIV test w informed consent since AZT rx will decrease fetal transmission from 25% to 8% (Jama 1995;273: 977); perhaps toxoplasmosis titer? (Nejm 1994;331:695) and TSH (Nejm 1999;341:549 vs 601)

At 16–20 wk, quadruple markers (AFP, HCG, inhibin, and estriol) for Down syndrome

At 24–28 wk: screen w 50 gm glucose, nonfasting, if 1-h blood sugar is >130–140 mg%, get full GTT; full GTT = 100 gm glucose, FBS <105, 1 h <190, 2 h >165 (but problems even if 120–165), 3 h <145; dx gestational DM by ≥2 values too high (Nejm 1986; 315:989,1025)

At 35–37 wk, group B strep culture (Nejm 2000;342:15)

Chem: Serum β-subunit tests positive within 2 wk of conception

Hem: Hgb drops by midtrimester from an average of 13.7 gm to 11.5 gm, then usually rises to 12.3 gm in 3rd trimester; if stays up, indicates plasma volume decrease and decr fetal weight (Ann Obgyn Scand 1984;63:245). Platelets average 322,000 in 1st trimester, 275,000 in 2nd, and 300,000 in 3rd (Jama 1979;242:2696)

Urine: Pregnancy tests now sensitive down to β-HCG of 50 U and hence 90% positive by 1st day of missed mense, 97% by 7th day (Jama 2001;286:1759)

Xray: Ultrasound at 4–6 wk for gestational sac, at 8–12 wk for crown/rump length, or 14–20 wk for biparietal diameter, if dates unclear; routine ultrasound for congenital anomalies not helpful? (Nejm 1993;329:821 vs 874)

Rx: Avoid teratogens, including antibiotics (list—Med Let 1987;29:61); safe meds list (Nejm 1998;338:1135); spina bifida caused by maternal vit A ingestion of [3]10,000 IU qd esp in 1st trimester (Nejm 1995;333:1369). See Table 14.4.1

Folic acid 1 mg qd and iron 325 mg qd supplements throughout pregnancy prevents deficiencies; folate periconception at 0.4 mg qd × 1 mo decreases neural tube defect risk by 71% (Peds 1993; 493:4), 4 mg po qd if pos family hx

Prenatal visits q 1 mo to 36 wk then q 2 wk if low risk, more if high risk (Jama 1996;275:847) to monitor fetal growth and maternal BP and education

of **hyperemesis gravidarum:** small feedings, stop Fe pills, give vit B_6 (pyridoxine) 25 mg po tid × 3 d (Rx Let 1999;6:68; Obgyn 1991;78:33); antihistamines like diphenhydramine (Benadryl) 25–50 mg po q 4–6 h, or trimethobenzamide (Tigan) 200 mg rectal suppos; or phenothiazines like prochlorperazine (Compazine) 25 mg po or pr qid, or 5 mg im, or promethazine (Phenergan) 25–50 mg po or pr qid, or chlorpromazine (Thorazine) 25–50 mg im q 4 h, or metoclopramide (Reglan) 5–10 mg po/im/iv; iv fluids and hospitalization for volume depletion and ketosis. Bendectin (contains pyridoxine) no longer available in US but sold as diclectin in Canada, and as Unisom sleep aid (pyridoxine + doxylamine) in US 1/2 tab po bid (Rx Let 2000;7:22), and probably is safe (Nejm 1998;338:1128)

of seizure disorders in pregnancy: seizure meds incr risk of congenital malformations (Nejm 2001;344:1132); cleft palate and spina bifida incr w all, least w phenobarb, more w valproate, and most w carbamazepine (Am J Publ Hlth 1996;86:1454) vs only carbamazepine? (Nejm 1991;324:674); phenobarb, esp if given in last trimester, impairs subsequent intelligence (Jama 1995;274: 1518); for phenytoin, one can predict which fetus will be deformed by an enzyme assay of amnion (Nejm 1990;322:1567)

of depression in pregnancy: TCAs and SSRIs probably ok (rv—Jama 1999;282:1264)

of hypothyroidism: monitor TSH, often need higher thyroid dose in pregnancy (Rx Let 1999;6:58)

Table 14.4.1 Selected Drugs That Can Be Used Safely During Pregnancy, According to Condition

Condition	Drugs of Choice	Alternative Drugs	Comments
Acne	Topical: erythromycin, clindamycin, benzoyl peroxide	Systemic: erythromycin, topical tretinoin (vitamin A acid)	Isotretinoin is contraindicated
Allergic rhinitis	Topical: glucocorticoids, cromolyn, decongestants, xylometazoline, oxymetazoline, naphazoline, phenylephrine, systemic: di-phenhydramine, dimenhydrinate, tripelennamine, astemizole		
Constipation	Docusate sodium, calcium, glycerin, sorbitol, lactulose, mineral oil, magnesium hydroxide	Bisacodyl, phenolphthalein	
Cough	Diphenhydramine, codeine, dextromethorphan		
Depression	Tricyclic antidepressant drugs, fluoxetine	Lithium	When lithium is used in first trimester, fetal echocardiography and ultrasonography are recommended because of small risk of cardiovascular defects
Diabetes	Insulin (human)	Insulin (beef or pork)	Hypoglycemic drugs should be avoided
Headache Tension	Acetaminophen	Aspirin and nonsteroidal antiinflammatory drugs, benzodiazepines	Aspirin and nonsteroidal antiinflammatory drugs should be avoided in third trimester

(continued)

607

Table 14.4.1 Selected Drugs That Can Be Used Safely During Pregnancy, According to Condition *(continued)*

Condition	Drugs of Choice	Alternative Drugs	Comments
Migraine	Acetaminophen, codeine, dimenhydrinate	β-adrenergic–receptor antagonists and tricyclic antidepressant drugs (for prophylaxis)	Limited experience with ergotamine has not revealed evidence of teratogenicity, but there is concern about potent vasoconstriction and uterine contraction
Hypertension	Labetalol, methyldopa	β-adrenergic–receptor antagonists, prazosin, hydralazine	Angiotensin-converting–enzyme inhibitors should be avoided because of risk of severe neonatal renal insufficiency
Hyperthyroidism	Propylthiouracil, methimazole	β-adrenergic–receptor antagonists (for symptoms)	Surgery may be required; radioactive iodine should be avoided
Mania (and bipolar affective disorder)	Lithium, chlorpromazine, haloperidol	For depressive episodes: tricyclic antidepressant drugs, fluoxetine, valproic acid	If lithium is used in first trimester, fetal echocardiography and ultrasonography are recommended because of small risk of cardiac anomalies; valproic acid may be given after neural-tube closure is complete

Nausea, vomiting, motion sickness	Diclectin (doxylamine plus pyridoxine) (same as Bendectin; available in Canada)	Chlorpromazine, metoclopramide (in third trimester), diphenhydramine, dimenhydrinate, meclizine, cyclizine
Peptic ulcer disease	Antacids, magnesium hydroxide, aluminum hydroxide, calcium carbonate, ranitidine	Sucralfate, bismuth subsalicylate
Pruritus	Topical: moisturizing creams or lotions, aluminum acetate, zinc oxide cream or ointment, calamine lotion, glucocorticoids; systemic: hydroxyzine, diphenhydramine, glucocorticoids, astemizole	Topical: local anesthetics
Thrombophlebitis, deep-vein thrombosis	Heparin, antifibrinolytic drugs, streptokinase	Streptokinase is associated with a risk of bleeding; warfarin should be avoided

Reproduced with permission from Koren G, Pastuszak A, Ito S. Drugs in pregnancy. Nejm 1998;338:1128–1137.
Data from Smith J, et al. Drugs of choice for pregnant women. In: Koren G, ed. Maternal fetal toxicology: a clinician's guide. 2nd ed. New York: Marcel Dekker, 1994:115–128.

LABOR AND DELIVERY

Cause:

Epidem: 60% go into labor between 39 and 41 weeks; rare to go >300 d unless anencephaly

Pathophys: (Nejm 1999;341:660)

Sx: Rhythmic pains radiate to small of back; bloody show; ruptured membranes w positive ferning and/or nitrazine paper testing

Si: Cervical effacement and dilatation. Presentations: vertex (96%), breech (4%), transverse lie and mental (<1%)

Crs:

Stage I: Onset of labor to full dilatation of cervix; usually 4–12 h

Stage II: Complete dilatation to infant delivery, median duration 50 min in nullips, 20 min in multips

Stage III: Infant delivery until placental delivery, usually 5–15 min

Cmplc: Many, especially pre-eclampsia, abruption, stillbirth, and fetal growth retardation, assoc w undetected clotting factor mutations, eg, Factor V Leiden (Nejm 1999;340:9)

• Endometritis

• Failure to progress, caused by cephalopelvic disproportion, or overmedication

• Mortality: maternal = 3–4/10,000; infant/perinatal = 3.5%, 2% stillborn, rates incr 3× in breech

• Perineal lacerations:

   1st degree: Superficial

   2nd degree: Tissue injury sparing rectal sphincter

   3rd degree: Partial or complete separation of rectal sphincter

   4th degree: Tear into rectum; even w good repair, many (>1/2?) 3rd and 4th degree lacerations pts have longterm fecal incontinence, especially if episiotomy or forceps used (Nejm 1993;329:1905)

• Premature labor, often due to bacterial chorioamnionitis (Nejm 2000;342:1500); due to short "incompetent" cervix predictable by transvaginal US at 24–28 WK (Nejm 1996;334:567)

• Premature rupture of membranes (PROM), >1 hr before onset of labor; w/u w sterile speculum exam and tests of vaginal fluid for ferning and nitrazine positivity, check fetal lung maturity (eg, L/S ratio) if <36 wk, group B strep chlamydia and gc cultures; rx (p 612)

- Prepartum bleeding in 3rd trimester: do digital exam of cervix only after ultrasound or set up to do immediate C/S because may be **placenta previa,** 1/150 deliveries, increases w maternal age and h/o previous praevia; caused by low implantation of placenta so it partially covers cervical os, those discovered in early pregnancy by ultrasound often migrate away by 3rd trimester; **placental abruption** (Jama 1999;282:1646), associated w HT and trauma but most are spontaneous, usually painful unlike praevia; can cause uterine enlargement and tenderness, fetal distress, maternal shock, rx by delivery; **vasa previa,** cord vessels scattered throughout membranes, 1/100 antepartum bleeders, pulsatile vessels at cervical os

- Presentation, abnormal: breech; rx w external cephalic version after 35 wks; ?moxibustion w herbs and acupuncture (Jama 1998;280:1580) at 33 wk

- Postpartum bleeding in mother: incr by aspirin use within 5 d of delivery (Nejm 1982;307:909); first examine for laceration or retained placenta, then oxytocin 10 U im or in dilute iv soln, eg, 10–30 U/1000 cc (not iv push), then vigorous bimanual massage of uterus, then methylergonovine (Methergine) 0.2 mg im (not iv), then 15-methyl prostaglandin $E_2\alpha$ (Hemabate) 250 mg im, may repeat in 15–90 min, then hysterectomy or hypogastric artery ligation

- Pulmonary embolus in 1/4000, a $10\times$ increase over baseline

- Shoulder dystocia; rx see below

Lab:

Chem: Amniotic fluid to test for lung maturity, if may be premature; false positives in diabetics

Noninv: Nonstress test (NST) for fetal movement and heart rate; oxytocin challenge stress test or nipple stimulation produces 3 or more contractions in 10 min to measure effect on fetal heart rate

Biophysical profile by ultrasound; calculate by scoring 0 if absent and 2 pt if present for fetal breathing movements, gross fetal body movements, fetal tone, reactive NST, and amniotic fluid volume in one pocket or total cm in each quadrant (amniotic fluid index) ≥ 2 cm; last 2 most important; 8/10 score is good (Am J Obgyn 1987; 156:527)

Fetal monitoring usually used in most deliveries now although abnormalities correlate w an already injured fetus and does prevent cerebral palsy (Ob Gyn 1995;86:613); repetitive late decels and decr variability both are assoc w a 2.5–3.5 incr incid of CP but 99.8% false pos rate (Nejm 1996;334:613); if use in all you increase C-section rate without any improvement in outcome (Nejm 1986;315:615)

Xray: Ultrasound, for gestational age, or for amniocentesis for fetal maturity if premature labor

Rx: Avoid peripartum ASA (Nejm 1982;307:909); and bupivacaine 0.75% for epidural or paracervical blocks since causes cardiac arrests, hard to resuscitate (FDA Drug Bull 1983;13:23)

Analgesia possible w local paracervical blocks, spinal, and/or continous epidural blocks, which may impair ability to walk and hence incr operative delivery rate (Nejm 1997;337:1715)

Spontaneous vaginal delivery; amniotomy (rupture of membranes) at 3^+ cm dilatation speeds labor by >2 h safely (Nejm 1993;328:1145); walking during early labor has no effect (Nejm 1998;339:76)

Vaginal birth after C/S (VBAC) successful in 60–80% if previous low horizontal incision; but ability to predict which pts works best is difficult (Nejm 1996;335:689); cmplc: uterine rupture (Nejm 2001;345:3) in 0.8% w/o but 2.5% w prostaglandin induction, compared to 0.15% if do repeat c/s and never goes into labor

Cesarean sections: current increase to 25% of all deliveries is fueled to some extent by "repeats" (Nejm 1984;311:887) but also by individual physician practice styles (Nejm 1989;320:706); in Ireland still only 5% C/S rate and perinatal mortality as good as US (Obgyn 1983;61:1); "active management of labor" by amniotomy within 1st h and pitocin at 6–36 mU/min to keep q 2 min contractions reduces C/S by 30% (Nejm 1992;326:450) vs no reduction in C/S rate though labor duration decr × 2 h plus less maternal fever (Nejm 1995;333:745)

of PROM (pathophys rv—Nejm 1998;338:663), w watching only vs induction w pitocin + protaglandin E (Nejm 1996;334:1005, 1053), antibiotics if fever, fetal tachycardia, pos grp B strep culture, if lasts >12–18 hr

of threatened premature delivery from PROM, premature labor, or preeclampsia (Jama 1995;273:413): β-methasone 12 mg im × 2, 24 h apart, or dexamethasone 6 mg im q 6–12 h × 4 once (Jama

2001;286:1581), between 24–34 wk gestation to reduce fetal risk of hyaline membrane disease and intraventricular hemorrhage

of premature labor, <34 wk (Nejm 1984;311:571; 1984;310:691):

- 1st: MgSO$_4$ 4 gm iv over 20 min, then 2 gm/h iv/im follow Mg levels, 5–7 mg/cc is therapeutic range (Clin Obgyn 1990;33:502), overdose can cause fatal respiratory depression;
- 2nd: Terbutaline or isoxsuprine (Ritodrine), but only delays delivery by 24–48 h without improving survival so use to buy time to transport or get steroids on board (Nejm 1992;327:308,349). Adverse effects: elevate blood sugar, cardiovascular risks (Med Let 1980;22:89), especially pulmonary edema (Ann IM 1989; 110:714).
- 3rd: Nifedipine 10 mg sl up to 40 mg/h then 20 mg q 6 h maintenance, safer than Ritodrine (Am J Obgyn 1990;163:105) but may impair uteroplacental bloodflow; or
- Indomethacin also works but infant cmplc's not worth it (Nejm 1993;329:1602)

of shoulder dystocia, all within 5 min:

1st: Episiotomy
2nd: Legs up (McRobert's maneuver)
3rd: Suprapubic pressure
4th: Wood's screw maneuver or disimpact anterior shoulder
5th: Remove posterior shoulder, fracture clavicle
6th: Cesarean section

of failure to progress: risk of neonatal intracranial bleed or othr damage elevated by use of forceps, vacuum or C/S so none preferable over the others (Nejm 1999;341:1709)

PREGNANCY-INDUCED HYPERTENSION, PRE-ECLAMPSIA/ECLAMPSIA, TOXEMIA

ACOG Tech Bull #219; Jan 1996, Nejm 1993;329:1265; 1992;326: 927; 1990;323:434,478

Cause: Unknown; genetic component, incid incr × 2 if maternal or paternal h/o pre-eclampsia (Nejm 2001;344:867)

Epidem: Incidence 1.5% of all private ob patients; 12% of teaching hospital patients; 20% in urban poor; 5–6% in primips who represent 85% of all pts w PIH/eclampsia; 25% of patients w chronic hypertension (Nejm 1998;339:667); 2nd most common cause of maternal deaths after pulmonary embolus, causes 15%

Pathophys: (Nejm 1996;335:1480, 1991;325:1439)

Sympathetic vasoconstrictor hyperactivity that abates w delivery (Nejm 1996;335:1480)

Normally, pregnancy induces a decrease in peripheral vascular resistance mediated by incr resistance to angiotensin; somehow this effect is lost via a trophoblast-dependent process w platelet dysfunction (Nejm 1990;323:478). Vasodilating prostacyclin (PGI2) level suppression present even in 1st trimester (Jama 1999;282:356)

CNS sx assoc w reversible brain edema and leukoencephalopathy, also seen in immunocompromised and renal failure pts (Nejm 1996; 334:494)

Sx: Pregnant, weight gain, edema, headache,* visual changes,* acute onset, abdominal pain* especially epigastric

Si:

- Hypertension, systolic >140 and/or diastolic >90 on 2 exams 6 h apart; before 20 wk = chronic HT, r/o molar pregnancy; after 20 wk gestation = PIH; diastolic >110* is ominous for eclampsia (seizures)
- Edema
- Proteinuria (= pre eclampsia), ≥300 mg/24 hr or 1⁺ proteinuria
- Hyperreflexia incidentally often but without prognostic significance

Crs: All sx disappear (in 95%) by 72 h postpartum; a small percentage may persist for weeks. If occurs in first trimester, must be mole or trophoblastic tumor

Cmplc: Preeclampsia: HT + proteinuria after 20 wk gestation, most in 3rd trimester; associated when severe but short of eclampsia, w a 1% maternal and 10% prenatal infant mortality; when severe evolves to eclampsia, without rx, in 25–50%

Eclampsia (toxemia; defined by seizures), predicted by number of findings above*; renal failure; CHF; CNS bleed; DIC; Sheehan's syndrome; fetal demise; hepatic hemorrhage and rupture (Nejm 1985;312:424); HELLP syndrome (p 616); newborn neutropenias, transient in 50%, associated w sepsis (Nejm 1989;321:557)

Fetal growth retardation

r/o other causes of hypertension in pregnancy: pheochromocytoma; more benign **transient hypertension of pregnancy;** and chronic hypertension in pregnancy (Nejm 1987;316:715)

Lab:

Chem: Uric acid elevated; creatinine elevations*

Hem: Hemolytic anemia* and thrombocytopenia,* which may be mild; platelet intracellular calcium markedly elevated by vasopressin in susceptibles (Nejm 1990;323:434); polycythemia indicating hypovolemia

Path: Renal, bx or at postmortem shows ATN, occasionally bilateral cortical necrosis, swollen glomerular endothelial cells containing fibrin. Placenta shows spotty necrosis w small vessel disease

Urine: 24 h protein >300 mg, may be >2 gm*; creatinine clearance decr (normally in pregnancy is 100–150 cc/min). 24-h calcium <100–150 mg, unlike benign hypertensives who excrete more calcium (Nejm 1987;316:715)

Rx: Preventive w: ASA 60–100 mg po qd by wk 12? (BMJ 2000;322:329 vs Nejm 1998;338:701); perhaps vit C 1000 mg qd + vit E 400 IU qd (Rx Let 1999;6:58); calcium controversial but probably not helpful (Nejm 1997;337:69 vs 1991;325:1399);

of HT during pregnancy (Can Med Assoc J 1997;157:1245): α-methyldopa (Aldomet) alone; or propranolol (Nejm 1981;305:1323); or α-methyldopa + hydralazine; or clonidine + hydralazine (Med J Aust 1991;154:378). But rx of PIH, unless severe, does not improve outcome. Avoid ACEIs, which are teratogenic (Jama 1997;277:1193)

of preeclampsia (Can Med Assoc J 1997;157:1245): bed rest; deliver when fetus mature; hospitalize for failure of home bed rest, diastolic BP ≥110, or proteinuria ≥2+ by dip or ≥500 mg/24 h; avoid diuretics and salt restriction; hydralazine 5–10 mg q 20 min iv to get diastolic BP < 105; or labetolol 10–20 mg iv q 10 min; or perhaps nifedipine 10 mg sl then po q 6 h (Obgyn 1991;77:331); follow w po hydralazine, α-methyldopa, or β blockers. Rx does not improve fetal outcome but does protect maternal CNS (Am J Obgyn 1990;162:960)

of eclampsia (seizures): stabilize, then deliver within 4–5 h of onset, may need D + C to get rid of all placenta; $MgSO_4$ 4 gm iv over 20 min, then 2 gm/h iv, or can give im, eg, 10 gm load then 5 gm q 4 h (Nejm 1995;333:201); follow Mg levels, 5–7 mg/cc is

therapeutic range; continue 12–24 h postpartum, may cause fatal
newborn respiratory depression, helped by iv calcium gluconate gm
for gm

HELLP SYNDROME (Hemolysis, Elevated Liver Function Tests, Low Platelets)

(Jama 1998;280:559)

Cause: PIH/preeclampsia

Epidem:

Pathophys: Unknown; overlaps w acute fatty liver of pregnancy (Ann IM
1987;106:703; Nejm 1985;313:367); both may be a manifestation
of a mitochondrial fatty acid metabolizing enzyme that also leads to
liver disease in the infants (Nejm 1999;340:1723)

Sx: Onset after 30th (usually >35th) week of pregnancy. Usually none but
may have any sx of PIH and/or headache, confusion; fatigue,
malaise; nausea and vomiting; abdominal pain, diffuse or right
upper quadrant

Si: Edema, hypertension, proteinuria, jaundice, encephalopathy, seizures,
coma; small liver; tender right upper quadrant; preeclampsia in all

Crs: 85% mortality without rx. Does not seem to recur in future
pregnancies

Cmplc: Hypoglycemia, DIC and hemorrhage, renal failure, eclampsia,
pancreatitis (back pain), fetal and/or maternal death

Lab:

Chem: AST (SGOT) and ALT (SGPT), uric acid, NH_3 all elevated;
bilirubin goes up later; hypoglycemia

Genetic testing of family (Nejm 1999;340:1723)

Hem: Wbc >15,000; microangiopathic anemia/DIC picture w
nucleated rbc's, rapidly falling platelet counts; elevated hct, PT, PTT,
and fibrin split products, and low fibrinogen levels

Path: Liver bx shows easily missed fat in microvesicles w central (not
peripheral) nuclei; r/o Reye's and tetracycline hepatotoxicity

Urine: UA shows proteinuria

Rx: Stabilize, stat delivery, transfuse platelets

HYDATIDIFORM MOLE (Molar Pregnancy)

Nejm 1996;335:1740

Cause: Gestational trophoblastic neoplasia; complete from a haploid sperm duplicating own chromosomes and inactivating ovum chromosomes, or partial w haploid karyotype

Epidem: 1/1500 pregnancies; 10% of all spontaneous abortions have mole changes (A. Hertig 1967). Increased incidence in Asians, women over age 40, and in women w h/o previous spontaneous abortion

Pathophys: Molar changes seen at junction of placenta and chorionic laeve when chorion is undergoing atrophy at 8–12 wk. Embryo portion dies at 3–5 wk, chorionic villi then accumulate fluid in connective tissue spaces from maternal circulation. Fetal circulation is absent, hence fluid accumulation. Invasive mole doesn't follow a normal pregnancy unless a twin was present

Range of disease exists from benign mole to choriocarcinoma (p 618)

Sx: H/o recent spontaneous abortion; severe morning sickness (hyperemesis gravidarum) lasting into 2nd trimester

Si: Vaginal bleeding in 1st trimester; uterus enlarged beyond dates although 10% may be small for gestational age

Crs:

Cmplc: Local invasion and/or benign metastases; choriocarcinoma or persistent gestational trophoblastic tumors (20–30%); thyrotoxicosis from a TSH-like protein present in 100% of moles (Ann IM 1975;83:307); pregnancy induced hypertension; tumor emboli

Lab:

Chem: HCG levels very high, does not decrease to normal within 6 wk of removal as a normal spontaneous abortion should

Path: Endometrial bx by D + C shows entire endometrium involved; volumes up to 3 L; translucent villi up to 1 cm diameter, appear like "grapes"; organized trophoblast (benign), to pleomorphic (potentially malignant)

Xray: CT and chest xray to look for mets; ultrasound done for abnormal bleeding detects most

Rx: Rhogam if Rh neg

Benign moles may be rx'd w simple D + E, followed by HCG levels q 2 wk

Invasive types or mets rx'd like choriocarcinoma (see below)

Good birth control to prevent new pregnancy while follow serial HCGs to 0 to be sure benign course

CHORIOCARCINOMA

Nejm 1996;335:1740

Cause: Fetal chorionic tissues of placenta; teratomas of ovary? (Nejm 1969;280:1439)

Epidem: 1/3 after spontaneous abortions, 1/3 after moles, and 1/3 after normal pregnancies; 500/yr in US; incidence incr × 10 in Asians and Hispanics

Pathophys: Local invasion and bloodborne metastases. In 50%, can't find primary lesion it's so small

Sx: Bleeding, excessive nausea and vomiting (morning sickness)

Si:

Crs: Without rx, die within 1 yr

Cmplc: Metastases, 80% to lung, 30% to vagina, 25% local, 10% to brain, 10% to liver, 5% to kidney; toxemia of pregnancy in late 1st or early 2nd trimester; perforated uterus; endometritis

Lab:

Chem: HCG levels very high, >100,000 IU/24-h urine (normal pregnancy, even at 28 d peak, is less than this, and later decreases to 5000 IU during most of pregnancy, and drops in last 2 wk at term). T_4 incr via TSH-like substance, and perhaps HCG. Liver function tests elevated if metastases

Path: Hemorrhagic central necrosis. Ovaries have large thecal cysts from HCG stimulation, but they will regress. On microscopic, syncytio-cytotrophoblasts w necrosis, hemorrhage, and inflammation

Xray: Head CT to r/o metastases. Ultrasound shows clumps of placenta

Rx: Surgical resection

Chemotherapy w methotrexate po or im and/or dactinomycin qd in 5-d bursts; 5-yr survivals w this rx are nearly 100% for intrauterine, 75% for extrauterine, 50% if CNS metastases, but 0% if hepatic mets

14.5 MISCELLANEOUS

Amenorrhea: Rx all anovulatory patients w medroxyprogesterone 10 mg po × 10 d q 3 mo to prophylact vs uterine cancer (D. Federman, 1985)
Primary amenorrhea (no menses by age 16–18) w/u: physical exam to look for imperforate hymen, vaginal agenesis, cervical stenosis, endometrial tbc, dwarfism (Turner's, get buccal smear or karyotype), pregnancy, virilized external genitalia (congenital adrenal hyperplasia, hemaphroditism, mixed gonadal dysgenesis, or androgen-producing ovarian tumor) (see Figure 14.5.1)

Anovulation causes: Stein-Leventhal syndrome, FSH/LH surge failure, eg, at times of menarche or menopause, w anorexia, et al.

Birth control (Med Let 1995;37:9—a rv of all methods, efficiencies, advantages, and disadvantages; Nejm 1989;320:777); 25–30% of couples having regular intercourse get pregnant each month (Nejm 1988;319:189)

MEDICATIONS (Med Let 2000;42:42; Nejm 1993;328:1543)

Estrogen/progesterone shots q 1 mo (Lunelle) (Rx Let 2000;7:66)
Birth control pills (P. Myers 5/91): combination pills of estrogen (usually ethinyl estradiol [EE]; or mestranol [ME] [50 μgm = 30 μgm of EE], or ethynodiol diacetate [EDA]); plus a progestin (usually norethindrone [NE], or norgestrel [NG], or levonorgestrel (LG), or norgestimate [NGE], or desogestrel [DG]) that suppresses LH surge and ovulation, maintain estrogen levels and mature endometrium regularly. Avoid (Jama 2001;285:2232) in pts w HT, migraine, DVT/PE, smokers over age 35
Estrogen side effects: thrombosis (venous, coronary, CNS) although low dose (≤35 μgm) estrogen pills may not incr CVAs (Ann IM 1997;127:596; Nejm 1996;335:8 vs Jama 2000;284:284:72 metanalysis) or other manifestations (Ann IM 1998;128:469) unless age >40 or smoke, no incr risk after stop smoking, but super-low dose estrogen pills (~20 μgm) may be slightly worse because of newer progesterone effect; nausea and lactation suppression
Progestin side effects: ASCVD via lipids, risk ends when discontinue pills (Nejm 1988;319:1313); hypertension; glucose intolerance; acne (androgenicity); depression; rarely liver adenomas (Nejm 1976;294:

Primary amenorrhea workup.

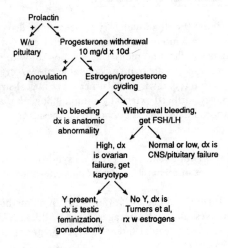

Secondary amenorrhea workup.

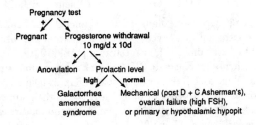

Figure 14.5.1

470); gallstones (Nejm 1976;294:189); all seem less w desogestrel as in Desogen 28 or Ortho-Cept 21 (Med Let 1993;35:73) including thromboembolism risks (Nejm 2001;345:1787).

No increase in breast cancer (Nejm 1986;315:405); no overall adverse effect of BCPs on mortality (Ann IM 1994;120:821) and may decrease ovarian cancer risk substantially

Androgenicity decreases as go from levoNG > NG > NE > NE acetate > EDA > DG. Triphasic oral contraceptives like Trinorinyl, Orthonovum 7/7/7, and Triphasil all increase, then decrease progesterone dose during cycle to try to decrease ASHD risk; questionable value (Med Let 1985;27:48; 1984;26:93)

Progesterone only

Levonorgestrel implant (Norplant) lasts 5 yr; pregnancy rate = 4/1000/yr, higher in obese and patients on seizure meds (Med Let 1991;33:17), good for adolescent mothers (Nejm 1994;331:1201)

Medroxyprogesterone (DepoProvera) 25–150 mg im q 3 mo; 25 mg probably enough (Fertil Steril 1984;42:216) even though 150 mg is recommended. Adverse effect: debatable small increase in breast cancer (Jama 1995;273:799)

Norethindrone (Micronor) 0.35 mg po qd

Norgestrel (Ovrette) 0.075 mg po qd

Moderate estrogen, low progestin

Modicon/Brevicon (NE 0.5 mg/EE 35 μgm)

Ortho 7/7/7 (NE 0.5–0.75–1/EE 35)

Ortho 10/11 (NE 0.5–1/EE 35)

Orthocept (DG 0.15/EE 30)

Orthocyllen (NGE 0.25/EE 35)

Ortho Tricyclen (NGE 0.18, 0.215, 0.25/EE 35)

Ovcon 35 (NE 0.4/EE 35)

Tri-Norinyl (NE 0.5–1–0.5/EE 35)

Triphasil and Tri-Levlen (levoNG 0.05–0.75–0.125/EE 30–40–30)

Low estrogen, moderate progestin

Loestrin 1/20 (NE acetate 1 mg/EE 20 μgm)

Alesse and Levlite (LevoNG 0.1/EE 20)

Moderate estrogen, moderate progestin

(*good first choices)

Demulen 1/35 (EDA 1 mg/EE 35 μgm)

Genora/Ortho/Norinyl 1/35 (NE 1/EE 35)

Genora/Ortho/Norinyl 1/50 (NE 1/ME 50)

*Levlen and *Levora (levoNG 0.15/EE 30)

Loestrin 1.5/30 (NE acetate 1.5/EE 30)

Lo-ovral (NG 0.3/EE 30)

*Nordette (levoNG 0.15/EE 30)

Nordette/Levlen (levoNG 0.15/EE 30)

Norinyl 1/35 (NE 1/EE 35)

Orthonovum 1/35 (NE 1/EE 35)

High estrogen, moderate progestin

Demulen 1/50 (EDA 1mg/EE 50 μgm)

Norinyl 1/50 (NE 1/ME 50) or 1/80 (NE 1/ME 80)

Norlestrin 1/50 (NE acetate 1/EE 50)
Orthonovum 1/50 (NE 1/ME 50) or 1/80 (NE 1/ME 80)
Ovcon (NE 1/EE 50)
Ovulen (EDA 1/ME 100)

Transdermal

Norelgestromin/ethinyl estradiol 150/20 (Evra [Ortho]) (Jama 2001;285:2347) q 1 wk, 3/4 wk; as effective and better compliance than BCPs

Maneuvers for birth control pill side effects

- Breakthrough bleeding: r/o infection; wait, since decreases from 30% to <10% after 3 cycles; increase progestin or go to monophasic if on tri; increase progestin androgenicity; increase estrogen if early in cycle
- Amenorrhea: r/o pregnancy; increase androgenicity or progestin; increase progestin; perhaps increase estrogen
- Nausea: take pill w food or at bedtime
- Acne: change to less androgenic progestin like Desogen 28 or Ortho-Cept 21 (Med Let 1993;35:73); Ortho Tricyclen is FDA approved
- Fluid retention, mastalgia, depression: decrease progestin; also estrogen?

OTHER METHODS

Postcoital contraception, "morning-after pill" (Nejm 1997;337:1058) decr pregnancy rate from 8% to 2% after single episode of intercourse, w:

- Oral birth control pills, eg 1 or 2 50 mg estradiol BCPs, or 2–4 35 mg estradiol BCPs po q 12 h twice, or as Preven emergency kit, $20 (Med Let 1998;40:102) within 72 h of unprotected intercourse has <2% failure rate (Med Let 1989;31:93), causes nausea and vomiting in 25–50%; repeat if vomits w/i 2 hr of dose or see pill in emesis; double doses if on antibiotics or seizure meds; consider giving all women a home supply (Nejm 1998;339:1)
- Levonorgestrel (Plan B) (Med Let 2000;42:10) 0.75 mg po × 2, 12 hr apart w/i 48 hr; better tolerated than estrogen/progestin combinations; $21
- Mifepristone (RU-486) 600 mg po; an antiprogesterone; <0.1% failure rate (Nejm 1992;327:1041); no nausea; not yet FDA approved
- IUD insertion esp if >72 hr but <5d since intercourse

Propranolol 80 mg vaginally qd (BMJ 1983;287:1245,1247); effective
for >10 h, inhibits sperm motility; 3 pregnancies/100 women/year,
comparable to diaphragm and IUD; highly absorbed

Mechanical Methods (in order of decreasing effectiveness):

- Vasectomy; reversals if vasectomy was <3 yr old resulting in a 76%
  pregnancy rate, if >15 yr old, 30% reversal pregnancy rate
- Tubal ligation; adv effects: ectopic pregnancy rate = 7/1000 in
  10 yr , higher (30/1000) when done by electrocoagulation (Nejm
  1997;336:762), no clear posttubal syndrome (Obgyn 1983;62: 673); no
  incr menstrual abnormalities (Nejm 2000;343:1681)
- Intrauterine devices (IUDs); Progestasert q 1 yr, Copper-T q 10 yr (Med
  Let 1988;30:25), or levonorgestrel (Mirena) (Med Let 2001;43:7) q 5 yr
  $500; cmplc: incr menstrual bleeding, dysmenorrhea
- Diaphragm; cervical caps no better and may be worse than diaphragms
  since dislodge (Am J Obgyn 1983;148:604), may increase cervical
  dysplasia (Med Let 1988;30:93)
- Condoms, male or female, polyurethane, which is as effective
  (2.6 pregnancies/100 women-years) as diaphragm and prevents herpes
  and HIV infection (Med Let 1993;35:123)
- Vaginal sponge (Med Let 1983;25:78) and/or spermicides; no increase in
  trisomies or birth defects (Nejm 1987;317:474, 478); spermicides don't
  help prevent STDs (Nejm 1998;339:504)

Domestic abuse/violence (Nejm 1999;341:886,1892,1899; Ann IM
1995;123:774)

Epidem: Incidence ~5%/yr, 20–33% of women have a pos hx (Jama
1998;280:433; Ann IM 1995;123:737). Highest risk in women
whose male partners abuse drugs or alcohol, are unemployed, and
have less than a high school education

Sx: Trauma; functional gi disorders (Ann IM 1995;123:782), anxiety,
depression, somatization

Si: Trauma in excess of hx + above

Rx: Screen by asking, "have you been hit, kicked, punched, or otherwise
injured in this past year, and if so by whom"; 70% sens, 85% specif
(Jama 1997;277:1357), but do it sensitively (Ann IM 1999;131:578)

Advocate for, offer choices, avoid blaming, assess danger; national
hotline: 1-800-799-SAFE

Dysfunctional uterine bleeding

Cause: Anovulatory cycles, eg, polycystic ovaries, androgen/cortisol excess, borderline pituitary or hypothalamic failure including menopause and menarche; uterine, eg, PID, cervical ectropion or polyp, cancer, fibroid, pregnancy; other medical illness, eg, bleeding disorder, hypothyroidism; Addison's disease

Sx: Menorrhagia, long and/or heavy periods; metrorrhagia, bleeding between periods

Si: Pelvic exam for mass, ovarian enlargement, fibroid, pregnancy, polyp

Cmplc: Anemia

Lab:

Chem: Pregnancy test, H + H

Path: Pap smear, endometrial bx if age ≥40 yr, hysteroscopy for failed medical rx after bx

Rx: For acute bleeding: 2–4 BCPs po × 1 or iv premarin 25 mg q 4 h until stop

Cycle w medroxyprogesterone (Provera) 10 mg qd × 10 d q 1–3 mo, or oral birth control pills

Surgical D + C; hysteroscopy; hysteroscopic resection of pathology; endometrial ablation w resectoscope, cautery, laser, or heat; hysterectomy

of anemia, iron

of pain, NSAIDS

Dysmenorrhea

Sx: Cramping, nausea, and vomiting w menses

Rx: Ibuprofen 400+ mg, better than ASA (Med Let 1984;26:67); oral bcps

Estrogen replacement therapy (Nejm 2001;345:34; Ann IM 1999;131: 605[rv]; Jama 1997;277:1140,)

ESTROGEN

• Conjugated estrogens from horse urine (Premarin) 0.625–1.25 mg qd (Obgyn 1984;63:759) and debatably even lower doses (Obgyn 1996;27:163) like 0.3 mg w adequate vit D and calcium enough to prevent osteoporosis (Ann IM 1999;130:897; Rx Let 1999;6:38), or
• Estradiol (Estrace) 1–2 mg po qd, both cost ~$20/mo; or patch bypasses liver, hence no beneficial cardiovascular/lipid effect (Ann IM 1992;117:85; Nejm 1997;336:683; 1991;325:756).

- Estropipate (Ogen), plus:

PROGESTERONE in woman w uterus (Jama 1996;275:370)

- Medroxyprogesterone (Provera) 10 mg qd last 10 d of each, q 2, or q 3 mo, must bleed 10 or more days after starting progesterone to be effective in preventing uterine cancer; or
- Micronized natural progesterone (Prometrium) (Rx Let 1998;5:39) 200 mg po 12/30 d or 100 mg po qd; or
- Continuous progestin, eg, 2.5 mg of medroxyprogesterone w continuous estrogen is just as effective and obviates periods (Jama 1996;276:1389, 1430), or
- Estrogen/progesterone combination pills; all ± $25/mo
  - Prempro (premarin 0.625 mg + progesterone 2.5 or 5 mg) (Rx Let 1998;5:16), or
  - FemHRT (Rx Let 2000;7:4) w 5 μgm estradiol + 1 mg norethindrone
  - Prefest (Rx Let 2000;7:16)
  - Activella (Rx Let 2000;7:40)

Estrogen adverse effects:

- Breast cancer risk (Nejm 1997;336:1769) incr over 4[+] yr, esp when combined w progesterone (Jama 2000;283:485, 534) vs no significant incr in women w positive family hx plus overall cause decr mortality (Ann IM 1997;127:973); decr mammography sens and specif (Jama 2001;285:171)
- Ovarian Ca (Jama 2001;285:1460; ObGyn 1998;92:472) possible slight incr
- Venous thromboembolic risk slightly incr, NNT-3 = 256 (Ann IM 2000;132:689), hence stop perioperatively, w hospitalization, w other risk factors
- Gall bladder disease incr (Jama 1998;280:605)
- Dry eye syndrome risk incr ×15–30% over yrs (Jama 2001;286:2114)

Definite improvement in:

- Bone loss and fractures (Jama 2001;285:2891; Ann IM 1995;122:9) including hip fractures decr by >1/2 (Nejm 1987;317:1169); improves bone density whenever initiated, even well after menopause, but must take ≥7 yr to have benefit (Framingham—Nejm 1993;329:1141,1192).
- ASHD?: conflicting studies (Ann IM 2001;135:1; 2000;133:933,999; Nejm 2000;343:572; 1999;340:1801), observational studies find a 50±% CAD reduction, perhaps direct effects as well as by lipid (lipoprotein A) improvements w estrogen alone or w progestins (Jama 2000;283:1845; 1998;280:605; Nejm 1997;336:683,1769) at least w micronized types but DBCTs find no significant decr in women w CAD

(Nejm 2000;343:522; Ann IM 1998;127:501) and perhaps incr risk in 1st yr (Ann IM 1999;131:463; Jama 1998;280:605) due to adv effects in those w low lipoprotein A levels to begin with (Jama 2000;282:1841) or genetic prothrombin mutations (Jana 2001;285:906); incr CVAs × 30% (Nejm 2001;345:1243; Ann IM 2000;133:933) esp in smokers (Nejm 1996;335:453; 1985;313:1038); also increases thromboemboli

- Rate of Alzheimer's disease incidence decr by 67% ? (Lancet 1996;348:429) vs no benefit in many other studies (Jama 1998;279:688)
- Colon cancer rates decr by 35–40% w concurrent use, revert after off × 5 yr (Ann IM 1998;128:705)
- Diabetes onset postmenopausally may be reduced (Rx Let 1998;5:51)

SELECTIVE ESTROGEN RECEPTOR MODULATORS (tamoxifen-like)

- Taloxifene (Evista) (Jama 1999;282:637; 1998;279:1445; Med Let 1998;40:29; Nejm 1997;337:1641,1686) 60–120 mg po qd, which helps bone (halves fx rates) and cholesterol w/o endometrial hyperplasia, and may decr breast Ca incidence (Jama 1999;281:2189) NNT-4yr = 126 (ACP J Club 1999;131:58) if detectable estradiol levels (Jama 2001; 287:216); but increases hot flashes and thromboembolic disease like DVT (1%) NNH-4yr = 155 (ACP J Club 1999;131:58); cost: $60/mo
- Tibolone (ACP J Club 1999;131:44) helps hot flashes, LDL, and bone density w/o endometrial or breast effects
- Phytoestrogens from soy, black cohosh, red clover, etc; probably cause no harm but efficacy unclear (Med Let 2000;42:17)

Gynecomastia in male or child, 40% are asx (Nejm 1993;328:490)
Cause: In adolescents, vast majority are transient and benign; Graves' disease (incr sex steroid-binding globulin); renal failure on dialysis; Klinefelter's; gonadotropin-producing tumors of lung or testicle (find w testicular ultrasound, or abdominal CT or MRI—Nejm 1991;324:334); malignant adrenal tumors; refeeding after starvation; local irritation; cirrhosis. Drugs: alcohol, α-methyldopa (Aldomet), amphetamines, captopril and other ACEIs, chemotherapy, cimetidine, diazepam, digitalis, estrogen minute amounts in foods or on fomites, haloperidol (Haldol), heroin, INH, marijuana, metronidazole (Flagyl), nifedipine, omeprazole (Prilosec), penicillamine, phenothiazines, phenytoin (Dilantin), ranitidine, reserpine, spironolactone (blocks androgen receptors), tricyclics, verapamil

Epidem: 25% are idiopathic, 25% pubertal, 10–20% drug-induced, 8% malnutrition or cirrhosis, 2% testicular tumor, 2% hypogonadism (Klinefelter's etc.), 1.5% hyperthyroidism, 1% renal disease

Pathophys: Increased estrogen and/or diminished androgens; many drugs cause it by displacing estrogen from binding protein

Lab:

Chem: HCG, LH, estradiol, testosterone, sTSH

Rx: Antiestrogens like 1st tamoxifen 10 mg po bid; clomiphene, cimetidine

Surgical resection

Hirsutism/hypertrichosis (Nejm 1990;323:909; Ann IM 1987;106:95; Med Let 1981;23:15)

Cause:

Isolated:

- Normal variation (Nejm 1992;327:194)
- Polycystic ovary

With assoc masculinization (voice, baldness, clitoromegaly)

- Adrenal carcinoma
- Cushing's syndrome
- Arrhenoblastoma
- Hilar cell adenoma or hyperplasia
- Luteoma
- Incomplete male pseudohermaphroditism
- Transvestitism/iatrogenic
- Mild congenital adrenal hyperplasia, 21-OH deficiency as well as 11β-OHase and 3β-OHase deficiencies (p 188), adult onset, HLA B14 and Aw33 linked (Nejm 1985;313:224), ~12% of adult female hirsutes

Lab:

Chem: Testosterone and dehydroepiandrostenedione levels to r/o testosterone-producing tumors; if ≥200 ng%, do 5 d dexamethasone suppression test (Nejm 1994;331:968,1015); 17-OH progesterone level <350 ng% in AM; if 350–1000, do ACTH stimulation test, should be <1000; and/or DHEA >800 μgm%

Rx: Cimetidine 300 mg 5x/d works by blocking androgen action at follicles (Nejm 1980;303:1042); spironolactone 75–200 mg qd; chronic steroids help 50%; bcps help 75%; electrolysis speeds responses. Topical eflornithine (Vaniga) (Med Let 2000;42:96) bid, slows hair follicle growth rate, helps hirsutism in women and pseudofollicultis barbae in men, takes 8 wk to help , <50% response rate; $42/mo (30 gm tube)

Infertility: No rx at all is as good as any of these in idiopathics (Nejm 1983;309:1201)

MALE INFERTILITY (Nejm 1995;332:312; Ann IM 1985;103: 906). Present in 50% of infertile couples:

1st: Physical exam, especially for varicocele (present in 40% infertile males and in 10% of fertile males); and scarred epididymis, vas deferens, and prostate. Avoid sulfasalazine, cimetidine, lead, arsenic, nitrofurantoin, marijuana, anabolic steroids, cocaine, heat exposure (eg, hot tubs), smoking

2nd: Sperm count (Nejm 2001;345:1388); normal >50 million/cc, >60% motile, >12% normal morphology; abnormal if <13 million/cc, and/or <50% motile, volume <10 cc, <9% normal morphology

3rd: FSH, LH, testosterone levels

if FSH is normal, and LH and testosterone low, dx is hypogonadotropic hypogonadism; get drug hx, sella MRI views and prolactin levels; withdraw drug if on any; rx w hCG-hMG or LHRH if both sella and prolactin normal; bromocriptine or surgery if big sella; bromocryptine and repeat films if sella normal and prolactin elevated

if elevated FSH and LH, and low testosterone, dx is primary panhypogonadism; or if FSH elevated, and normal testosterone and LH, dx is isolated germinal compartment failure; rx both w adoption or artificial insemination

if normal FSH, and elevated LH and testosterone, dx is partial androgen resistance; no rx known except adoption or artificial insemination

if normal FSH, LH, and testosterone and is oligospermic (not azoospermic), dx is varicocele or idiopathic; rx w surgery for varicocele; steroids? for measurable sperm antibodies, male or female (Nejm 1980;303:722); tetracycline for *Ureaplasma* infection? (Nejm 1983;308:505); split ejaculate insemination

if normal FSH, LH, and testosterone, and is azoospermic, get seminal fructose; if positive get postejaculation UA, if sperm present dx is retrograde ejaculation and needs a neurology w/u; if fructose-negative, get vasograms, bx and/or exploration looking for obstruction (majority) and rx with microductal surgery, most of such men have idiopathic obstructive azoospermia assoc w cystic fibrosis gene defects but lack other CF manifestations (Nejm 1998;339:687); if negative, dx is germinal compartment failure, rx with adoption and insemination, in vitro fertilization

FEMALE INFERTILITY

1st: Regular intercourse × 1 yr without birth control if normal anatomy; avoid nitrous oxide and other anesthetic exposures (Nejm 1992;327:993)

2nd: Do basal body temperature, increases in 2nd half of the cycle if ovulating; can confirm w serum progesterone levels or endometrial bx. Pregnancy occurs from intercourse 6 d prior to ovulation (10% chance) to day of ovulation (33% chance) and day of conception has no effect on fetal viability or gender (Nejm 1995;333:1517)

3rd: If no ovulation and partner normal by exam and testing, consider ovulation-inducing drug rx (Med Let 1988;30:91) w intrauterine insemination (Nejm 1999;340:177,224). Adverse effects: multiple births, 20% w some regimens; pathologic ovarian enlargement and ovarian cancer if used >1 yr (Nejm 1994;331:771)

- Clomiphene (blocks hypothalamic estrogen receptors so human chorionic gonadotropin releasing hormone (HCGRH) is stimulated, 30–40% effective
- Clomiphene + HCG in sequence; 66% pregnancy when above fails
- Clomiphene + dexamethasone; 75% of failures w clomiphene alone, get pregnant
- FSH + LH (Pergonal), then HCG if low basal gonadotropins and estrogens; 25% pregnancy rate, increases to 33% w clomiphene
- HCG and buserelin (LHRH agonist) (Nejm 1989;320:1233)
- Gonadorelin, HCGRH analog, given in q 90 min bursts iv over 3 wk results in a 60% pregnancy rate (Med Let 1990;32:70)

MALE OR FEMALE INFERTILITY

- Adoption help guidelines (Am Fam Phys 1985;31:109)
- Infertility support group = Resolve, Box 474, Belmont, MA 02178
- In vitro fertilization (embryo transfer), after estrogen/progesterone cycling in ovarian failure (Nejm 1986;314:806); cost = $50,000–100,000/delivery (Nejm 1994;331:239)
- Surrogate parenting or in vivo fertilization and uterine transfer

Menopausal sx/hot flashes (Nejm 1994;330:1062, I. Schiff 1988)
- Estrogens (p 624) help hot flashes, osteoporosis, vaginal atrophy, and

sleep; contraindicated in uterine or breast cancer or men w prostate cancer on GRH antagonist rx (Rx Let 2000;7:44)
- Progesterone alone as pills or topically (Pro-Gest) (Rx Let 1999;6:54) helps hot flashes and sleep; may worsen for 1–2 d before improving in women on tamoxifen; megesterol (Megace) 20 mg po bid (Nejm 1994; 331:347); or DepoProvera 150 mg im q 3 mo
- Veniafaxine (Effexor) 12.5 mg po bid
- Fluoxetine (Prozac) 20 mg po qd or other SSRI
- Clonidine 0.1 mg po qd helps 40% (Ann IM 2000;132:788)
- Gabapentin (Neurontin) 100 mg po hs up to 300 mg tid
- Testosterone transdermally 300 μgm/d improves sexual function significanlty in post BSOO premenopausal women (Nejm 2000;343:682)

Placenta accreta
Cause: Unknown
Epidem: 1/1500 deliveries
Pathophys: Invasion into myometrium
Sx: Pain; antepartum hemorrhage
Si: Can't completely extract on manual removal of placenta
Cmplc: Uterine rupture w subsequent pregnancy
Rx: Manual removal of placenta; if fail, D + C; but gravid uterus easily perforated. May need D + C under direct vision (laparotomy) or hysterectomy if extensive

Premenstrual syndrome: (Nejm 1995;332:829,1534 (RC trials by Hamilton, Ont); 1991;324:1208)
Epidem: 3–8% prevalence in all US women
Pathophys: All due to abnormal response to normal estrogen/progesterone changes during menstrual cycle (Nejm 1998;338:209)
Sx: Last 7 d of menstrual cycle; tension, irritability, dysphoria, bloating, edema, emotional lability, headache, breast swelling (imprecisely defined); r/o depression by at least 1 wk/mo without sx
Rx: Exercise works (endorphins)
Tricyclics: clomipramine (Anafranil) po qd
SSRIs (Med Let 2001;43:5):
- Fluoxetine (Prozac/Sarafem) 20 mg po qd continuously helps by double blind randomized trials, reduces sx × 50%
- Paroxetine (Paxil) (Neuropsycho Pharm 1995;12:169)
- Sertraline (Zoloft) 50–100 mg po qd prevents by RCTrial (Jama 1997;278:983)

Benzodiazepams: aprazolam (Xanax) 0.25–1 mg po qid day 18 to 1st day
of menses helps modestly (37% better compared to 30% in controls)
(Jama 1995;279:51)

Pyridoxine (B$_6$) (Bmj 1999;318:1375) 50 mg po qd-bid,

Others often tried: Progesterone (no good evidence that helps—Med Let
1984;26:101); calcium, eg Tums ii bid (Rx Let 1998;5:53); evening
primrose? (prostaglandin precursor) 750 mg po bid; BCPs?;
spironolactone; danazol; gonadotropin-releasing factor blocking
analog like leuprolide (Nejm 1998;338:209); surgical oophorectomy
(Nejm 1984;311:1345,1371)

Rape exam (Nejm 1995;332:234)

w/u:

- Medical hx
- Evaluate and rx physical injuries; use only saline as speculum
  lubricant
- Culture for cervix, rectum, throat (gc only) for gc and chlamydia;
  sperm sample aspirate; test for hep B, syphilis, HIV, pregnancy,
  blood type
- Clothing, Wood's lamp exam for semen, then ask victim to place
  in plastic bag; pubic hair combings, subungual samples

rx:

- Prophylactic antibiotics if indicated or requested (Rx Let 1998;
  5:12): ceftriaxone 125–250 mg im or spectinomycin 2 gm im; plus
  doxycycline 100 mg po bid × 7 d, or azithromycin 1 gm po × 1
  plus metronidazole 2 gm po × 1
- Immunize w hep B vaccine and HBIG unless contraindicated
- Prevent pregnancy if appropriate w:
  50 µgm estradiol BCPs, or
  35 µgm estradiol BCPs po q 12 h × 2
- Psychiatric support/counseling
- Report to police

F/u in 2–4 wk

Vaginitis causes (Nejm 1997;337:1896)

Infectious:

- *Gardernella vaginalis* and other bacteria (p 407), 50%
- Monilia (25%) (p 143)

- *Trichomonas* (p 476) (20%)
- Foreign body, eg, tampon

Noninfectious:
- Atrophic in postmenopausal women
- Chemical irritant or traumatic
- Allergic, hypersensitiviy or contact

Chapter 15
Ophthalmology

D. K. Onion

ACUTE ANGLE CLOSURE GLAUCOMA

Nejm 1978;299:182

Cause: Genetic predisposition, hyperopia (farsightedness)

Epidem: ~0.2% of population; especially in middle aged and elderly

Pathophys: Normally, aqueous humor is secreted in posterior chamber by the ciliary body, then goes through the pupil to the anterior chamber and out the trabecular meshwork at the scleral-iris junction. Congenital predisposition of a smaller eye and shallow anterior chamber w close apposition of iris and lens so that fluid is trapped where it is made behind the iris, which bows forward to cover the trabecular meshwork, blocking outflow. Secretion of aqueous humor then causes pressure to build, compressing first the optic nerve where the scleral cribosa is the weak point, leading to cupping and atrophy when chronic.

Sx: Onset usually age >50 yr. Precipitated by mydriatics, antacids, anesthesia, darkness. Rainbow halos often first sx, due to corneal edema; eye pain, sudden, often bilateral; headache, nausea and vomiting, scotomas in nasal fields causing blindness

Si: Red eye, especially circumcorneal; partially dilated fixed pupil. Corneal edema, blistered and hazy; corneal pressure >30 mm Hg, pressures >18 mm Hg have a 65% sens/specif (Nejm 1993;328:1097)

If chronic or recurrent attacks, optic disc is pale and cupped

Tonometry: 8–22 = normal; 20–30 = probably normal (only 3.5% will go on to glaucoma in 5 yr); >30 mm Hg much higher % go on to glaucoma

Crs:

Cmplc: Blindness; other eye affected within 5–10 yr in 40–80%, and use of pilocarpine does not protect

Lab:

Rx: Surgical laser iridotomy under local (Med Let 1984;26:52); may need pilocarpine 1–2% gtts q 5–10 min until relieved + systemic carbonic anhydrase inhibitor (acetazolamide 1 gm iv or 0.5 gm po stat) to lower pressure enough to allow laser rx

OTHER GLAUCOMAS: OPEN ANGLE, SECONDARY, CONGENITAL

Nejm 1998;339:1298; 1993;328:1097 (open angle)

Cause:

Open angle: Gene on chromosome #1 (Nejm 1998;338:1022); often precipitated over 2–3 wk by systemic or topical steroids, including high but not low- or medium-dose nasal or inhaled steroids (Jama 1997;277:722). Some may evolve out of the 10% over age 40 who have intraocular HT

Secondary: Multiple (see pathophys)

Congenital: Genetic

Epidem:

Open angle: 2% of population age >40 yr; most prevalent form in US; more frequent in myopics, diabetics, relatives of pts w it, and the elderly; incidence in blacks is 6–8 × that in whites (Nejm 1991;325:1418)

Congenital: Associated with big eyes (except microcornea); Sturge-Weber syndrome; neurofibromas; Marfan's syndrome; Pierre Robbin syndrome; tumors of eye; rubella syndrome; oculocerebrorenal syndrome (Lowe's)

Pathophys:

Open angle: Gradual meshwork occlusion decreases fluid movement.

Secondary: Uveitis inflammation; traumatic bleeding in anterior chamber; diabetic neovascular membranes; postoperative; exfoliation; elevated venous pressure; pigmentary; tumors; mature lens induced; ghost cells (old rbc's)

Sx:

Open angle: Transient visual blurring; slow loss of bilateral visual sensitivity; no pain, no halos

Secondary: Red eye, pain

Congenital: Photophobia, manifest in child by tears and eye rubbing

Si:

Open angle: Tunnel vision; cupped disc w cup/disc ratio >0.3, usually >0.7; intraocular pressures may be elevated or normal

Secondary: Debris in anterior chamber; red eye; corneal edema

Congenital: Big hazy cornea, frequently bilateral

Crs:

Open angle: 1–3% visual field loss/year

Cmplc: Blindness in all if untreated

Lab:

Xray:

Rx:

Secondary: Rx the primary disease, eg, steroids for uveitis, laser rx of neovascularization, evacuate clot for acute traumatic

Congenital: Surgical goniotomy or trabeculotomy by age 6 yr at latest, results in 90% success

Open angle (Rx Let 1999;6:4; Med Let 1996;38:100): All meds may have systemic side effects even though delivered locally (Ann IM 1990;112:120)

1st, β blockers

- Timolol 0.25–0.5% i gtt bid, or Timoptic XE qd. Adverse effects: may have significant systemic absorption and effects, especially if pt is a genetically slow metabolizer or there is coincident po drug use like quinidine (Jama 1995;274:1611); $10/mo/eye
- Betaxolol (β-1 selective)
- Levobunolol (Med Let 1986;28:45)
- Metipranolol (Optipranolol) i gtt bid, cheapest (Med Let 1990;32:91)

2nd, Prostaglandins, 2nd: latanoprost (Xalatan) 0.005% i gtt qd; cmplc: brown pigmentation of iris; $25/mo/eye

α-Adrenergic agonists: brimonidine tartrate (Alphagen) i gtt bid; cmplc: beware in pts w arterial insufficiency

Cholinergics: pilocarpine at i gtt qid
Carbonic anhydrase inhibitors
- Acetazolamide 500 mg po bid or 250 mg qid
- Brinzolamide (Azopt) 1% i gtt tid
- Dorzolamide (Trusopt) (Med Let 1995;37:76) 2% i gtt tid, for chronic topical rx; or w timolol as Cosopt
if fail, laser trabeculoplasty; or if not enough, surgery

OPTIC NEUROPATHIES: ISCHEMIC AND NEURITIS

Nejm 1992;326:634—neuritis; 1978;299:533

Cause:
Ischemic: Arteritis
Optic neuritis: Half are idiopathic, half due to multiple sclerosis
Epidem:
Ischemic: More common over age 50
Optic neuritis: F:M >2:1, between menarche and menopause
Incidence = 6/100,000/yr
Pathophys:
Ischemic: Arteritis of posterior ciliary arteries
Sx:
Ischemic: Sudden blindness
Optic neuritis: Sudden uniocular, visual loss; painful eye on movement
Si:
Ischemic: Edema of disc and predisc, hemorrhages; pale disc later
Optic neuritis: Normal disc becomes pale and edematous but often normal if retrobulbar neuritis only; impaired color plate acumen; diminished pupillary reaction to light (Marcus Gunn pupil)
Crs:
Ischemic: 42% recover in 6 mo (Jama 1995;273:625)
Optic neuritis: 70% recover in 8 wk; up to 60% later develop MS over next 40 yr (Neurol 1995;45:244). See Fig. 15.1
Cmplc:
Ischemic: 2nd eye often involved days to years later. r/o common nonarteritic type under age 50, associated with diabetes, hypertension

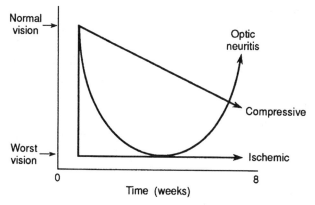

Figure 15.1

Optic neuritis: r/o MS (30–50% risk of it); compressive infiltrative neuropathies from metastases pituitary adenoma, meningioma, glioma, internal carotid aneurysm, craniopharyngioma; all of which have gradual visual loss and pale disc, shunt vessels

Lab:

Hem:

Ischemic: ESR increased

Path:

Ischemic: Temporal artery bx within 1 week of starting steroids

Noninv:

Optic neuritis: Visual evoked responses decreased

Xray:

Optic neuritis: CT of optic canals if no improvement in 6 wk to r/o compressive nerve lesion

Rx:

Ischemic: Stat steroids if ESR elevated or positive temporal artery biopsy; optic nerve surgical decompression may be harmful (Jama 1995;273:625)

Optic neuritis: (Neurol 2000;54:2039): 3 d of q 6 h iv 250 mg methylprednisolone, perhaps followed by 1 mg/kg po × 10 d, speeds resolution, slightly reduces recurrences, and decreases rate of MS over the next 2 yr (Nejm 1993;329:1764 vs 1993;329:1808) but not over 5 yr

CATARACTS
Ann IM 1985;102:82

Cause: Age; occasionally steroids, even inhaled types incr risk slightly (Jama 1998;280:539; Nejm 1997;337:8); diabetes, etc.; genetic predisposition, accounts for 50% of incidence variance (Nejm 2000;342:1786)

Epidem: Increased with UVB (320–390 nm wavelength) exposure throughout life (Jama 1998;280:714; Nejm 1988;319:1429)

Pathophys: Cortical and nuclear types associated with UVB, posterior types not. Posterior types related to steroid use

Sx: Blurred vision

Si: Opacity in lens seen with naked eye or in red reflex

Crs: Slowly progressive

Cmplc:

Lab:

Rx: UV protection, eg, brimmed hat and glasses (Nejm 1988;319:1429)
Cataract extraction and intraocular artificial lens implantation very successful (Med Let 1982;24:102)

MISCELLANEOUS

Corneal Burns

Acid/alkali burn
Sx + Si: Coagulation of corneal epithelium; acid superficially, alkali deeply
Rx: Irrigate/flush at pH 7, for hours with alkali burn even if looks ok; then long-term lubricants; steroids w ophthalmology consult

Tear gas, eg, Mace (Nejm 1969;281:413)
Sx + Si: Pain, can cause permanent corneal damage
Rx: Irrigate as above

UV burn
Sx + Si: Pain, h/o UV exposure; pitted cornea
Rx: Mydriatics, pressure eye patch × 24 h

Blepharospasm
Rx: Botulism toxin im (Med Let 1990;32:100)

Chalazion (cyst of meibomian gland in eyelid)/**hordeolum** (inflamed cyst, stye)
Rx: Chalazion w surgical excision; hordeolum (stye) w hot packs and topical antibiotics

Coping with blindness, devices available (Nejm 1981;305:458); reading machines (Med Let 1992;34:13); diurnal rhythms may be retained if retinohypothalamic tracts preserved (Nejm 1995;332:6)

Diplopia: Image is displaced maximally in direction of paralyzed muscle's pull. Oculomotor CN innervations; straight up and down are combinations of muscles; pure muscle movements are up and out, up and in, etc.

Foville's syndrome: Part of posterior inferior cerebellar artery syndrome; paralysis of horizontal gaze, ipsilateral V impairment including taste on anterior tongue, VII dysfunction, VIII deficits, and ipsilateral Horner's

Internuclear ophthalmoplegias: Lesions of medial longitudinal fasciculus (MLF), so that conjugate gaze impossible, medial rectus responds only on convergence; seen often in MS

Macular degeneration (age-related type)
Nejm 2000;343:483
Cause: Unknown
Epidem: Most common cause of severe visual loss in developed countries; present in 30%, 7% symptomatic prevalence over age 75. Assoc w: smoking (incid incr × 2.4—Jama 1996;276:1141, 1147); positive fam hx; low antioxidant vitamins, and zinc intake; whites
Pathophys: Atrophic and neovascular forms
Sx: Decr visual acuity
Si: Drüsen >63 µM, retinal pigment epithelial atrophy or clumping in macula
Rx: Laser rx of neovascular lesions; perhaps for neovascular type, marginally beneficial photodynamic rx w verteporfin (Visadyne) (Med let 2000;42:81)

OPHTHALMOLOGY

Muscles Affecting Right Eye Movements and Their Innervations (Facing Patient)

Table 15.1

Lateral		Medial
superior rectus (CN III)		inferior oblique (CN III)
lateral rectus (CN VI)		medial rectus (CN III)
inferior rectus (CN III)		superior oblique (CN IV)

Parinaud's syndrome: Paralysis of upward gaze, convergence retraction, nystagmus, pupillary light/near dissociation, papilledema, lid retraction; seen in lesions of pineal and hydrocephalus

Red eye, acute (Nejm 2000;343:345)

1. Foreign body (FB)
Epidem: Most common
Sx + Si: Foreign body under lids or in cornea
Rx: Remove FB, then antibiotic cream and patch eye × 24 h

2. Conjunctivitis (Med Let 1990;32:71)
Cause: Viral, especially adenovirus; allergic; bacterial, mostly pneumococcus in colder climates, in warmer places *Haemophilus* (including Koch-Weeks bacillus), chlamydia, some staph
Epidem: 95% of remainder after FB. Viral type highly contagious
Sx + Si: Feeling of sand in eye, morning secretions; palpebral and bulbar conjunctival injection, PERRLA and normal vision; preauricular lymph node in chlamydial type; itching is predominant sx in allergic type
Crs: Infectious types start in 1 eye, spread to the other; viral type is contagious for >10d
Cmplc: r/o gc infection if hyperacute
Rx: Sulfacetamide 10%, Tm/S (Polytrim) gtts cidal rather than static and stings less than sulfa but costs 10× as much, or neomycin/polymyxin qid, or tobramycin or gentamicin 0.3% gtts qid × 10 d. Not chloramphenicol which can lead to aplastic anemia. Oral tetracycline or macrolide for chlamydial type
For allergic (Med Let 2000;42:39), topical:
• NSAID ketorlac (Acular) 0.5% I gtt qid (Med Let 1993;35:88); or
• H$_1$ antihistamine levocabastine (Livostin) (Med Let 1994;36:35) 0.05% i gtt qid, costs $22/2 wk, or similar emedastine (Emadine) I gtt qid (Rx Let 1998;5:29); or

- Mast cell stabilizers, cromolyn (Crolom) 4% i–ii gtts ou qid, $15/2wk; or lodoxamine (Alomide) (Med Let 1994;36:26) 0.1% i–ii gtts qid, costs $14/2 wk; or nedocromil (Alocril); or pemirolast (Alamast)
- Mast cell stabilizer/H_1 antihistamine combos: olopatadine (Patanol) 0.1% i–ii gtts ou bid, $17/2 wk; or ketotifen (Zaditor) (RxLet 2000;7:15)

3. **Iritis,** a form of uveitis

Causes: Of anterior and posterior uveitis (Nejm 1978;299:130) (uvea = choroid, iris, and ciliary body): idiopathic (1st), tbc, syphilis, histoplasmosis (often no bug in lesion), sarcoid, coccidioidomycosis, toxoplasmosis, rheumatoid arthritis especially in children or any inflammatory arthritis, anti-DNA and -RNA antibodies perhaps viral-related (Nejm 1971;285:1502), h. simplex and zoster, *Candida,* hypermature cataract, trauma, intraocular tumor, Whipple's disease bacterium (Nejm 1995;332:363)

Epidem: 2% of remainder after FB

Sx + Si: Photophobia, eye ache, tenderness, tearing without exudate, visual blurring, turbid aqueous humor (wbc's and protein) or hypopyon, low pressure (5–10 mm Hg), miosis (constricted pupil), circumcorneal injection

Rx: Steroids topically, mydriatics like Cyclogyl to prevent iris-lens synechiae

4. **Keratitis:**

Cause: H. simplex (50%) and other viruses (h. zoster, adenovirus), contact lenses especially overnight use (Nejm 1989;321:773, 779), exanthems, bacterial, chronic topical anesthetic use (Nejm 1968;279:396)

Epidem: 1% of remainder after FB

Sx + Si: Photophobia, FB sensation; corneal ulcer (dendritic if herpetic), mixed type injection, PERRLA, corneal wbc infiltrates

Cmplc: Achronic corneal neurotrophic ulcers

Rx: When h. simplex: 1st, trifluridine (Viroptic) 1 gtt 1% solution q 2 h; or 2nd, Ara A; then consider prophylaxis w acyclovir 400 mg po bid × 12 mos which decr recurrence rates from ~35% to <20% (Nejm 1998;339:300)

When bacterial, appropriate antibiotics; mydriatics to relax ciliary spasm in chronic corneal neurotrophic ulcers: corneal transplant and/or perhaps topical nerve growth factor (nejm 1998;338:1174, 1222)

5. **Acute glaucoma** (p 633)

Epidem: 1% of remainder after FB

Sx + Si: Halos, blurred vision, severe pain, headache and vomiting; steamed cornea, semidilated pupils, circumcorneal injection, hard eye (50–60 mm Hg)

Rx: Miotics, β blockers, and acetazolamide while waiting surgery to keep angles open. Laser iridotomy

Retinitis pigmentosa

Cause: Genetic, autosomal dominant or recessive

Pathophys: Rhodopsin gene on chromosome #3 is mutated (Nejm 1990;323:1302)

Sx: First night blindness, then tunnel vision. Late loss of color vision, and blind eye by age 50–60 yr

Si: Optic nerve pallor, pigmentaton of retinal fundus, attenuated arteries

Subconjunctival hemorrhage (Nejm 2000;343:345)

Cause: Trauma (often minor) or coughing/vomiting, bleeding disorders

Sx: Usually just noticed, no pain

Si: Unilateral localized circumscribed hemorrhage obscuring underlying sclera; no conjunctivitis

Crs: Resolves in <3 wk

Chapter 16
Pediatrics

D. K. Onion

16.1 NEWBORN DISORDERS

NEONATAL JAUNDICE

Cause: (Nejm 2001;344:581)

Indirect bilirubin elevations:
- Glucuronyl transferase deficiency
  - normal in premature infant, especially if incr enterohepatic circulation
  - congenital deficiency (Crigler-Najjar syndrome) rarely; rx w phototherapy, perhaps hepatocyte transplantation (Nejm 1998; 338:1422)
- ABO and Rh incompatibility
- Breast milk (pregnane-3α, 20β-diol)-induced jaundice, never needs rx no matter how high (Peds 1993;91:470)
- Hypothyroidism (cretinism)
- Drug induced, eg, by excess vit K, or chloramphenicol (gray baby syndrome)

Direct bilirubin elevations:
- Infections
  - Bacterial sepsis
  - Intrauterine infections like syphilis, and TORCH (Toxoplasma, rubella, CMV, herpes) infections, which typically elevated LFTs and direct bilirubin
  - Perinatally acquired infections like herpes, enteroviruses, hepatitis B
- Biliary obstruction

Epidem: Physiologic jaundice more common in Asians

Pathophys: More bilirubin production from incr rbc turnover and limited amounts of glucuronyl transferase, which attaches glucuronic acid to unconjugated, poorly water-soluble bilirubin so it can be excreted

Sx: Jaundice in newborn

Si: Icterus

Crs: Usually benign; Crigler-Najjar rapidly fatal though some variants can survive

Cmplc: Kernicterus (brain damage) with retardation and basal ganglia degeneration

Lab:

Chem: Elevated bilirubin, indirect elevation > direct; up to 17 mg% in term infants in 1st wk of life can be normal

Rx: None at term if under 25 mg% unless prematurity, sick child, or hemolysis from G6PD or other cause where should rx >20 mg% (Peds 1992;89:809; 1983;71:660)

Feeding on demand, breast or bottle, decr the enterohepatic recirculation of bilirubin

Bilirubin lights (fluorescent white, blue or green) isomerize bilirubin to hepatically excretable benign products (Med Let 1971;13:11), if >15 mg% at age 25–48 hr, >18 mg% at 44–72 hr, >20 mg% at >72 hr

Exchange transfusions if lights not enough

RESPIRATORY DISTRESS SYNDROME
(Hyaline Membrane Disease)

Cause: Immature lungs from premature delivery, often exacerbated by maternal diabetes (Nejm 1976;294:357)

Epidem: Prematurity associated with familial asthma in mother and child (Nejm 1985;312:742)

Pathophys: Surfactant deficiency or inhibition allows collapse of alveoli; plasma exudate forms membrane (Nejm 1971;284:1185)

Sx: Onset 0–4 h postpartum

Si: Grunting respirations, tachypnea, intercostal retractions, atelectasis, ductus murmur, flaring

Crs: Worsens over first 24–28 h, then resolves over 5–7 d

Cmplc: Bronchopulmonary dysplasia chronic lung disease in many from O_2 rx with scarring, and barotrauma (Nejm 1990;323:1793), perhaps helped w inhaled steroids (Nejm 1999;340:1005,1036); pneumothorax; diaphragmatic hernia; patent ductus arteriosus, especially with fluid overload (Nejm 1983;308:743), rx with indomethacin (Nejm 1984;310:565); retrolental fibroplasia, especially in low birth weight (<1 kg) premies exposed to high light levels in NICUs (Nejm 1985;313:401) or 100% O_2 levels w pO_2 levels >80 mm Hg for >12 h (Nejm 1992;326:1050)

r/o TTN (transient tachypnea of newborn), a benign and common condition; group B strep and other infections; congenital heart disease and other anomalies

Lab:

Chem: Blood gases show respiratory acidosis, hypoxia

Xray: Chest shows air bronchograms, "ground glass" appearance

Rx: Prevent w steroids between 28–32 weeks if threatened premature delivery; but not helpful for low birth weight infants (Nejm 2001;344:95)

Surfactant prophylaxis endotracheally (Med Let 1990;32:2; Nejm 1988;319:476) at least in infants ≤26 wk is better than waiting for sx to start (Nejm 1991;324:867; 1991;325:1696); long term, at 1 yr, use shows no benefit (Nejm 1991;325:1696; 1989;320:959) in morbidity but survival is 30% better and costs less (Nejm 1994;330:1476). Ligation of ductus arteriosus prophylactically if <1 kg (Nejm 1989;320:1511). Inositol in TPN of premature infants ×5 d helps (Nejm 1992;326:1233)

Support by keeping warm (hypothermia causes bronchoconstriction); D10W at 80–160 cc/kg/24 h to maintain glucose homeostasis, may need volume infusions to maintain BP or perfusion; continuous positive airway pressure (CPAP) breathing via ET tube with surfactant (Nejm 1994;331:1051) or liquid perflubron (Nejm 1996;335:761)

16.2 CONGENITAL SYNDROMES

CLEFT PALATE AND LIP

Cause: Genetic plus perhaps in utero environmental factors (vitamin deficiencies cause in rats); autosomal recessive; recurrence in subsequent siblings ~3%, much lower if different father, no change if mother changes town of residence, hence genetic not environmental (Nejm 1995;333:161)

Epidem: 1/1000 white births, 1/5000 black births; 3rd most common congenital anomaly after club feet and radiologic spina bifida. Increased incidence in inbred populations; associated (25%) with other anomalies too

50% are lip and palate, 25% lip alone (male > female), 25% palate alone (female > male)

Pathophys: Failure of maxilla and nasal fusion in midline

Sx: Poor suck

Si: Cleft

Crs:

Cmplc: Social; malocclusion; chronic otitis and hearing loss from eustachian tube dysfunction; mechanical speech problems; FTT from poor caloric intake or associated anomalies

Lab:

Rx: Test hearing and refer to ENT, or state cleft lip program available in most states

Feed with special nipples; speech rx postop emphasizing hard consonants; blowing exercises through mouth (pinwheel, wind instrument)

Surgical timing is controversial, some say repair at age 6 wks if lip alone; at age 14 weeks if palate involved too; but must repair before start speech

Dental prosthesis

DOWN SYNDROME

Cause: Defective chromosome #21; new translocation (3% of all), or congenital trisomy (97%); of the latter, 95% are maternal, 5% paternal (Nejm 1991;324:872)

Epidem: 1/650 live births; incr in mothers age >35 yr. Associated Alzheimer's disease in families, especially premature Alzheimer's (Ann IM 1985;103:566) and correlates with amyloid A4 protein excess production and deposition (Nejm 1989;320:1446)

Pathophys: Usually group G trisomy of chromosome #21 (97% overall, 90% when mother age <35 yr). Translocations: 50% are #21 to a D (#13–#15), associated with parental chromosome abnormalities most of the time, mother is carrier 95% of time, father 5%; or 50% are to a G (#20–#22) and in that circumstance <5% of time do parents have abnormal chromosome prep. In mothers age <35 yr, 10–15% are such G translocations

Short 5th finger and toe due to middle phalanx failure to calcify normally and late onset maturation arrest (P. Gerald 1968)

Sx: Mongoloid appearance, floppy, retarded

Si: Findings subtle at birth and become more apparent later: hypotonia; developmental delay; short, brachycephalic with excess skin on the back of the neck; hypoplastic midface bones; single palmar crease, epicanthal fold (50%); Brushfield's spots (white) on iris (present in 10% normals too); short 5th finger and toes; duodenal obstruction in many, especially from atresia and ring pancreas; low-set, hypoplastic ears; heart murmurs and congenital heart disease, especially atrial septal defect (in 25%); imperforate anus (3%); umbilical hernia; tachycardia and pupillary sensitivity to atropine (Nejm 1968;279:407)

Crs:

Cmplc: Odontoid ligament laxity causing C_1 on C_2 dislocation as in rheumatoid arthritis (Peds 1992;89:1194); leukemia; incr infection rates; incr Hashimoto's thyroiditis (get TSH q 1 yr)

r/o D-1 (#13–#15) trisomies with elevated fetal hgb, decr A_2 hemoglobin, polydactyly, cleft palate, eye defects (Nejm 1967;277:953); E (#17–#18) trisomy with many mongoloid-type changes and associated with congenital biliary atresia; perhaps a viral etiology (Nejm 1969;280:16)

Lab:

Hem: Chromosome prep shows trisomy or translocation

Serol: SPEP shows diffuse incr globulin

Xray: Hip films show horizontal acetabulum. Skull films, facial and sphenoid views show hypoplasia; bronchogram show "pig bronchus," ie, one ending in a blind pouch

PEDIATRICS

Down Syndrome, continued

Rx: Prevention (Am J Publ Hlth 1998;88:551); many of these tests can be used in combination (Nejm 1999;341:461,521) to incr sens and specif:
- α-Fetoprotein (low in Down's) under age 35 yr, w 2nd trimester, alone, or as "triple test" w
- HCG β subunit and
- Unconjugated estriol
- Protein (inhibin) A levels perhaps, in first trimester (Nejm 1998; 338:955; 1996;334:1231)
- Karyotype analysis by amniocentesis if over 35 or when risk calculated from these results is >1/250 (equivalent to risk at age 35 yr); this strategy equalizes risk of Down's vs abortion from amnio (Nejm 1994;330:1114, 1151)
- Ultrasound in 2nd semester, which can detect 60–75% by neck skin thickness but specif ~25% (Nejm 1997;327:1654) or as low as 0.00015% in normal women or 0.002% in high risk women! (Jama 2001;285:1044); and by femur length (Nejm 1987; 317:1371)
- Chorionic villus sampling now almost as safe as amnio, and abortion can be done much earlier, eg, in 1st trimester (Nejm 1989;320:7)

Then w 2nd trimester abortion (Nejm 1979;300:157—useful table of incidence by maternal age); amniocentesis has a 0.3% false-positive (error) rate. Half of fetuses with Down's at 15 wk gestation will spontaneously abort or die perinatally; 1.5% abort after amniocentesis (Nejm 1979;300:118—ethics discussion)

Primary care: of newborn, confirm clinical suspicion w karyotype; cardiac consultation on all; hearing screen, thyroid studies, CBC; early intervention program and parental support group referral of child, annual thyroid screen, cervical spine films at 3 and 12 yr prn long tract si's or sx; periodic hearing and ENT assessment; periodic ophthalmologic exam; dental visits begin at age 2 yr

HIRSCHSPRUNG'S DISEASE

Cause: In familial forms, inactivation mutation in REI proto-oncogene, like type II MEN (Nejm 1995;335:943)

Epidem: Usually in infants; male:female = 1:4

Pathophys: Aganglionic segment of colon, variable in length from a few cm in rectum to all rectum and descending colon. No sympathetic neurons in this segment resulting in constant contractions and no relaxation, which is necessary for effective peristalsis, and this results in intestinal obstruction, acute (infants) or chronic (children and teenagers)

Sx: Abdominal pain, chronic constipation without the occasional "huge stools" typical of retentive encopresis

Si:

Crs:

Cmplc: Enterocolitis, most common cause of death

r/o Chagas' disease; chronic idiopathic intestinal obstruction (Nejm 1977;297:233); other malfunction of sphincters with which patients can be operantly conditioned to control stool (Nejm 1974;290:646)

Lab:

Path: Rectal bx aganglionic

Rx: Surgical excision of affected segments or bypass that segment

PHENYLKETONURIA (PKU)

Nejm 1980;303:1336, 1394

Cause: Genetic, autosomal recessive; several different mutations, each with different severity implications (Nejm 1986;314:1276) from mild asx phenylalaninemia to severe PKU

Epidem: 1–7/100,000 newborns (Peds 2000;105:e10); 1.2/100,000 adults (Nejm 1970;282:1455)

Pathophys: Deficiency of hepatic phenylalanine hydroxylase (converts phenylalanine [Phe] to tyrosine [Tyr]) causes buildup of Phe in all body tissues which in turn leads somehow to mental retardation

Sx: Mental retardation; seizures; behavior problems

Si: Retarded, pale, eczema, blond hair; in adult, psychoses often, even if mentally normal (Nejm 1973;289:395)

Crs:

Phenylketonuria, continued

Cmplc: Mental retardation in 100% of offspring of affected women unless level kept <10 mg% (Jama 2000;283:756; Nejm 1983;309:1269)

Lab:

   Chem: Phenylalanine level >20 mg% is diagnostic; if >2 mg%, repeat it; if <2 mg%, no need for further testing, even if done on first day of life and not having eaten yet (Nejm 1981;304:294). Persistent, low (<12 mg%) elevation has no intelligence-impairing effect (Nejm 1971;285:424)

Rx: Prevent by screening heel blood samples for Phe once at age 1–3 d (Nejm 1979;300:606); counsel treated PKU girls at age 12 to keep level <10 during pregnancy, to avoid having children with mental retardation (Am J Pub Hlth 1982;72:1386; Nejm 1980; 303:1202). Refer all positive screens to tertiary care center

   Diet low in Phe, commercially prepared; the earlier it is started, the less the retardation; can stop at age 4 except during pregnancy? (Nejm 1980;303:1341; 1975;293:1121) vs restriction up to age 8 or 10 yr results in higher IQs (Nejm 1986;314:593)

PYLORIC STENOSIS

Cause: Genetic?; sex-linked?

Epidem: Males > females; 10% of affected fathers' offspring will have, 50% of affected mothers' children will have; 1/100–1/600 births

Pathophys: Concentric muscular hypertrophy of pyloric smooth muscle, in which nitric oxide synthetase deficiency precipitates the disease (Nejm 1992;327:511)

Sx: Well and gaining weight for first 3–5 wk of life, then develop projectile vomiting without bile in it

Si: "Olive" in right upper quadrant by palpation in 70%

Crs: Benign with surgical repair

Cmplc: r/o annular pancreas (rx with duodenojejunostomy); duodenal atresia; Addisonian crisis due to congenital adrenal hypoplasia; antral diaphragm

Lab:

   Chem: Lytes show hypochloremic, hypokalemic alkalosis

Xray: Ultrasound; UGIS only if mass not seen or felt, to confirm dx

Rx: Surgery

UNDESCENDED (Cryptorchid) TESTICLE

Nejm 1986;314:510

Cause:

Epidem: 2–3% of term babies, decreases to 0.7% at age 1 without treatment, then prevalence is flat thereafter

Pathophys:

Sx:

Si: Unilateral in 75%, bilateral in 25%; most have associated inguinal hernia

Crs: Sterility, questionably prevented by early operation

Cmplc: Cancer in affected and contralateral testicles, incr 20–40×; higher with higher inguinal canal location even postoperation; cellular changes w/i 6–12 mo of nondescent

r/o retractile (normal) nonscrotal testicle that can be manipulated to bottom of scrotum; virilized female prepubertally w serum Müllerian inhibiting substance level, which is present in boys but not girls w 92/98% sens/specif (Nejm 1997;336:1480)

Lab:

Rx: Surgery by age 1 yr

Hormonal rx with HCG or GnRH not much help (Nejm 1986;314: 466, 510)

16.3 ORTHOPEDICS

CONGENITAL DYSPLASIA OF HIP
(Developmental Dysplastic Hip)

Peds 1964;34:554

Cause: Perhaps a genetic defect, autosomal dominant

Epidem: <5/1000 births; female:male = 8:1; winter incidence twice summer incidence by birthdays; positive family hx in 1/3; incr incidence in Mediterraneans and Scandinavians, in first borns, and × 8 if breech delivery

Pathophys: Acetabular defect with shallow, vertically sloping roof and infolded glenoid; weight bearing results in anteversion of femoral neck which progresses to DJD and eventually to subluxation and/or dislocation

Sx: H/o breech delivery (12–20%). Limp

Si: In newborn, only finding may be positive subluxation provocation test
(Barlow test; subluxation of femoral head with adduction and
posterior pressure on femur); Ortolani test, relocates with a "clunk"
w hips flexed 90° abducted and anterior pressure up on greater
trochanters; telescopic femoral movement with hip at 90° (<1%
false neg, 80% false pos). May have short leg unilaterally;
asymmetric buttock folds; wide perineum; hip abduction often is
limited (normal is 90° at birth when hip flexed)
  In walking child, limp and positive Trendelenburg's test unilaterally

Crs: 95% resolved with only conservative rx at 3 yr f/u

Cmplc: Adductor contractures; DJD
  r/o similar hip dysfunctions caused by meningomyelocele and cerebral
  palsy adductor spasm/contractures

Lab:

Xray: Ultrasound under 3 mo age since no secondary center of
  ossification yet
  Plain films will miss dx in 25%. Femoral epiphysis ossification center
  smaller, higher, and more lateral relative to acetabular center;
  acetabular roof obliquity pronounced, >30°; neck/shaft angle
  widened, ie, becomes more vertical

Rx: <1 mo age: abduction splint or brace (Pavlok Harness) × weeks or
  months until xray shows improvement or can no longer dislocate.
  Best to rx if any doubt; will have 80% false positive by clinical
  exam. Double diapering inadequate
  Older child: spica cast in abduction after closed reduction
  Adult: wait until sx's, then crutches, corset, decr activity, then surgical
  total hip

LEGG-PERTHES DISEASE (Coxa Plana)
  Nejm 1992;326:1473

Cause: Unknown
Epidem: Children age 4–9; males > females
Pathophys: Avascular necrosis of proximal femoral epiphysis for
  unknown reason

Sx: Vague h/o intermittent ache around thigh and/or knee (think of in any child c/o knee pain); limp; avoids running; occasionally bilateral

Si: Internal rotation limited; pain with motion; positive Trendelenburg's test; limp; late, muscle atrophy and leg shortening

Crs: With rx, resolves over many months

Cmplc: DJD of hip; r/o slipped capital femoral epiphysis in same age group

Lab:

Xray: Widened, irregular epiphyseal line; later increased density of femoral epiphysis; then flattened femoral head ossification center; then sclerotic head with cystic appearance, fragmentation, revascularization, and finally bone abnormalities of coxa magna and flattened articular surface

Rx: In incomplete femoral head involvement, observation and limited activity is usually all that is done

With whole-head involvement, place in abduction/internal rotation brace while revascularizes

In severe cases, eliminate weight bearing × 2–3 yr while revascularizes. If unilateral, "Perthes sling" = ischial weight bearing with built-up shoe; rarely used now

SCOLIOSIS

Bull Rheum Dis 1987;37(6):1; Nejm 1986;314:1379

Cause: Genetic, at least in 30% (positive family hx); autosomal dominant; polygenic

Epidem: Female:male = 4:1. 10% of population have minor abnormalities, 1.5% have significant abnormalities, 0.5% need rx. Worldwide. Increased in ballet trained children (Nejm 1986;314: 1348,1379)

Pathophys: Perhaps due to unequal development of vertebral growth plates, or unequal muscle and ligamentous balance

Sx: Onset age 9–13, usually asx

Si: Most have thoracic curve convex to R, lumbar to L; hump appears on one side when bent over (razor back deformity) with high, usually R shoulder; asymmetric scapulae; plumb line from posterior neck when standing misses gluteal cleft; when standing, space between arm and body is asymmetric comparing R to L

Screen for lateral hump when bent over using leveling device across
back (scoliometer; measures rib rotation); refer to orthopedist if
>15° and still in early puberty; screening efficacy unclear (Jama
1999;282:1427; USPTF—Jama 1993;269:2667)

Crs: Gradual progression in curvature until skeletal maturity by age 18

Cmplc: Deformity; respiratory compromise

r/o leg length discrepancy

Lab:

Xray: Rarely indicated, can be used to follow care despite radiation

Rx: Minor (<15–20° by scoliometer): recheck q 3 mo

Intermediate (20–30°): to prevent increase esp in preadolescent girls,
thoracolumbarsacral orthosis or Milwaukee brace; adverse effects:
protrusion of incisors

Severe (30–40°): surgical placement of Harrington rods

16.4 INFECTIOUS/ACQUIRED DISEASES

ATTENTION DEFICIT/HYPERACTIVITY DISORDER (ADHD)

Nejm 1999;340:40,780; NIH Consensus Conf 1998;16(2); Jama
1998;280:1086 (adult type); 279:1100; 1995;273:1871

Cause: Genetic? Multifactorial? 25% of cases have h/o ADHD in a parent

Epidem: 3–5% of children; male:female = 2:1 in children, 1:1 in
adolescents, 1:2 in adults; high (50%) prevalence in special
education students (Am J Publ Hlth 1998;88:881)

Associated with lead burden, poverty, familial chaos, Tourette's
syndrome (60% of Tourette's have ADHD), and positive family hx

Pathophys: Perhaps metabolic dysfunction in the brain. Decreased glucose
metabolism in brain areas associated with attention and motor
activity by PET (Nejm 1990;323:1361). Neurotransmitter
imbalance? Sugar or aspartame in diet does not correlate w
worsening behavior (Nejm 1994;330:301). Worsened by
psychosocial deprivation

Sx: Inattention, hyperactivity, impulsivity, aggression. In trouble with peers, parents, and/or school; underachievers in school from poor self-esteem

Si: Short attention span; poor inhibitory control; aimless restlessness

Crs: Onset usually before school age at least before age 7; 8–10% (Jama 1995;273:1871) continue to have problems in adulthood

Cmplc: Learning disabilities in 25%; conduct (lying, stealing, fights) or oppositional disorders (disobedience, defiance, rule breaking) in 40%, but only if other comorbid dx's. Parental discord/divorce r/o abuse/neglect

Lab:

Rx: Very complicated teacher/parent/child psychosocial dynamics usually present; best strategy when requested to prescribe meds is to request a school "individual education plan" evaluation, which will pay for a multidisciplinary clinic eval and result in less unnecessary medication (S. Sewall 10/95)

Behavioral modification strategies not clearly helpful (Nejm 1999;340:780). Training in social skills. Remedial education. Parental support systems; sugar intake does not increase hyperactivity in normal or ADHD child (Jama 1995;274:1617)

Avoid melatonin for sleep (Rx Let 1997;4:21)

Medications (Nejm 1999;340:780; Med Let 1994;36:109), clearly help short-term (JAMA 1998;279:1100), many believe are useful into adulthood; response to meds does not prove dx

- Amphetamines, racemic mixture (Adderal)
- Methylphenidate (Ritalin) 2.5–10 mg po q-tid, slow release tabs available (Ritalin SR, Concerta) and useful (Med Let 2000;42:80), $30/mo
- Dextroamphetamine (Dexedrine) 2.5–5 mg po q-tid or as qd spansules, $20/mo
- Pemoline (Cylert) 5–6 mo po qd; unpredictable significant risk of severe hepatotoxicity even if safely used × yrs; get consent and q 2 wk LFTs (Rx Let 1999;6:39); $40/mo
- Other adjunctive meds:
  - Antidepressants (tricyclics) like desipramine (Norpramin) but potential sudden death and other cardiac toxicity esp when used w stimulants; or
  - Bupropion (Wellbutrin) 100–200 mg SR bid esp in adults (Rx Let 2001;8:23); but lowers seizure threshold; or

PEDIATRICS

- Clonidine po or patch (Med Let 1996;38:109); but also has sudden death risk, as well as OD potential in younger sibs w even one 0.1 mg pill (Rx Let 1999;6:33)

CROUP (Acute Laryngotracheobronchitis)

Nejm 1994;331:285, 322

Cause: Parainfluenza virus most commonly, respiratory syncytial virus (p 662), and others

Epidem: Incidence 3/100 under age 6 yr, most age 1–3; 1.3% must be hospitalized; M > F (Jama 1998;279:1630)

Pathophys: Perhaps 2 types, or may be just 2 ends of a spectrum:
1. Acute laryngotracheitis follows 2–3 d of cold/cough
2. Spasmodic croup, sx without antecedents and probably represents a hypersensitivity reaction to a virus (Am J Dis Child 1983;137:941)

Sx:

Si: Barking cough, tachypnea, hoarseness, inspiratory stridor, intercostal muscle retractions; when severe, cyanosis and/or altered level of consciousness

Crs: Vast majority are self-limited

Cmplc: r/o foreign body, epiglottitis, bacterial tracheitis especially diphtheria, congenital anomaly (vascular ring etc.), whooping cough (p 402)

Lab:

Rx: Mist tent or just humidified O_2, racemic epinephrine by neb or IPPB q 2 h but watch for rebound

Steroids (Bmj 2000;319:595; Jama 1998;279:1630; Peds 1995;66:220), at least for hospitalized pts or to prevent hospitalization
- Dexamethasone 0.3–0.6 mg/kg im/iv/po single dose
- Budesonide (Pulmicort) 2–4 mg in 4 cc neb; only half as effective as dexamethasone but still much better than placebo (Nejm 1998; 339:498)

KAWASAKI'S DISEASE
Nejm 1992;326:1246; 1991;324:1664

Cause: Unknown

Epidem: Incidence = 5–8/100,000/yr

Pathophys: A vasculitis of medium sized vessels and a mucocutaneous lymph node disease

Sx: Prolonged high fever, variety of rashes, red eyes, nodes

Si: Fever in children age 1–8 yr, nonpitting edema, cervical lymphadenopathy, and desquamation of skin especially palms, perineal area, trunk, lips, as well as nonexudative conjunctivitis, and "strawberry" tongue (pictures—Nejm 1995;333:1391)

Crs:

Cmplc: 25% get coronary artery aneurysms later

r/o measles, scarlet fever, RMSF, leptospirosis, EBV, JRA

Lab:

Hem: ESR, platelets, and wbc elevated

Rx: IgG to prevent complications (Nejm 1986;315:342, 388), 2 gm/kg iv over 10 h × 1 (Nejm 1991;324:1633)

NEUROBLASTOMA AND RETINOBLASTOMA
Nejm 1991;325:1608; 1991;324:464; 1985;312:1500

Cause: Retinoblastoma, in 10–15%, is genetic, autosomal recessive; other neuroblastoma is rarely genetic

Epidem: Both, like Wilms' tumor of childhood, associated with in utero radiation exposure (Nejm 1985;312:541)

Other neuroblastoma, male:female = 33:23

Pathophys: Retinoblastoma originates in retina; acts autosomal dominant but really is recessive; develops tumor when normal arm of #13 is dropped (Nejm 1984;310:550) ("2-hit" theory)

Adrenal medulla origin

Malignancy correlates with the number of N-*myc* oncogene chromosome copies (Nejm 1996;334:231; 1993;328:847; 1985;313:1111) as well as allelic loss of chromosome 1p (Nejm 1996;334:225)

Sx: Positive family hx in 10% w retinoblastoma

In other neuroblastomas, 50% are under age 1 yr; 75% are <3 yr (75%)

Si: In retinoblastoma, strabismus; "cat's eye" light reflex; bilateral in 30%
   In other neuroblastomas, abdominal mass; Horner's syndrome;
      thoracic mass; hepatomegaly
Crs: In retinoblastoma, peak mortality at age 2–3 yr; 81% survival; rarely
      metastatic
   In other neuroblastoma: stage I: localized to organ of origin; stage II:
      node negative or ipsilateral node positive beyond organ or origin;
      stage III: beyond midline; stage IVS: small primary tumors and
      metastases in liver, bone, skin often spontaneous regression;
      stage IV: mets to bone or distant nodes, survival <15% (Onc 1997;
      11:1857,1869,1875)
Cmplc: In retinoblastoma, osteosarcoma in 30% of genetic type from the
      same oncogene (Ann IM 1990;113:781); overall 2nd primary
      incidence is 50% in 50 yr, contrast controls where = 5% (Jama
      1997;278:1262)
Lab:
   Chem: Urine VMA and HVA elevation in neuroblastomas if distant
      metastases present often (Nejm 1972;286:1123)
   Path: Recombinant DNA studies in retinoblastoma to predict if is in
      the 40% with chromosome #13 abnormalities who have bilateral
      recurrent disease (Nejm 1988;318:151; 1986;314:1201)
Xray: MRI helps distinguish neuroblastoma stage IV from IV-S stages
Rx: (rv—Ann IM 1982;97:873)
   of retinoblastoma: if no mets present, surgical excision or radiation; if
      mets present, partial surgical excision; 6% operative mortality, then
      radiation rx and chemo rx, eg, with cyclophosphamide, prednisone,
      actinomycin D, vincristine, and chlorambucil
   of neuroblastoma: chemo rx with "second-look" operations; in
      stage IV, aggressive radiation, chemo and marrow transplant
      (Nejm 1999;341:1165)

16.5 MISCELLANEOUS

NEWBORNS

Apgar score (Nejm 2001;344:467): 5 min score predicts survival (not neurologic outcome), bad (about 1/3 die) if ≤3, great if 7–10; score = 0–2 pts for pulse rate, respiratory effort, muscle tone, reflex irritability, and color

Birth defects: Increased 7× in 2nd child after an affected 1st; this risk is reduced by changing city of residence (environmental) but not by changing fathers (genetic) (Nejm 1994;331:1)
Increased w: organic solvent exposure ×13, esp in 1st trimester (Jama 1999;281:1106); 1st trimester exposure to folate antagonists (Nejm 2000;343:1608) like Dilantin, primodone, Tegretol, phenobarbital, Tm/S, and triamterene; possibly aspirin? (Nejm 1985;313:347 vs 1989;321:1632)

Breast feeding: drugs of choice, see Table 16.5.1

Cerebral palsy: Controversy if most cases are associated with congenital malformations (Nejm 1996;334:613; 1994;330:188; 1986;315:81, 124) or intrauterine exposure to maternal infection (Jama 1997;278:207), or birth asphyxia
20% incid in infants <1500 gm at birth, improved if $MgSO_4$ given prepartum, unclear why (Jama 1996;276:1805,1843)
Physical therapy not clearly helpful in rx, at least in infants (Nejm 1988;318:803)
Associated w low T_4 levels in premies (Nejm 1996;334:821)

Circumcision: Debate of utility with minimal benefits, but, probably because is low risk and traditional, they continue to be performed (Nejm 1990;322:1308); some effect on adult sexual practices (Jama 2000;284:1417; 1997;227:1052)
Slightly (2–4×) lower gc and syphilis rates in circumcised adult males (Am J Pub Hlth 1994;84:197) but no decrease in warts or chlamydia
Anesthesia with dorsal nerve lidocaine (Nejm 1987;317:1321,1347); topical lidocaine-prilocaine (Nejm 1997;336:1197); or circumferential ring block w <1cc 1% lidocaine at penile mid shaft is most effective anesthesia of all (Jama 1997;278:2157)

PEDIATRICS

Table 16.5.1 Drugs of Choice for Breast-Feeding Women*

Drug Category	Drugs and Drug Groups of Choice	Comments
Analgesic drugs	Acctaminophen, ibuprofen, flurbiprofen, ketorolac, mefenamic acid, sumatriptan, morphine	Sumatriptan may be given for migraines. For potent analgesia, morphine may be given.
Anticoagulant drugs	Warfarin, acenocoumarol, heparin (regular and low-molecular-weight)	Among breast-fed infants whose mothers were taking warfarin, the drug was undetectable in plasma and the bleeding time was not affected.
Antidepressant drugs	Sertraline, tricyclic antidepressant drugs	Other drugs such as fluoxetine may be given with caution.
Antiepileptic drugs	Carbamazepine, phenytoin, valproic acid	The estimated level of exposure to these drugs in infants is less than 10% of the therapeutic dose standardized by weight.
Antihistamines (histamine H_1 blockers)	Loratadine	Other antihistamines may be given, but data on the concentrations of these drugs in breast milk are lacking.
Antimicrobial drugs	Penicillins, cephalosporins, aminoglycosides, macrolides	Avoid the use of chloramphenicol and tetracycline.
β-Adrenergic antagonists	Labetalol, propranolol	Angiotensin–converting-enzyme inhibitors and calcium-channel–blocking agents are also considered safe.
Endocrine drugs	Propylthiouracil, insulin, levothyroxine	The estimated level of exposure to propylthiouracil in breast-feeding infants is less than 1% of the therapeutic dose standardized by weight; the thyroid function of the infants is not affected.
Glucocorticoids	Prednisolone and prednisone	The amount of prednisolone that the infant would ingest in breast milk is less than 0.1% of the therapeutic dose standardized by weight.

*This list is not exhaustive. Cases of overdoses of these drugs must be assessed on an individual basis.

Reproduced with permission from Ito. Drug therapy for breast feeding women. Nejm 2000; 343:118–126. Copyright 2000, Mass. Medical Society. All rights reserved.

Diarrhea, especially rotaviral type

Fetal defect detection (rv—Nejm 1986;315:305) by ultrasound, and amniocentesis

Fever (T ≥100.4°F [≥38°C]) under age 2 mo (Peds 1993;92:1)
<28 d, w/u and hospitalize
1–3 mo: w/u w blood culture, LP, UA + urine culture, chest xray; and rx w antibiotics, unless looks ok, wbc <15,000, <5 wbc in UA; admit and rx if any positive; ok to send home without antibiotics if negative as long as can see q 1–2 d until well (Nejm 1993;329:1437)
3$^+$ mo, if nontoxic, w/u only if T >102.2°F (>39°C)

Hemorrhagic disease (Am J Publ Hlth 1998;88:203): GI, dermal, or intracranial; onset age 5–12 wk; caused by low vit K levels, especially in breast fed infants; rx w im vit K at birth, perhaps po q 1 mo

Immunizations (p 684)

Low birthweight (<2500 gm)/**Very low birthweight** (<1500 gm) (Nejm 1998;:339:313; 1993;327:969)
Cause: Small for gestational age (SGA)/intrauterine growth retardation (IUGR), and/or premature birth causes like PROM w chorioamnionitis, idiopathic preterm delivery, HT, abruption, and tobacco, marijuana, or cocaine use (Nejm 1989;320:762); more rarely IUGR, incompetent cervix, cord prolapse fetal distress
Epidem: Increased in (Nejm 1995;333:1737)
  • US blacks × 2–3× (13% of deliveries in blacks vs 4–6% for other groups), probably due to poor socioeconomic status and/or shorter (<9 mo) interpregnancy intervals (Nejm 1995;332:69)
  • Teenage pregnancy even up to age 19 (Nejm 1995;332:1113)
  • H/o previous preterm (<37 wk) delivery (Nejm 1999;341:943)
  • Pre-pregnancy maternal wgt <50kg
  • H/o previous sibling or mother w low birth wgt (Nejm 1995; 333:1744)
Crs: (Nejm 2000;343:378)
  Prematurity: At 22 wk gestation, no survival without severe morbidity
    At 23 wk, <10% survive, 5% w/o disability
    At 24 wk, 26% survive, 12% w/o disability
    At 25 wk, 45% survive, 23% w/o disability

PEDIATRICS

SGA/IUGR: At <600 gm or <24 wk gestation, survival is ≤10–20% although NICU use increases the time to death and morbidity of survivors is severe

At 700 gm or 25 wk gestation, survival is 70–80% (Nejm 1993;329:1597,1649)

Rx: Prevent w metronidazole + erythromycin rx of bacterial vaginosis at 24 wk, reduces risk in high risk women from 50% to 30%? (Nejm 1996;333:1732 vs 2000:342:581)

NICU improves survival of low birthweight children if born in NICU hospital from 165 to 128/1000 mortality (Nejm 1982;307:149) vs. these rates are no different than survival without NICU use

Indomethacin decr PDAs and CNS hemorrhage but does not improve 18 mo survival w/o neurologic deficit (Nejm 2001;344:1966)

Ophthalmia neonatorum (Nejm 1995;332:600)
Cause: Gonorrhea, chlamydia
Epidem: Onset in 1st 28 d of life
Pathophys: Conjunctival infection from maternal genital infection
Si: Exudative conjuctivitis in neonate
Cmplc: Blindness, common w gc, rare w chlamydia
r/o herpes simplex if ulcerations
Lab:
Bact: Gram stain will show gc, not chlamydia
Rx: Prevent w prepartum culture screens, and/or prophylaxis at birth w 2.5% povidone iodine (5% soln diluted 50:50) (Nejm 1995;332:562) which is less toxic and more effective than 1% silver nitrate, 1% tetracycline ointment, or 14% erythromycin
of disease: systemic erythromycin (Med Let 1999;41:85), along w topicals

Respiratory syncytial virus bronchiolitis
Epidem: Peak incidence December–April. Big problem in immunocompromised (Nejm 1986;315:77), premature infants and ones w cardiopulmonary disease under age 2 yr
Si: Bronchiolitis w wheezing
Cmplc: Otitis media (Nejm 1999;340:260)
r/o parainfluenza virus (Nejm 2001;344:1917), asthma, adenovirus, and cystic fibrosis if recurs

Lab: Nasopharyngeal swab antigen test

Rx: Prevent w isolation, which decreases nosocomial spread (Nejm 1987; 317:329). RSV immune globulin q 1 mo (Nejm 1993;329:1524) or expensive monoclonal antibody, Palivizumab q 1 mo (Med Let 2001;43:13) may decrease incidence in high-risk infants. Eventually vaccination (Nejm 2001;344:1917; 1999;340:312)

O_2, iv fluids, albuterol up to 3 mg/kg q 20 min by neb, possibly steroids. Aerosolized ribavirin if on ventilator speeds improvement (Nejm 1991;325:24) as it may for sick newborns not on ventilator (Jama 1985;254:3047)

Spina bifida, anencephaly, and other neural tube and ventral wall defects Nejm 1999;341:1509

Cause: Idiopathic usually; seizure medication toxicity (1/100) only from carbamazepine (Nejm 1991;324:674); maternal vit A ingestion ≥10,000 IU q d esp in 1st trimester (Nejm 1995;333:1369)

Epidem: 1/1000 births in US; similar in Southern China, but in N China, rate is 6/1000 (Nejm 1999;341:1485). Risk incr × 2 w maternal obesity (Jama 1996;275:1089,1093)

Pathophys:

Si: Meningocele, myelomeningocele, etc

Lab:

Chem: α-Fetoprotein, HCG, and estriol levels at 15–18 wk gestation from last menstrual period; if elevated, then get ultrasound; amniocentesis not needed if ultrasound ok (Nejm 1990;323:557); but maternal AFP elevations are associated w incr fetal loss, levels 2–3× normal w a 2.5× increase, levels >3× w 10× increases (Nejm 1991;324:662)

Rx: Prevent w folic acid >0.4 mg qd periconception, 0/2000 births vs 6/2000 (Jama 1995;274:1698; Nejm 1998;338:1060; 1992;327: 1832 vs 1989;321:430); dramatically decreases neural tube defect risk (Nejm 1999;341:1485; Peds 1993;493:4); perhaps 4 mg po qd if pos family hx; now added to all US grain products, eg, flour (Nejm 1999;340:1449) and had decr overall incid by 20% (Jama 2001; 285:2981)

Consider abortion

In utero repair (Jama 1999;282:1819, 1826)

Delivery by cesarean section may result in less motor deficit? (Clin OBGyn 1998;41:393 vs Nejm 1991;324:662)

Sudden infant death syndrome (SIDS) and near SIDS

Epidem: 1.4 deaths/1000 live births in US. Runs in families; no association w DPT immunizations (J Peds 1991;119:411); incr incidence by sleeping prone and by deformable mattress, swaddling, warm room, URIs (Nejm 1993;329:377, 425), and children exposed to passive cigarette smoke (Jama 1995;273:795)

Incidence decr by 40% to <1/1000 w public education against sleeping prone (Pediatr Ann 1995;24:350) but message hardest to get to lower socioeconomic groups (Jama 1998;280:329,336,341)

Pathophys: Probably several sleep apneas (>15 s) precede fatal event. URI and nasal obstruction precipitate? Some may be assoc w long QTc > 0.44 on EKG (Jama 2001;286:2264; Nejm 1998; 338:1709)

Cmplc: r/o trauma/smothering asphyxia (Nejm 1991;324:1858; 1986; 315:100,126)

Lab: May be associated with elevated Hgb F levels (Nejm 1987;316:1122 vs 1989;321:1359), and some subset of cases w long QT interval (Nejm 2000;343:262; 1987;317:1501)

Rx: Prevent by positioning children on sides or supine (on back; "back to sleep" campaigns) (Jama 2001;285:2244; 1995;273:818; 1994; 272:1646) for 1st 6 mo of life (BMJ 1991;303:1209), doing so reduced incidence in Tasmania from 3.8 to 1.5 deaths/1000 (Jama 1995;273:783) and by 90% in Norway (J Ped 1998;132:340) but no difference found in southern California (Jama 1995;273:790); avoid soft bedding under infant. Apnea monitors not effective (Jama 2001;285:2199, 2244)

Temperature control in newborn is poor; higher ambient temperature may precipitate apnea (Nejm 1970;282:461); hypothermia immediately postpartum decreases with plastic swaddle in both newborn premie and term babies (Nejm 1971;284:121)

Diaper rash (S. Sewall, 10/94)

Cause: Irritation by stool/urine

Pathophys: Debate if ammonia from urea-splitting bacteria plays a role, also about role of stool enzymes and bile salts

Cmplc: Secondary candidiasis, may be associated w oral thrush, and often precipitated by antibiotic use, appears as confluent erythema w 1–3 mm satellite macule/papules

r/o seborrheic dermatitis, well-demarcated fiery red confluent rash, responds quickly to steroid creams; psoriatic diaper rash w shiny scales, responds slowly to topical steroids; staph infection often causing bullous impetigo lesions that resemble cigarette burns, rx w antibiotics; rarely Jacquet's ulcers of vulva or buttocks, zinc deficiency (acrodermatitis enteropathica), herpes simplex, scabies, and Kawasaki's disease (high fever)

Rx: (Contemp Peds 4/86)

Frequent diaper change keeping skin clean and dry; avoid strong soaps; avoid occlusive diapering, put disposables on loosely and/or tear some holes in plastic, omit rubber pants; zinc oxide ointment helps protect skin (Vaseline, A + D ointment, Desitin, Eucerin, etc.)

Nystatin cream for monilial type (satellite lesions)

Failure to thrive w/u: 1st CBC, lead levels, UA/culture, lytes, BUN; and TSH if height much less than weight

Febrile seizures (Nejm 1993;329:79; 1992;327:1122)

Epidem: Age of onset usually 6 mo–3 yr. Incidence higher w positive family hx; 1/3 under age 2 yr caused by roseola? (Nejm 1994;331: 432), but still need w/u under age 1 w LP etc. 2–4% of children under age 5 have at least one

Si: 1/2 are partial complex, 1/2 are grand mal. Fever usually closer to 101°F (38.3°C) than 105°F (40.5°C)

Crs: 33% recur, more often if age <18 mo; 50% recur within 6 mo, 75% within 1 yr, 90% within 2 yr if going to. No long term intellectual/behavioral deficits later (Nejm 1998;338:1723)

Rx: No prophylaxis; or perhaps, at 1st si of fever, acetaminophen or diazepam (Valium) 0.33 mg/kg q 8 h

PEDIATRICS

Food allergies including milk allergy (Jama 1997;278:1888)
Cause: Proteins in cow's milk, egg whites, peanuts, soybeans, fish, shrimp, et al.
Epidem: 6% prevalence under age 3, 2/5% prevalence of cow's milk allergy alone in children <2
Pathophys: IgE-mediated types cause classic skin, gi, and systemic histamine reactions
   IgA-mediated types cause dermatitis herpetiformis type skin changes and gastroenteritis
   Cell-mediated types cause hypersensitivity reactions, eg, to gluten causing sprue
Sx: Histaminic sx including wheezing and rhinitis, or gastroenteritis, or malabsorption, or constipation due to perianal inflammation (Nejm 1998;339:1100)
Crs: 85% "outgrow"
Cmplc: r/o non-allergic cow's milk toxicity leading to gi bleeding in children
Lab: RAST test, skin testing
Rx: Elimination diets

Malformations: Rv of all types and causes (Nejm 1983;308:424; Jones KL, ed, *Smith's Recognizable Patterns of Human Malformations.* Philadelphia: WB Saunders, 1996)

Nutrition: Cow's milk ok after 12 mo if give iron, gi bleeding insignificant (Med Let 1983;25:80); perhaps supplement either breast or cow's milk w FeSO$_4$ from birth to age 2 yr to prevent permanent impairment of school performance from iron deficiency (Nejm 1991;325:687). Breast milk can contain ethanol if mother drinking and can result in psychomotor impairment at age 1 (Nejm 1989;321:425)

Shaken baby syndrome (Nejm 1998;338:1822)
Cause: Non-accidental trauma
Epidem: Infants <3 yr, most <1 yr; 24% of all trauma in under age 2 children. Assoc w poverty and low socioeconomic status
Pathophys: Subdural and subarachnoid bleeds from torn bridging vessels
Sx: Lethargy, decr tone, seizures (40–70%), bruises, burns; facial bruises w any nonspecific set of sx under age 3 should prompt queries, CT, and skeletal series (Jama 1999;281:621, 657)
Si: Hydrocephalus

Xray: CT, maybe MRI; plain films (skeletal survey) for fractures
Rx: Hospitalize, child protection

Viral exanthems:
- Measles (rubeola) (p 516)
- Scarlet fever (p 399)
- 5th disease (parvovirus) (p 508)
- Chickenpox (p 501)
- Rubella (p 509)
- Roseola, exanthem subitum, or 6th disease (p 524)

Waiting room exposure to sick children does not increase infectious
disease risk (Nejm 1985;313:425)

CHILDREN

Anesthesia/sedation: (Nejm 2000;342:938)
Topical w:
- Lidocaine, epinephrine + tetracaine mixture (LET) for open wounds;
  takes 20 min to work
- EMLA (2.5% lidocaine + 2.5% prilocaine); takes 60 min to work
Parenteral w: Fentanyl iv or ketamine iv/im
- Sedation w: Midazolam (Versed) 0.025–0.05 mg/kg up to 0.4 mg/kg
  max iv; or 0.1–0.15 gm/kg im; or 0.5–0.75 mg/kg po or pr
- Pentobarbital 1–6 mg/kg iv/im; or 1.5–4 mg/kg po/pr

**Autism, pervasive developmental disorders (PDDs),
   Asperger syndrome:**
Epidem: (Jama 2001;285:3093,3141) prevalence of autism = 17 and
   PDDs = 46/10,000 in preschool children
Pathophys: Severe developmental disorder w delayed language and/or
   communication skills, social interactions and reciprocity, and
   imaginative play
Rx: Secretin injection no help (Nejm 1999;341:1801)

Benign pediatric murmurs (Fam Pract Recert 1986;8:51) Echo if systolic murmur radiates to carotids (J. Love 12/94). See Table 16.5.2

Table 16.5.2

Murmur	Location	Character	Differential Dx
Still's	LLSB to apex	Coarse, vibrating early systolic; S_2 splits and closes normally, murmur diminishes w sitting or deep inspiration	VSD, MVP, IHHS
Basal ejection (pulmonic flow)	ULSB	Base only, no click (unlike real PS), S_2 splits and closes normally	PS (click), ASD, Anomalous venous return
Physiologic	UL and RSB	To back and axilla	AS, PS, PDA
Supraclavicular bruit	Supraclavicular area	Teenagers	AS
Venous hum	Neck, USB	Continuous, gone when supine	PDA, AVMs

Child abuse (Nejm 1990;332:1425; Ped Clin N Am 1990;37(4): 791–1012): Physical, sexual in both boys (Jama 1998;280:1855) and girls, emotional/neglect

Sx: Sleep disorders, nightmares, sexualized play, school problems, phobias, depression

Si: Patterned bruises/burns, fractures, head injuries; in infant, shaken baby syndrome (p 666)

Cmplc: Mortality, greatest in first year of life, esp if 2nd or more child of teenage mother (Nejm 1998;339:1211); FTT; in adulthood, more physical sx, depression, drug and alcohol abuse, psych problems (Jama 1997;277:1362)

Xray: (Nejm 1989;320:507)

Rx: Prevention with home visits (Nejm 1989;320:531)

Hospitalize, report suspect cases

of sexual offenders, gonadotropin releasing hormone analog im q 1 mo, medically castrates (Nejm 1998;338:416)

Enuresis (bedwetting) (S. Sewall 7/98; Med Let 1990;32:38; Ann IM 1987;106:587)

Epidem: M:F = 2:1

Rx: Patient education available on web at http://www.drynights.com
  Only consider rx after age 6; 15%/yr resolve after age 6 yr
  Alarms 75% effective?; compliance tough, though improved w DDAVP
    given for 1st 3 wk; cost $60–75
  Desmopressin (DDAVP) 10–20 μgm in each nostril hs, or
    200–400 μgm po hs; may help a little especially when combined
    with other rx, effectiveness ~65% at 6 mo but wears off to 10% at
    1 yr. Adverse effects: hyponatremia, seizures, and rare sudden death
    (Med Let 1990;32:53); costs $3–6/night
  Imipramine 25–50 mg (75 mg over age 12); helps 25–35%; check QT
    interval on EKG before starting; cheap but OD risk

Hypertension (Nejm 1996;335:1968); upper limits of normal
  (see Table 16.5.3); most HT under age 19 is secondary and a cause
  can be found

Table 16.5.3   95th Percentile of Blood Pressure in Boys and Girls 3 to 16 Years of Age, According to Height[*]

Blood Pressure	Age	Height Percentile for Boys				Height Percentile for Girls			
		5th	25th	75th	95th	5th	25th	75th	95th
	(yr)	(mm Hg)				(mm Hg)			
Systolic	3	104	107	111	113	104	105	108	110
	6	109	112	115	117	108	110	112	114
	10	114	117	121	123	116	117	120	122
	13	121	124	128	130	121	123	126	128
	16	129	132	136	138	125	127	130	132
Diastolic	3	63	64	66	67	65	65	67	68
	6	72	73	75	76	71	72	73	75
	10	77	79	80	82	77	77	79	80
	13	79	81	83	84	80	81	82	84
	16	83	84	86	87	83	83	85	86

[*]The height percentiles were determined with standard growth curves, Data are adapted from those of the Task Force on High Blood Pressure in Children and Adolescents. Reproduced with permission from Silnaiko AR, Hypertension in children. Nejm 1996;335:1969.

Intussception:
Epidem: Peak incidence age 1–5; assoc w rotavirus vaccine, which may
  hypertrophy Peyer's patches that then act as sleeving mass (Peds
  1999;104:575)

Sx: Crampy pain and strikingly normal between cramps, though can eventually develop stupor (Peds 1980;65:A1057); bloody "currant jelly" stool

Si: Normal exam between cramps

Rx: Barium enema to dx and rx

Short stature: Dwarfism (p 223)

Idiopathic short stature (<3%tile) (Nejm 1999;340:502, 557) can be rx'd w recombinant HGH × 5–10 yr to normal adult heights; but expensive ($20K/yr) and of questionable ethics to do so

Constitutional delay in growth and development in adolescent males can be rx'd without loss of final height with testosterone × 1 yr? (Nejm 1988;319:1563)

Chapter 17
Prevention and Health Maintenance

D. K. Onion

17.1 SCREENING AND PREVENTION

References:

Ann IM 1997;127:910—nice historical rv, no recipes

P. Frame, J Fam Pract 1996;22:341,417,511; 1986;23:29

US Preventive Services Task Force's Guide, 1995, Williams and Wilkins (1-800-638-0672)

Jama 1995;273:1030—Group Health, Seattle; when done over time, decreases death and/or disability, eg, breast cancer, immunizations, bike accidents, smoking

H. Sox, Nejm 1994;330:1589—good summary tables

Ann IM 1992;116:593—discusses how reasonable people may come to opposite conclusions re a screening strategy

Ann IM 1991;114:758—best, most concise summary disease by disease

GENERAL ISSUES

Types of prevention
- Primary prevention: prevention of a disease before it exists, eg, immunization against H. flu
- Secondary prevention: detection and reversal (cure) of a disease after it already exists but before it is symptomatic

Metanalysis results agree w subsequent controlled trials only 65% of the time (Nejm 1997;337:536)

Number needed to treat (NNT) (Nejm 1988;318:1728; Ann IM 1992; 117:916): the reciprocal of the absolute risk reduction; the number of patients to whom an intervention must be applied over a fixed period, usually 1–5 years, in order to confer a benefit for one of them, eg, dietary and cholestyramine rx of men with cholesterols over 265 mg % over 5 yr causes an absolute risk reduction of 1.12% from 12% to 10.88%, which means that 1/0.012 or 89 must be treated for 5 years to cause one patient to benefit. Ann IM 1992; 117:916 suggests "TNT" = "tons needed to treat," eg, 10.3 metric tons of cholestyramine to prevent one death in Helsinki trial; = NNT-5 = 77. Nice example of how to present such data to pts using finasteride rx of BPH as an example where NNT-4 = 16 (Nejm 1998;338:612)

Statistical calculations (T = true, P = positive, F = false, N = negative):

$$\text{Sensitivity} = \frac{TP}{(TP + FN)}$$

$$\text{Specificity} = \frac{TN}{(TN + FP)}$$

$$\text{Positive predictive value} = \frac{TP}{(TP + FP)}$$

$$\text{Negative predictive value} = \frac{TN}{(TN + FN)}$$

Criteria for justifiable preventive intervention
- For a primary prevention intervention:
  1. Significant disease with a defined and substantial morbidity and/or mortality
  2. The intervention (treatment, education, etc.) is:
     a. Effective, ie, improves prognosis and the result is superior to waiting for the disease to appear
     b. Acceptable to patients
     c. Low risk
     d. Available (financing, facilities, and providers to provide)

- For a secondary intervention, the above must be true, plus:
  1. An asx phase of significant duration must exist
  2. A screening test must be available that is
     a. Acceptable (financing, comfort, risk) to patients
     b. Sensitive and specific at the projected disease prevalence and does not detect a lot of subclinical conditions that may never be clinically relevant (Nejm 1993;328:1237), eg, 40% of men in their 60s may have prostate cancer but less than 1% will ever be clinically affected (Ann IM 1993;118:793,804)

Problems with prevention in primary care practice
- No or little feedback for a job well done; lots of negative feedback when primary care doctor deals with the complications of preventive rx or works up the false positives
- Without tough rules to follow, primary care doctor may be quickly overwhelmed by off-hand, incorrect, and/or inappropriate specialist recommendations ("if you primary care docs would just screen for UTIs, glaucoma, etc.")
- A doctor's sense of responsibility makes him or her assume too much responsibility rather than devolving some onto the community or the individual patient
- Overzealous specialty society (eg, American Cancer Society) recommendations impair our ability to seek informed consent (Nejm 1993;328:438)
- Elimination of wellness through false positives and illness labeling of normal variation (Nejm 1994;330:440)

Goals of the periodic health exam (annual physical, though frequently done, is a waste of time and inconsistently done—P. Frame, J Fam Pract 1995;40:543, 547)
- Prevention
- Patient-doctor rapport building to improve future access
- Elicitation of sx (rv of systems) or risk factors that deserve further study and that the patient may have not felt important enough to volunteer
- Maintenance of doctor's skills, eg, Babinski testing, funduscopic exam, thyroid exam, heart sounds, etc.
- Fulfill patient expectations, eg, of touching, of a heart-lung exam being part of a full exam, etc.

17.2 ADULTS

Reasonable preventive interventions in adults for practicing physicians; * = good evidence for; for others fair evidence or only expert consensus; alphabetically organized by disease; primary or secondary intervention indicated by (1° prevention) or (2° prevention). In all cases, presumption is of an asx patient; sx should always be investigated.

Abdominal aortic aneurysm (Can Task Force—Can Med Assoc J 1991; 145:783; P. Frame, Ann IM 1993;119:411)
Group: All age >65 yr
Screen: Abdominal exam for aneurysm >5–6 cm q 1 yr; perhaps ultrasound esp in male relatives over age 60, 18% incidence (Ann IM 1999;130:637)
Intervention: Resection (2° prevention)
Issues: Appropriate size to operate on; borderline cost-benefit ratios

Alcoholism
Groups: All
Screen: Take history q 1 yr or with accidents or h/o hypertension
Intervention: AA referral, Antabuse (2° prevention)
Issues: Intervention efficacy

Anemia, iron-deficiency
Groups: Low socioeconomic status or institutionalized elderly
Screen: Hematocrit
Intervention: Iron po (2° prevention)
Issues: Debatable efficacy (Ann IM 1992;116:44)

ASHD/CVAs
Groups: All
Intervention #1: *Detect and rx hypertension (1° prevention) (Ann IM 1995;122:937)
  Freq: <q 1 yr
  NNT: 3 if diastolic >115 mm Hg; 141 if diastolic 90–109 mm Hg
  Issues: Treatment goals?

Intervention #2: *Detect and rx elevated cholesterols (1° prevention), not of value over age 70 (Jama 1994;272:1335,1372) or in women unless established ASCVD (Jama 1995;274:1152)

Freq: <q 4 yr

NNT: In men over 40 w LDL >150, NNT-5 = 40 (Nejm 1995; 333:1301)

Issues: Compliance; risks, morbidity, and costs of medications

Intervention #3: *Estrogen replacement rx in peri- and postmenopausal women

Freq: Continuous

NNT:

Issues: Breast cancer risk

Breast cancer

Groups: (Ann IM 1997;127:1029,1035; Sci 1997;275:1056, Ann IM 1995;122:534,539,550; 1994;120:326); in summary, clearly helpful age 50–70$^+$, hotly debated between age 40–50 if low risk (nice summary—Jama 1999;281:1470), none promote under age 40. 33% overall false pos mammogram or clinical breast exam in 5 exams over 10 yr, 50% w 10 mammograms between age 40–50 (Nejm 1998;338:1089) or less (Nejm 1998;339:560)

Of elderly women age 70$^+$, marginally beneficial up to age 85 if 5–10 yr lifespan likely and esp if have normal bone mineral density (Jama 1999;282:2156; Ann IM 1992;116:722)

Of women age 50–70$^+$ yr mammography w clinical breast exam clearly increases survival done q 1–2 yr (Rand summary—Jama 1995;273: 142, 149; Nejm 1992;327:323; Ann IM 1994;120:326 vs Can Med Assoc J 1992;147:1459, 1477); Swedish meta-analysis of 5 studies also finds benefit (30% relative risk mortality reduction) between age 50–70 yr but not younger (Lancet 1993;341:973); NNT = 270 (Ann IM 1997;127:955)

Of women age 40–50 yr q 1 yr (not q 2 yr), if high risk (positive family history, cancer in opposite breast [Nejm 1984;310:960; J Fam Practice 1983;16:481], or h/o mammoplasties), clearly benefit

Less clearly helpful if low risk; false pos mammograms over 10 yr in 1/3 of the women; mammography saves 2.3/1000, while clinical breast exam alone saves 1.5/1000, so mammography helps 1/1250 in that age group (Nejm 1993;328:438; 1993;329:276), or NNT = 2500 (Ann IM 1997;127:955); discuss risk/benefit ratios w women age 40–50 who frequently think cancer incidence much higher than is, and don't understand risks of f/u of false-pos tests; psychological effects of false-positive mammograms are real, even after all found to be ok (Ann IM 1991;114:657)

Screen:
Physician breast exam* q 1 yr, 54% sens 94% specif (Jama 1999;282: 1270); self-breast exam monthly

Mammography (Ann IM 1995;122:534,539,550) 75% sens, 90% specif; interpretations, 80% agreement intra- and interobserver (Nejm 1994;331:1493) q 1–2 yr (q 2 yr adequate—J Natl Ca Inst 1993;85:1644) over age 50, q 1 yr under age 50 if do at all

Intervention: Excise when small (2° prevention)

NNT: Age 40–50 yr, mortality (20 yr delayed) NNT-10 = 1000–2500 w only 4% true pos mammograms; age 50–60 yr, NNT-10 = 400 w 9% true pos mammograms; age 60+, NNT-10 = 150 w 17% true pos mammograms

Issues: Cost/access, test sens/specif, safety, periodicity

Car accidents
Groups: All
Intervention: Encourage seatbelt use (1° prevention)
Freq: <q 1 yr
Issues: Efficacy of physician intervention?

Cervical cancer (Nejm 2001;344:1603)
Group: Women age 20–70 yr with cervix
Screen: Pap* smear q 1 yr if <35 and/or multiple partners; q 5 yr if >35 and <8 lifetime partners (Canadian Walton Rep—Can Med Assoc J 1982;127:581) and no h/o abnormal paps or STDs in pt or partner; alternatively at least q 3 yr at age 20–65 (Ann IM 1990;113:214); and in elderly >65, get 2–3 paps 3 yr apart if not previously done then stop (Ann IM 1992;117:520). Unnecessary if s/p hysterectomy for benign disease (Nejm 1996;335;1559,1599; Jama 1996;275: 940). 5–10% false neg rate in best labs. Atypical squamous cells uncertain significance (ASCUS), should be <5% of paps
Intervention: Excise, ablate (2° prevention)
Issues: False-negative Paps

Colon cancer (Nejm 2000;343:1603,1641; Ann IM 1997;126:808, Nejm 1998;338:1153; 1995;332:861)

Groups: All age >45 or 50 yr; at age 35–40 yr if at higher risk (Jama 1999;281:1611) from IBD, familial polyposis, >1 first degree relative w colon cancer (Nejm 1994;331:1669), or one first degree relative w cancer under age 55

1° Prevention #1: NSAID use, eg, ASA po b-tiw (Ann IM 1994;121:241)

1° Prevention #2: Hormone replacement rx in women decreases risk by 30–40% (Ann IM 1998;128:705)

1° Prevention #3: Calcium 1200 mg po qd as milk or direct supplement (Nejm 1999;340:101; Jama 1998;280:1070)

Screen #1: Stool guaiacs 3× annually by Hemoccult (Nejm 2001;345:555; 1998;338:1153 nice summary of the debate; Ann IM 1997;126: 808). Some studies use rehydration of guaiac card, but not done in other studies that also show benefit (Ann IM 1997;126:808)

    Intervention: Adenomatous polyp detection and removal, and early cancer excision (2° prevention) NNT-18 = 143 (Nejm 2000; 343:1603)

    Issues: Test sensitivity (81%) and positive predictive value (5.6%); when colon w/u neg, UGI endoscopy yields ~13% dx's including 1% cancers, esp indicated if anemic (RR = 5×) (Am J Med 1999; 106:613). 50–90% sens for cancer and about 30% for polyps; workups of positives will demonstrate a cancer or polyp in about 1/3 and an upper GI source (benign) in many (~1/3) (Nejm 1998; 339:653); false-neg rate increased from 20% to 40% with time (2–8 d) between obtaining and doing the test (Ann IM 1984;101: 297). Such annual (not biannual) testing decreases 5-yr mortality by 1/3 (Ann IM 1993;118:1), or from 8% to 5% over 13 yr but overall mortality the same in all groups (Lancet 1996;348:1467,1472, Minn. guaiac study—Nejm 1993;328:1365,1416). Costs, physician skill

Screen #2: Flexible sigmoidoscopy (Jama 2000;284:1954) q 5–10 yr w quaiacs q 1 yr w colonoscopy if either positive, as good as or better than

    Colonoscopy (Ann IM 2000;133:573,647; Nejm 2000;343:162,169, 207) q 10 yr over age 50 since sig misses 25% of cancers (Nejm 2001;345:555,607); no need for quaiacs with it

    Intervention: Polyp (villous, tubulovillous, debatably tubular adenomas—Jama 1999;281:1611) detection and removal w colonoscopy of whole bowel, and early cancer excision (2° prevention)

NNT: 1000
Issues: Costs, physician skill

Deafness
Groups: Occupationally exposed
Intervention: Encourage ear noise protection (1° prevention)
Freq: <q 1 yr
Issues: Efficacy of physician education

Dental caries
Groups: All
Interventions/Freq: *Dental prophylaxis q 1 yr (1° prevention);
    *brush/floss qd (1° prevention)

Depression (Ann IM 2001;134:345, 418)
Screen: Various instruments like "are you depressed," and "have you lost
    interest in things"; together 95% sens
Intervention: Antidepressants
Frequency: Maybe once
Issues: Cost ($30,000/quality-adjusted life year); rx efficacy

Diabetes (Jama 1998;280:1757)
Groups: Family hx, grossly obese, h/o gestational diabetes, black, age 25+
Screen: FBS vs. hgb A1C >7.0% (Jama 1996;276:1246,1261)
Intervention:
    Diet and exercise at impaired glucose tolerance stage decreases 5 yr
        conversion rate to overt DM from 35% to 15% (Nejm 2001;344:
        1343)
    Diet and hypoglycemic agents (1° prevention of cmplc's)

Diphtheria/tetanus
Groups: All
Intervention: *dT immunization (1° prevention)
Freq: Once ~age 50 yr if had full pediatric series including booster at age
    14 (Ann IM 1994;121:540)

Hepatitis B
Groups: High risk (health workers, iv drug users, prostitutes, gay males)
Intervention: Vaccine (1° prevention); HBIG postexposure (1° prevention)

Freq: Once
NNT: 8 in gay males, higher w other groups

Hypothyroidism
Groups: Women >50 yr with vague sx (ACP) or >60 yr (USPTF); or both
sexes over age 35–40 (Jama 1996;276:285)
Screen: TSH
Intervention: Thyroid replacement (2° prevention)

Influenza (Med Let discussion annually in Sept)
Groups: High risk at least, or all >65 yr, or over age 50 per CDC 2000;
but not usually worthwhile in age 18–65 work forces (RCT—Jama
2000;284:1655)
Intervention: Immunization (1° prevention)
Freq: q 1 yr
Issues: Immunization efficacy (not bad—Nejm 1994;331:778)

Lung cancer, COPD, ASHD, strokes (Jama 1993;269:232)
Group: All smokers
Intervention:
> **#1:** Smoking cessation instruction (1° prevention) after asking 3
> questions (Ann IM 1991;115:59): (1) What do you know about
> smoking's impact on your health? (2) Are you ready to quit?
> (3) What would it take for you to stop? Plus transient nicotine
> replacement rx (BMJ 1994;308:21)
> **#2:** CT or chest xray; insufficient data; being studied but unlikely
> (Nejm 2000;343:1627); low dose spiral CT screening of smokers
> >60 found 23% w nodules, followed q 3 mo and bx'd ones that
> grew (10%), and 27/28 were cancer but cost high (Med Let 2001;
> 43:6)

Freq: Smoking cessation try q 1 yr
Issues: Efficacy of intervention? Weight gain of 5–10 lb after quitting a
disincentive (Nejm 1991;324:739)

Melanoma
Group: All
> **Screen:** Self-exam q 1 yr?
> **Intervention:** Excision (2° prevention); sunscreen use (1° prevention)
> **Issues:** Low incidence

Group: Those with family hx of melanoma or atypical (dysplastic) nevus syndrome
    Screen: Self-exam q 6 mo? Physician exam q 6–12 mo?
    Intervention: Excision (2° prevention)

Neural tube defects/spina bifida: Folic acid peripartum to prevent (p 663)

Obesity
Groups: All
Screen: Weight q 1 yr?
Intervention: Diet, exercise (2° prevention)
Issues: Intervention efficacy makes screening for of questionable value (Can Med Assoc J 1999;160:513)

Osteoporosis (of asx pts very debatable—NIH CDC-Jama 2001; 285:785)
Group: Perimenopausal women and elderly men
    Intervention: Calcium + vit D po (1° prevention) (Nejm 1997;337:670)
    Freq: Continuous
Group: Perimenopausal women
    Screen: Bone mineral density by various techniques
    Intervention: Estrogen rx (1° prevention) (p 624); alendronate 5–10 mg po qd if low bone mineral density (Jama 1998;280:2077 vs 2119) and esp if can't take ERT and/or have already had fx's
    Freq: Continuous
    Issues: Risks and cmplc of estrogen rx

Pelvic inflammatory disease (Amer J Prev Med 2001;20 (3S):90—Nejm 1998;339:739,768)
Group: Young (<25) asx women, and? men
Screen: 1st void urine ligase chain reaction test for chlamydial DNA (89% sens, 99% specif)
Intervention: Azithromycin 1 gm po ×1

Pneumococcal infections
Groups: High risk, eg, asplenics; all age >65 yr?
Intervention: Immunization (1° prevention)

Freq: Once, unless 1st dose before age 65, then revaccinate after 5 yr × 1
  (Jama 1999;281:243)

Prostate cancer: Unclear if helpful (M. Barry—Nejm 2000;344:1373);
  most major preventive medicine groups recommend against; may be
  premature and harmful if undertaken before prospective trials (Jama
  1997;277:467 vs ok if life expectancy >15 yr—1997;277:497; 1996;
  276:1976; 1996;275:1976; 1994;272:773 vs 813, Ann IM 1997;126:
  394,468,480; 1993;119:914 vs 948, Nejm 1995;333:1401), but is
  being done more and more without such trial results (Med Let 1992;
  34:93). Let pt decide after education (Wennberg—J Genl Int Med 1996;
  11:342)
Group: Males age >50 yr; ? age 40 and 45 (Jama 2000;284:1399) esp if
  black and/or positive fam hx at young age
Screen: Rectal and PSA level >4 μgm/L (87% sens for aggressive tumors
  and 55% sens for nonaggressive ones; 91% specif—Jama 1995;
  273:289), w f/u transurethral ultrasounds of abnormals? (Nejm
  1991;324:1156 vs Ann IM 1993;119:948) vs >10 μgm/L with
  ultrasound follow-up of abnormals (Med Let 1992;34:93; Nejm
  1991;324:1161) q 2 yr if initial level <2, q 1 yr if 2–4 μgm/L (Jama
  1997;277:1460). If free PSA level <25%, higher cancer risk (Jama
  1998;279:1542)
Intervention: Prostatectomy, radiation, or antiandrogen rx; but is unclear
  that prognosis can be changed (Jama 1992;267:2191) esp if
  localized disease (Jama 1998;280:969,975,1008), although 1995
  data from Mayo Clinic area suggests may be improving incidence
  (Jama 1995;274:1445) (2° prevention)
Issues: 30% of males age >50 yr have latent clinically insignificant cancer
  at incidental postmortem exams and 40% of men in their 60s may
  have prostate cancer but less than 1% will ever be clinically relevant
  (Ann IM 1993;118:793,804); need long-term follow-up data;
  >25% of tumors found w rectal exam and PSA strategy are small
  ones found serendipidously so significance unclear (Jama 1997;
  278:1516)

Rubella syndrome in children
Group: All women age <35 who are potential childbearers
Intervention: Titers and immunization (1° prevention)

PREVENTION AND HEALTH MAINTENANCE

Sexually transmitted diseases

Group: Prostitutes, gay males, multiple-partner patients, contacts of cases, iv drug users

Screen #1: Culture for gc; enzymatic test for chlamydia; VDRL for syphilis

    Intervention: Antibiotics (2° prevention)

Screen #2: HIV serology

    Intervention: Counseling re transmission (1° prevention)

    Issues: Counseling same whether positive or negative test

Sudden death in athletes (Ann IM 1998;129:379)

Group: Teenagers and older

Screen: Sports physical, school PE, athletic exam for:

    Family h/o sudden death or premature heart disease

    Personal h/o HT, fatigue, syncope, DOE

    Physical exam for murmurs supine and standing, femoral pulses, Marfan's stigmata, BP

    Echocardiogram if abnormalities

Intervention: Avoidance of sports, possible preventive interventions medically or surgically

Suicide/homicide

Group: All

Intervention: Handgun control via physician support of legislation decreases both by 25% (Nejm 1991;325:1615) (1° prevention)

Testicular cancer

Group: Men age 15–40 yr

Screen: Self-exam q 1 mo?; or physician exam when see <q 1 yr?

Intervention: Excision (2° prevention)

Issues: Low incidence

Uterine cancer

Group: Women with an intact uterus especially those with h/o obesity or unopposed estrogen stimulation

Screen: H/o vaginal bleeding, ask q 1 yr; or endometrial sampling in high risk groups q 1 yr?

Intervention: Hysterectomy (2° prevention)

PROPOSED BUT NOT OF PROVEN HELP

- Heart disease by EKG and/or ETT
- Ovarian cancer by pelvic, ultrasound, or Ca-125, mainly because prevalence so low (Jama 1995;273:491; Ann IM 1994;121:124; 1993;119:838,901)
- Scoliosis by back exam of early teenagers not clearly effective (USPTF—Jama 1993;269:2667)
- UTI by UA, urine culture

ELDERLY (Age > 65 Yr)

   Rv of all issues and literature (J Fam Pract 1992;34:205,320; Am J Pub Hlth 1991;81:1136); must balance benefits w projected life expectancy (NNT estimates—Jama 2001;285:2750)

- Hearing screening by hx, PE, otoscopy for cerumen, and possibly audiometry (w portable Welch-Allyn audioscope—Am J Med Sci 1994;307:40) for presbycusis
- Smoking hx
- BSE instruction, exam, mammogram for breast cancer up to age 75 or to estimated life span minus 10 yrs (Ann IM 1992;116:722)
- BP for hypertension
- Visual acuity for refractive error
- Skin exam for cancer, infection, dry skin
- Dental exam
- Pap q 3 yr until 2–3 negatives, then stop (Ann IM 1992;117:520)
- Immunizations: dT q 10 yr or initial series if not previously done, yearly influenza, debatably pneumovax

ADULT IMMUNIZATIONS

   (Ann IM 1994;121:540; Guide for Adult Immunizations, Am College Phys 3rd ed. 1994; Nejm 1993;328:1252; Med Let 1990;32:54)

- Td at age 50 yr
- Pneumococcal vaccine at age $60^{+} \times 1$; repeat if given >6 yr earlier

- Influenza q 1 yr (see Sept. Med Let discussion annually)
- Hep B if at high risk for exposure

17.3 CHILDREN

Newborn:
- Screen for toxoplasmosis, PKU
- Eye prophylaxis vs gonorrhea and chlamydia: tetracycline 1% ointment once or erythromycin is better than silver nitrate (Nejm 1988;318:657)
- Vitamin K to prevent hemorrhagic cmplc; no increase in childhood cancers by using it (Nejm 1993;329:905)
- Hearing loss, bilateral: screening of questionable benefit though mandated in 32 states (Jama 2001;286:2000)

Infants/Children:
- Lead screening of all children, with serum lead levels, at 6–12 mo and q 6–12 mo to age 24 mo, screen older children only if high risk. See Table 17.3.1

Table 17.3.1

Level	Plan
<10 µg %	Repeat per above schedule
10–25 µg %	Repeat, improve environment, give po Fe, which decreases Pb absorption
25–45 µg %	Aggressive rx of environment, po Fe, consider chelation
45+ µg %	Refer for chelation

- Dietary fluoride supplement dosage schedule in mg/d. See Table 17.3.2

Table 17.3.2

Age (years)	Home Water Fluoride Concentration (ppm or mg/L)		
	<0.30 ppm	0.3–0.6 ppm	>0.60 ppm
6 mo–3yr	0.25 mg qd	0	0
3–6	0.50 mg qd	0.25 mg qd	0
6–16	1.0 mg qd	0.5 mg qd	0

- **Scoliosis (p 653);** screening in schools in preteens is controversial

Immunization Schedules: (Jama 1995;273:693; Nejm 1992;327:1794; for Hib, Med Let 1991;33:5; for DTaP [acellular pertussis] and hep B, Med Let 1992;34:69):

General rules:

Give when due, as long as temperature ≤100°F (≤37.7°C) (debatable—Jama 1996;275:704; Jama 1991;265:2095).

Give dT, DPT, Hib and Hep B im; give MMR sc

Hib in protocol below is for MSD 3 shot series; other types require additional dose at 6 mo but using any of the 3 available Hib vaccines at 2, 4, 6, and 12–15 mo is ok (Jama 1995;273:849)

Egg allergies no contraindication to measles vaccination (Nejm 1995; 332:1262)

Conjugate pneumococcal 7-valent vaccine in children now being recommended routinely (Med Let 2000;42:25; Rx Let 2000;7:14; Jama 2000;283:1460)

Routine (Mmwr 1999;48(1):12–6; Jama 1997;277:203), at age:
- Birth: Hep B #1 (Jama 1995;274:1201), perhaps eventually in combo w Hep A vaccine
- 2 mo:
    DTaP #1 (Nejm 1995;333:1045) +
    Hib #1
    Hep B #2
    IPV #1
    Pneumo #1
- 4 mo:
    DTaP #2
    Hib #2, or all 4 (DTaP + Hib) as TriHIBit
    IPV #2
    Pneumo #2
- 6 mo:
    DTaP #3
    Hib #3, or all 4 as TriHIBit
    IPV #3
    Pneumo #3
- 15 mo:
    DTaP #4

Hib #4, or all 4 (DPT + Hib) as Tetramune (Med Let 1993; 35:104)

MMR #1

Hep B #3

Varicella vaccine (Varivax) (Jama 1997;278:1529) 0.5 cc sc ×1

- 4–6 yr:

  DTaP #5

  IPV #4

  MMR #2

- 11⁺ yr:

  dT q 10 yr

  MMR #2 if not given at age 4–6

  Hep B #4

  Possibly varicella vaccine if no previous immunization or h/o chicken pox (Jama 1997;277:203)

Catch up under age 7:

- 1st:

  DTaP #1

  OPV #1

  MMR

  Hib #1 if <5 yr

  Heb B # 1, ped dose (Rx Let 2000;7:9)

  Pneumo #1

- 2 mo:

  DTaP #2

  OPV #2

  Hib #2 if <15 mo when started

  Heb B # 2

  Pneumo #2 if <2 yr

- 4 mo:

  DTaP #3

  Heb B # 3

- 6–12 mo: OPV #3

Catch up over age 7:

- 1st:

  Td #1

  OPV #1

  MMR #1

Heb B # 1, 2, 3 q 1 mo pediatric doses, or, if over age 10,
2 adult doses 6 mo apart (Rx Let 2000;7:9)
- 2 mo:
  Td #2
  OPV #2
  MMR #2 (optional)
- 6 mo:
  Td #3
  OPV #3

Chapter 18
Psychiatry

D. K. Onion

18.1 MEDICATIONS/TREATMENTS

Med Let 1997;39:33

TRANQUILIZERS/SLEEPING TREATMENTS
Med Let 2000;42:71; rv of insomnia dx and rx—Nejm 1997;336:341

Benzodiazepines: Nejm 1993;328:1398; Med Let 1991;33:43; 1988;30:26
Many have long half lives; withdrawal sx × 1–4 wk after chronic use
(Nejm 1986;315:854); safest hypnotics available unless combined w
alcohol abuse, but none alone work long term for sleep (Jama
1997;278:2170). All increase the likelihood of accidents (Am J Pub
Hlth 1990;80:1467), especially in elderly, and especially the
long-acting ones in the first week of use (Jama 1997;278:27); thus if
use at all, use 1/2–1/3 normal dose
Benzodiazepines in roughly equivalent po doses:
*Indicates short half-life, thus good hypnotic/sleep meds
  - Alprazolam* (Xanax) 0.5 mg; may work for panic attacks without
    tolerance developing but hard to withdraw (must very slowly) and
    recurrences are frequent (Med Let 1991;33:30)
  - Chlorazepate (Tranxene) 7.5 mg
  - Chlordiazepoxide (Librium) 10 mg
  - Clonazepam (Klonopin) 0.5 mg; binds similar site but since long
    acting, less of a "high" and preferable; can also be used to
    withdraw from alprazolam by switching to clonazepam for 2–3 wk
    while tricyclic started (J. Dreher 7/91)
  - Diazepam (Valium) 5 mg, also available im/iv

- Estazolam (ProSom) 1–2 mg
- Flurazepam (Dalmane) 30 mg
- Lorazepam* (Ativan) 1–2 mg; ok for sleep if used occasionally (Med Let 1989;31:23), effective im, renal excretion
- Meprobamate (Miltown) 60 mg
- Midazolam* (Versed) iv use, syrup also available; used for sedation/anesthesia only
- Oxazepam* (Serax) 15–30 mg; ok for sleep if used occasionally (Med Let 1989;31:23), hepatic glucuronidation preserved even w liver disease so often used for DTs
- Temazepam* (Restoril) 15–30 mg; may be best for sleep (Med Let 1991;33:91)
- Triazolam* (Halcion) 0.125–0.25 mg; higher incid of "blackouts"
- Zaleplon* (Sonata) (Med Let 1999;41:93) 5 mg; very short acting
- Zolpidem* (Ambien) 10 mg; may be best for sleep (Rx Let 1999; 6:49); $1.50/tab

Others
- Antihistamines like diphenhydramine (Benadryl) 25–50 mg po hs; anticholinergic side effects
- Barbiturates; substantial OD risk
- Buspirone (BuSpar) 5–10 mg t-qid, for chronic anxiety, not a benzodiazepine, no abuse potential or interactions with driving or alcohol; not for panic disorder or sleep; takes several weeks to work like tricyclics (J Dreher 7/91); levels increased a lot by erythromycin and itraconazole (Rx Let 1998;5:1); $10/wk (Med Let 1986;28:117)
- Chloralhydrate (Noctec) 500 mg po hs; OD risk, rapid entry into CNS increases dependence and abuse, tachyphylaxis
- Ethchlorvynol (Placidyl); substantial OD risk, and rapid entry into CNS increases dependence and abuse
- Antidepressants like trazodone or amitriptyline; but OD risk, anticholinergic side effects w latter
- Zolpidem (Ambien) 10 mg hs (5 mg in elderly); not a benzo but binds brain benzo receptors; no tolerance develops, ODs aren't bad and can be rx'd w flumazenil (Mazicon). Adverse effects: nausea and vomiting, rare psychotic reactions; $1.50/tab

Non-rx/Herbal Hypnotics: (Rx Let 2000;7:46)
- Kava root extract, herbal equivalent of benzodiazepines (Rx Let 2001;8:16, 1998;5:20); adv effect: hepatotoxicity

- Melatonin (Nejm 1997;336:186; Med Let 1995;37:962) 2 mg sustained release, or 1–5 mg po hs; helpful to allow chronic hs benzo taper (Rx Let 1999;6:69), 5 mg po qd × 2$^+$d helps jet lag (ACP J Club 2001;135:97) and useful to entrain blind people in a 24 hr cycle (Nejm 2000;343:1070,1114). Adverse effects: hypothermia, gonadal inhibition
- Valerian root 200–900 mg po hs; sold as Alluna w hops

Cognitive Behavioral rx: (Jama 2001;285;1850)
- Educate re normal age-specific sleep patterns
- Sleep in bed; not reading/TV etc
- Establish standard wake-up time
- Get up during extended awakenings
- Stop daytime naps
- Set time in bed = avg sleep time + 30 min; incr or decr × 15 min q 1 wk if sleep efficiency >85% or <80%

ANTIPSYCHOTICS
Med Let 1991;33:47; Nejm 1996;334:34

Older types: (see Table 18.1.1)

Table 18.1.1

Name	Equivalent mg Potency
Phenothiazines	
Chlorpromazine (Thorazine)	100 mg
Thioridazine (Mellaril)	100 mg
Perphenazine (Trilafon)	10 mg
Thioxanthines	
Trifluoperazine (Stelazine)	5 mg
Thiothixene (Navane)	4 mg
Chlorprothixene (Taractan)	100 mg
Other	
Haloperidol (Haldol)	2 mg
Clozapine (Clozaril) (see below)	50 mg
Molindone (Moban)	10 mg

Common adverse effects:
- Acute dystonic reactions, rx with antihistamines, barbiturates, or antiparkinsonism meds

- Akathisia (restlessness, inability to sit still)
- Neuroleptic malignant syndrome (p 526);
- Parkinsonism, rx with anticholinergics like benztropine (Cogentin), trihexyphenidyl (Artane), etc.
- Tardive dyskinesia (p 577)

Atypical Antipsychotics: All have fewer extrapyramidal side effects than do older antipsychotics, and often cause weight gain (Rx Let 2000;7:45)

- Clozapine (Clozaril) (Jama 1995;274:981; Med Let 1993;35:16) 12.5 mg po qd gradually increasing to 300–400 mg qd; a tetracyclic, works without increasing prolactin or causing parkinsonism so can use in those pts (Nejm 1999;340:757), but can cause seizures and fatal agranulocytosis (Nejm 1993;329:162) that recur if rechallenged, so with q 1 wk CBC monitoring for 1st 6 mo costs $9000/yr (Nejm 1991;324:746; 1990;323:827; Med Let 1990;32:3); rare tardive dyskinesia; drug alone costs $5000/yr + costs of CBCs; interacts w lithium and phenytoin by decreasing blood levels, with benzodiazepines by causing respiratory arrest, and with carbamazepine (Tegretol) by worsening agranulocytosis risk

- Olanzapine (Zyprexa) (Med Let 1997;38:5) 5–20 mg po qd; 1st choice now for schizophrenia. Adverse effects: postural hypotension, somnolence, constipation, wgt gain, incr LFTs; no agranulocytosis, rare tardive dyskinesia

- Quetiapine (Seroquel) (Rx Let 1997;4:65); adv effect: cataracts (must check eyes q 6 mo)

- Risperidone (Risperdal) (Med Let 1994;36:33), start at 0.5–1 mg po bid, increase to 3 mg po bid in 3 d; helps negative sx of schizophrenia (eg, apathy) much better than phenothiazines or haloperidol but not as well as clozapine, yet also helps the positive sx, with only rare tardive dyskinesia and no agranulocytosis. Adverse effects: asthenia, sedation, occasional orthostatic hypotension, weight gain, prolactin elevations, sexual dysfunction; cost: $313/mo for 3 mg bid

- Ziprasidone (Geodon) (Med Let 2001;43:51) 20–80 mg po bid, im form coming; less wgt gain than w others. Adverse effects: long QT, more than others in class. Cost $250/mo

PSYCHIATRY

ANTIDEPRESSANTS

Nejm 2000;343:1942; Ann IM 2000;132:738,743; Med Let 1999;41:33

All types of roughly equal efficacy and have similar dropout rates (Am J Med 2000;108:54); taper shorter acting ones over 2–4 wk to avoid withdrawal side efects (Rx Let 1999;6:31)

Mixed Serotonin and Norepinephrine Reuptake Inhibitors:

Tricyclics: Start low and increase by 25 mg q 4–5 d; give 2–3 h before hs; 80% improve sleep within 1st wk; check levels 10–12 h after last dose; if asx after 6 mo, taper by halving dose × 4 mo, then tapering by 25 mg/wk to avoid cholinergic hyperactivity w abrupt withdrawal. Safe in pregnancy (Nejm 1997;336:258). Levels incr by aging, weight loss, inflammatory diseases, cimetidine, morphine, steroids, alkaline urine; depressed by smoking, hyperlipidemia, barbiturates, anticonvulsants, acid urine, and antipsychotics hence BEWARE use w phenothiazines, which incr TCA levels, especially Mellaril, which lengthens QT intervals as well and thus can cause ventricular arrhythimias (Med Let 1978;20:49). Appetite stimulated by amoxapine, amitriptyline, and doxepin; suppressed by protriptyline, imipramine, and desipramine. Adverse effects: all can worsen heart block and incr arrythmias like class I antiarrythmics slightly (Am J Med 2000;108:2); overdose; anticholinergic effects of dry mouth, urinary retention, blurry vision, and sexual dysfunction

- Amoxapine (Asendin); quite stimulating especially of appetite, cf Ritalin. Adverse effect: metabolite can cause tardive dyskinesia
- Amitriptyline (Elavil); start at 50 mg hs, increase by 25 mg q 2–3 d to 150 mg qd; much lower doses in elderly, eg, 10 mg po qd
- Clomipramine (Anafranil) 50–150 mg po qd, also helps obsessive/compulsive behaviors especially trichotillomania (Nejm 1989; 321:497). Adverse effects: seizures, much anticholinergic effect, weight gain, sexual dysfunction
- Cyclobenzaprine (Flexeril) 10 mg po qd-tid, esp for muscle and neuropathic pain, rarely used for depression and no studies to show it is an effective antidepressant
- Desipramine (Norpramin); same dosing as amitriptyline; least sedating, fewer anticholinergic side effects

- Doxepin (Sinequan); sedating; use this or trazodone (Desyrel) in elderly (UCLA 1/92)
- Imipramine (Tofranil) 200 mg po qd
- Nortriptyline (Pamelor, Aventyl) 100 mg po qd, titrate to blood levels of 50–150 ngm/cc
- Protriptyline (Vivactil) 5 mg tid–10 mg qid po
- Venlafaxine (Effexor) 25–100 mg po bid or as Effexor XR (Jama 2000;283:3082) 37.5 mg gradually incr to 75–225 mg po qd; effective for anxiety, better than buspirone (Rx let 1999;6:22). Adverse effects: activation and hypertension, also occur × 3 d w cessation of drug (Rx Let 1998;5:9)

Tetracyclics:
- Maprotiline (Ludiomil)

Serotonin Antagonists:
- Mirtazapine (Remeron) (Med Let 1996;38:113) 15–45 mg po hs. Adverse effects: sedation, wgt gain, rarely agranulocystosis; $60/mo for 30 mg qd

MAO Inhibitors: (Rarely prescribed, because of food restrictions and many drug interactions, especially bad ones w tricyclics):
- Phenelzine (Nardil) 15 mg qd × 1, 30 mg qd × 3 d, then 30 mg b-tid, avoid specific foods (Med Let 1980;22:38); BEWARE concomitant use of meperidine (Demerol) and all opiates, which cause severe sedation; sexual dysfunction
- Tranylcypromine (Parnate); no drowsiness or sedation

Selective Serotonin Reuptake Inhibitors (SSRIs): Except for fluvoxamine, all useful for panic d/o, depression, bulimia, and OCD; all free of anticholinergic side effects, safer if taken in OD than but equal in efficacy to the tricyclics (BMJ 1993;306:683); safe in pregnancy (Jama 1998;279:609; Nejm 1997;336:258) in 1st and 2nd trimesters but at least w fluoxetine, incr perinatal cmplc in 3rd trimester as well as low birth wgt (Nejm 1996;335:1011); and safer to use post-MI than tricyclics (Jama1998;279:287); all have half lives <24 hr except fluoxetine, which is 90 hr (Mayo Cl Proc 1994;69:1069). Adverse effects: nausea, diarrhea, sleepiness, bruxism (Rx Let 2000;7:16), sexual dysfunction in 70% of both men and women (Rx Let 1997;4:31), weight loss esp w fluoxetine; drug interactions: incr TCAs, haloperidol, clozapine, warfarin, metoprolol, serotonin syndromes esp w fluoxetine (anxiety, restlessness, diarrhea, sexual dysfunction, insomnia, and nausea; all decrease w continued use) worse w MAOIs; all ~$66±/mo

- Citalopram (Celexa) (Med Let 1998;40:113) 20–80 mg po qd; adv effects: interacts w MAO inhibitors, incr levels of β blockers, TCAs; levels incr by cimetidine; long QT at high doses
- Fluoxetine (Prozac, Sarafem) (Nejm 1994;331:1354; Med Let 1990;32:83) 20–40 mg po qd in am, 60 mg q 1 wk may work, long-acting forms not worth it (Med Let 2001;43:27); 7 d half-life, takes 3 wk to plateau, hence after started can go to 40–60 mg q 1 wk (Rx Let 1999;6:27); an "upper," even 20 mg qd may be too much for some patients; not too useful in the elderly; generic in late 2001
- Fluvoxamine (Luvox) (Med Let 1995;37:13) 50–200 mg po hs; for obsessive-compulsive disorder. Adverse effects: serotonergic ones as above, dangerous ODs w hypotension and seizures, toxic epidermal necrolysis (Lancet 1993;342:304), slows metabolism of benzodiazepines, warfarin, phenytoin, propranolol, theophylline, tricyclics, etc.
- Sertraline (Zoloft) (Med Let 1992;34:47) 50–150 mg po qd, or even 200 mg (Jama 1998;280:1665); used often in elderly
- Paroxetine (Paxil) (Med Let 1993;35:24) 20–40 mg po qd

Serotonin Antagonists and Reuptake Inhibitors:
- Netazodone (Serzone) (Med Let 1995;37:33) 100–300 mg po bid; similar to trazodone. Adverse effects: sedating, atropine effects
- Trazodone (Desyrel) 100–300 mg qd, 25–100 mg in elderly for sleep; mixed serotonergic effects; no anticholinergic problems; can use w SSRIs especially if sleep disturbance, 3.5 hr half life. Adverse effects: priapism (Med Let 1984;26:35); more sedating than tricyclics; may increase phenytoin, digoxin levels; appetite suppression; postural hypotension sometimes; w *Ginko,* can cause coma (Rx Let 2000;7:53)

Dopamine and Norepinephrine Reuptake Inhibitors:
- Bupropion (Wellbutrin) (Med Let 1993;35:25) 100 mg po tid; no anticholinergic side effects. Adverse effects: agitation, insomnia; sometimes anticholinergic sx; seizures, esp at doses >450 mg qd and esp if h/o bulimia

Other:
- Carbamazepine (Tegretol) ~1000 mg po qd; used for hypomania especially in rapid cycling bipolar pts; $37/mo generic, $52/mo trade
- Lithium (Eskalith) (Nejm 1994;331:591) 0.3–0.6 gm po tid to serum level = 0.8–1.0 mEq/L 12 h after last dose (Nejm 1989;

321:1489); usually used for bipolar patients with prominent manic component to illness, good response for acute mania in 70%. Adverse effects: teratogenic; many drug interactions; goiter in 15%, lowered T_3T_4 with elevated TSH in 5%, similar to I_2 load; worsens COPD (Nejm 1983;308:319); nephrogenic DI in 20–70%, rx with amiloride 5–10 mg bid (Nejm 1985;312:408) or other thiazide; hypokalemia and PVCs (Nejm 1972;287:867); elevated calcium and PTH (Ann IM 1977;86:63); tremor; NV + D; $8/mo generic, $20/mo for Eskalith at 1200 mg qd

- Valproate (Depakote)/divalproex (Depakene) (Med Let 1994; 36:74) 250–750 mg po b-tid to level of 50–125 μgm/cc; 1st choice for prevention of manic sx and used for hypomania especially in rapid cycling. Adverse effects: nausea and vomiting, wgt gain, rash, alopecia, ataxia. $94/mo for 1500 mg qd

- St. John's wort?? (Med Let 1997;39:107) 300 mg po tid; potency and efficacy still unclear, but meta-analysis suggests as efficacious as TCAs (ACP J Club 1999;130:60) for mild depression, vs no effect in RDBCT (Jama 2001;285:1978); a MAO inhibitor (Pharmacopsychiatry 1997;30:supplmnt 2:108). Adverse effects: photosensitivity and secondary neurotoxicity can cause neuropathic pain in sun exposed areas (Rx Let 1998;5:68); incr cataracts (Rx Let 1999;6:51); drug interactions (Med Let 2000; 42:56; Rx Let 2000;7:18) w digoxin, warfarin, SSRIs, indinavir; possibly w oral contraceptives (decr effect), losartan, theophylline, tricyclics

18.2 DISEASES

ALCOHOLISM AND WITHDRAWAL

Nejm 1998;338:592; 1989;321:442; Ann IM 1984;100:405

Cause: Multifactorial including genetic (cross-fostering studies—Nejm 1988;318:180) and/or behavioral characteristics leading to addiction

Epidem: M:F = 4:1. Acute and chronic complications of alcohol may occur more often in women than men due not to size differences but to gastric mucosa alcohol dehydrogenase activity (Nejm 1990; 322:95)

Pathophys: GI and pancreatic acute and chronic toxicity (Ann IM 1981; 95:198). Withdrawal sx due to incr noradrenergic activity (Ann IM 1987;107:875) and long-term changes in GABA and glutamate receptors

Sx: H/o significant trauma (70%—Ann IM 1984;101:847), eg, motor vehicle accident (Nejm 1987;317:1262)

Standardized questionnaires (Ann IM 1998;129:353; Jama 1998; 280:166; 1994;272:1782) like MAST, AUDIT, TWEAK (*T*olerance measured by ability to "hold" ≥6 drinks or "high" on ≥3 drinks; *W*orried friends; *E*ye openers; *A*mnesia hx; *K*ut down plans), and the short test CAGE questions (have you tried to *C*ut down; are you *A*nnoyed by criticism of your drinking; do you sometimes feel *G*uilty about your drinking; and do you sometimes have an *E*ye-opener drink in the morning?—Jama 1984;252:1905). TWEAK score ≥2 is 87% sens and specif in women, 95% sens and 56% specif in men; scores ≥3, less sens and more specific. CAGE score ≥2 has 74% sens, 91% specif (Jama 1994;272:1782; Ann IM 1991;115:774).

Upper limit of alcohol consumption not assoc w problems is <4 drinks qd and <14–17/wk for men, and <3 drinks qd and <7–12/wk for women (Jama 1995;276:1964; Am J Pub Hlth 1995;85:823)

Si:

Crs:

Cmplc: Hypokalemia, hypomagnesemia, hypocalcemia, hypoglycemia, hypophosphatemia, ketoacidosis, respiratory alkalosis (Nejm 1993; 329:1927)

Increased mortality from cirrhosis, accidents, cancer, respiratory illness when >4 drinks qd (Am J Pub Hlth 1993;83:805; Ann IM 1984; 101:847); smoking-related mortality continues even if stop drinking (Jama 1996;275:1097)

Pneumonia, due to diminished macrophage function, ciliary action, and polymorphonuclear wbc responses (Nejm 1970;282:123)

Sudden death (arrhythmias) and strokes (Curr Concepts Cerebro Dis 1986;21:24; Nejm 1986;315:1041)

Delirium tremens (DTs) including prior h/o often, agitation, tremor, disorientation, delirium, hallucinations, seizures, hyperthermia (rectal temp); 10–20% mortality

Wernicke's encephalopathy and Korsakoff's psychosis (p 240)

Seizures, as often during drinking as in withdrawal? (Nejm 1988;319:666) whenever alcohol levels are rapidly falling

Vitamin A deficiency causing impaired night vision (Ann IM 1978;88:622)

Lab:

Chem: Blood alcohol level >0.08 mg% = legal intoxication, but levels often >0.02% in alcoholics w few overt si of intoxication; fatty acid ethyl esters pos up to 24 h later (Jama 1996;276:1152)

LFTs up, acutely GGTP, chronically AST (SGOT), GGTP, alk phos

Xray: CT scan of head for alcohol seizures only if evident head trauma or focal si's (Ann IM 1981;94:519)

Rx: Primary prevention: screen with GGTP, if >50 U/L, educate once, repeat in 1 month and 1 yr (Prev Med 1991;20:518); or ask re number of drinks/wk, if >14 for men, >11 for women, then educate q 1 mo × 2, this strategy decr alcohol intake by 1/3 = 1/2 over 1 yr (Jama 1997;277:1040)

Secondary prevention (Am J Med 2000;108:263; Jama 1998;279:1230): structured treatment program should include anticipatory guidance by primary doctor, "12-step" program (AA), and perhaps prophylaxis (Nejm 1999;340:1482) w

- Naltrexone (ReVia) (Med Let 1995;37:64) 50–100 mg po qd; an opiate antagonist, hepatic metabolism; not effective by DBCT (Nejm 2001;345:1734); $5/d for ReVia
- Disulfiram (Antabuse) 250 mg qd (Ann IM 1989;111:943), cheap
- Acamprosate (Campral) (Jama 1999;281:1318) 1300–2000 mg po qd divided; cheap
- Odansetron (Zotran) (Jama 2000;284:963,1016) 4 μgm/kg po bid helps if alcoholism onset <25 yr old by blocking 5-HT receptors
- Tiapride (not yet available)

Alcoholics Anonymous (AA), detoxification programs, etc.; prognosis for rehabilitation better after motor vehicle accident (Nejm 1987;317:1262). W safe stable home situation, outpatient rx as good as inpatient (Nejm 1989;320:358). Nonhospital residential programs adequate and cheaper (Nejm 1990;323:844, Institute of Medicine recommendations re drug and alcohol rehab policies). Later controlled drinking controversial, <2% can safely pull it off (Nejm 1985;312:1678)

PSYCHIATRY

Rx any depression (p 692) (Jama 1996;275:761) w SSRIs
of withdrawal (Jama 1997;278:145):
 of DTs: hospitalize, iv diazepam 1mg/min, or lorazepam 1mg/5 min
  until BP and agitation decr
 of lesser degrees of withdrawal:
 • Thiamine 100–200 mg im/iv bid × 2 d +
 • Benzodiazepines:
  Lorazepam (Ativan) 2 mg im q 1 hr or po q 2 hr to control si and
   sx, to 12 mg max
  Chlordiazepoxide (Librium) 100 mg po/im q 6 h × 4 doses, then
   q 8 h × 3 doses, then q 12 h × 2 doses, then hs once, then
   stop; or 25–100 mg po q 4–6 h prn scoring system like below
   results in hospital d/c >2 d sooner (Jama 1994;272:519);
   beware oversedation that takes days to recover from since has
   a 36+ h half-life, or
  Oxazepam (Serax) 30 mg po q 6 h × 7 d (Am J Psych 1989;146:
   617); or 30 mg po q 4 h × 6 doses, then q 6 h × 4 doses, then
   q 8 h × 3 doses, then q 12 h×2 doses, then hs once, then
   stop; or 0–45 mg po q 4 h (q 2 h if no improvement after last
   dose) based on various scoring systems (Br J Addict 1989;84:
   1353) that rate tachycardia (>100), hypertension (>140/90),
   sweating, tremor, fever (99.6°F [37.6°C]), insomnia,
   agitation, disorientation, and hallucinations (Clin Pharmacol
   Ther 1989;34:822), or
  Diazepam (Valium) (Clin Pharmacol Ther 1983;34:822)
   0–15 mg iv/im/po q 2–4 h based on a scoring system as above;
   long half-life like chlordiazepoxide
 • Ancillary meds:
  Atenolol 50–100 mg po qd (Nejm 1985;313:905)
  Carbamezepine
  Clonidine (Ann IM 1987;107:874)
  MgSO$_4$ 50% solution, 2 cc iv/im q 8 h × 2 d
  Thiamine 100 mg po/im tid × 3d
of seizures: lorazepam (Ativan) 2 mg iv after 1st seizure reduces 25%
 recurrence rate within next 6 hr to 3% and over 48 hr from 32% to
 4% (Nejm 1999;340:915)

ANXIETY

Jama 2001;286:450; 2000;283:2573; Nejm 1993;329:631; 1989;321:1209

Cause: Genetic component perhaps; incr in families w h/o alcoholism

Types:
- Generalized anxiety (most common)
- Panic disorder (PD)
- Phobias
- Obsessive-compulsive disorder
- Posttraumatic stress disorder from severe stress in adult life or childhood

Epidem: Panic disorder lifetime prevalence = 1.5–3.5%; 2/3 of the time pts have another primary psychiatric dx, especially depression

Pathophys: In PD, dysfunctional brain neurotransmitter alarm system (Jama 2000;283:2573)

Sx: Generally onset in 20's; sx include hyperventilation, palpitations, pains, fears, flushes; h/o long medical workups, agoraphobia (in 50% if ots w OD)

Panic attack: unfounded sudden fear, terror, sense of impending doom with associated somatic manifestations; defined as 3 such attacks within 3 wk

Post-traumatic stress disorder: onset either immediate within 1–2 d of event or delayed mos–yrs, manifest by numbing and avoidance sx (Oklahoma bombing—Jama 1999;282:755); seen especially in wounded veterans and incest/abuse victims; manifest by hyperalertness and difficulty falling asleep (Nejm 1987;317:1630); often associated w confounding chemical abuse

Si: Sympathomimetic si's; obsessive-compulsive actions (Nejm 1989;321: 540) in OCD types

Crs: Often chronic and disabling

Cmplc: Suicide in panic disorder debatably

r/o alcohol and/or substance abuse; **caffeine addiction/withdrawal,** especially with headache and fatigue (Jama 1994;272:1043,1065; Nejm 1992;327:1109)

Lab:

Rx: (Nejm 1993;328:1398; Med Let 1991;33:43)

SSRIs in low doses: sertraline (Zoloft) or fluvoxamine (Luvox) (only FDA approved SSRI in children) for generalized anxiety (Rx Let

2001;8:28), panic d/o, OCD even in children and adolescents
(Nejm 2001;344:1279; RCT—Jama 1998;280:1752), PTSD, and
social phobias

Psychotherapy only if significant intercurrent psychological issues
present

Kava (J Clin Psych 2000;20:84) for generalized types

Buspirone 5–10 mg t-qid to 60 mg/d max; can prevent emergence of
but not acute sx; only for generalized types

Venlaxatine (Effexor)

of social phobias:

> Propranolol for stage fright type of anxiety, 40 mg 1.5 hr before
> stress, can improve performance (Med Let 1984;26:61); also
> helps violent outbursts in the elderly (M. Beers UCLA 1/92)
>
> SSRIs (Brit J Psych 1999;175:120; Jama 1998;280:708) like
> paroxetine (Paxil) 20–50 mg po qd
>
> Phenelzine (Nardil)
>
> Cognitive behavioral rx

of simple phobias (eg, of animals): desensitization

of OCDs:

> SSRIs in incr doses
>
> Clomipramine (Anafranil) 50–250 mg po qd, which helps obsessive/
> compulsive behaviors especially trichotillomania (Nejm 1989;
> 321:497) as do SSRIs

of panic disorder:

> Cognitive-behavioral therapy helps, adds to imipramine rx (Jama
> 2000;283:2529)
>
> Antidepressants like:
>
> > Fluoxetine (Prozac) or other SSRI in low, not usual, doses (Med
> > Let 1994;36:89), perhaps w buspirone
> >
> > Monoamine oxidase inhibitor is as effective as benzodiazepines
> > for some anxious patients even if no depression
> >
> > Benzodiazepines, eg, alprazolam (Xanax) or clonazepam
> > (Klonopin) for panic disorder, but addicting so taper (pts
> > often resistant) after tricyclics, SSRIs, or MAOIs on board
> > (Rx Let 1998;5:52)

ANOREXIA NERVOSA

Ann IM 2001;134:148; Nejm 1999;340:1092; Ann IM 1986;105:790

Cause:

Epidem: Women:men = 20:1; associated with bulimia and depression; prevalence of bulimia + anorexia = 5–10% of young women; prevalence incr w family h/o addictive disorders

Pathophys: Amenorrhea, from wgt loss-induced hypopituitarism with low LH and FSH (D. Federman 3/85); develops when <90% ideal body wgt (IBW = 100 lb at 60 in, + 5 lb for each inch over that)

Sx: Over 25% weight loss; onset before age 17; laxative use; diuretic use; excessive exercising; amenorrhea; always think selves too fat no matter how thin; secretive eating

Si: Lanugo hair; thin to cachectic

Crs: 50% progress to chronic bulimarexia; 9% mortality

Cmplc: Suicide (2–5%); depression; osteoporosis/bone loss (Ann IM 2000; 133:790); CHF (starvation—Nejm 1985;313:1457)

r/o Addison's disease (Nejm 1996;334:46)

Lab:

Chem: Hypokalemia; amylase elevated, sometimes due to pancreatitis, but many times due to salivary origin (lipase and pancreatic fraction normal—Ann IM 1987;106:50); hypophosphatemia

Noninv: EKG at regular intervals (Ann IM 1985;102:49) to detect myocardiopathy; long QT

Rx: Inpatient or OP behavioral program only effective rx;
Adjunctive:

Metoclopramide (Reglan) 10 mg ac and hs may return gastric emptying to normal and help psychiatric state (Ann IM 1983;98:86)

Vitamin D and calcium to prevent osteoporosis

BULIMIA

Nejm 1999;340:1092; Ann IM 1987;107:71

Cause: Self-induced vomiting; often use emetine and other meds

Epidem: Women:men >20:1; usually associated with anorexia; prevalence among young women = 4–8%; 2% of college women are bulimic (Am J Pub Hlth 1988;78:1322)

Associated w childhood sexual abuse in 1/3 (Am J Publ Hlth 1996; 86:1082)

Pathophys: Diminished cholecystokinin production causes decr satiety (Nejm 1988;319:683)

Sx: Onset later than anorexia; compulsive eating binges followed by intense anxiety/guilt leading to purging

Si: Callus on back of hand from emesis induction; dental caries from gastric fluids on teeth; enlarged salivary glands; thin or normal weight

Crs:

Cmplc: CHF from starvation and ipecac myocardiopathy and myopathy (Nejm 1985;313:1457); aspiration pneumonias and Mallory-Weiss tears; hypokalemia and sudden death due to long QT syndrome (Ann IM 1985;102:49)

Lab:

Chem: Amylase elevated, sometimes due to pancreatitis, but often due to salivary origin (lipase and pancreatic fraction normal—Ann IM 1987;106:50); urinary emetine levels (Nejm 1996;334:47); lytes show: hypoK$^+$, high HCO_3, normal anion gap acidosis w laxative use

Noninv: EKG at some regular interval (Ann IM 1985;102:49)

Rx: Metoclopramide (Reglan) 10 mg ac and hs may return gastric emptying to normal and help psych state (Ann IM 1983;98:86)

Imipramine; may work by increasing pc cholecystokinin and therefore satiety (Nejm 1988;319:683)

Fluoxetine (Prozac)

Psychotherapy

SCHIZOPHRENIA

Nejm 1994;330:681; 1993;329:555

Cause: Polygenic; significant genetic component by twin studies (Ann IM 1969;70:107), 10% for fraternal twins, 50% for identical twins; also multifactorial nongenetic contributors that cause abnormalities in neural circuits and cognitive mechanisms (Njem 1999;340:645)

Epidem: (Nejm 1999;340:603) <1% of general population; incidence incr × 10 if parent or sibling has schizophrenia; incr urban prevalence may be artifact of care source distribution; and, controverially, if born in Feb or March?

Pathophys: Psychosis (hallucinations, delusions, disorder in form of thought) linked to incr brain dopaminergic activity; incidence and symptomatology similar across cultures

Limbic and temporal lobe subtle atrophy (Nejm 1992;327:604; 1990; 322:789) specifically demonstrable by MRI in the L hippocampus-amygdala and L posterior superior temporal gyrus (Nejm 1992; 327:604)

Sx: Bizarre, irrational behavior

Si: Inappropriate affect, though may be entirely appropriate to delusions and hallucinations; loose associations; primary process (nonrational, magical, childlike); diminished sociality, drive, and emotional responsiveness; ambivalence, love-hate oscillations

Crs: Recurrent psychotic episodes usually beginning at age 17–24 yr, with residual sx between psychotic episodes

Cmplc: r/o chemical abuse and/or dependence, delirium (p 573), prescription drug toxicy (long list—Med Let 1998;40:21), bipolar manic disorder, brief reactive psychosis, dissociative disorders including very rare **dissociative identity disorder** or multiple personality disorder (voices are those of the other personalities); metachromatic leukodystrophy

Lab:

Rx: (p 690) (Ann IM 2001;134:47; Nejm 1996;334:34; Med Let 1991;33:47)

1st:
- Olanzapine (Zyprexa) 10–20 mg/d
- Risperidone (Risperdal) (Med Let 1994;36:33), start at 0.5–1 mg po bid, increase to 3 mg po bid in 3 d
- Quetiapine

2nd: Other antipsychotics (p 690) like chlorpromazine (Thorazine), fluphenazine (Prolixin), etc., and haloperidol (Haldol)

3rd: Clozapine (Clozaril) (Med Let 1993;35:16) 12.5 mg po qd gradually increasing to 300–400 mg qd, overall costs similar to usual antipsychotics but benefits a little better (Nejm 1997; 337:809)

PSYCHIATRY

DEPRESSION/BIPOLAR DISORDERS
(Manic-Depressive Illness)

Ann IM 2001;134:47; Nejm 2000;343:1942; 1993;329:628; 1991;325:633

Cause: Genetic, autosomal dominant suggested by strong family correlations in major and bipolar types, HLA-linked on chromosome #6 (Nejm 1981;305:1301; Jama 1972;222:1624) at least in some bipolar types

Epidem: Increased incidence in postpartum female, late middle age and elderly, pts w family h/o alcoholism. Major depressive disorder onset in teens and 20s w recurrence in adulthood in 2/3 (Jama 1999;281:1707). Lifetime incidence 15–25%

Pathophys: ACTH, TSH, sleep studies, and neurotransmitter abnormalities to explain cause keep being proposed and discounted

Sx: 2+ wk of function impairing sx including depressed mood or loss of interest, plus changes in at least 3 of the following: weight, sleep w early morning awakening, activity level, energy, ability to think, or suicidal ideation

Somatic complaints alone or w complaints of depression, guilt, and other psychological sx (Nejm 1999;341:1329)

Ask re: suicidal thoughts (no incr risk of precipitating those thoughts if ask), previous suicide attempts, sleep disturbance lasting ≥2 wk, guilt feelings ≥2 wk, hopelessness (1 or more such sx have an 84% sens—Jama 1994;272:1757)

Si: Flat affect, sad, irritable, panic attacks; mania in bipolar d/o

Crs: Variable; may be chronic relapsing

Cmplc: Suicide, alcoholism, mania; lower bone mineral density in women (Nejm 1996;335:1176)

r/o secondary causes like stress, bereavement, illness, alcohol/drug use; **seasonal affective disorder** (SAD) (Jama 1993; 270:2717); M/F:1/3–4, especially in northern climates in winter; sx of lethargy, incr sleep, decr libido, weight and appetite changes; rx w half hr tid 10,000 lux light box ($400), × 2 h qd (Am Fam Phys 1988;38:173), or get outdoors at noon; many pts may have latent bipolar d/o and rx may precipitate mania

Lab:

Rx: Preventive evaluation of alcohol use, suicidality (Nejm 1997:337:910)

Brief, focused cognitive behavioral analysis, psychotherapy as good as meds and also provides additive benefit to drug rx? (uncontrolled trials: Nejm 2000;342:1462, Arch Gen Psych 1999;56:829) but probably not for severe or bipolar types

Medications (Ann IM 2001;134:47) (see p 692); rx for 6 mos after remit (Am J Psych 1998;155:1247):

1st: SSRIs, after 6–9 mo successful rx, maintenance reduces recurrence from 25% to 5% (NNT-1 = 5 by DBRCT—Jama 1998;280:1665), adjunctive benzo's for 1st 4–6 wk helpful (J Affect Disord 2001; 65:173)

2nd: Buproprion (Welbutrin); nefazodone (Serzone), Venlataxine (Effexor), TCAs

3rd: Combinations of TCAs, SSRIs, and MAOIs

4th: Electroshock therapy q 2–3 d × 2–3 wk is most effective antidepressant especially if suicidal or elderly (Nejm 1984;311:163); very safe; follow w lithium + nortriptyline to maintain (Jama 2001;285:1299); only relative contraindication is intracranial mass; adv effect: transient memory loss

Others: Trazodone or buspirone 10–20 mg po bid possibly as adjunct to SSRIs

T_3 (Cytomel) 25–50 µgm po qd as adjunct to SSRIs or tricyclics

Pindolol (Visken) 2.5 mg po tid perhaps as adjunct to SSRIs

Gabapentin (Neurontin) (Rx Let 1999;6:41) perhaps

Topiramate (Topamax), low dose 25–75 mg po qd esp in obese

of mania (Med Let 2000;42:114), in order of choice:

1st: Valproic acid to levels 12 hr after last dose of 50–125 µgm/cc probably more effective than lithium, certainly as prophylaxis

2nd: Carbamazepine

3rd: Lithium 6–900 mg po qd titrated to therapeutic blood levels, if manic component, or augmentation of primary antidepressants if they alone fail (J Clin Psychopharm 1999;19:427)

4th: Lamotrigine (Lamictal) perhaps for mania and depression in bipolar d/o

SOMATIZATION DISORDER
("Hysteria," "Neuresthenia")

Ann IM 1997;126:747; Jama 1997;278:673; Nejm 1986;314:1407

Cause:

Epidem: 0.2–2% of women and assoc w positive family h/o same; <0.2% in men

Pathophys:

Sx: Onset before age 30 yr; depressive sx; lifetime h/o 12$^+$ (in male) or 14$^+$ (in female) unexplained sx, often pain. Often include or merge w multiple functional GI disorders like globus hystericus, dysphagia, dyspepsia, irritable bowel syndrome, etc. (Ann IM 1995;123:668)

Si: Normal exam

Crs: Lifelong

Cmplc: Hospitalization, procedures, and false-positive test results

  r/o **hysteria,** a manifestation of psychosomatic or somatiform illness including conversion reactions like hysterical paralysis or blindness, manifest by a single bizarre sx unlike the polysymptomatic pattern of somatization d/o; **somatiform disorder** which has fewer sx and later onset, patient will not accept reassurance and is associated with alexithymia, an inability to discern or describe feelings (Nejm1985;312:690); **hypochondriasis** (Nejm 1981;304:1394), which does respond at least transiently to reassurance; other functional somatic syndromes (p 834)

Lab: Minimal

Rx: Patient reassurance, see frequently, avoid testing as much as possible

PERSONALITY DISORDERS

  Jama 1994;272:1770

Cause: Genetics and environment

Epidem: Prevalence 6–10% of general population, ~50% of psych hospital pts

Pathophys: Pervasive lifelong character styles not viewed as pathological by patient (except in obsessive compulsive personality d/o), unlike neurotic sx, which are. Several may have less extreme pathology of axis I disorders, eg, schizophrenia, manic depressive disorders, etc.

Sx: Odd/eccentrics cluster: paranoid, schizoid, and schizotypal types

  Dramatic/emotional/erratic cluster: antisocial, borderline, histrionic, and narcissistic types

  Anxious/fearful cluster: avoidant, dependent, ob/compulsive types

Si:

Crs: Onset in adolescence

Cmplc: r/o active axis I disorders, neurosis (pt can identify problem and complains about it), and chemical dependency chronic or in early recovery

Lab:

Rx: Time-limited benzodiazepines for anxiety

of self-sacrifice (dependent, passive-aggressive, and depressive types): listen to sx and anticipate pt ambivalence re improvement; plus antidepressants and carbamazepine for borderlines

of manipulative/antisocial types: firm limits

of dependency and overdemandingness (dependent and borderline types): empathetic recognition of pt's need for reassurance and anxiety about being alone; plus limit-setting consistency, clarity and structure, and impulse-stabilizing meds like lithium

of obsessive/compulsiveness: respect need for control by providing information, eg, test results ASAP, plus engaging pt in rx plan; meds: SSRIs, clomipramine not effective unlike in OCD

of dramatization (histrionic type): disallow inappropriate familiarity w a respectful professional manner without shortening time w pt

of self-importance (narcissistic type): nondefensive acceptance of earlier consultation and referral

of detachment and paranoia (schizoid, schizotypal, avoidant types): allow privacy, plus antipsychotics

PSYCHIATRY

Chapter 19
Pulmonary Diseases

D. K. Onion

19.1 INFECTIONS

PNEUMONIA
(Nejm 1995;333:1618)

Cause:
Age <1 month, commonly: *Escherichia coli,* group B strep
  less commonly: *Staphylococcus aureus,* RSV, *Enterobacter* spp.
1 mo–5 yr, commonly: RSV, parainfluenza virus, adenovirus
  less commonly: *Streptococcus pneumoniae, Chlamydia*
5–15 yr, commonly: influenza A, adenovirus
  less commonly: *Mycoplasma, S. pneumoniae*
Adults (%'s from Nejm above): *S. pneumoniae* (50%), viral including
  influenza A (10%), aspiration (8%), H. flu (6%; others feel much
  higher, up to 30%, depending on group), *S. aureus* (4%), gram
  negatives (6%), atypicals (15%) including *Mycoplasma* (4%) and
  Chlamydia (5%), which are higher >20%) in young adults, and
  Legionella (5%)
In elderly, prognosis bad if elevated BUN, hypotensive, respiratory rate
  >30 (Ann IM 1991;115:428)

Epidem: Much more common in immunosuppressed pts who constitute
  60% of hospital adm's for pneumonia

Sx: Cough, fever, dyspnea, sputum production, pleurisy

Si: T° (80%); RR >20 in adults; RR >40 age 1–5, >50 age 2–12 mo, >60
  under 2 mo, in children, 70% sens and specif (Arch Dis Child
  2000;82:41, 46); rales (80%), consolidation changes (30%),
  bronchial breath sounds, dullness, E to A changes

Cmplc: Empyema

Lab:

ABGs: Admit if pO$_2$ <60

Bact: Blood cultures (pos in 11% overall, in 67% w *S. pneumoniae*), sputum gram stain (50% pos *in S. pneumoniae*)

Hem: CBC

Xray: Chest, infiltrate, although false negs esp in 1st 24 h or w neutropenia or w PCP (10–30% neg); effusions (40%)

Rx: (Med Let 2001;43:65)

Outpts: erythromycin, azithromycin, or clarithromycin; or 2nd, tetracycline at least under age 60 w/o complicating illness (Jama 1997;278:32); or a 3rd generation fluoroquinolone w good antipneumococccal activity like levofloxacin, moxifloxacin, or gatifloxacin, especially if > age 60

Inpts: 3rd generation cephalosporin like ceftriaxone or cefotaxime w a macrolide; or a 3rd generation fluoroquinolone

ICU pts: imipenem + aminoglycoside if *Pseudomonas* possible (Med let 1996;38:25)

Aspiration (Nejm 2001;344:665): levofloxacin 500 mg qd, or ceftriaxone 1–2 gm qd

19.2 ASTHMA AND INTERSTITIAL LUNG DISEASE

ACUTE RESPIRATORY DISTRESS SYNDROME (Shock Lung)

Nejm 2000;342:1334

Cause: Direct injury: multiple agents including pneumonia, aspiration, inhalation injury (30–40% risk), salicylate poisoning (Ann IM 1981;95:405), fat emboli, drowning (p 15), hantavirus infection in southwestern US (Nejm 1994;330:949)

Indirect injury: bacterial sepsis (30–40% risk) most often from intra-abdominal gi perforation, pancreatitis, neurogenic (head trauma), drug OD, transfusions, bypass

Epidem: Incidence incr by risk factors (See Table 19.2.1):

If multiple risk factors, 25% get (Petty—Ann IM 1983;98:593); most develop within 48 h of getting risk factors; hypotension precedes in

Table 19.2.1

Risk	% with Risk Who Get ARDS
Disseminated IV coagulopathy	22
Cardiopulmonary bypass	2
Burns	2
Bacteremia	4
Hypertransfusion	5
ICU pneumonia	12
Aspiration	35

90%. Chronic alcohol abuse doubles risk and mortality (Jama 1996; 275:50)

Pathophys: Normal pressure pulmonary edema from capillary leak (Nejm 1982;306:900). Assoc w decr levels of pulmonary urokinase, which causes increased fibrin deposition and scarring (Nejm 1990;322: 890), elevated cytokines and other inflammatory proteins, depressed interleukins and interleukin receptor availability

Sx: Dyspnea

Si: Hypoxia, tachypnea; PCWP <18 mm Hg

Crs: Substantial mortality ~45% (Jama 1995;273:306), usually not respiratory

Cmplc: Barotrauma, especially if peak pressures >70 cm water for more than a day. Pulmonary fibrosis in 30%

r/o CHF, *Pneumocystis carinii* and other overwhelming opportunistic infections

Lab:

ABGs: Hypoxia; $P_aO_2/F_iO_2 \leq 200$

Bact: Bronchopulmonary lavage for pathogens

Xray: Chest shows diffuse bilateral pulmonary infiltrates starting perihilar within 24 h, often looks like CHF; may progress to "white out"

CT shows patchy involvement, the extent of which correlates w ABGs; also can show occult abscesses or barotrauma

Rx: Treat underlying disease; Swan-Ganz monitoring of PCWP and cardiac output; avoid fluid overload

Newer ventilator modes like lower volumes and permissive hypercapnia, inverse I/E, pressure control; PEEP when on ventilator, 0–30 cm water, can't use preventively (Nejm 1984;311:281,323);

debate re max and minimal settings parameters (Nejm 1998;338: 341,347,355,385); increases in PEEP cause decreases in cardiac output due to left shift of interventricular septum (Nejm 1981; 304:387) as well as diminished venous return and elevated pulmonary vascular resistance, which increase R to L shunt in 15% of the population w a potential ASD (Ann IM 1993;119:886)

Nitric oxide inhalation improves V/Q mismatch and arterial pO_2, but unclear if improves survival (Nejm 1993;328:399,431)

Steroids (Nejm 1987;317:1565) and aerosolized surfactant (Nejm 1996;334:1417) no help

ASTHMA (Chronic Eosinophilic Bronchitis)

Jama 1997;278:1855; Nejm 1992;327:1928; 1992;326:1540

Cause: Innumerable allergens including house dust mites, animal dander, actinomyces in car air conditioners (Nejm 1984;311:1619) and other mold spores, cockroach allergens (Nejm 1997;336:1356), and soybean dust (Nejm 1989;320:1097)

Genetic autosomal dominant susceptibility on chromosome #5, co-inherited w atopy susceptibility (Nejm 1995;333:894), as well as various mutations of interleukin 4 and its receptor (Nejm 1997; 337;1720:1766)

Epidem: 4–5% of US population increasing overall (Nejm 1994;331: 1584) and greater prevalence in low income groups (Nejm 1994; 331:1542)

Pathophys: Airway inflammation. Multiple types including exercise-induced (Nejm 1994;330:1362), cholinergic; as well as older distinctions between "extrinsic/familial atopic" plus exposure by age 1 to house mite antigens (Nejm 1990;323:502); and intrinsic/ idiopathic or infectious type associated with h/o bronchiolitis (10–30% will go on to asthma—Peds 1963;31:859), bronchiectasis, chronic bronchitis, and eventually COPD and emphysema. Some argue that all are really allergic (extrinsic) (Nejm 1989;320:271)

Morning wheezing due to circadian decrease in epinephrine and perhaps steroids as well (Nejm 1980;303:263). In extrinsics, IgE is sensitizing. ASA sensitivity is a direct action on kinin receptors by leukotrienes (Ann IM 1997;127:472). Food sulfites precipitate (Med Let 1986;28:74) as does first- and second-hand cigarette smoke (Nejm 1993;328:1665)

Sx: Quadrad of dyspnea, wheezing, cough, and sputum production; exercise and/or cold induction caused by respiratory tract heat loss directly and through evaporation in dry air (Nejm 1979;301:763) w pattern of bronchoconstriction lasting 20^+ min, 3–8 min after cessation of exercise (Nejm 1998;339:192); URI induction often; h/o occupational irritants; h/o allergen induction

Si: Wheezing, though may only have dyspnea on exertion or cough (Nejm 1979;300:633); dyspnea; cyanosis late; papilledema with acutely increased pCO_2; nasal polyps (30% of extrinsics); paradoxical pulse from "tethered heart" within the mediastinum, correlates with severity (Nejm 1973;288:66)

Crs: Annual decrement in FEV1% twice as great in asthmatics as in normals (Nejm 1998;339:1194). Overall mortality not incr (Nejm 1994;331:1537); acute attack prognosis worse if have diminished sensitivity to hypoxia (Nejm 1994;330:1329)

Cmplc: Respiratory arrest with respiratory acidosis, not arrhythmia, is most common mode of death (Nejm 1991;324:285); may be precipitated by exposure to airborne spores of *Alternaria alternata,* an IgE-producing allergen (Nejm 1991;324:359); NSAID, esp ASA, induced exacerbations in 5–10%, especially those with nasal polyps

Multifocal atrial tachycardia associated with hypoxia, aminophylline, and catechol rx (Nejm 1968;279:344)

In pregnancy (rv of management—Jama 1997;278:1865); associated with premature labor and RDS of newborn (Nejm 1985;312:742)

r/o vocal cord dysfunction, a frequent mimicker; conversion reaction? (Nejm 1983;308:1566); pulmonary emboli rarely (Nejm 1968;278:999); CHF, gastroesophageal reflux disease trigger

Lab:

Chem: Theophyllin levels to optimize dose

Hem: Eosinophil elevation correlates with severity (Nejm 1990;323:1033); sputum eosinophils also helpful to tell from COPD

Path: Mucous metaplasia of ciliated epithelial cells into goblet cells

PFTs: Before and after bronchodilators; FEV_1 % reductions. Intrinsics are rarely normal between attacks, but extrinsics are. Peak flows done at home by pt are useful in management

Skin testing: Basically documents if is atopic or not

Xray: Chest to r/o pneumothorax (Nejm 1983;309:336) and pneumonitis; atelectasis

Rx:

ACUTE (Med Let 1993;35:11):

Catechols (Med Let 1999;41:51), β2 selective, via inhaler with spacer or via nebulizer q 1 hr × 3; all equi-effective and similar cost ($30/mo) at 2 puffs q 3–6 h (Med Let 1987;29:11); use prn sx, not prophylactically:
- Albuterol (Proventil, Ventolin, and others) 0.1–0.15 mg/kg/dose up to 5 mg/dose if >40 lb q 2 h (Guidelines for Asthma, National Asthma Education Program, NIH 1991)
- Bitolterol (Tornalate)
- Terbutaline (Brethine) 250 μgm/puff

Steroid bolus, eg, 100–300 mg iv hydrocortisone, then q 6–8 h help (Nejm 1986;314:150), or prednisone 2 mg/kg po; but takes 6+ h, so no rush (Ann IM 1990;112:822); follow up with 8+ d of tapering prednisone to prevent acute recurrence (Nejm 1991;324:788) or 10 d level (40 mg po qd) rx w no taper (Lancet 1993;341:324); not inhaled steroids (Nejm 2000;343:689)

Fluids, depending on initial hydration status, as much as 360 cc/m^2 in first h, then 1500 cc/m^2/24 h; too much can cause pulmonary edema (Nejm 1977;297:592); with 2 meq Kcl/kg /24 h, 3 meq Na/kg/24 h, and NaCO$_3$ if pH < 7.35 and/or it takes >1 h to decrease pCO$_2$; O$_2$

Bipap or respirator if pH low and pCO$_2$ up and stays there despite initial efforts

Occasionally:
- Iprotropium 500 μgm (2.5 cc) neb clearly helps w severe exacerbations (Am J Med 1999;107:363; Ann Emerg Med 1999; 34:8; Nejm 1998;339:1030)
- MgSO$_4$ iv, perhaps (ACP J Club 1999;131:36)
- Aminophylline (Nejm 1993;119:1155,1216; Ann IM 1991;115: 241,323) 5.6 mg/kg load over 20–30 min then 0.5 mg/kg/h; but efficacy and safety in doubt (ACP J Club 2001;134:97)
- Anesthesia for status asthmaticus when all else fails

CHRONIC (Med Let 2000;42:19; 1999;41:5; Nejm 1989;321:1517):

Spacers with all inhalers; commercial or homemade w 500 cc plastic soda bottle (Lancet 1999;354:979), although may reduce compliance due to bulkiness and inconvenience

Monitor with peak flow meters at home and have pt take short crs of steroids anytime peak flow falls >2 std deviations below mean for 2 out of 3 consecutive days (Ann IM 1995;123:488)

Dust-free bedroom if skin test shows sensitive to dust or house mites; cover pillows and mattress, damp-mop, cover hot air vents, all produce dramatic effects (Peds 1983;71:418); and rarely, if this fails, desensitization to house dust mite antigens, danders, and pollens like ragweed (Am J Respir Crit Care 1995;151:969), which has minimal (Nejm 1996;334:501,531) to no benefit (Nejm 1997; 336:324)

Influenza vaccine safe and effective in adults and children (Nejm 2001; 345:1529)

Medications (NIH 1997 Guidelines—Rx Let 1997;4:20)

- Step 1 for mild, intermittent sx, short-acting β agonist (Nejm 1996;335:841; 1995;333:499) inhaler prn, like those listed above; associated with 2× increased death rates or even higher if use >2 canisters/mo (Nejm 1992;326:503; BMJ 1991;303:1426); in nebulizers, or metered dose inhalers and with inhaler devices for kids and uncooperative adults (Nejm 1986;315:870)

- Step 2 for mild persistent sx, prn short-acting β agonist inhaler as above + low dose inhaled steroids (Nejm 1995;332:868) like:

- Beclomethasone (Beclovent, Vanceril), triamcinolone (Azmacort), or flunisolide (Aerobid) metered dose inhaler (MDI) 2 puffs b-tid (Nejm 1991;325:388; 1989;321:1517; Med Let 1985;27:5) and safe long-term in children (Nejm 1993;329:1702) and adults? (Nejm 1994;331:700 vs 737), or

- Budesonide (Pulmicort, Turbuhaler) dry powder inhaler (DPI) (Med Let 1998;40:15) 200 µgm (low dose) to 800 µgm (high dose) qd-bid, also available in a very expensive nebulizer form (Med Let 2001; 43:6); adrenal suppression at 800 µgm bid (Am J Med 2000;108:269), and stunts growth for at least 1st yr in children (Nejm 2000;343:1054,1024,1113; 1997;337:1659)

- Fluticasone (Flovent) (Med Let 1996;38:84) MDI or as Flovent Rotadisk DPI (Med Let 1998;40:15) in 44 (low), 110, (med) and 220 µgm/inh doses

- Cromolyn canister (Med Let 1994;36:37) inhaler best choice in children (Nejm 1992;326:1540) and good in some adults, esp those w eosinophilia and incr IgE levels; $65/canister

- Nedocromil (Tilade) (Med Let 1994;36:37; 1993;35:62), similar to cromolyn; $37/canister

- Step 3 for moderate persistent sx, prn short acting inhaled β agonist as above + medium dose (2–3 puffs t-qid) inhaled steroids as above +
  - Long-acting β agonist like
    - Salmeterol (Serevent) (Med Let 1994;36:37) 2 puffs or 1 puff of powder form (50 μgm) bid; safe and effective in children (though not as effective as beclomethasone—Nejm 1997;327:1669) can be used w other prn short-acting catechols (Am J Med 1999;107:209); dangerous if used by pts as an acute rx drug (Jama 1995;273:967) and not as good as inhaled steroids for monoRx (Jama 2001;285;2583,2594,2637); $60/canister unlike most others, which are $20–30/canister. Also available combined w fluticasone 100, 250, or 500 μgm as Advair Diskas powder inhaler bid (Med Let 2001;43:31), $103/mo
    - Formoterol (Foradil) (Med Let 2001;43:39; Nejm 1997;337:1405) 1 puff pwdr (12 μgm) inhalation bid, or as needed (Lancet 2001;357:257)
  - Theophylline (Nejm 1997;337:1405,1412,1996;334:1380; Ann IM 1984;101:63) low dose therapy w only 250–375 mg bid despite low blood levels, used w inh steroids as good as long acting β agonists; cause bronchodilatation and incr diaphragmatic strength (Nejm 1989;320:1521); long-acting forms like Theo-dur etc., 400 mg qd, can be increased to 600–800 mg qd in q 3 d increments, monitor levels (Nejm 1983;308:760). Long duration of action so especially helpful for hs use (Ann IM 1993;119:1216). Levels are increased by BCPs, erythromycin, flu shots, allopurinol, cimetidine, coffee; decr by phenytoin, nicotine, phenobarbital. Toxic sx: seizures, tachycardia, NVD, tremor (Ann IM 1991;114:748); no impairment of school performance (Nejm 1992;327:926)
- Step 4 for severe persistent sx, high dose inh steroids like budesonide or others above + whatever it takes including po steroids.

Other meds:
- Leukotriene receptor antagonists (LRAs), perhaps as a Step 2 drug instead of inhaled steroids (Ann IM 1999;130:487; Nejm 1999;340:197):
  - Montelukast (Singulair) (Jama 1998;279:1181; Med Let 1998;40:71; Rx Let 1998;5:15) 5 mg (child over 6) chewable or 10 mg po (adult) tab hs, cost $70/mo

- Zafirlukast (Accolate) (Ann IM 1997;127:472; 1997;126:177, Med Let 1996;38:111) 20 mg po bid, not under age 12; less effective than inh steroids to decr inflammation; use esp for ASA induced asthma and exercise exacerbations in pts already on β agonists. Adverse effects: many drug interactions, causes or unmasks (Jama 1998;279:455) Churg-Strauss eosinophilic vasculitis, rare severe hepatitis (Ann IM 2000;133:964). $60/mo
- Zileuton (Zyflo) (Med Let 1997;39:18; Jama 1996;275:931; Ann IM 1993;119:1059) 600 mg po qid; $82/mo
- Ipratropium (Atrovent) inhaler alone or w albuterol (Combivent), esp in elderly or for β blocker induced disease
- Antibiotics if acute or chronic infection, like tetracycline, erythromycin (beware theophylline levels), Tm/S
- Proton pump inhibitor (Rx Let 2000;7:5) like omeprazole 40 mg po qd if any reflux sx or if is resistant to rx, although studies don't show benefit (ACP J Club 2000;132:15)
- Experimental: methotrexate po qd, experimental; allows lower doses of steroids in steroid-dependent patients (Ann IM 1990; 112:577; Nejm 1988;318:603) but no improvement in outcome (Ann IM 1991;114:352); chiropractic rx no help (Nejm 1998; 339:1013)

of exercise-induced asthma (Nejm 1998;339:192)
- Chronic inhaled steroids
- Inhaled albuterol, cromolyn, or nedocromil 15 min before exercise
- Salmeterol inhalation bid (Nejm 1998;339:141), but effect several hours out lost w continuous use
- LRAs like montelukast 10 mg po qd (Nejm 1998;339:147), better long term than salmeterol (Ann IM 2000:132:97)
- Heparin inhalation? (Nejm 1993;329:90)

OCCUPATIONAL ASTHMA (Byssinosis, Mill Fever, etc.)

Nejm 1995;333:107; Ann IM 1984;101:157

Cause: Byssinosis (Nejm 1987;317:805), bacterial endotoxin in cotton dust, hemp and flax dust, redwood sawdust, isocyanates, castor bean dust, etc. Occupational airborne exposures in factories that process raw products

Epidem: Very common, especially in cotton mill carding rooms where 70% of all workers will react within 1 yr of employment, 40–50% develop sx

Pathophys: Acute pulmonary bronchoconstriction starts on first work day of the week; later in the disease course, sx's persist further into the week. Occupational asthma is in contrast to allergic alveolitis where predominant inflammation is in alveoli (see below); mill fever may be a variant of allergic alveolitis; nylon flock workers' lung (Ann IM 1998;129:261)

Sx: Tight chest, dyspnea, cough for a day or 2 after a weekend off or other rest. Fever with mill fever

Si: Decreased ventilation capacity during the work day

Crs: Progressive bronchospasm may lead to irreversible obstruction

Cmplc: Pulmonary hypertension; severe COPD, even if leave work (Ann IM 1982;97:645)

Lab:

PFTs: Decreased FEV_1/FVC

Xray: Chest often normal, or shows hyperinflation

Rx: Prevent by improving dust removal. Pre- and post-Monday work FEV_1 checks

of sx, inhaled bronchodilators; avoid dust

ALLERGIC ALVEOLITIS/PNEUMONITIS

Ann IM 1976;84:406; Nejm 1973;288:233

Cause: Actinomycetes, rarely other fungi (cryptococcus, aspergillus), or any organic dust

Epidem: Occupational/recreational exposures in several possible ways: eg, exposure to wood dust (Nejm 1972;286:977); mushroom picker's disease; cork dust (suberosis); pigeon breeder's disease (Ann IM 1969;70:457); farmer's lung disease (distinct from silo filler's disease, which is caused by NO_2 direct toxicity causing pulmonary edema, rx with steroids); maple bark stripper's disease from cryptococcus under bark or in pulp wood (Ann IM 1970;72:907); bagassosis (moldy cane); air conditioners (Nejm 1970;283:271); aspergillosis, although more commonly causes a predominantly bronchoconstrictive disease rather than alveolitis (Ann IM 1970;72:395)

Pathophys: An individual is sensitized to 1–2 μm-sized antigens. Compared to allergic asthma, more alveolar and less bronchiolar involvement

Sx: Cough

Si: Fever, no sputum

Crs: Often reversible with withdrawal of source often; but may be chronic

Cmplc: Chronic interstitial pneumonitis, occasionally is apical and thus can look like tbc

r/o nitrofurantoin acute allergic type pneumonitis (Nejm 1969;281: 1087); nematode asthma

Lab:

PFTs: Low normal FEV_1 % and FVC if interstitial disease, especially in chronic forms

Serol: Specific antibody testing

Xray: Chest shows pulmonary alveolar infiltrates that look like pulmonary edema

Rx: Avoidance of allergen; masks for farmers if they can use during brief exposures; steroids for brief courses

COPD/CHRONIC BRONCHITIS/EMPHYSEMA

Nejm 2000;343:276

Cause: Bronchitis/hyperreactive airways from smoking, recurrent infections; cystic fibrosis (p 721); $α_1$-antitrypsin deficiency ($α_1$-ATD) (Nejm 1993;328:1392), autosomal recessive (Nejm 1977;296: 1190), and usually combined with smoking in heterozygote, occurs even w/o smoking in homozygote

Epidem: Smoker-type onset usually after age 50 yr; males > females; incr prevalence in cold damp climates. Maternal smoking may increase incidence in offspring (Nejm 1983;309:699). $α_1$-ATD type: gene incidence ~5% in US (Nejm 1969;281:279); onset by age 45

Pathophys: Proteases, especially elastase from polys and macrophages, are balanced by $α_1$-antitrypsin, the primary anti-elastase; hence functional deficiencies cause loss of lung elasticity; and smoke both inactivates it (Ann IM 1987;107:761; Nejm 1983;309:694) and increases the polys in the lung capillaries (Nejm 1989;321:924). Thus elasticity is decreased, causing loss of connective tissue support that normally keeps bronchioles open; when expiratory pressure is incr, that loss of elastic support causes bronchiole collapse and resulting "ball valving" entrapment of air and hence emphysema, along with V/Q imbalances, end-stage hypoventilation, and incr pCO_2. Goblet cell hyperplasia may contribute to bronchiolar plugging and initiate more of above

Sx: Dyspnea on exertion of arms more than legs (Nejm 1986;314:1485); chronic productive cough with bronchitis not emphysema; see Table 19.2.2

Table 19.2.2

Sx (J Gen IM 1993;8:63)	Sens (%)	Specif (%)
Orthopnea	19	88
Smoker	94	24
Dyspnea	82	33
Cough	51	71
Wheezing	51	84
Chronic sputum	42	89

Si: Barrel chest. Two extremes: "blue bloater" (CHF, hypoxia, and hypercarbia), to "pink puffer" (weight loss, low pCO_2, moderate decrease in pO_2 at rest and left-sided CHF, which may be occult (Nejm 1971;285:361))

Forced expiratory time over trachea >6 sec (75% sens/specif—Jama 1993;270:731). See Table 19.2.3

Table 19.2.3

Si (J Gen IM 1993;8:63)	Sens (%)	Specif (%)
Diminished breath sounds	29	85
Wheezing	14	99
Cough	14	93
Subxyphoid PMI	4	99
Rales	1	99

Crs: Pink puffer has better prognosis than blue bloater because pulmonary hypertension is less (Nejm 1972;286:912)

Cmplc: Polycythemia; pulmonary hypertension (p 723), peptic ulcer disease (Nejm 1969;281:279), acute respiratory failure; lithium worsens (Nejm 1983;308:39); hypophosphatemia, especially on ventilator, <1 mM/L (<1.5 mg%) impairs diaphragmatic contractility, treatable (Nejm 1985;313:420)

Lab:

Bact: Chronically infected sputum with bronchitis

Path: Emphysema, centrilobular of secondary and tertiary respiratory bronchioles most commonly; in α_1-ATD, panlobular of primary lobules and PAS-positive staining inclusions in hepatocytes (Nejm 1975;292:176)

PFTs: Diffusion capacity decr in emphysema, not bronchitis or asthma alone, due to loss of total alveolar/capillary membrane surface area; <55% of predicted correlates with hypoxia on exercise (Nejm 1984;310:1218); incr total lung capacity; decr FEV_1/FVC; 7-min nitrogen washout with O_2 is prolonged

Serol: In α_1-ATD, SPEP shows decr α_1 peak <0.2 gm (no false pos—Ann IM 1970;73:9)

Rx: Stop smoking (p 737) to prevent or stabilize progression, steroid inhalers not much help if don't (Nejm 1999;340:1948); pulmonary rehab programs (Lancet 1996;348:1115; Ann IM 1995;122:823; Lancet 1994;344:1394) clearly improve quality of life and endurance (Chest 1997;111:1077; J Respir Crit Care Med 1995; 152:S77). Cardioselective β blockers safe if needed for ASHD (ACP J Club 2001;135:87)

Vaccination vs influenza, pneumococcus, and eventually maybe RSV and para-influenza (Jama 2000;283:499)

O_2: 1–2 L/min nasal prongs hs safe even if pCO_2 chronically elevated (Nejm 1984;310:425), but round-the-clock O_2 only method shown so far to increase survival (Ann IM 1983;99:519). CHF rx with digoxin, if L- but not if R-sided failure, helps (Ann IM 1981;95:283)

Meds:

1st: Catechol bronchodilators including salmeterol up to ii inhalations bid, often used as an alternative to or w iprotropium (Rx Let 1998;5:15); via nebulizers not IPPB (Ann IM 1980;93:612) or inhalers; used prn is not safe routinely (Nejm 1992;326:560)

2nd: Steroid inhalers (Nejm 1992;327:1413), help sx but don't slow progression, and incr osteoporosis (Nejm 2000;343:1902)

3rd: Theophylline preparations; acutely of questionable benefit (Ann IM 1987;107:305) but help ~50% of chronics (Chest 1993;104:1101) via incr diaphragmatic muscle strength and by dampening sense of dyspnea as can opiates (Nejm 1995;333:1547)

Anticholinergics such as ipratropium (Atrovent) 2–3 puffs qid (Nejm 1988;319:486; Med Let 1987;29:71); or tiotropium pwdr inhaler qd may be better (not yet FDA approved—Thorax 2000;55:289)

Antibiotics prophylactically: Tm/S, tetracyclines, or amoxicillin at first si of cold, fever, or change in sputum (Jama 1995;273:957; Med Let 1980;22:68)

Perhaps α_1-proteinase inhibitor for α_1-ATD (Med Let 1988;30:29) iv weekly or monthly

Surgical resection of bullae and/or severely impaired areas (Nejm 2000;343:239; 1996;334:1095,1198), can improve diaphragm and accessory muscle effectiveness; may help only pts w low inspiratory resistances, ie, those w/o a lot of intrinsic airway disease (Nejm 1998;338:1181); still considered experimental by Medicare in 1998

of acute exacerbation (Ann IM 2001;134:595,600; Nejm 1999;340:1941): O_2, antibiotics, bronchodilators, steroids × 1–2 wks maximum; no chest PT, mucolytics, or theophyllines

CYSTIC FIBROSIS (Mucoviscidosis)

Nejm 1997;336:487; 1996;335:179; 1993;328:1390; 1976;295:481, 534; Ann IM 1977;87:188

Cause: Genetic mutations of the CF gene on chromosome #7; autosomal with variable penetrance (Nejm 1993;329:1308; 1990;323:1517)

Epidem: Whites have 98.4% of all cystic fibrosis; 1/30,000 whites in US; heterozygotes about 5% of population. Blacks have a 1.4% prevalence of heterozygote; all other racial groups have a prevalence <0.2%; only 1 reported case in Asian (Nejm 1968;279:1216)

Pathophys: Deficient Cl^- secretion and excessive Na^+ resorption across epithelial surfaces (Nejm 1991;325:533). Exocrine gland fibrosis in homozygote; pancreatic duct obstruction causes pancreatic insufficiency (Nejm 1985;312:329). Bronchi obstructed, leading to secondary infections especially with staph and *Pseudomonas*, COPD, and pulmonary failure. Vas deferens obstruction/absence causes male sterility (98%) (Nejm 1972;287:586); nothing analogous in female. Sweat glands obstructed, causing an inability to lose heat

Sx: COPD; heat exhaustion; malabsorption sx; sterility, esp male (90%) which may be only sx (Nejm 1995;332:1475)

Si: Meconium ileus at birth (15%); no sweat; malnourished; severe chronic bronchitis and pulmonary insufficiency

Crs: Depends on age of onset and complications; 2-yr mortality >50% once FEV$_1$ % becomes <30% of predicted, PaO$_2$ <55 mm Hg or pCO$_2$ >50 mm, so begin planning lung transplant then (Nejm 1992;326:1187)

Cmplc: COPD, bronchiectasis, pneumothorax (20% lifetime incidence), massive hemoptysis (7% get in lifetime); growth retardation; pancreatic insufficiency (80%); diabetes mellitus (20%) without vascular lesions (Nejm 1969;281:451); rectal prolapse, may be presenting sx; gallstones, in 50% by age 26, w common bile duct obstruction (15–20%) (Nejm 1988;318:340); modest increase in gi cancers in adulthood (Nejm 1995;332:494); osteoporosis w fx's and kyphosis in adulthood (Ann IM 1998;128:186)

Lab:

Bact: S. aureus in sputum and/or nasal pharynx; in sputum, *Pseudomonas* or *E. coli,* both of which produce a mucoid material almost pathognomonic of CF (Nejm 1981;304:1445)

Chem: Sweat tests with or without pilocarpine stimulation; characteristically Cl >60 mEq/L, usually >80, r/o Addison's, atopic dermatitis, malnutrition, hypothyroidism, and a few rare others (Nejm 1997;336:487). Duodenal aspirate shows diminished pancreatic enzyme secretion and pH <8 even after secretin stimulation

Noninv: PFTs show diminished vital capacity, incr residual volume

Semen analysis: Azoospermia

Xray: Sinus films show opacified paranasal sinuses

Rx: Prevent by carrier detection with tissue culture (Nejm 1981;304:1); but not practical to screen entire white population yet (Nejm 1990;322:328). In affected families, in-vitro fertilization and preimplantation testing possible (Nejm 1992;327:905)

Screen newborns maybe w blood trypsinogen levels since may eventually be reasonable to institute dietary and pulmonary interventions early (Nejm 1997;337:963)

of cmplc:
- Pulmonary, rx same as COPD, consider:

  Prophylactic antibiotics like ciprofloxacin or antibiotic aerosols like tobramycin (Nejm 1999;340:23) for *Pseudomonas* (Nejm 1993;328:1740); but antibiotic management complex esp in end stages

  Amiloride (Midamor) inhaler qid slows progression, perhaps by blocking Na resorption and thus thinning mucus (Nejm 1990;322:1189)

  Avoid smoke exposure, eg, in home (Nejm 1990;323:782)

  Acetyl cysteine (Mucomyst) DNAase inhaler qd-bid significantly thins secretions (Nejm 1994;331:637; 1992;326:812) and modestly improves PFTs, and decreases infections, but inhaler without medication costs $2000 and total cost/yr used qd is $12,000 (Med Let 1994;36:34)

  Ibuprofen 25 mg/kg qd chronically slows progression (Nejm 1995;332:848)

  Lung transplant helps severely affected (Jama 2001;286:2683)
- Pancreatic (p 259)
- Intestinal obstruction w Gastrografin enema, which increases gi fluid

---

19.3 PULMONARY HYPERTENSION

PULMONARY HYPERTENSION (Primary and Secondary)

Nejm 1997;336:111 (primary type); Ann IM 1987;107:216

Cause: Primary types due to autosomal dominant gene in 6% (Nejm 2001;345:319) including ones assoc w HAT (Nejm 2001;345:325)

Secondary causes: COPD w hypoxia (most common), recurrent pulmonary emboli (Nejm 2001;345:1465; Ann IM 1988;108:425), silicosis, sarcoid, CHF, mitral stenosis, L-to-R shunts, most of which worsen w vasodilator rx (Ann IM 1986;105:499), HIV infection, cocaine and/or iv drug use, cirrhosis, and fenfluramine-type anorexic drugs (Nejm 1996;335:609), collagen vascular diseases like scleroderma (Ann IM 2000;132:425)

Epidem: In primary, female:male = 1.7:1; peak onset between age
30–40 yr; associated w positive family hx

Pathophys: (Nejm 1992;327:70)

Excess platelet thromboxane A and deficient endothelial cell
prostaglandin productions are associated w both primary and
secondary pulmonary HT, cause or effect? Endothelin-1 peptide
may cause (Nejm 1993;328:1732)

Sx: Onset over 1–3 yr, see Table 19.3.1

Table 19.3.1

Sx	As 1st sx (%)	Present Sometime During Crs (%)
Exertional dyspnea	60	98
Fatigue	20	73
Chest pain	7	47
Syncope or near-syncope	13	77
Edema	3	37
Palpitations	5	33
Raynaud's	?	10

Si: $P_2 \geq A_2$; RV heave; R-sided S_3; pulmonary systolic and diastolic
murmur

Crs: Progressive; median survival is 2.8 yr; 68% survive 1 yr, 50% survive
3 yr, and 34% survive 5 yr, worse if mean PA pressure ≥ 85 mm Hg,
mean RA pressure >20, or cardiac index <2 L/min/m^2 (Ann IM
1991;115:343)

Cmplc: Cor pulmonale, sudden death (7%)

Lab:

ABGs: Low pCO_2 often is the only abnormality; hypoxia later in
course, first exertional, then at rest

Rx: of secondary types, rx the cause if possible; thrombectomy successful
in chronic embolus patients even after yr (Nejm 2001;345:1465;
Ann IM 1987;107:560); O_2 critical if hypoxic etiology

of primary type: avoid indomethacin and other prostaglandin
inhibitors that increase pressure (Ann IM 1982;97:480)

of both types:

Warfarin anticoagulation increases survival (Nejm 1992;327:76)

Vasodilator rx:
- Prostacycline epoprostenol (Flolan) iv continuous pump infusions (Ann IM 2000;132:425,500; 1999;130:740; 1990;112:485; Nejm 1998;338:273,321; 1996;334:296; Med Let 1996;38:14), or perhaps as inhaled iloprost (Ilomedia) 25 μgm 6–12 × qd (Nejm 2000;342:1866; Ann IM 2000;132:435), $60,000/yr;
- Calcium channel blockers help 25%, and in those 25%, the 5-yr survival is improved to 94% (Nejm 1992;327:76), eg, diltiazem and nifedipine 40–120 mg po qd (Ann IM 1983;99:433)

Lung transplant (p 734)

ACUTE MOUNTAIN SICKNESS (High Altitude Cerebral and Pulmonary Edema)
Nejm 2001;345:107; Med Let 1992;34:84

Cause: Acute change in elevation above at least 7000–8000 ft, by going up mountains, or in unpressurized airplanes (commercial airlines pressurized at 9000 ft); and usually w associated exertion

Epidem: Increased incidence with exercise and cold weather; increased in teenagers (Nejm 1977;297:1269) and patients with congenital aplasia of right pulmonary artery (Nejm 1980;302:1070). Inhabitants of high altitudes can get just with 1–2 d at low altitudes and return. Physical conditioning before ascent has no effect on acute mountain sickness, pulmonary edema, or cerebral edema incidence. 22% incid at 7000–9000 ft, 42% at 10,000 ft

Pathophys: Cerebral edema from either cytotoxic vascular dilatation or change in blood-brain barrier permeability (Jama 1998;280:1920). Normal pulmonary capillary wedge pressures; increased atrial natriuretic factor; increased capillary permeability (Ann IM 1988; 109:796)

Sx: Onset in 6–48 h; headache (62%); fatigue (26%) and lassitude; anorexia (11%), nausea, and vomiting; insomnia (31%); dyspnea (21%); dizziness (21%)

Si: Dyspnea; dry cough; Cheyne-Stokes respirations, especially at night. Acute pulmonary edema (4% of nonacclimatized people at 12,000–14,000 ft) without warning si's; cerebral edema w ataxia and confusion; asymptomatic retinal hemorrhages (Ophthalm 1992;99:739; Nejm 1970;282:1183)

Crs: Spontaneous resolution in 3–4 d

PULMONARY DISEASES

Cmplc:
Lab:
  ABGs: Mild respiratory alkalosis
Xray: MRI of head in cerebral edema type shows white matter edema, esp of corpus callosum
Rx: Prevent by avoiding exertion for several days or acclimatize at 6000–8000 ft for 2–4 d; O_2 at 4–10 L/min, hs and at first sx. Acetazolamide 250 mg po b-tid 24–48 h, decreases incidence by 50%; dexamethasone 4 mg po q 6 h before and during exposure; perhaps decreases cerebral edema (Nejm 1984;310:683) and mountain sickness but not the physiologic consequences, ie, it may mask the sx (Nejm 1989;321:1707)
  of sx: most importantly, descend at least 1000 ft at 1st sx; O_2
  of pulmonary edema: prophylactic nifedipine 20 mg SR po q 8 h; decrease PA pressures (Nejm 1991;325:1284), eg, w nitric oxide 10% inhalations (Nejm 1996;334:624); morphine im to relieve anxiety and pool peripheral blood; rest and descend
  of cerebral edema: dexamethasone 8 mg po/iv, then 4 mg q 6 h; O_2; immediate descent

PULMONARY EMBOLUS
  Nejm 1998;339:93

Cause: Embolic clots to pulmonary arteries via systemic venous return
Epidem: Very common; probably incidence correlates best with thoroughness of postmortem exam
  Associated with: estrogen-containing bcps, esp 2nd ($<50\mu$gm estrogen + norgestrel, levonorgestrel, or norgestrienone), or worse 3rd generaton (desogestrel, gestodene, or norgestionate) types, pregnancy (Nejm 1996;335:108), and postmenopausal replacement rx; occult cancers, 15% of cancer patients will have within 2 yr (Ann IM 1982;96:556); DVT and its genetic precipitants (p 112); surgery, especially of legs; cramped air travel (Nejm 2001;345:779), end of trip incid = 1.5/million for trips >3100 mi, 4.8/million if >6200 mi
Pathophys: Thrombophlebitis causes thrombus, which breaks free and migrates to the lungs; many pts have many small emboli chronically

rather than one big one. Rarely are calves the source; most from thigh and pelvic veins (Ann IM 1981;94:439); no si or sx of DVT in 50%

Sx: Sudden or chronic dyspnea; pleuritic chest pain w infarct; hemoptysis; fever; syncope with large emboli

Si: All uncommon; elevated JVP; high diaphragm on one side by percussion; basilar atelectasis; pleural effusion; wheezing (Nejm 1968;278:999); BP cuff test for calf pain; $P_2 > A_2$; cyanosis

Crs: (Nejm 1992;326:1240)

Resolves over 10–30 d (Nejm 1969;280:1194); 80% overall survival; 60% without rx, 90% with rx; 75% of deaths occur in first 2 h; DVT clinically resolves in 1/3 after 3 d of heparin rx

Fatalities <2% in yr following dx if rx'd × 3–6 mo (Jama 1998; 279:458)

Cmplc: "Milk leg" from incompetent leg veins; chronic pulmonary hypertension (Ann IM 1988;108:425)

r/o air embolism (Nejm 2000;342:476)

Lab: (McMaster's Univ rev—Ann IM 1991;114:300; 1983;98:891)

ABGs: pO_2 <80 mm Hg, 10% false negative; <90 mm Hg, 0% false negative

Hem: Elevated fibrin split products/D-dimer (SimpliRED), 84% sens, 68% specif (Ann IM 1998;129:1006); combined w abg criteria above, if D-dimer negative and pO_2 >80 on RA, no false negs for PE (Thorax 1998;53:830); or combined w alveolar dead space fraction ≤20%, 98% sens 50% specif (Jama 2001;285:761)

Noninv: EKG may show $S_1Q_3T_3$, very specific but only w massive emboli (Am J Emerg Med 1997;15:310); anterior T wave inversions (68% sens) (Chest 1998;113:850); or ≥3 of the following (70% sens) (Am J Cardiol 1994;73:298): RBBB or pRBBB, S in I and aVL ≥15mm, poor R progression, Q in III and F not II, RAD >90°, voltage <5 mm in limb leads, T inversions in II + F or $V_1 - V_4$

Xray: All doable even in pregnancy (Nejm 1996;335:108)

Chest shows infiltrates, effusions, high diaphragm, lucency

V/Q scan to look for multiple mismatched defects (87% sens, 97% specif), but even if all defects are matched, odds of pulmonary embolus still are substantial (case—Nejm 1995;332:321; Ann IM 1983;98:891), ie, 40% (PIOPED—Jama 1990;263:2753)

Spiral (helical) CT, need prospective studies because sens 50–100% and specif 80–100% in various studies (Ann IM 2001;135:88; 2000;132:227; Arch IM 2000;160:293)

MR angiography 75% sens, 95% specif (Nejm 1997;336:1422)
Pulmonary arteriography is diagnostic and the gold standard
To find DVT, B-mode duplex ultrasound now as good or better (Ann
IM 1989;111:297) than IPGs; ultrasound positive in only 1/3 of
documented pulmonary embolus cases (Ann IM 1997;126:775);
venograms (Nejm 1981;304:1561; Ann IM 1978;89:162);

Rx: Prevent w warfarin or sc unfractionated q 12 h or qd low molec wgt
heparin (p 35)

Screen for reversible causes w factor V (Leiden), homocysteine, and
lupus anticoagulant (which requires more intense anticoagulation)

Heparin (p 35), low molecular weight or unfractionated for at least 5 d
if start warfarin on day 1 (Nejm 1990;322:1260). Used long term in
pregnancy, keeping PTT 1.5× control at 6 h

Warfarin to an INR of 2–3 (p 36) × 6 mo (Nejm 1995;332:166)

Thrombolysis maybe if severe, w streptokinase (cheap but allergenic),
speeds clearing and return to better PFTs and vein function (Nejm
1980;303:842; Ann IM 1980;93:141,629); or TPA if right heart
failure w acute embolus

Surgical IVC plication, or umbrella without anesthesia (Nejm 1972;
286:55); embolectomy (50% survival) rarely needed

FAT EMBOLI

Nejm 1993;329:926,961; 1967;276:1192

Cause: Fat globules, from bony fractures, via the circulation to the
pulmonary arteries and other vessels? Often seem w total hip
replacement (94%—Clin Orthoped Related Research 1999;355:23)

Epidem: Symptomatic emboli in 3% of all femoral shaft trauma; cause of
death in 5% of all trauma deaths; but 90% of emboli cause no sx or
are undetected

Pathophys: Fat from marrow or from tissue enter veins to inferior vena
cava, or enter the lymphatics and from there go to the thoracic duct
via the superior vena cava to the lungs and beyond to the systemic
circulation; there the fat emboli are broken down by lipoprotein
lipase into triglycerides and free fatty acids, which are toxic
molecules

Sx: 24–48 h latent period after femoral, pelvic, tibial, humeral, or other trauma; then nonlateralizing CNS sx's of confusion/acute brain syndrome; dyspnea and respiratory distress

Si: Fever; tachycardia; skin petechiae (85%), mantle distribution over chest, neck, and conjunctiva; cyanosis; confusion

Crs: Of those with sx, 10–20% mortality if no coma; 85% mortality if coma present

Cmplc: Adult respiratory distress syndrome (p 709)

Lab:

Chem: Lipase elevated in 3–5 d, peaks at 5–8 d

Hem: Thrombocytopenia

Noninv: Transesophageal cardiac echo shows emboli themselves during fx repair (Clin Orthoped Related Research 1999;355:23)

Path: Bx of petechiae or kidney show fat in capillaries with platelets about them; use frozen section, which avoids formalin dissolution of the fat. Sputum stained for fat, 80% false negative; bronchial lavage shows intracellular fat in >33% of cells (8/8 patients—Ann IM 1990;113:583)

Urine: Fat stain positive in 60% with acid-washed glass

Xray: Chest shows bilateral fluffy infiltrates, ARDS

Lung scans show mismatched V/Q defects

Rx: Methylprednisolone 1^+ mg/kg q 6 h × 3 d at first si in likely patient; prevents without complications (Ann IM 1983;99:439)

Supportive rx of ARDS (p 709)

19.4 PULMONARY TUMORS

MESOTHELIOMA

Ann IM 1982;96:746; Nejm 1980;303:200

Cause: Neoplasia from asbestosis

Epidem: 2.5 cases/million population/yr. Most (all?) from asbestos exposure (Nejm 1969;280:488)

Pathophys: Quite malignant; ~20% are abdominal (peritoneal), which are all associated with heavy asbestos exposures, unlike often transient exposures of pulmonary types

Sx: Nonpleuritic pain and/or dyspnea (95%). Pulmonary osteoarthropathy arthritis pain (distal extremities with periosteal new bone formation), often severe; benign types of mesothelioma have pulmonary osteoarthropathy 100% of the time, and it goes away with surgical rx

Si: Clubbing; ascites with peritoneal type

Crs: Rapid demise in <12 mo, usually about 4 mo after dx; die from primary lesions, not metastases usually. 0–10% 5-yr survival with rx

Cmplc: Pericardial effusions; small bowel obstructions with peritoneal types

Lab:

Chem: Pleural fluid hyaluronic acid level >0.8 mg/cc is diagnostic but >50% false negatives

Path: Pleural fluid cytology often hard to interpret because normal mesothelial cells can appear malignant; pleural bx usually diagnostic

Xray: Chest shows pleural plaques (calcified); pulmonary fibrosis in 20% of pulmonary types, 50% of abdominal types; pleural effusions usually

Rx: Debatable (Ann IM 1977;87:618) if anything helps

LUNG CANCER

Ann IM 1975;83:93

Cause: Types: alveolar cell, small (oat) cell, bronchogenic (squamous and adeno-), and large cell undifferentiated

Neoplasia; viral origin with alveolar? (cf. sheep "yagshikta") though still smoking induced; carcinogens with bronchogenic types

Epidem: Epidemic now in US; leading cause of cancer death in males and females although male > female w squamous type; male = female w adenocarcinoma

All are increased in smokers and those exposed to smoke as a child (Nejm 1990;323:632); asbestos-exposed workers (incidence is about 20%!) but not people living in mining areas (Nejm 1998; 338:1565); radon-exposed uranium miners (Nejm 1984;310:1481, 1485) and home owners (Nejm 1994;330:159). Smoking multiplies the radon effect

Pathophys: Alveolar type is multicentric in origin; rarely metastasizes, rather presents as pneumonitis from its local invasion. Oat or small cell type is extremely malignant. Bronchogenic types are of endobronchial origin, then locally invade and eventually metastasize via the lymphatics

Sx: Hemoptysis, often intermittent but late in course may be massive; pain, pleuritic or simply a deep sense of abnormality often when cancer is in the mediastinum; weight loss; cough; dyspnea; arthritis (pulmonary osteoarthropathy)

Si: Wheeze unilaterally; clubbing; hoarseness from recurrent laryngeal nerve paralysis; pulmonary osteoarthropathy (10%); Pancoast's syndrome (Nejm 1997;337:1359,1370): Horner's syndrome, shoulder and arm pain from C_8 T_1T_2 root compression in brachial plexus that radiates down ulnar nerve with vasomotor changes in the hand, plus first rib erosion on chest xray

Crs: (Chest 1986;89:225S) Coin lesions found incidentally have a 30% 5-yr survival. See Table 19.4.1

Table 19.4.1

Stage	At Presentation (%)	5-yr Survival (%)
I- $T_1N_0M_0$	10%	75
- $T_2N_0M_0$		57
II- $T_2N_0M_0$ or $T_1N_1M_0$	20	52
- $T_2N_1M_0$		39
III A- $T_3N_{0-2}M_0$ or $T_1N_2M_0$	70 (III+IV)	15
- $T_2N_2M_0$		15
III B- $T_{1-3}N_3M_0$ or $T_4N_{1-3}M_0$		<10
IV-$T_{1-3}N_{0-3}M_1$		0

T_1 <3 cm, T_2 >3 cm, T_3 to chest wall

N_0, no nodes; N_1, peribronchial and ipsilateral hilar; N_2, ipsilateral mediastinal and subcarinal nodes; N_3, supraclavicular and contralateral mediastinal nodes

M_0, no mets; M_1, distant mets

Cmplc: Pneumonia and effusions; superior vena cava syndrome; CNS metastases; hormone production, especially with small cell types, eg, of ADH, PTH (also common with squamous cell), ACTH, gonadotropins causing gynecomastia (Nejm 1968;279:640); neuropathies and myopathies including autonomic dysfunction leading to pseudo-small bowel obstruction (Ann IM 1983;98:129); Eaton-Lambert syndrome (myasthenia-"resistant" or unresponsive to neostigmine), caused by antibodies to calcium channels that trigger Ach release at nerve endings (Nejm 1995;332:1467); in small cell types, rare paraneoplastic limbic encephalitis (Nejm 1999; 340:1788) w seizures, dementia, irritability, depression, which may precede cancer discovery in 60%, 20% of time assoc w testicular Ca, due to shared antigens btwn tumor and limbic neuronal proteins

Lab:

Path: Cytologies on sputa or bronchoscopy specimen; bronchoscopy bx, mediastinoscopy bx; supraclavicular node bx, often find on left with left upper lobe lesions, on right with all other locations

Xray: Chest xrays even with cytologies not worth doing as screening test (Ann IM 1989;111:232). Bone invasion usually means it is a squamous cell type. Anterior segment upper lobe infiltrates are cancer (90⁺%) until proven otherwise. Paralyzed diaphragm if phrenic nerve involvement

CT scans can help define a coin lesion as benign by finding central calcium; stable plain films over 2 yr also can reassure that lesion is benign; expensive PET scans also helpful for 1–4 cm nodules (Jama 2001;285:922)

Rx: Prevent by stopping smoking, though takes 3–20 yr for risk to decrease to that of a nonsmoker (Am J Pub Hlth 1990;80:954)

Surgery to try to cure, unless: nerve involvement, massive lesion or distant metastases, bad pulmonary functions, oat cell type, malignant pleural effusion, contralateral mediastinal nodes, or ≥ stage IIIa. Results best at hospitals doing >67 lung Ca resections/yr (Nejm 2001;345:181)

Radiation and chemoRx no better than rad alone (Nejm 2000;343: 1217, 1261) vs combo rx helpful adjuvant vs (Nejm 1992;327: 1434) cures some small cell types (44% 5 yr suvival—Nejm 1999;340:265) and some small % of stage III non-small cell types (Ann IM 1996;125:723; Nejm 1990;323:940), eg, 25% survival at 4 yr with radiation and cisplatin (Nejm 1992;326:524); temporary remission rates higher, especially if pre-op chemo rx given (Nejm 1994;330:153)

Palliative radiation to rx bronchial obstruction, or to give pain relief when in brachial plexus; radiation alone can never cure (Ann IM 1990;113:33)

19.5 MISCELLANEOUS

Bronchitis, acute (Ann IM 2001;134:518,521)
Cause: Usually viral esp influenza; *Bordetella pertussis, Mycoplasma,* and
   TWAR (*Chlamydia pneumoniae*) are all <10%
Sx: Productive cough
Si: No T°, tachycardia, tachypnea, or focal lung findings
Xray: Chest if cough >3 wk
Rx: Symptomatic

Cough, chronic idiopathic in adults (Ann IM 1993;119:977)
Cause: Postnasal drip from sinusitis; asthma; gastroesophageal reflux;
   medications, especially ACE inhibitors
Si: Methacholine challenge test positive if asthmatic origin
Xray: Sinus films, chest xray
Rx: Asthma or GE reflux if either present
   1st: Decongestant/antihistamine bid, helps 39/45; perhaps w codeine or
      dextromethorphan (Med Let 2001;43:23)
   2nd: Nasal steroids bid
   3rd: Albuterol inhaler; or terbutaline 2.5 mg po tid or inhale, cures 2/3
      (BMJ 1983; 287:940); or aminophylline, and a po β agonist like
      terbutaline

Diving (Scuba) accidents: Barotrauma causes pneumothorax and air
   emboli to brain and all organs including muscles and heart; CPK
   elevations, which correlate w severity (Nejm 1994;330:19). Bends
   (gas forming in vessels as ascend) causes pain and various organ
   impairments. Rx w hyperbaric O_2 (call divers alert network,
   919-684-8111)
   Also 5× incr in strokes if patent foramen ovale (Ann IM 2001;134:21)

Expectorants, none thought clinically useful in adults now:
Acetylcysteine; via inhalation; breaks S-H bonds of mucous glycoproteins;
   used for trach care and in CF patients
Glyceryl guaiacolate (Robitussin) po; vagal stimulation of secretions?
Iodides (SSKI); 10–20 gtts in water po; increases glandular secretions and
   proteolytic enzymes, which decrease viscosity; but out of favor due to
   long-term toxicity concerns
Deoxyribonuclease aerosol qd-bid (Nejm 1994;331:637; 1992;326:812)

Hemoptysis, differential dx (Ann IM 1985;102:833):
• Chronic bronchitis: viral/bacterial infection, coughing
• Pulmonary vascular changes: telangiectasias, emboli, mitral stenosis
• Nonpulmonary source: nasopharynx, gi, mouth
• Bronchiectasis
• Tbc
• Cancer
• Coagulation abnormalities: drug-induced or acquired

Lung transplant: Unilateral without heart transplant and using cyclosporine rather than steroids 40% 5 yr survival (Nejm 1999;340:108)

Physical therapy to chest is of no value unless lots of secretions (Nejm 1979;300:1155) or neuromuscular lung disease is present

Pleural effusion analysis (Ann IM 1985;103:799)
Transudates caused by CHF; hypoproteinemia; chronic renal failure; cirrhosis; normal vaginal delivery, 2/3 have in first 24 h (Ann IM 1982;97:852)
Exudates, sensitivities, and specificities, see Table 19.5.1

Pleurodesis (Ann IM 1994;120:56), for recurrent pneumothorax or malignant effusions; use tetracycline (Jama 1990;264:2224), or doxycycline 500 mg, or minocycline 300 mg; talc even better but requires thoracoscopy, or bleomycin

Pneumothorax (Nejm 2000;342:868)
Spontaneous occurs usually in male smokers age 10–40
Secondary occurs in COPD and pneumocystis infected AIDS pts

Positive airway pressure ventilation (Nejm 1997;337:1747)
Continuous positive airway pressure (CPAP) via endotrach tube or mask over mouth and/or nose; for acute or chronic respiratory failure, pulmonary edema, and chronic CHF
BiPAP, mask administered, 2 level pressure systems w higher inspiratory and lower positive end expiratory pressures (PEEP); for acute or chronic respiratory failure

Table 19.5.1

Lab Test	Pos Value	Sens (%)	Specif (%)
For exudates in general			
1. LDH	>200 U (if normal in serum is [2]300)	70	100
2. Fluid/serum LDH	>0.6	86	98
3. Protein	>3 gm	89	91
4. Fluid/serum protein	>0.5	90	98
#1 + 2 or 4		99	98
Necessity of surgical drainage of exudate			
pH	<7.0	70	100
	<7.2	90	87
LDH	>1000 U	100	80
For tbc			
Culture	positive	24	100
Culture and pleural bx	either positive	90	100
For carcinoma			
Cytologies and pleural bx	either positive	68	100

Pulmonary function tests

Arterial blood gases: spuriously low pO_2 when high numbers of platelets or WBCs (Nejm 1979;301:361)

Carbon monoxide diffusion capacity, specif but not sens in predicting exertional hypoxia (Nejm 1987;316:1301)

Pulmonary toxins

O_2: tracheobronchitis develops with 95% O_2 within 6 h in normals (Ann IM 1975;82:40)

Radiation toxicity, acute reaction in 4–6 wk; rx with steroids; creates scarring in 4–12 mo (Ann IM 1977;86:81)

Radiographic pneumoconiosis (diffuse interstitial changes on chest xray): Differential dx

• Alveolar proteinosis (Ann IM 1976;85:304): fatty substance accumulates in alveoli. Death from restrictive disease though some spontaneous remissions. Rx with pulmonary lavage (Nejm 1972;286:1230). Steroids contraindicated because of fungal superinfections

- Asbestosis: lower lobe predominant; fine streak pattern; pleural effusions (21%) (Ann IM 1971;74:178); incr incidence of mesothelioma and carcinoma
- Berryliosis: acute or chronic for yr after exposure; looks like sarcoid (Ann IM 1988;108:687); a hypersensitivity pneumonitis (Nejm 1989;320:1103)
- Chronic occupational asthma (p 716) and allergic pneumonitis/alveolitis (p 717)
- Cystic fibrosis (p 721) when end stage
- Eosinophilic granuloma
- Idiopathic pulmonary fibrosis
- Interstitial carcinomas: alveolar cell, breast
- Lymphangiomyomatosis: in women age 15–40 yr, and both sexes w tuberous sclerosis; usually progressive and fatal; rx w lung transplant (Nejm 1996;335:275), or medroxyprogesterone? (Nejm 1980;303:1461)
- Lymphocytic interstitial pneumonitis: associated with hypoglobulinemia, Sjögren's, etc. (Ann IM 1978;88:616)
- Pulmonary thesaurosis (Nejm 1974;290:660): seen in hairdressers Patchy infiltrates. Clears when avoid hair sprays. Nodes look like sarcoid. Lung looks like idiopathic pulmonary fibrosis
- Sarcoid (p 821)
- Silicosis: eggshell calcified nodes
- Talcosis: incr density of pattern
- Tuberculosis (p 431)
- Tungsten carbide maker's exposure: rx'able by stopping dust exposure? from cobalt involved in process (Ann IM 1971;75:709)

Respirator weaning by qd trials of spontaneous breathing rather than multiple trials, intermittent mandatory ventilation, or decreasing pressure-supported ventilation (Nejm 1995;332:345)

Sick building syndrome
Cause: 25% due to exhaust; 75% to anaerobes, etc.
Sx: Fatigue, headache, inability to concentrate
Rx: Increase outdoor air to 20^+ ft^3/min/person (Nejm 1993;328:821)

Smoking cessation (Jama 1999;281:72; Med Let 1995;37:6; Nejm 1995;333:1196)

Nicotine, either patch or gum formulation w concomitant education results in a 33% 2-yr discontinuation rate (Nejm 1988;318:15) vs 10–15% w placebo

- Patch (Habitrol, Nicoderm, Prostep) (Nejm 1991;325:311; Arch IM 1991;151:749) 24 h/day in decreasing doses from 21 mg × 2–3 wk, then 14 mg × 2–3$^+$ wk, then 7 mg × 2–3$^+$ wk, then stop. Best 6 mo outcomes = 28% cessation, 44 mg patches may or may not be safe and effective (Jama 1995;274:1347 vs 1353); can use gum, inhaler, or nasal spray for added jolt w the patch (Rx Let 1999;6:22). May also be ok even in ischemic heart disease (Nejm 1996;335:1792, Arch IM 1994;54:989); coincident smoking w patch not advisable but also not dangerously risky (Nejm 1996;335:1792); cost for 8 wk = $220; or can use 16 h 15/10/5 mg patches (Nicotrol)
- Gum (Nicorette) 2–4 mg/piece, 9–12 pc/d, max 20 pc/d; tough on teeth (Med Let 1984;26:98; Ann IM 1984;101:121); cost $100 (2 mg)–$200 (4 mg) per mo
- Inhaler (Nicotrol) (Rx Let 1998;5:21) 6–16 cartridges qd × 3 mo, then taper over 3 mo; predominant mouth absorption; adverse effect: asthma exacerbation. $45/42 cartridges
- Nasal spray 10 mg/c up to 5×/hr, <40 sprays qd; effective used w patch (Bmj 1999;318:285)

Bupropion (Welbutrin, Zyban is long acting formulation) (Rx Let 1997;4:34) 150 mg LA qd, incr to bid after 1 wk × 6–8 wk; start 1 wk before quit date to build level; success at 8 wk = 45% and at 1 yr = 23%, double control rates and weight gain less (Nejm 1997;337:1195); use w nicotine formulations (Addiction 1998;93:907), eg, 21 mg patch wks 2–7, 14 mg wk 8, 7 mg wk 9 produced a 36% 1 yr quit rate (Nejm 1999;340:685)

Antidepressants (Nejm 1997;337:1230): nortriptyline, doxepin, fluoxetine (Prozac)

Clonidine po or patch may also help

Chapter 20
Renal/Urology

D. K. Onion

20.1 FLUID/ELECTROLYTES/ACID-BASE

If hypovolemic, initial bolus of NS: 250–500 cc in adult, 10–20 cc/kg in child

24 Hr REQUIREMENTS

• Basal requirements/24 h. See Table 20.1.1

Table 20.1.1

Age	Water	Na[1]	K[+]	Calories
Adult	2500 cc	100 mEq	20 mEq	4–800[2]
Child <2 yr	120 cc/kg	2–3 mEq/kg	1–2 mEq/kg	125/kg[3], 150/kg for premie
Child >2 yr	80 cc/kg	2–3 mEq/kg	1–2 mEq/kg	125/kg

• Loss requirements: Typical adult potential 24-h losses beyond basal by source. See Table 20.1.2
• Deficit calculations; adult body spaces of fluid and lytes for calculating deficits to be made up, usually within 24 h

K^+: female = 35 mEq/kg, male = 45 mEq/kg presuming normal pH of 7.40

Water: 60% of body weight in kg; water deficit = 0.6 (ideal body wgt) (1–140/Na); (Nejm 1977;297:1444)

Table 20.1.2

	Saliva	Sweat	Gastric	Pancreatic	Large + Small Bowel
Water (cc)	1500	variable	2500	700	3000
Na (mEq/L)	variable	10–50	45	110–150	100–140
K (mEq/L)	variable	10	10	2.5–7.5	5–35
HCO_3 (mEq/L)				90–110	20–50
Cl (mEq/L)			100	50–55	
Organic anion (mEq/L)					174

ORAL REHYDRATION SOLUTIONS (ORS)

(Nejm 1990;323:891; Med Let 1987;29:63; contents—Postgrad Med 1983;74:336.) In mild-moderate dehydration, give at 10–25 cc/kg/h replacement rate, then 100–150 cc/kg/d maintenance. See Table 20.1.3

Table 20.1.3

	WHO Oral Rehydr Soln	Rehydralyte	Pedialyte/Lytren
Na (mEq/L)	90	75	50
K (mEq/L)	20	20	20
Cl (mEq/L)	80	65	40
HCO_3 (mEq/L)	30	30	30
Glucose (gm/L)	20	25	20
Form	powder	liquid	liquid
Cost/qt	$0.35	$4	$3

- Homemade ORS: Sugar:salt = 8:1; for instance,
  2 tsp sugar + 1/4 tsp salt + a squeeze of lime in 8-oz glass of boiled water; or 8 tsp sugar, 1 tsp salt + citrus in 1 L (three 12-oz coke cans); or
  4-finger scoop sugar, 3-finger pinch salt, + citrus in 1 L boiled water; or 8 bottle caps sugar, 1 cap salt, + citrus in 1 L boiled water
  Cereal (rice, corn, or wheat) starches 50–80 gm/L (Nejm 2000;342: 308,345; 1991;324:517; 1988;319:1346) or as rice syrup; ferment in colon, help Na pumps there; better than glucose/sucrose; but can't measure out, plus they ferment quickly in field unless contained in a commercial powder or syrup

RENAL/UROLOGY

Table 20.1.4

Clinical State	Result	Differential dx
Volume depletion	Na 0–10 mEq/L	Extrarenal Na loss
	>10	Renal salt wasting, Addison's
Acute oliguria	Na 0–10	Prerenal azotemia
	>30	ATN
Hyponatremia	Na 0–10	Intravascular volume depletion
	^{3}intake	SIADH vs Addison's
Hypokalemia	K 0–10	Extrarenal K loss
	>10	Renal K wasting
Metab alkalosis	Cl 0–10	Cl-responsive alkalosis
	^{3}intake	Cl-resistant alkalosis

From Wallach, *Interpretation of Diagnostic Tests*. 4th ed. New York: Little, Brown; 1980:165, with permission.

OSMOLARITY

- Calculated mOsm = 2(Na) + glucose/18 + BUN/2.8 (Ann IM 1989; 110:854)
- Unmeasured osmoles or osmolar gap (measured minus calculated) seen with ethylene glycol (0.05 gm% = 22 mOsm), ethanol, and abnormally elevated serum lipids or proteins, but also inexplicably in lactic acidosis and diabetic ketoacidosis (Ann IM 1990;113:580)

ANION GAP CHANGES

Nejm 1977;297:814

- Calculation: (Na) − (Cl + CO_3) = gap, or R fraction
- Low anion gap (<10): Multiple myeloma, hypoalbuminemia, bromism, hypernatremia, hyperkalemia, hypermagnesemia, hypercalcemia, lithium
- High anion gap (>15): Most metabolic acidoses, nonketotic hyperosmolar coma, hypomagnesemia, hypokalemia, hypocalcemia

- Seen in renal failure patients, hemolysis, freshwater drownings, Addison's disease, ACE inhibitor use, NSAID use, Tm/S use especially in AIDS pts (Nejm 1993;328:703); r/o "pseudo"-hyperkalemia due to thrombocythemia, incr white cells, or fist clenching when draw blood (Nejm 1990;322:1290)
- EKG shows tall peaked Ts, evolves to wide QRS and loss of P waves, then evolves to sine wave as K increases
- Rx w CaCl ampule iv; and/or insulin + glucose drip; and/or HCO_3 iv; and K-resin binder (Kayexalate) po; and/or dialysis, hemo- or peritoneal; or albuterol via nebs (Ann IM 1989;110:426)

ACIDOSIS

- pH effect on O_2 hemoglobin dissociation: decr pH leads to immediate R shift of hemoglobin/O_2 curve, ie, easier dissociation
- K^+ shifts = 0.6 mEq/10 nEq of H^+; pH nEq: pH 7.7 = 20 nEq, 7.6 = 25, 7.5 = 32, 7.4 = 40, 7.3 = 50, 7.2 = 63, 7.1 = 79, 7.0 = 100. Thus a K^+ of 5.1 at a pH of 7.0 is really a K^+ of 1.5 at a pH of 7.4

Respiratory acidosis (Nejm 1998;338:26)

Cause: Respiratory failure, inability to breath adequately; rapid onset of coma relative to pH, compared to metabolic acidosis, since CO_2 penetrates CSF readily and raises pH rapidly (F. Plum—Nejm 1967;277:605); CO_2 also diffuses into all tissues including myocardium, rapidly leads to electromechanical dissociation (EMD), hence HCO_3 rx of arrest unwise no matter what blood gases are; arterial gases are misleading too (Nejm 1986;315:153)

Rx: Respiratory support

Metabolic acidosis (Nejm 1998;338:26)

Cause: Ketosis from DKA, isopropyl alcohol poisoning, lactic acidosis (alcohol, septic shock, metformin rx, hypotension, or short bowel *Lactobacillus* overgrowth [Ann IM 1995;122:839]); salicylate, methanol (formic), paraldehyde, ethylene glycol, or toluene glue

RENAL/UROLOGY

poisoning; severe diarrhea,[*] D-lactate produced by gut flora (Nejm 1979;301:249), pancreatic fistulas[*]; uremia, RTA

[*]Indicates cause of low anion gap acidosis

Lab: Salicylates, lytes, ketones, alcohol level, measured vs calculated osmoles, lactate level (Jama 1994;272:1678)

Rx: Rx of the primary disease; rx with any alkali, even HCO_3 may paradoxically worsen even if pH < 7.2 (Ann IM 1990;112:492) although helpful in "low" (normal) anion gap acidoses (* above). Dichloroacetate no help in lactic acidosis (Nejm 1992;327:1564)

Acid–Base Nomogram Bands = Mean ±2 SD Response in Normals

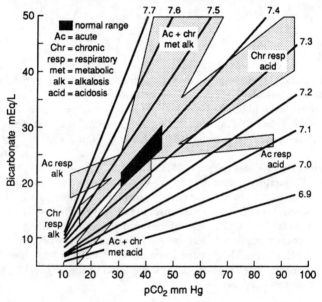

Figure 20.1.1 Reproduced with permission from Petersdorf et al, eds. Harrison's principles of internal medicine. 12th ed. New York: McGraw-Hill, 1991:290.

Respiratory alkalosis (Nejm 1998;338:107)
Cause: Hyperventilation, voluntary or iatrogenic
Sx: Tetany
Cmplc: Rare since most never incr pH >7.55
Rx: Increase dead space, eg, with bag breathing; or slow rate and/or depth

Metabolic alkalosis (Nejm 1998;338:107)
Cause: Vomiting, diuretics (renal H^+ loss to save K^+ and Na^+)
Pathophys: Sx and cmplc when pH > 7.6, which causes decr ionized calcium levels
Sx: Headache, tetany, seizures, delirium, stupor
Si: Depressed respirations
Cmplc: Supraventricular and ventricular arrhythmias; angina induction
Lab: Alkalosis, hypo K^+
Rx: KCl and NaCl repletion, not K-gluconate; NH_4Cl 10 gm = 180 mEq iv as 1–2% soln, or arginine HCl in extreme or resistant cases. See Fig. 20.1.1

HYPOPHOSPHATEMIA
T. Bigos 1991

Cause: Malnutrition; aluminum-binding antacids; iv glucose, which drives intracellularly; renal tubular damage from hypokalemia, osmotic diuresis, or Fanconi's. In types without cell injury like acute DKA, hyperalimentation, or acute respiratory alkalosis, no bad consequences occur because total body PO_4 depletion has not occurred (Nejm 1985;313:447)
Epidem:
Pathophys:
Sx: Confusion, weakness
Si:
Crs:
Cmplc: Bleeding (impaired platelet function), infections (impaired granulocyte function), rhabdomyolysis
Lab: PO_4 low
Rx: 2.5 mg elemental phosphorus/kg in NS over 12-h iv, or po w NeutroPhos

HYPONATREMIA

Nejm 2000;342:1581; Ann IM 1990;113:417

Cause:

- Elevated ADH from:
  Syndrome of inappropriate ADH (SIADH), most commonly, or tumor (Ann IM 1985;102:165)
  Drugs: vincristine, cytoxan, clofibrate, narcotics, nicotine, isoproterenol
  Hypovolemia
- Increased renal ADH sensitivity: Chlorpropamide and other 1st but not 2nd generation hypoglycemics, NSAIDs especially ibuprofen and indomethacin (Nejm 1984;310:568), thiazides, carbamazepine
- Lab error (pseudohyponatremia) due to elevated proteins (Nejm 1984;310:568), glucose, mannitol, or post TURP glycine
- Free water replacement of isotonic emesis, diarrhea, blood, serum; or idiopathically postop (Nejm 1986;314:1529)
- Hypothyroidism, Addison's disease
- Psychiatric pts with polydipsia, SIADH, and decr renal free water excretion (Nejm 1988;318:397)
- Postop (1–3 d), equal sex ratio, 1% incidence; caused by high vasopressin (ADH) levels and hypotonic or sometimes even isotonic (Ann IM 1997;126:20) iv fluids, but respiratory arrest and mortality much higher in menstruating women (Ann IM 1992;117:891)

Epidem: Females > males; seen in premenopausal marathon-running women from free water replacement of sweat loss (Ann IM 2000;132:711)

Pathophys: Cerebral edema causes CNS sx

Sx: Confusion, HA, N + V, muscle cramps

Si: Seizures/confusion, depressed reflexes

Crs:

Cmplc: Mortality incr ×60 in hospitalized patients when Na <130 (Ann IM 1985;102:2164)

r/o adrenal insufficiency, hypothyroidism

Labs:

Chem: Na <125 mEq/L; uric acid <5 mg% with ADH-producing tumor or SIADH (Nejm 1979;301:528)

Rx:

Acutely stop drugs; give saline and furosemide (Lasix); if developed
slowly, correct at <2.5 mEq/h, not >10 mEq/day (Ann IM 1997;
126:57) with iso- or perhaps hypertonic (3% NaCl, thus 3×
normal) saline and, possibly iv furosemide, then go slowly to avoid
pontine demyelination (Ann IM 1997;126:57; Nejm 1987;317:
1190); or go slowly over days, no benefit from rushing or using
twice normal saline even when Na <110 (Ann IM 1987;107:656)
unless symptomatic or is very acute. Dialysis (hypertonic,
intraperitoneal)

Estimate effect of change in serum Na by 1 L fluid =

$$\frac{(\text{infusate Na} + \text{infusate K}) - \text{serum Na}}{\text{Total body water (p 738)} + 1}$$

Chronic (Na <130 >2d):

if neurologic si: avoid hypoxia, then iv saline or hypertonic saline as
above to improve outcome (Jama 1999;281:2342)

if no neurologic si: 1st, restrict water and, if SIADH, give liberal salt
diet or salt tablets; 2nd, salt tablets + loop diuretic; 3rd,
demeclocycline (Declomycin, a tetracycline) 0.6–1.2 gm/day
(Nejm 1978;298:173); 4th, lithium 300 mg po t-qid; perhaps,
vasopressin antagonists in the future (Nejm 1985;312:1121)

HYPERNATREMIA/HYPEROSMOLAR STATES

Nejm 2000;342:1493

Cause:

- Central diabetes insipidus (p 746)
- Nephrogenic DI (p 746), including drug induced by lithium,
  demeclocycline (Declomycin), foscarnet
- Dehydration from:
  Inability to drink
  Betadine rx of burns
  Diminished urine concentration and diminished thirst in elderly
  (Nejm 1984;311:753) especially when have adult onset
  diabetes and leads to nonketotic hyperosmolar coma (Nejm
  1977;297:1452)

Epidem: Most common in infants and debilitated elderly
Pathophys:
Sx: Confusion

Si: Confusion, stupor, coma; hypotension, dehydration
Crs:
Cmplc: Mortality >40% in elderly (Ann IM 1987;107:309); seizures
Lab:
 Chem: Na >150 mEq/L or >300 mOsm/L, measured or calculated
   (p 740)
Rx: Acutely replace water, but not >12 mEq/24 h (brain swelling),
    w D5W, 1/4-normal saline (0.225%), or 1/2-normal saline (0.45%);
    water deficit calculation (p 739), or
 estimate effect of change in serum Na by 1 L fluid =
   $$\frac{(\text{infusate Na}+\text{infusate K})-\text{serum Na}}{\text{Total body water (p 738)}+1}$$
 Chronically rx w thiazides and/or carbamazepine, which increase renal
    sensitivity; or vasopressin nasal or im (p 747)

DIABETES INSIPIDUS (Central and Nephrogenic)

Cause:
 Central: idiopathic (30%); pituitary tumor (Nejm 2000;343:998),
    sarcoid or eosinophilic granuloma; any CNS insult, eg, tumor,
    trauma, surgery; alcohol ingestion, transient, aggravates all other
    causes
 Nephrogenic:
  • Genetic, the "Hopewell hypothesis," the ship on which two Scots
    came to US and spread via sex-linked recessive gene (Nejm 1988;
    318:881); but now know at least 2 different genes involved and
    may not be true (Nejm 1993;328:1534)
  • Drug-induced: Lithium (occurs in 20–70% who take); demethyl-
    tetracycline
  • Transient in pregnancy (Nejm 1984;310:442), due to incr
    vasopressinase (Nejm 1987;316:1070)
  • Renal tubular damage from hypercalcemia, hypokalemia, chronic
    pyelonephritis, chronic partial obstruction, sickle cell anemia,
    aging, lead poisoning, renal tubular acidosis
Epidem: Pregnancy may unmask (Nejm 1991;324:522)
Pathophys: Vasopressin (ADH) deficiency or resistance; normally it dilates
    splanchnic arterioles, increases renin, and stimulates factor VIII

clotting factors; in kidney cause water resorption (Nejm 1988; 318:881)

Idiopathic central DI associated w lymphocytic infiltration of neuro-hypophyseal area and probably immune in etiology (Nejm 1993; 329:683)

Sx: Excessive thirst and urination

Si: Hypovolemia

Crs:

Cmplc: Mental retardation due to infantile dehydration

r/o **psychogenic water drinker** who can partially concentrate urine with fluid restriction (Nejm 1981;305:1539)

Lab:

Chem: Na >145, at least when limit water po. Serum vasopressin (Nejm 1981;305:1539) decr a little in psychogenic water drinker, markedly in central DI; elevated significantly in nephrogenic DI. 24-h urinary ADH in U/h is decr in central DI, and elevated in nephrogenic DI (Ann IM 1972;77:715). Uric acid elevated, why? (Nejm 1971;284:1057)

Urine: Specific gravity <1.019. If complaining of incr thirst but serum Na normal, then water-restrict and thereby dehydrate until q 1 h urine specific gravities plateau; then compare this specific gravity with that after ADH (vasopressin) injection; or water-restrict to hypernatremia, getting coincident urine and serum osmoles. True DI patient will not get urine osmoles much >300, unlike psychogenic water drinker who can get urine osmoles ≥600

Xray: IVP shows dilated collecting system in genetic nephrogenic DI
MRI of pituitary in central type

Rx: Acutely replace water deficit (p 739) at less than 12 mEq Na increase/24 h

of central type, desmopressin (vasopressin analog) 5–20 μgm nasal, sq, or iv q 4–20 h for complete type (Ann IM 1985;103:229; Med Let 1978;20:26). Desmopressin is resistant to vasopressinase (Nejm 1987;316:1070). For incomplete type, treat the same or treat like nephrogenic

of nephrogenic type: thiazides, carbamazepine (Nejm 1974;291:1234), or chlorpropamide (Nejm 1970;282:1266); amiloride 5–10 mg bid helps at least lithium type (Nejm 1985;312:408)

RENAL/UROLOGY

20.2 ACQUIRED RENAL DISEASES

RENAL STONES

Nejm 1992;327:1141; Ann IM 1989;111:1006; 1977;87:404

Cause: Calcium oxalate (75%), from hyperparathyroidism (10^+%) but probably mostly (>50%) idiopathic (rarely sarcoid) hypercalciuria, which is genetic in most cases with autosomal dominant inheritance; struvite (10–15%), from UTIs w urease-producing organisms; urate (5%); hydroxyapatite or brushite (5%), cystine (1%)

Epidem: Incidence = 100/100,000 men, 36/100,000 women; 3–5% of US population will get sometime in life; incidence higher in SE US

Pathophys: 80% of stones are calcium type, associated with a red blood cell and probable renal tubular oxalate excretion defect (Nejm 1986; 314:599) or a deficit of the Ca/Mg pump (Nejm 1988;319:897); another 10% are associated with hyperparathyroidism

Increased calcium absorption may also play a role, either primary or by bringing out deficits like those above, eg, in sarcoid (Nejm 1984; 311:116). Uric acid stones may also precipitate calcium on themselves

Calcium oxalate stones are increased in colectomy, blind loop syndrome, and intestinal bypass pts due to bacterial breakdown of bile salts leading to absorption of glycolytic acid (Ann IM 1978;89:594)

Struvite stones are caused by ammonia from urea-splitting *Proteus* in pts with chronic UTIs due to indwelling Foley and/or quadraplegia

Sx: Pain radiating into groin; hematuria gross and/or microscopic; especially in children, the latter may be the presenting finding (Nejm 1984;310:1345)

Si:

Crs: Recurrence after first stone is 15% at 1 yr, 35% at 5 yr, 50% at 10 yr (Ann IM 1989;111:1006)

Cmplc: r/o renal artery embolism pain (Ann IM 1978;89:477); and rare primary hyperoxaluria w oxalosis as renal failure develops (Nejm 1994;331:1553)

Lab:

Chem: Serum calcium and uric acid w 1st stone

For recurrent stone, 24 hr urine for creatinine clearance, Na, calcium, urate, citrate, oxalate; or spot urine ratios

24-h urine calcium ≥300 mg in men, ≥250 mg in women

Ca/creat ratio ≥0.2 mg/mg creat
Uric acid >1 gm/24 h; or

$$\frac{\text{urine urate} \times \text{serum creat}}{\text{urine creat}} > 0.7$$

24-h urine oxalate >40 mg (Nejm 1993;328:880)

Path: Stone analysis

Urine: Rbc's, crystals (pictures—Nejm 1992;327:1142)

Rx: Dietary: drink 2$^+$ L of fluid qd, especially coffee and wine but not grapefruit juice (Ann IM 1998;128:534); reduce salt and protein intake; avoid calcium supplements but further decr in dietary calcium intake is not beneficial because calcium decreases oxalate and urate absorption (Ann IM 1997;126:497; Nejm 1993;328:833, 880); avoid phosphoric acid-containing soft drinks (J Clin Epidem 1992;45:911)

Thiazides help renal tubular/absorptive type, eg, hydrochlorthiazide 50 mg qd, or amiloride 5 mg po qd (Nejm 1986;314:599; 1984;311:116)

Allopurinol 300 mg po qd decreases calcium oxalate stone recurrence if there is an increased 24-h urine urate (Nejm 1986;315:1386)

Polycitra K 30–80 mEq po qd (Ann IM 1986;104:33) or citrate in lemon juice as lemonade (J Urol 1996;156:907) by creating a soluble complex w calcium; tablet type may cause gi bleed (Med Let 1986;28:48); works by increasing stone inhibitors

Na cellulose PO$_4$ 5 gm po qd-tid to get 24-h urine calcium <300 mg (Med Let 1983;25:67); blocks gi calcium uptake

Pyridoxine 2 gm po qd for oxalate stones? (Nejm 1985;312:953)

Cholestyramine po for secondary oxalic aciduria (Nejm 1972; 286:1371)

Surgical percutaneous dissolution of renal pelvis stones over 1–3 wk (Nejm 1979;300:341); basketing via cystoscope; or surgical excision. Extracorporeal shock wave lithotripsy, $2 million machine, requires anesthesia (Ann IM 1985;103:626) but very effective especially for calcium oxalate stones

RENAL/UROLOGY

RENAL FAILURE
Nejm 1970;282:953

Cause: Multiple, especially diabetes and hypertension (Nejm 1996;334: 13); chronic acetaminophen or ASA use (Nejm 2001;345:1801)

Pathophys:

- Acidosis from decr renal ability to secrete hydrogen ion
- Ca/P imbalances (Nejm 1987;316:1573,1601) from uremic suppression of vit D effect and decr renal conversion to active forms, decr degradation of PTH; decr phosphate clearance leads to CaP precipitation in vessels, skin, kidneys, heart, and further hypoCa; all these lead to osteomalacia or secondary hyperparathyroidism. Aluminum antacids decrease vit D effect (Nejm 1982;307:709) and cause Al deposition in bones, increasing fractures
- Potassium high or low depending on intake alone, since distal tubular excretion by remaining nephrons is already maximal
- Anemia, mostly from decr erythropoietin, bleeding from impaired clotting (Nejm 1986;315:731) and dialysis losses
- BP changes: Hypertension from Na overload, incr sympathetic tone and/or incr renin (Nem 1992;327:1912); hypotension due to end-organ resistance to ADH and aldosterone
- Neuropathies, peripheral and autonomic, from demyelination due partly to incr PTH (Nejm 1978;298:1000), reversible (Nejm 1971;284:170)
- Delayed hypersensitivity immune suppression
- Pruritus probably caused by histamines (Nejm 1992;326:969)

Sx: Lassitude, pruritus, nausea/vomiting, anorexia, muscle cramps, sleep disturbance

Si: Distinctive breath (Nejm 1977;297:132), incr pigmentation, anemia, volume reversible pulmonic valve insufficiency (Ann IM 1985;103: 497), postural hypotension (Nejm 1974;290:650) or hypertension, absent tendon reflexes and other peripheral neuropathies

Cmplc: Fractures and osteomalacia, acidosis, metastatic calcifications, infections especially viral pericarditis (Nejm 1969;281:542), rarely goiter (uremic suppression—Ann IM 1976;84:672), renally excreted drug toxicities; sleep apnea, helped by nocturnal hemodialysis (Nejm 2001;344:102)

Lab:

Rx:

of bleeding (Nejm 1998;339:245): estrogens (Nejm 1986;315:731) as conjugated estrogens 0.6 mg/kg iv qd × 4–5 d or 50 mg po qd; desmopressin sc or nasally (p 350), erythropoietin

of drug dosing: Ann IM 1980;93:62—table for all

of edema: furosemide up to 500 mg any route; 0.5–2 gm can be used but risk of transient or permanent nerve damage, especially auditory; or bumetanide 2–6 mg bolus q 12 h; or either, in similar doses as continuous infusions, eg, bumetanide 1 mg/h safer and as effective (Nejm 1991;115:360)

of hyperkalemia: (p 741); beware of alkalosis with chronic use along with milk of Mg (Nejm 1972;286:23)

of malnutrition/fatigue: androgens like nandrolone 100 mg im q 1 wk (Jama 1999;281:1275)

of pruritus: antihistamines; erythropoietin rx helps (80%) (Nejm 1992; 326:969); ultraviolet tan (Ann IM 1979;91:17; Nejm 1974;291: 136); iv lidocaine (Nejm 1977;296:261); activated charcoal (Ann IM 1980;93:446); parathyroidectomy

of HT: ACEIs preferable to calcium channel blockers (Nejm 1999;340: 1322); keep BP <125/80 to slow worsening renal function and proteinuria (Ann IM 1995;123:754)

of calcium/phosphate abnormalities (Nejm 1995;333:166): parathyroidectomy (Nejm 1968;279:695) now rarely needed; $CaCO_3$ (Tums) binds PO_4 and improves Ca × P product better than AlOH binders (Nejm 1991;324:527), which increase aluminum levels, leading to anemia, dementia, and bone changes (Nejm 1997;336: 1557, 1982;307:709), rx with deferoxamine (Nejm 1984;311:140; Ann IM 1984;101:775); low-phosphate diets plus $CaCO_3$ or Ca acetate po given with meals to minimize absorption of dietary PO_4 (Nejm 1989;320:1110); vit D as calcitriol 0.25 μgm po qd if Ca <10.5 and PTH high (Med Let 1982;24:92) to prevent secondary hyperparathyroidism

of anemia: recombinant erythropoietin iv tiw (Ann IM 1991;114:402) or sc just as good (Nejm 1998;339:578; Am J Med 1990;89:432) to maintain hct at 30–35%, higher not necessary even if heart disease (Nejm 1998;339:584); adequate iron replacement and dialysis facilitate erythropoetin response to keep hct >30% (Nejm 1996;334:420)

RENAL/UROLOGY

of azotemia:

- Diet: Protein restriction to <0.4–0.6 gm/kg/day (BMJ 1992;304: 214; Nejm 1989;321:1773) but is controversial because malnutrition predicts poor prognosis, and phosphates to 1 gm qd together (Nejm 1991;324:78) along w tight BP control, slow renal failure progression (Nejm 1994;330:877); and tight lipid control?
- ACE inhibitors slow progression (Nejm 1996;334:939) esp if used early when creatinine clearance = 40–60 cc/min and if proteinuria present; even in polycystic disease; unrelated to decr in BP
- Dialysis (Nejm 1998;338:1428):

  Peritoneal (Nejm 1969;281:945)

  Hemo: survival not as good as cadaveric transplant (Nejm 1999; 341:1725) and dialysis significantly worsens renal transplant survival (Nejm 2001;344:726). Adverse effects: folate deficiency (Nejm 1968;279:970), EKG artifacts with fistula/ cannula arm (Nejm 1978;298:1439); mortality = 10–20%/yr; Zn deficiency causes primary gonadal impairment, reversible with 25 mg po qd (Ann IM 1982;97:357); amyloidosis; rare antacid Mg intoxication (Nejm 1969;280:981), rare Cu intoxication from tubing (Ann IM 1970;73:409), Fe deficiency; incr ASHD (Nejm 1974;290:697); gynecomastia; hepatitis B rarely a cause now w immunization avaiable but still seen w hepatitis C chronic hepatitis. For-profit dialysis centers have lower survival and transplant rates (Nejm 1999; 341:1653,1691)

  Hemofiltration for transient support (Nejm 1997;336:1303)
- Transplantation graft survival 90+% at 1 yr and 80+% at 5 yr and rapidly improving still (Nejm 2000;342:605): HLA typed matched or mismatched from living or cadaver donors, 50% 10 yr survival (Nejm 2000;343:1078). Immunosuppression with cyclosporine, nephrotoxic though (Nejm 1986;314:1219, 1293), then prednisone + azathioprine (Nejm 1988;318:1499) or mycophenolate (CellCept) in 1st yr. Adverse effects: incr tumors (decr surveillance) including squamous cell carcinomas of skin (Nejm 1991;325:843), incr ASHD (Ann IM 1979;91:554), CMV infections prevented w valacyclovir (Nejm 1999;340:1463) or gangcyclovir

ACUTE TUBULAR NECROSIS
Nejm 1996;334:1448

Cause: Often multiple
- Shock, simple or that associated with: muscle breakdown/ myoglobinuria, eg, traumatic crush injury (Nejm 1991;324:1417), exercise, or hypothermia; open heart surgery (1/3 get some, 3% get full ATN, correlates with pump time—Ann IM 1976;84:677), abdominal aneurysm repair with aortic cross-clamping, etc. (Ann IM 1976;85:23; Nejm 1974;291:807)
- Nephrotoxins including heavy metals, CCl_4 and other organic solvents, drugs (eg, gentamicin, amphotericin), snake venom
- Intravascular hemolysis
- IVP or CT contrast material especially in elderly whose creatinine is >2 mg% (Nejm 1989;320:143), or patients with multiple myeloma

Epidem:

Pathophys: GFR decreases before tubular function decreases; fortunate, otherwise would dehydrate quickly. Tubular necrosis → interstitial edema → more oliguria due to increased extratubular pressure

Sx:

Si: Oliguria usually, though nonoliguric form very common now with rapid fluid rx

Crs: Recovery in 10–30 d if maintain with dialysis; 30–40% will be left with a diminished GFR or concentrating ability so can't concentrate urine >3× plasma (Ann IM 1970;73:523)

Cmplc: (p 750); CHF

r/o other causes of acute oliguria (Nejm 1998;338:671) like: obstructive disease; other intrinsic renal diseases like acute GN and interstitial nephritis especially drug (NSAID)-induced type; and prerenal causes including hypovolemia and low cardiac output syndromes

Lab:

Path: Gross shows swollen kidney; congested medullary pyramids with pale cortex; microscopic shows tubular necrosis especially proximally with poisons; interstitial edema; regenerating tubules by day 3

Urine: Smell absent, unlike prerenal azotemia (Nejm 1980;303:1125) Urine osmoles <350 in contrast to prerenal azotemia where >500; osmole/plasma osmole ratio <1.7; Na >40 mEq/L unlike <20 in prerenal azotemia; urea nitrogen <3× plasma unlike >8 in prerenal azotemia; creatinine <20× plasma unlike >40 in prerenal azotemia; volume <400 cc/24 h, 50% false neg but that's more benign type anyway

UA sediment shows tubular casts

Rx: Prevent

in myoglobinuria from rhabdomyolysis after crush injury (Nejm 1991;324:1417), w iv fluids + mannitol to keep output >100cc/hr + alkalinize urine w iv NaHCO3; or w iv fluids + furosemide

when radiocontrast used in pt w creat >1.2 or creat clearance <50 cc/min (Rx Let 2001;8:13): d/c NSAIDs × 3–4 d, hold metformin × 2d, stop diuretics, give 1/2-NS at 1 cc/kg/h × 12 h just before and for 12 h after angiography (11% incidence using this regimen), or combined w acetylcysteine 600 mg (3 cc of 20% soln) taken w soft drink po bid day before and day of, decr incid to <2% (Nejm 2000;343:180, 210). Prophylactic dopamine infusion no help (Ann IM 1994;120:744), mannitol and furosemide of equally doubtful help (Nejm 1994;331:1416)

Anaritide (atrial natiuretic peptide) iv acutely may help oliguric form but may worsen dialysis-free survival in anuric cases (Nejm 1997; 336:828)

Supportive with protein limitation to <30 gm/day; water to 400 cc plus urine output + insensibles; watch K^+ by avoiding old blood if transfuse, and treat elevations with Na polystyrene (Kayexalate); peritoneal or hemodialysis, especially if muscle breakdown

NEPHROTIC SYNDROME

Nejm 1998;339:894, 338:1202; 1994;330:61

Cause:

Primary types:

- Membranous GN (p 758); the cause in 7% of children with nephrotic syndrome, and in 40% of adults
- Minimal change GN (p 758); the cause in 76% of children and 20% of adults
- Chronic proliferative GN (40%); in 4% of children and 7% of adults

- Focal, segmental GN; in 8% of children and 15% of adults
- Other: in 5% of children and in 18% of adults

Secondary types:
- SLE and other collagen vascular diseases
- Amyloid (especially in rheumatoid arthritis; multiple myeloma; familial Mediterranean fever; chronic infections like SBE, hepatitis B, and HIV)
- Bee stings and snake venom
- Diabetic Kimmelstiel-Wilson disease
- Heavy metal drug rx, eg, gold
- Chronic iv heroin use (Nejm 1974;290:19; Ann IM 1974;80:488)
- Cancer, eg, lung, probably by paraneoplastic antibody-antigen complexes (Nejm 1993;328:1621), colon, prostate, breast

Epidem:

Pathophys: Protein losses in urine lead to all si and sx's and lab abnormalities. Caused by two types of pathologic processes: generalized uniform basement membrane thickening or damage as seen in membranous GN, and minimal lesion types caused by an elutable small protein deposited on the glomeruli (Nejm 1994;330:7); and spotty deposition of immune complexes as seen in poststreptococcal nephritis, SBE, SLE, and serum sickness

Elevated lipids are due to the hepatic response to decr albumin oncotic pressure (Nejm 1985;312:1544). LDL is increased by slowed metabolism and an increase in apoprotein B production (Nejm 1990;323:579).

Sx: Edema, periorbital in the morning and pedal in the afternoon

Si: Edema, anasarca

Crs: Nephrotic syndrome due to secondary causes, may reverse after rx of primary disease (Nejm 1970;282:128)

Cmplc: Infections, if IgG loss; acquired factor IX deficiency (Ann IM 1970;73:373); renal vein thrombosis (Ann IM 1976;85:310); hypercoagulable states in 50% lead to pulmonary emboli, etc; malabsorption of food and meds due to bowel wall edema; accelerated ASHD

r/o myeloma and primary renal (AL) amyloidosis w urinary immuno-electrophoresis

Lab:

Chem: LDL cholesterol is increased (Ann IM 1993;119:263); hypoalbuminemia

Path: Renal biopsy usually shows etiology (pictures—Ann IM 1972; 76:479), foot process fusion by electron microscopy in minimal lesion GN; "wire loops" by light microscopy in membranous GN; incr mesangial cells without polys in proliferative GN

Serol: Serum protein electrophoresis (SPEP) shows decr IgG in membranous GN type ("big holes" let IgG leak out); decr complement; incr α_2- and β-lipoprotein

Urine: 24-h protein >3–3.5 gm; "oval fat bodies" (fat-laden tubular cells in sediment). Protein/creatinine ratio on random urine as good or better than 24-h urine; <0.2 is normal, ≥3.5 is nephrotic (Nejm 1983;309:1543)

Rx: Diuretics and severe Na restriction

Captopril and other ACE inhibitors improve lipids (Ann IM 1993;118:246) and lower protein excretion

Antihyperlipidemia rx

Anticoagulation w warfarin or at least ASA

Specific rx to etiologic diagnosis

ACUTE PROLIFERATIVE GLOMERULONEPHRITIS

Nejm 1998;339:891

Cause:

- Idiopathic
- Circulating immune complexes (Nejm 1976;295:185), eg, antithyroglobulin-thyroglobulin type in Graves'? (Nejm 1981;304:1212,1230);
- Poststreptococcal (Ann IM 1979;91:76), types 4, 12, 57, and Redlake (Nejm 1970;283:832) from skin lesions or throat; these types never cause acute rheumatic fever (Nejm 1970;283:561);
- Postviral including coxsackie B, echo, influenza A and B, and adenovirus pharyngitis infections; cause 4% (Ann IM 1979; 91:697)

Epidem: In adults, <50% are poststreptococcal; more commonly due to skin infections when does occur; in children >95% are poststrep, often in epidemics. Males > females among children

Pathophys: Circulating ag/ab complexes deposited in "lumpy" way in basement membrane

Sx: History of strep infection 10–14 d before; abrupt onset; malaise; headache; facial edema; flank pain; cloudy urine

Si: Hypertension, periorbital facial edema, hematuria, oliguria

Crs: Correlates with anuria and biopsy; best when strep cause; better with younger age; once healed no later deterioration (Nejm 1982;307: 725); microhematuria can persist for up to year afterward

Cmplc: Hypertensive crisis

r/o SBE, hypersensitivity angiitis, polyarteritis nodosa, Goodpasture's (Ann IM 1975;83:734), SLE, anaphylactoid purpura

Lab: (Nejm 1983;309:1299)

Chem: Elevated creatinine and BUN; proteins normal

Hem: ESR elevated; factor VIII increase correlates with poor recovery (Ann IM 1975;83:337)

Path: Renal biopsy shows grossly swollen "flea-bitten" kidneys; microscopically, focal or diffuse (SLE) glomerular involvement, diagnostic infiltration by polys, and lumpy deposition of immune complexes; rapidly progressive GN in anti-BM antibody (Goodpasture's) or small vessel vasculitis (p 833) etiologies has diagnostic crescent formation, and linear immunofluorescent antibody deposition in antibasement membrane type

Serol: ASO titer >400 Todd U is diagnostic of strep, >125 U is suggestive; C_3 <100 mg% via alternate pathway and in contrast to normal CH_{50} and C_4 (Nejm 1992;327:1366)

Urine: Hematuria with rbc casts; r/o collagen vascular disease, SBE, vasculitis, severe hypertension, ATN, vascular occlusion, trauma, hereditary nephritis, **idiopathic focal proliferative glomerulo-nephritis** (benign, recurs with sore throats, and has normal complement levels—Ann IM 1970;73:921); **Goodpasture's syndrome** w anti-basement membrane antibodies and hemoptysis, rx'd w plasma exchange, Cytoxan and steroids (Ann IM 2001; 134:1033)

Proteinuria >30 mg but <6 gm/24 h; resolution doesn't guarantee no permanent damage

Creatinine clearance low

Rx: Penicillin × 2 wk acutely, no value as prophylaxis; supportive of renal failure

MEMBRANOUS GLOMERULONEPHRITIS

Nejm 1974;290:313

Cause: Idiopathic, or associated with BM deposition of antibody seen with *Staphylococcus albus*-infected hydrocephalic shunts (Nejm 1968;279:1077), hepatitis B (Nejm 1979;300:814), especially in children with chronic HBsAg (Nejm 1991;324:1457; Ann IM 1989;111:479), captopril use (Sci Am Text Med 1986), NSAID use (Jama 1996;276:466), malignancy (Am J Kid Dis 1993;22:5)

Epidem: Primarily in adults

Pathophys: Increased BM thickness in glomerular tuft by electron and light microscopy

Sx: Few, feel well, insidious onset

Si: Of nephrotic syndrome (p 754)

Crs: 80% 5-yr survival

Cmplc: Nephrotic syndrome; renal failure

Lab:

Path: Renal biopsy shows incr BM thickness on light microscopy, especially with PAS stain, and on electron microscopy

Urine: Hematuria (40%)

Rx: No rx beyond diuretics and antihypertensives justified, no renal failure in 88% after 5 yr, 73% after 8 yr, and 65% recover in 5 yr (Nejm 1993;329:85)

Steroids and cytotoxic drug roles controversial, usually reserved for pts w 24-h urine protein >10 gm, and/or elevated but not progressive creatinine elevations; methylprednisolone, or alternate with chlorambucil q 1 mo × 6 mo (Nejm 1992;327:599); or cyclophosphamide + prednisone × 1 yr (Ann IM 1991;114:725); or prednisone alone as good (Ann IM 1992;116:438)

In hepatitis B glomerulonephritis, α interferon (very expensive) for 4 mo (Ann IM 1989;111:479) although recurs off rx and side effects substantial

MINIMAL CHANGE ("Lipoid") NEPHRITIS

Cause: Unknown

Epidem: Children, rare in adults

Pathophys: Increased podocyte processes and fusion (Ann IM 1968; 69:1171)

Sx:

Si: Of nephrotic syndrome

Crs: Most resolve completely in both adults (Ann IM 1974;81:314) and children

Cmplc:

Lab:

> *Path:* Renal biopsy shows no abnormalities on light microscope; on electron microscopy, incr number and fusion of foot processes
>
> *Urine:* Proteinuria enough to diagnose nephrosis (ie, >3.5 gm)

Rx: Prednisone 60 mg/m²/d, taper over 2⁺ mo

> Cyclophosphamide 2.5 mg/kg/d × 8 wk; safe, effective if steroids alone inadequate or relapses occur (Nejm 1984;310:415)

CHRONIC GLOMERULONEPHRITIS

Nejm 1998;339:895

Cause: Sequel of membranous and proliferative glomerulonephritis (GN) and idiopathic

Epidem: 50% probably membranous GN, 20% probably proliferative GN, 30% unknown etiology including IgA nephropathy, 10% of all end stage renal disease, higher in older men

Pathophys: Gradual progression of initiating disease leads to glomerular hyalinization with secondary tubular atrophy and interstitial fibrosis leads to renal failure

> IgA deposits are presumed immune complexes

Sx: Nephrotic syndrome (p 754)

Si: Of nephrosis, HT

Crs: Slowly decreasing renal function over many years, usually >20 yr

Cmplc: of renal failure (p 750)

Lab:

> *Chem:* BUN and creatinine elevated
>
> *Path:* Renal biopsy shows scarring, focally or diffuse
>
> *Urine:* Proteinuria

Rx: Supportive (p 750) including aggressive ACE inhibitor rx of HT of IgA nephropathy: fish oil, 12 gm qd may slow progression by preventing damage by mediators like prostaglandins etc.

RENAL/UROLOGY

IgA NEPHROPATHY

Nejm 1998;339:890; 1994;331:1194

Cause: Altered regulation of production or structure of IgA

Epidem: High prevalence in western Pacific Rim, low in US and Europe; M > F, esp under age 25; most common form of GN worldwide, most common cause of asx hematuria

Pathophys: IgA immune complexes deposited in glomeruli, diffuse mesangial deposits; Henoch-Schönlein purpura similar morphologically, maybe etiologically

Sx: Goss hematuria, esp assoc w URI or gastroenteritis

Si: Hematuria (60%), asx (30%); AGN, or nephrotic syndrome (10%)

Crs: 20–40% progress to chronic renal failure

Cmplc:

Lab:

Serol: Elevated IgA levels

Rx: Fish oil; ACE inhibitors

20.3 INHERITED RENAL DISEASES

POLYCYSTIC KIDNEY DISEASE

Nejm 1993;329:332; 1990;323:1085; Ann IM 1984;101:238

Cause: Genetic, autosomal dominant; at least 2 different gene sites (Nejm 1988;319:913), most commonly (90%) on chromosome #6

Epidem: Most diagnosed in early adulthood although infantile type does occur and presents as large kidneys at birth, die within months. Peak onset at age 45; 100% get by age 90; F = M; prevalence = 1/400–1000

Pathophys: Tubular cysts increase in size by secretion of solutes, and compromise renal function (Nejm 1969;281:985) and thereby increasing renin-aldosterone systems that cause hypertension (Nejm 1990;323:1091); also occur in liver

Sx: Flank/back pain (61%); positive family hx (60%); dysuria (8%); gross hematuria (12%); nocturia (8%); headache (20%); nausea (5%)

Si: Hypertension (62%); palpable kidney (52%); palpable liver (27%); abdominal tenderness (20%); peripheral edema (10%); systolic murmur (10%)

Crs: 5–10 yr after BUN starts to increase

Cmplc: Hepatic cysts (40%), increasing incidence with age; also in pancreas and spleen; berry aneurysm (4%), screen pts w family h/o aneurysm w CT or MRI and operate if >10 mm (Nejm 1992;327: 916, 953); aortic and mitral valve dilatations (Nejm 1988;319:907); colonic diverticulosis (Ann IM 1980;92:202); Na wasting, occasionally renal tubular acidosis

r/o other renal cystic disease (Ann IM 1978;88:176):
- Multicystic renal disease, which consists of benign, common retention cysts
- Multicystic dysplasia: Compatible with life if unilateral, most not hereditary, associated with urethral atresia, rarely autosomal dominant and associated w deafness and hypoparathyroidism (Nejm 1992;327:1069)
- Medullary cystic disease (Nejm 1981;305:1334) with anemia, severe Na wasting, renal failure, and death in teens; X-linked recessive
- Medullary sponge kidney with tubular ectasia, benign except for stones and pyelo, worst in women (Nejm 1982;306:1088), small stones in cysts (r/o nephrocalcinosis and tbc), associated with Ehlers-Danlos syndrome, also with autosomal recessive renal-retinal dysplasia with retinitis pigmentosa (Ann IM 1976;84:157)
- Hypokalemia-induced medullary cysts, reversible (Nejm 1990; 322:345)

Lab:
Chem: BUN and creatinine increase late in course
Path: Dilated nephrons and tubules lead to cysts
Urine: AM specific gravity <1.015; proteinuria, pyuria
Xray: IVP shows large cystic kidneys
Ultrasound is most sensitive test, and can look for hepatic cysts too (40%); most abnormal by age 20 in carriers (J. Engel 2/92)
Rx: of renal failure
Tight BP control may retard progression, ACE inhibitors can be used cautiously but precipitate acute renal failure (Ann IM 1991;115: 769); avoid catheterization at all costs since can lead to rapidly fatal infection; avoid hypokalemia, which can increase cyst growth rate
Occasionally need surgical relief of pressure from bloody cystic compression of adjacent structures

RENAL TUBULAR ACIDOSIS

Nejm 1969;281:1405

Causes: Types I (classic) and II, both types may be genetic, autosomal dominant, or induced in a renal transplant (Ann IM 1973;79:352; 1969;71:39); type IV is the most common

Of type I: amphotericin B, dose-related (Nejm 1968;278:124); hyper-IgG states especially with collagen vascular diseases; hepatic cirrhosis (Nejm 1969;280:1); toluene glue sniffing (Ann IM 1981; 94:758; Nejm 1974;290:765); nephrocalcinosis

Of type II: sulfonamides; old tetracycline; carbonic anhydrase inhibitors; Fanconi syndromes

Of type IV: diabetes via hyporeninemia/hypoaldosteronism

Epidem:

Pathophys: Type I is caused by distal tubular damage, which causes an inability to acidify urine, which then leads to general cation loss, hyperchloremic acidosis, calcium loss, renal stone formation. "Complete" syndrome is continuous acidosis no matter what the po intake is; "incomplete" syndrome requires an acid load to bring out

Type II is caused by a proximal tubular defect in bicarbonate resorption so that there is a lowered serum threshold for bicarbonate loss in the urine (T_{max}) but no problem otherwise even with an acid load

Hyperchloremia maintains ionic balance of blood. In most other acidotic states another anion such as lactate, acetate, or formate takes place of depleted HCO_3

Sx: Hypokalemic weakness, hypocalcemic tetany

Si: Hyperventilation and other signs of metabolic acidosis

Crs: Genetic types have onset at school age

Cmplc: Ricketts and osteomalacia; nephrolithiasis and calcinosis

Lab:

Chem: Acidosis, hypokalemia, and hyperchloremia, but r/o other causes (Nejm 1977;297:816) of hyperchloremic metabolic acidosis with normal anion gap (p 740), like diarrhea, NH_4Cl intake, acetazolamide (Diamox), or other carbonic anhydrase inhibitors, and obstructive uropathy (Nejm 1981;304:373); or with a low anion gap as seen in multiple myeloma (Nejm 1977;296:858), and aldosterone deficiency

Urine: Elevated phosphates, potassium, calcium; and in type II, glucose. Urinary pH in type I always >5, even after 0.1 gm NH_4Cl/kg po; watch urine over 8-h period (Nejm 1971;285:501);

r/o Na depletion, which will prevent kidney from excreting enough H^+, ie, Na^+ distal absorption takes priority over H^+ and K^+ absorption (Nejm 1987;316:140). Urinary pH in type II <5 in severe acidosis but >5 when serum bicarbonate is still <20 mEq/L, eg, after the above NH_4Cl load

Urinary anion gap (gap = Na + K − Cl) is positive, unlike negative gap seen in diarrhea (Nejm 1988;318:594)

Rx: K-gluconate or other potassium-containing replacement without chloride, to absorb excess body acid (Nejm 1969;280:671); or $NaHCO_3$; or Shohl's solution of citric acid and sodium citrate

20.4 INFECTIONS

FEMALE CYSTITIS/URETHRITIS

J Am Ger Soc 1996;44:1235 (elderly), Nejm 1993;329:1328; Ann IM 1989;111:906

Cause (K. Holmes—Nejm 1980;303:409): 70% due to coliforms at >10^5/cc in urine; 11%, coliforms at <10^5/cc in urine; 5%, *Chlamydia trachomatis;* 1%, *Staphylococcus saprophyticus* (often misread as *S. epidermidis* or *albus* by labs) 4% (Jama 1999;281:736); gc; herpes simplex

Epidem: Incidence, up to perhaps 20% of all women get each year; incr with catheters, mostly from perimeatal invasions of urethra along outside of catheter (Nejm 1980;303:316); $\geq 10^2$ organisms are significant in catheterized patients (Nejm 1984;311:560); incr with sexual activity, history of previous episodes, and spermicides + diaphragm use (Nejm 2000;343:992; 1996;335:468); not prevented by various hygiene habits except voiding after sex (Ann IM 1987; 107:816)

Pathophys: Recurrent disease, due to a possible inherent defect in epithelial cell membrane leading to easier adherence by bacteria (Nejm 1986;314:1208; 1981;304:1062)

Sx: Dysuria, frequency; stuttering onset over days with chlamydia type OTC home kits specific but quite insens, many false negs (Rx Let 1997;4:21)

RENAL/UROLOGY

Si:

Crs: Many resolve without rx and many are subclinical (asx) (Nejm 2000;343:992); catheter-induced UTIs have 2–4 times the mortality of non-catheter-induced UTIs (Nejm 1982;307:637) and only 1/3 resolve after removal without rx, 90% will with single dose or 10 d rx (Ann IM 1991;114:713)

Cmplc: r/o vaginitis, herpes, and subclinical pyelo, which can dx when it relapses eventually; reflux nephropathy in children w renal US + VCUG w 1st documented UTI; chronic interstitial (idiopathic) cystitis (Med Let 1997;39:56)

Lab:

Bact: Culture of midstream urine (clean catch unnecessary—Nejm 1993;328:289), $>10^5$ organisms in only 50% of truly infected women with sx; 10^2 a better criterion when sx (Ann IM 1993; 119:454; Holmes—Nejm 1982;307:463)

Urine: UA shows pyuria, >5–6 wbc/hpf (10% false neg, 50% false pos when have sx—Nejm 1982;307:463); hematuria (often not with chlamydia); dipstick nitrite tests have high false-pos rates so cultures much better (Ped Infect Dis J 1991;10:651). Sens/specif of all such tests vary greatly by pretest likelihood, eg, w <5 wbc's/hpf, sens/specif both = 60%, if >5 wbc, sens is 100%, specif 22% (Ann IM 1992;117:135)

Xray: IVP and cystoscopy of no value to workup recurrent UTIs in adult women (Nejm 1981;304:462)

Rx: (Med Let 1981;23:69)

Prevent in postmenopausal women w recurrent UTIs w estriol 0.5 mg cream (Ovestin) qd × 2 wk then biw, helps without significant estrogen absorption (Nejm 1993;329:753)

Prophylaxis w Tm/S 1/2 a single strength (40/200) pill qd hs (Nejm 1974;291:597), or postintercourse; is cost effective if ≥3 UTIs/yr (Ann IM 1981;94:250)

Antibiotics (Med Let 1999;41:98):

- Regular rx of a UTI: Tm/S single strength bid, ciprofloxacin 250 mg po bid or other fluoroquinolone, or amoxicillin 250–500 mg po tid × 7–10 d, if no gonorrhea, chlamydia, or vaginitis (Nejm 1981;304:956; 1980;303:409,452). 20% resistance to cephalothin, sulfa, amoxicillin (Jama 1999;281:736)

- 3-day regimens in uncomplicated patients also reasonable (Ann IM 1989;111:906), eg Tm/S DS bid × 3d gives 82% cure vs 67% cure for amoxicillin 500 mg po bid × 3d (Jama 1995;273:41); or a fluoroquinolone
- Single-dose regimens: Tm/S 160/800 (DS), 1–2 pills (1st choice—Ann IM 1988;108:350), as good when take prn at home as prophylactic use (Ann IM 1985;102:302); amoxicillin 2–3 gm po; or sulfasoxazole 1–2 gm po

Bladder anesthetics: phenazopyridine (Pyridium) 200 mg po tid × 2 d; stains urine dark orange

of asx bacteriuria, no rx indicated, although it correlates w worse prognosis, rx does not improve (Ann IM 1994;120:827)

of catheter-associated UTI: d/c catheter if can, rx if sx; can't clear UTI if catheter still in place

ACUTE PYELONEPHRITIS
Ann IM 1989;111:906

Cause: Gram-negative rods (95%), most commonly *E. coli* (especially a few uropathic strains—Nejm 1985;313:414), and next most frequently, *Proteus* spp; more rarely, gram-positive cocci (5%), staph and *Enterococcus*. Possibly ascend from a cystitis, or come from hematogenous seeding

Epidem: High prevalence at postmortem, especially in women; but <30% of these patients had sx in life

Increased incidence in patients with urinary retention; females age <18 mo and of childbearing age; patients with gu instrumentation (Nejm 1974;291:215); and with papillary necrosis in sickle cell disease and diabetes

Pathophys: Possible predisposition to infection of renal medulla due to incr osmotic pressures, which cause white cell inhibition, decr blood flow, and NH_3 inhibition of C'4 complement

Sx: Fever, flank pain; frequency, urgency, dysuria, and hematuria

Si: CVA punch tenderness

Crs: Of significant bacteriuria: 1/3 have sx; 80% recurrence over 2 yr with new organism, then stable; later, with marriage and pregnancy may recrudesce (Nejm 1970;282:1443)

Cmplc: Renal failure, chronic pyelo (perhaps in 40%—Jama 1970; 224:585)

Acute Pyelonephritis, continued

    r/o cystitis, intercourse-induced incr bacteriuria (Nejm 1978;298:321),
        cystitis with congenital vesicoureteric reflux by doing a voiding
        cystourethrogram, acute interstitial nephritis (Ann IM 1980;93:735)

Lab:
    Bact: Urine culture $\geq 10^2$ col/cc; antibody-coated bacteria may
        distinguish from cystitis, but unreliable and not available (Ann IM
        1989;110:138)
    Gram stain of unspun urine show ≥ 1 bacterium/oil immersion field

Xray: IVP shows dilated calyces and ureter acutely, r/o peritonitis (Nejm
    1972;287:535)

Rx: Repair of vesicoureteral reflux, but may not alter course (BMJ 1983;
    287:171)
    Antibiotics: ciprofloxacin (Jama 2000;283:1583) × 1 wk, or
        gentamicin + ampicillin or Tm/S (J Infect Dis 1991;163:325)
        × 2 wk or until have sensitivities since 30% of *E. coli* now are
        resistant to amoxicillin alone

CHRONIC INTERSTITIAL NEPHRITIS AND CHRONIC PYELONEPHRITIS

Cause: (Ann IM 1975;82:453)
- Drug-induced (20%) analgesic nephropathy (Nejm 2001;345:1801; 1998;338:446), direct toxicity with papillary necrosis, from acetaminophen (Nejm 1989;320:1238) and other NSAIDs (Nejm 1994;331:1675), especially men age >65 yr (Ann IM 1991;115:165); often ongoing clandestine use even after dx (J Clin Epidem 1991;44:53)
- Vascular disease causing nephrosclerosis (10%)
- Hypercalcemia and hyperuricemia (11%) w or w/o stones
- Idiopathic (10%—Ann IM 1975;82:453)
- Infectious: Rarely (Ann IM 1975;82:453) in women with asymptomatic bacteriuria renal failure even with many recurrences (Nejm 1979;301:396); same is true in elderly, though bacteriuria is a marker for other potentially fatal illness (Nejm 1986;314:1152); bacteria are usually *E. coli* and *Proteus* spp
- Diabetic or sickle cell-induced papillary necrosis

- K^+ depletion, especially due to incr aldosterone (Nejm 1990; 322:345)
- Sjögren's syndrome (Ann IM 1968;69:1163)
- Hereditary nephritis
- Reflux nephropathy

Epidem:

Pathophys:

Sx: Often none until end-stage renal failure; hypertension

Si:

Crs:

Cmplc: Renal failure; bladder cancer in phenacetin type (Ann IM 1980; 93:249)

r/o Allergic reactions w fever and/or rash, to penicillin (Nejm 1968;279: 1245), furosemide (Nejm 1973;288:124), NSAIDs esp naproxen (Nejm 1979;301:1271), cimetidine (fever and acute sx—Ann IM 1982;96:180), methoxyflurane anesthesia (Jama 1970;223:1239); only in NSAID induced type, proteinuria and eosinophils in urine by Hansel's stain (90%) (Wright's stain doesn't work on urine); rx w steroids if drug cessation not enough

Lab:

Urine: UA shows low specific gravity (present in all diseases that affect tubules, including hydronephrosis and infection; is reversible—Ann IM 1971;75:49); pyuria and casts; never significant proteinuria except in Sjögren's (Ann IM 1968;69:1163)

Xray: IVP shows calyceal clubbing; CT shows characteristic changes in analgesic nephropathy (Nejm 1998;338:446)

Rx: Discontinue any potential drug cause; rx associated disease; rx bacterial infection with appropriate antibiotic but no benefit in rx of asx bacteriuria in elderly males (Nejm 1983;309:1420); if sx, then Tm/S 1/2 tab qd (Nejm 1977;296:780), nitrofurantoin 50 mg qid or methenamine 1 gm qid with vitamin C 500 mg

MALE PROSTATITIS/CYSTITIS

J Am Ger Soc 1996;44:1235 (elderly), Ann IM 1989;110:138

Cause: *E. coli* (25%); other gram negatives (25$^+$%), including *Proteus* and *Providencia;* enterococci and *S. epidermidis* (20%)

RENAL/UROLOGY

Epidem: Rare unless obstruction by BPH, foreign body like catheter or
   stone, bladder tumors, or urethral strictures
   Increased incidence in elderly, mainly due to BPH, so that by age 65
   UTI incidence is same as in women
Pathophys:
Sx: Urethritis syndrome: dysuria, frequency, and urgency
   Obstructive syndrome (with prostatic involvement): hesitancy,
      nocturia, dribbling, slow stream, and terminal dysuria to penile tip
Si: Fever with prostatitis, not cystitis
   Rectal shows tender swollen prostate in prostatitis
Crs:
Cmplc: Pyelonephritis, chronic prostatitis, epididymitis (p 769)
   r/o gonorrhea, chlamydia, orchitis
Lab: No workup of occult urinary tract lesions indicated with first UTI in
   adult men; first episode should be worked up in boys and male
   infants w renal US and VCUG to r/o urethral valves and reflux
   Bact: Culture of urine, $>10^3$ col/cc with single or predominant
      organism (97% sens/specif); $>10^5$ col/cc if taken from condom
      catheter, reliable if clean glans, new catheter, and take urine within
      2 h of placing catheter. "4-glass" (first, mid, terminal void, and
      postprostatic massage specimens) cultures showing $>10\times$ higher
      colony counts in last 2 compared to first 2 is diagnostic of
      prostatitis
Rx: of asymptomatic bacteriuria, no rx indicated; although it worsens
   prognosis in elderly, rx doesn't improve prognosis (Ann IM 1994;
   120:827)
   of cystitis and acute prostatitis: Tm/S 160/800 bid; or if resistance
      suspected, ciprofloxacin; all for 7–10 d first time, but for 6–12 wk
      for recurrence
   of chronic prostatitis: Tm/S, ciprofloxacin especially if *Pseudomonas
      aeruginosa* (Nejm 1991;324:392), doxycycline, or aminoglycoside;
      all × 6–12 wk; still have 30–40% failure rates probably because
      much chronic prostatitis is abacterial and unresponsive to rx (Ann
      IM 2000;133:367)

EPIDIDYMITIS

Causes: Under age 35–40, most are due to chlamydia, occasionally gonorrhea or *Ureaplasma* spp spread venereally; over age 35–40, most due to gram-negative bacterial infections (Nejm 1978;298:301) caused by reflux of infected urine

Epidem: Rare under age 18 yr; peak incidence at age 32

Pathophys: Inflammation localized to epididymis only, testes spared

Sx: Gradual onset, although may first notice when hit lightly and report traumatic etiology

Si: Swollen epididymis with normal testicle in middle

Crs: May last 7–10 d with rx, longer without bedrest

Cmplc: Abscess, chronic pain, infertility

   r/o orchitis, usually viral; **testicular torsion** (usually under age 18, average age 14, often have had episodes in past, and more acute onset; must operate within 4–5 h to save 70%, only 15% saved at 10 h—Nejm 1977;296:338)

Lab:

   Bact: Urine culture

   Urine: UA to r/o infection

Rx: (Med Let 1999;41:86)

   Antibiotics: same under or over age 35–40; ofloxacin 300 mg po bid × 10 d; or ceftriaxone 250 mg im × 1 then doxycycline 100 mg po bid × 10d

   Bedrest, scrotal support, perhaps a NSAID, lidocaine block of spermatic cord in extreme pain cases

20.5   TUMORS/CANCERS

BENIGN PROSTATIC HYPERTROPHY

Cause:

Epidem: Common, 30% prevalence by physical exam at age 40–50, 35% of all men eventually will have sx requiring meds or surgery (Prostate suppl 1996;6:67); 50% over age 70 though only 25% have sx

Pathophys: Usually lateral and median lobes around the urethra lead to obstructive sx by a ball valve effect

Sx: Urgency and urge incontinence; obstructive sx like: hesitancy, decr stream, nocturia, postvoid dripping

Am Urol Assoc scoring system (Nejm 1995;332:99): 5 pts = always, 4 = >1/2 the time, 3 = 1/2 the time, 2 = <1/2 the time, 1 = <1/5 the time, 0 = never for each of the following sx:

1. Incomplete emptying
2. Frequency >q 2 h
3. Stop/start voiding
4. Urgency
5. Decreased flow
6. Strains to void
7. Nocturia, 0–5$^+$/noc

Classification: mild = 0–7 total pts, moderate = 8–18 pts, severe 19–35 pts

Si: Enlarged prostate, median furrow filled in on rectal exam

Crs:

Cmplc: Obstructive uropathy, chronic cystitis, bladder calculi; no incr risk of prostate cancer except that incurred by age (Ann IM 1997; 126:480)

Lab:

Noninv: Peak urine flows: >20 cc/sec = WNL, 15–20 cc/sec = mild, 10–15 cc/sec = moderate, <10 cc/sec = severe (Nejm 1995;332:99)

Rx: (Nejm 1995;332:99)

Medical: Avoid caffeine, alcohol, antihistamines, and OTC meds w ephedrine; relaxed voiding; possibly saw palmetto (*Serenoa repens,* and *Sabal serrulata*) herbal rx (ACP J Club 1999;130:61; Med Let 1999;41:18; Jama 1998;280:1604), but preparation compositions vary; may inhibit testosterone production (Nejm 1998;339:785)

1st: α blockers hs like

- Terazosin (Hytrin) (Nejm 1996;335:533,586), start w 1 mg, go to 5–10 mg po qd, improves flow within 2 wk. Adverse effects: runny nose, impaired ejaculation, dizziness and postural hypotension (Med Let 1994;36:15), $45/mo
- Prazosin
- Doxazosin (Cardura) 2–8 mg po qd, $30/mo
- Tamsulosin (Flomax) (Med Let 1997;39:96) 0.4–0.8 mg 1/2 hr pc po qd; less hypotensive effect than others; $40–80/mo

2nd:
- Finasteride (Proscar) 5 mg po qd (Med Let 1992;34:83; Nejm 1992;327:1185,1234); prevents conversion of testosterone to dihydrotestosterone; may or may not (Nejm 1996;335:533,586) be worth a 6-mo trial if moderate or worse sx and large gland; if works continue it since improvement continues over >4 yr; for prevention of acute retention or surgery, NNT-4 = 16 (Nejm 1998;338:612); cmplc: impotence and decr libido in 6–8% vs half that in controls, better after 1 yr (men w these sx dropped out); $63/mo

3rd:
- Nafarelin 400 μgm sc qd suppresses testosterone by blocking LH release; works but requires continuous use and it medically castrates

Surgical:

TURP, required in 10%, if retention and/or severe sx; cmplc = 4% incontinence, 5% impotence at 1 yr (J. Wennberg—Jama 1988;259:3010,3018,3027) but later VA study found incontinence and sexual dysfunction same in watchfully waiting pts as in operated pts and thus operation for pts w moderate sx may make sense although no harm in waiting (Nejm 1995;332:75); and unexplained 2.5× incr death rate after TURP compared to open, mostly MIs (J. Wennberg—Nejm 1989;320:1120, controversial—Nejm 1989;320:1142)

Suprapubic prostatectomy

TUNA (transurethral needle ablation)

Transurethral microwave thermotherapy possible (Lancet 1993;341:14; BMJ 1993;306:1293) though much less effective than TUR (Med Let 1996;38:53)

Laser prostatectomy

Balloon dilatation simpler less effective (Med Let 1990;32:64)

Simple incision

Stenting

TESTICULAR CARCINOMAS (Seminoma, Embryonal [Germ] Cell Carcinoma, Teratoma, Choriocarcinoma)

Nejm 1997;337:242

Cause: Neoplasia

Epidem:

Seminoma: Peak incidence age 35–45. Increased in undescended testicle even after operative repair; lifetime incidence of some malignancy is 1/80 for inguinal undescended testicles, 1/20 for abdominal testicles

Nonseminoma types: Peak incidence age 20–40; incr in Klinefelter's syndrome and in undescended testicles even postrepair; malignancy occurs in 1/80 inguinal, 1/20 abdominal undescended testicles over lifetime

Pathophys:

Seminoma: Rarely highly invasive; metastasizes via lymphatics to retroperitoneal nodes and lung

Nonseminoma: Includes teratomas and choriocarcinomas; highly malignant; hematogenous and lymphatic spread. Probably the source of a significant number of "undifferentiated" tumors found metastatic in body without primary located

Sx: Testicular mass, but not always palpable in non-seminoma types

Si: Testicular mass; gynecomastia if incr HCG or estrogen production (Nejm 1991;324:317) in nonseminoma types; reactive hydrocoel sometimes

Crs:

Seminoma: Excellent prognosis even with distant mets

Cmplc: Paraneoplastic limbic encephalopathy (p 732)

r/o orchitis and epididimytis, which improve in 7–10 d of antibiotic rx

Lab:

Chem:

- *In nonseminoma types:* HCG levels incr in 40% esp chroio, embryonal cell and seminoma; can use as way to follow success of chemo Rx (Ann IM 1984;100:183); α-fetoprotein incr in embryonal, teratoCa, and yolk sac types

Path:

- *In nonseminoma types:* Grossly looks irregular and cystic; micro-scopically shows many tissue types and totally undifferentiated cells; teratomas have all 3 germ layer types; choriocarcinomas have syncytiotrophoblasts with pleomorphic nuclei

- *In seminoma:* Gross shows lobulated, smooth tumor; microscopic shows irregular, round nuclei, clear cytoplasm, lymphocytic infiltration with granuloma formation

Xray: CT for retroperitoneal nodes

Rx:

Seminoma: Surgical excision, rarely need node exploration; + radiation (very radiosensitive); 90% 5-yr survival

Nonseminoma:

Radical orchiectomy, often w retroperitoneal node exploration for staging, esp if present by CT

Chemotherapy w adjuvant course × 2 if positive nodes; prevents recurrence in 1/2 (Nejm 1987;317:1433); or curative (Ann IM 1981;94:181). Cisplatin, bleomycin, and vinblastine or etoposide (Nejm 1987;316:1435); or ifosfamide with others, after failure with first course (Ann IM 1988;109:540)

PROSTATIC CARCINOMA

Nejm 1995;333:1401; 1994;331:996; 1991;324:236; Ann IM 1996; 125:118,205

Cause: Neoplasia

Epidem: 10% of all male cancer deaths, 40,000 deaths/yr in US 2nd after lung; peak incidence at age 60–70. Histologic prevalence at postmortem = 10% at age 50 increasing up to 70% at age 85; since lifetime chance of clinical prostatic cancer is only 6–8%, most must remain asx; histologic cancer is equally present in all races and environments, but clinical incidence very variable (Ann IM 1993; 118:793), so blacks > whites > Asians; racial survival by tumor grade is equal (Jama 1995;333:1599)

If present in a first and a 2nd degree relative, risk is incr × 8; risk may also be elevated in pts w BRCA-1 gene mutation (Nejm 1997;336: 1401). No incr risk in BPH (Ann IM 1997;126:480)

Pathophys: Peripheral origin in gland (androgenic zone); slow growth, local invasion first, later metastasizes. High testosterone levels may make latent cancer clinical

Sx: Obstructive sx (p 770)

Si: Mass on rectal exam in prostate, very firm to rock hard, nontender (30% found this way)

RENAL/UROLOGY

Crs: Correlates with presence of *ras* oncogene P21 (Nejm 1986;314:133), age at dx, tumor volume (Jama 1996;275:288), and Gleason grade (Jama 1998;280:978; 1995;274:626)

Stage A_1: Well differentiated and single site, found at BPH surgery

Stage A_2: Poorly differentiated and/or multiple sites, found at BPH surgery

Stage B: Nodule without bone or epididymal invasion, or incr acid phosphatase; 80% 5-yr survival

Stage C: Extracapsular extension; acid phos ok and no bone mets; 60% 5-yr survival; C1 to seminal vesicles, C2 fixed to pelvic wall

Stage D_0: Elevated acid phosphatase

Stage D_1: ≤3 pelvic nodes

Stage D_2: Distant bony and soft tissue mets; 15% 5-yr survival

Cmplc: Local invasion; mets to bone (blastic and clastic) often, lung, etc.

Lab:

Chem: Acid phosphatase, prostatic fraction incr in 67% with metastatic disease; false positive with hepatic impairment (Nejm 1980;303:497,499)

Prostate specific antigen (PSA) as screen (p 681); or to monitor disease, like CEA for bowel cancer; rectal exam may transiently elevate

Path: Needle biopsy. Histologic/cytologic grades (Jama 1995;274:626); Gleason score (sum of 2 most common types scored up to 5 each) 2–4, best; 5–7 progressively worse; 8–10, worst) correlate w survival when overlaid on staging system (Nejm 1994;330:242)

Stanford alternative scoring system (Jama 1999;281:1395): total % tumor Gleason grade 4 or 5; if <10%, prognosis excellent

Xray: Bony mets, blastic and clastic; look like Paget's. Ultrasound transrectally as a bx directing or perhaps as a screening tool. Neither MRI nor urologic ultrasound is useful in staging (Nejm 1990;323:621)

Rx: Preventive interventions (p 681)

of advanced disease and metastases esp if Gleason grade score ≥5 may be worthwhile, need studies (Jama 1999;281:1642; 1997;277:467)

of Stage A-B: Localized disease (Jama 1998;280:969,975,1008; Nejm 1994;330:242 vs opinion in Ann IM 1996;125:118): prognosis depends on age, Gleason score, and whether tumor was found by PSA or nodule detection on rectal. Correct strategies unclear, await RCT; watchful waiting may be enough (Jama 2000;283:3258)

Radical prostatectomy, radiation implant, external beam radiation, and/or anti-androgen rx all promoted, but survival over 10–15 yr periods is not improved by aggressive rx and cmplc of rx on sexual, bladder, and bowel functions are significant (Jama 1995;273:129), eg, 65% impotence rate, 8% incontinence rate 18 mo after radical prostatectomy (Jama 2000;283:354)

Stage B: Radical prostatectomy after pelvic node exploration; perhaps less if low Gleason score

Stage C: Radiation to control sx, helps in 90%; hormonal rx as below

Stage D: Anti-androgen rx, certainly if disease progression, perhaps immediately (Nejm 1999;341:1781,1837)

- Castration and/or diethylstilbestrol 1 mg suppresses testosterone to castration level in 75% (3 mg suppresses in nearly 100% but increases cardiovascular risk beyond cancer risk—Ann IM 1980; 92:68)

- Leuprolide, antigonadotropic releasing hormone since it is a gonadotropic releasing hormone (LHRH) analog, $10/day (Med Let 1985;27:71; Nejm 1984;311:1281,1313) or buserelin (Nejm 1989;321:413), or goserelin sc q 1 mo (Med Let 1990;32:102); all are as effective as castration (Ann IM 2000;132:566), all cause transient (1 week) increase in testosterone; improve 5 yr survival, when given before or w radiation, from 50% to 85% in locally advanced disease (Nejm 1997;337:729)

- Antiandrogens like flutamide (Eulexin) (Med Let 1996;38:56), $300/mo; or ketoconazole 600 mg qd, especially used with leuprolide (Nejm 1987;317:812); or bicalutamide (Casodex); or nilutamide (Nejm 1989;321:413), also used with antiGnRH rx (leuprolide) (Nejm 1989;321:413,419) to eliminate adrenal androgens and to mitigate initial testosterone flare; but no added benefit after medical (Lancet 2000;355:1491) or surgical orchiectomy (Nejm 1998;339:1036). Adverse effects: hepatotoxicity (Ann IM 1993;119:860), gynecomastia, gi sx

of bone pain from osteoblastic mets, strontium-89 (Metastron) or samarium-153 (Quadramet) (Med Let 1997;39:83)

Herbal: PC-SPES combo of 8 herbs has strong estrogenic effects (Med Let 2001;43:15; Nejm 1998;339:785)

RENAL/UROLOGY

BLADDER CARCINOMA

Nejm 1990;322:1129

Cause: Transitional cell carcinoma (90%) in bladder or rarely from ureter or kidney pelvis; squamous cell carcinoma (5%); adenocarcinoma (5%)

Epidem: Carcinogens: smoking (incr incidence × 2—Nejm 1971;284: 129); cyclophosphamide (Cytoxan) rx (5% risk at 10 yr, 10% at 12 yr, 16% at 15 yr), esp if had hemorrhagic cystitis (Ann IM 1996;124:477; Nejm 1988;318:1028); occupational aniline dye exposure, phenacetin users (Nejm 1985;313:292), pelvic xray therapy, and schistosomiasis, which causes squamous cell type only.

Possible carcinogens include cyclamates and saccharin (Nejm 1980; 302:537), and chronic infections and stones

Male:female = 3:1; most over age 50

Lifetime incidence: 20/100,000

High fluid intakes decr incidence (Nejm 1999;340:1390)

Pathophys: In some patients IgG-induced killer T-lymphocyte control of the cancer occurs locally (Nejm 1974;291:637)

Sx: Intermittent hematuria, painless, often with only last drops of urine; obstructive sx if low in bladder; fever and pain of pyleonephritis

Si:

Crs: 80% 5-yr survival with superficial type, 20% with invasive type.

Table 20.5.1 Invasive Type 5-yr Survival Breakdown by Stage and Type of Rx

Stage	Radiation Rx (%)	Cystectomy (%)
T_1/A	72	70
T_2/B_1	40	65
T_3/B_2, C	30	30
T_4/D	15	15

Cmplc: Pyelonephritis; metastases locally, often without si or sx. Often misdiagnosed as UTI since 1/3 are infected when present

Lab:

Path: Urine cytologies useful to pick up carcinoma in situ or high grade tumors when are hard to see on cystoscopy (Nejm 1972;287:86); may be helpful to screen high-risk groups; 20% or more false negatives, 5% or more false positives.

Cystoscopy and biopsy indicated for gross hematuria and/or in older smokers

Urine: Hematuria, gross (cancer more likely than if only microscopic) or microscopic (2% will have bladder cancer, 0.5% will have renal cell cancer)

Survivin (an inhibitor of apoptosis) levels present, 100% sens 95% specif (Jama 2001;285:324)

Xray: IVP to r/o upper tract disease; chest xray to r/o mets

Rx:

of superficial, transuretheral resection. Adjuvant intrabladder chemotherapy, eg, BCG (Nejm 1991;325:1189; Med Let 1991;33:29) (beware of tbc skin testing, which will show severe reactions), or mitomycin or doxorubicin, or intrabladder valrubicin (Valstar) (Med Let 1999;41:32) in pts w high-grade tumors, CIS, or recurrent superficial disease

of invasive, radical cystectomy w radiation and w cisplatin chemotherapy (Nejm 1993;329:1377,1420)

RENAL CELL CARCINOMA

Nejm 1996;335:865

Cause: Neoplasia, possibly from carcinogens like phenacetin (Ann IM 1980;93:249); rarely genetic and familial (Ann IM 1993;118:106)

Epidem: 4 (women)–10 (men) per 100,000/yr incidence (Jama 1999;281: 1628); peak incidence age 60–80; incr incidence in Lindau-von Hippel disease, smokers, obesity and HT (Nejm 2000;343:1305) Male:female = 3:1

Pathophys: Frequent vascular metastases

Sx: Hematuria (70%); renal colic due to clots (50%); costovertebral angle pain; left varicocele due to left spermatic vein obstruction (2%)

Si: Flank mass (30–60% on presentation); anemia (41%); fever (17%); polycythemia (4%); hypertension; accessory nipples (20%) (Ann IM 1981;95:182)

Crs: Without metastases, 75% 5-yr survival; with single resected met, 35% 5-yr survival; with multiple mets, 4% 5-yr survival

Cmplc: Hypercalcemia due to incr parathormone, amyloidosis

Lab:

Chem: Alkaline phosphatase incr (produced in tumor)

Renal Cell Carcinoma, continued

Xray: IVP or CT, mass; only 6% will be cancers (Rad 1974;113:153); noninvasive (CT) workup 90% accurate (Am J Roentgenol 1987; 48:59)

Occasionally ultrasound with diagnostic tap if complex cystic lesion; if solid, do angiography or CT

Rx: Surgical resection; resection of multiple mets doesn't improve survival; no chemotherapy or radiation rx helpful

of metastatic disease: after resection of primary, interleukin γ-2b (Nejm 2001;345:1655); or α-2a (Nejm 1998;338:1272); not interferon γ-1b (Nejm 1998;338:1265)

20.6 MISCELLANEOUS

Acute renal failure, vascular causes: See Table 20.6.1

Foley catheter use: Foley for less than 24 h with orthopedic surgery better than intermittent catheterization (Nejm 1988;319:321)

Hematuria: Associated with hypercalcemia (possibly through micro-stones) especially in children (Nejm 1984;310:1345); when asymptomatic, unassociated with another abnormality (proteinuria or HT), and under age 40 not worth pursuing (Sci Am Text Med 1985). Differential dx: GN, infection, clotting disorder, stones, exercise-induced, drugs, trauma, cancer, benign familial, sickle cell disease, HUS, HSP

Impotence (erectile dysfunction; sexual dysfunction) Nejm 2000; 342:1802; male and female—Jama 1999;281:537

Cause: Drugs including thiazides, β blockers, clonidine, α-methyldopa (Aldomet), cimetidine, psychiatric medications, chemotherapy of cancer, and a long list of others that occasionally do it (Med Let 1987;29:65; Ann IM 1976;85:342); diabetes (Nejm 1989;320: 1025); other endocrine etiologies (Ann IM 1983;98:103), prolactin tumors, male menopause, hypogonadism (high FSH and LH, low testosterone)

Table 20.6.1 Diagnosing Vascular Causes of Renal Failure

Condition	Clinical Clues	Confirmatory Evidence
Vasomotor disorder	Hypercalcemia, sepsis	Treat cause $\rightarrow\downarrow$ Scr
	NSAIDs, converting enzyme inhibitors, cyclosporine	Stop drug /$\downarrow$ dose $\rightarrow\downarrow$ Scr
Contrast nephropathy	Contrast exposure	Observe 3–5 days $\rightarrow\downarrow$ Scr
Hepatorenal syndrome	Liver failure	$\downarrow$urine sodium concentration; fluids $\rightarrow$ no effect Scr
Atheroembolic disease	Atherosclerosis, ischemic feet	Eosinophilia
	Recent angiogram	(Calf biopsy?)
Scleroderma renal crisis	Scleroderma, abrupt $\uparrow$ BP and Scr	Normal urine analysis or 1–2 + proteinuria
Malignant hypertension	Diastolic blood pressure >130 mm Hg, papilledema	$\downarrow$ Blood pressure $\rightarrow\downarrow$ Scr
	Encephalopathy	
Hemolytic-uremic syndrome	Post-partum period	$\downarrow$ Platelets, $\uparrow$ LDH
	Mitomycin C, bloody diarrhea	Hemolysis, schistocytes
	Hemorrhage, weakness	$\downarrow$ Platelets, $\uparrow$ LDH
Thrombotic thrombocytopenic purpura	Fever, central nervous system changes	Hemolysis, schistocytes
Acute cortical necrosis	Shock, disseminated intravascular coagulation, prolonged acute tubular necrosis	Computed axial tomography$\downarrow$
	Complicated pregnancy	Cortical ischemia/calcifications
Ischemic nephropathy	Atherosclerosis	Arteriogram $\rightarrow$ stenosis
	Unusual hypertension	Correction $\rightarrow\downarrow$ Scr
	Asymmetric renal size	
Renal infarction	Atrial fibrillation	$\uparrow$ LDH, abnormal scintigraphy
	Recent myocardial infarction, flank pain	Angiogram $\rightarrow$ embolism

BP = blood pressure; LDH = lactic dehydrogenase; NSAIDs = nonsteroidal anti-inflammatory drugs; Scr = serum creatinine concentration.
Reproduced with permission from Abuelo G. Diagnosing vascular causes of renal failure. Ann IM 1995;123:608.

RENAL/UROLOGY

Epidem: Prevalence = 39% at age 40, 67% at age 70 (J Urol 1994;151:
  54); vs 7% at age 25, 11% at age 45, 18% at 555 (Jama 1999;
  281:537)
Cmplc: r/o ejaculatory failure, decr libido
Lab:
  Chem: Testosterone, prolactin, LH, FSH
Rx: (Jama 1997;277:7)
  Testosterone 200 mg im q 2 wk, or patch (Nejm 1996;334:710, Med
  Let 1996;38:49) as scrotal (Testoderm) 4–6 mg, or nonscrotal
  (Androderm) 2.5–5 mg patch q 24 hr, or Androgel (Med Let
  2000;42:49); above in men if testosterone deficient, but also helps
  women w post BSOO sexual dysfunction at 300 μgm/d? at least
  short term (Nejm 2000;343:682,730)
  Bupropion (Rx Let 2001;8:34) 150 mg po qd-bid helps 30% including
  women; often used w antidepressants, which decr sexual function
  Yohimbine (Yocon) 5.4 mg po tid said to help but studies equivocal
  and it may cause hyperadrenergic states (Med Let 1994;36:115)
  Vasoactive drugs:
  • Alprostadil (MUSE) (prostaglandin E) 250–1000 μgm intra-
    urethral pill, works 2/3 of the time (Nejm 1997;336:1); or 5–
    20 μgm intracavernously, or w papaverine and phentolamine
    (Trimix); cmplc: local pain (33%), hypotension (3%); $20/dose
  • Papaverine up to 60 μgm intracavernous, along with phentola-
    mine, or alprostadil (prostaglandin E_1) (Nejm 1996;334:873, Med
    Let 1995;37:83) at 1.25 μgm if neurogenic, 5–10 μgm usually
    enough except higher doses to 60 μgm needed often in vascular
    impotence, erections should last <60 min, ≤1/d, <3/wk, cost
    $20/shot (10 or 20 μgm/cc), help 86%; self-administered with
    insulin syringe; cmplc: priaprism (Med Let 1987;29:95), and
    penile fibrotic nodules, which are less with alprostadil but
    transient testicular pain is common; costly (Med Let 1990;32:116)
  • Triple vasodilator cream (BMJ 1996;312:1512) (3% amino-
    phylline, 0.25% isosorbide dinitrate, 0.05% co-dergocrine
    mesylate) possibly, esp for psychogenic type
  • Sildenafil (Viagra) (Med Let 1998;40:51; Nejm 1998;338:1397;
    Rx Let 1998;5:19) 50–100 mg po (25 mg if on erythromycin,
    ketoconazole, or itraconazole, or in renal or hepatic failure)
    1 hr before anticipate intercourse, helps 70$^+$% (50–60% of
    diabetics—Jama 1999;281:421) by blocking enzyme that metabo-
    lizes vasodilating nitric oxide via cyclic quanosine monophosphate

(cCMP). Adverse effects: transient visual changes, severe hypotension if given w nitrates or HIV protease inhibitors (Rx Let 1999;6:41), mild headache, facial flushing, indigestion, ok w other (non nitrate) anti-anginal and HT meds (Nejm 2000;342:1622); $10/tab but all 3 strengths cost same so can buy 100 mg pills and break in half (Rx Let 1998;5:25)

Vacuum/constriction devices: vacuum devices (Erectaid), or adjustable bands (Actis or Rejoyn) work but are clumsier

Prostheses, permanent or inflatable, surgically inplanted

Prerenal azotemia and compensatory mechanisms (Nejm 1988;319:623)

Proteinuria (Ann IM 1983;98:186), <2 gm/24 h

Transient in 10% with severe medical disease or stress (Nejm 1982; 306:1031)

Orthostatic proteinuria: none with first morning urine; benign even over 50 yr (Ann IM 1982;97:516; Nejm 1981;305:618)

Obesity-associated: due to focal GN, decreases w wgt loss or ACEI rx (Nephron 1995;70:35); or due to sleep apnea w no GN and reversible w rx of sleep disorder (Arch IM 1988;148:87)

Sexually transmitted diseases (STDs), causes, see Table 20.6.2

Table 20.6.2

Viruses	Bacteria
HIV	*Neisseria gonorrhoeae*
Hepatitis A, B, and C	*Treponema pallidum*
Human papilloma virus	*Ureaplasma urealyticum*
Herpes simplex viruses	*Shigella sp*
Cytomegalovirus	*Campylobacter sp*
Molluscum contagiosum virus	*Group B strep (?)*
	Chlamydia trachomatis
Protozoans	*Mycoplasma hominis*
Trichomonas vaginalis	*Haemophilus ducreyi*
Giardia lamblia	*Calymmatobacterium granulomatis*
Entamoeba histolytica	*Gardnerella vaginalis (?)*
	Mobiluncus sp
Ectoparasites	
Phthirus pubis	
Sarcoptes scabiei	

RENAL/UROLOGY

24-h urine collection adequacy: Total creatinine should be 20–26 mg/kg/d (J.B. Henry, Clinical Diagnosis and Management by Laboratory, Philadelphia: WB Saunders 1984:1439)

Vasectomy: Reversal even when successful leads to fertility only about half the time because of permanent testicular damage (Nejm 1985; 313:1252,1283) and perhaps sperm antibodies. But in-vitro fertilization possible at least in cases of congenital absence of vas (Nejm 1990;323:1788)

Chapter 21
Rheumatology/Orthopedics

D. K. Onion

21.1 PAIN/ANTI-INFLAMMATORY MEDICATIONS

Pain—Med Let 1998;40:79

NSAIDS

Med Let 2000;42:57,73; Nejm 1991;324:1716)

All inhibit prostaglandin synthetase (cyclo-oxygenase) types 1 and 2 (COX-1 and -2); most cmplc are associated w COX-1 inhibition and future NSAIDs will probably have less (J Clin Rheum 1996;2:135, Semin Arth Rheum 1996;26:435). All except for salicylates are associated w Na retention, 2–8× increase in end stage renal disease (Nejm 1994;331:1675), and membranous GN nephrotic syndrome (Jama 1996;276:466); all but nonacetylated salicylates cause platelet dysfunction that is irreversible w ASA but reversible w all others; all cause gastric irritation to varying degrees (Nejm 1999;340:1886):
Low risk: nonacetylated salicylates, nabumetone, sulindac, etodolac
Mod risk: ibuprofen, naproxen, ASA, ketoprofen, tolmetin, diclofenac
High risk: piroxicam, indomethacin, flurbiprofen, fenoprofen, meclofenamate

SALICYLIC ACIDS

Acetylsalicylic acid (ASA) 1–3 gm po qid, therapeutic serum level = 20–30 mg%, 3–8-h half-life; analgesic effect potentiated by caffeine

(Arch IM 1991;151:733); for all arthritis except septic and gout as well as for anticoagulant effect at 75–300 mg po qd doses. Adverse effects: tinnitus, delirium/confusion, asthma/anaphylaxis esp in pts w eosinophilia and nasal polyps, increased bleeding time for 2 d, platelet dysfunction for 7–10 d. Cheap

Nonacetylated salicylates (Trilisate, Dolobid, Disalcid) 0.4–1.2 gm po qid; for all arthritis except septic. Adverse effects: similar to ASA but no effect on platelets or gastric mucosa. Generic, $8–50/mo, $100/mo for trade names

PROPIONIC ACIDS

Fenoprofen (Nalfon) 600 mg po b-tid, 3-h half-life; for all arthritis except septic. Adverse effects: usual + rash, immune nephritis unlike the prostaglandin-induced increased BUN of other NSAIDs, platelet dysfunction for 1 d. $32/mo

Flurbiprofen (Ansaid) (Med Let 1989;31:31); no better than others; more expensive, $38/mo generic, $102/mo trade name

Ibuprofen (Motrin, Advil) 0.4–1.2 gm po qid, 3-h half-life; in children (Med Let 1989;31:109) as antipyretic, 5 mg/kg for fever <102°F (<38.9°), 10 mg/kg for fever >102°F (>38.9°) (no Reye's reported); for all arthritis except septic, as strong an analgesic as Tylenol #3. Adverse effects: diarrhea, gi intolerance but lowest of all NSAIDs (BMJ 1996;312:1563), renal failure (Ann IM 1990;112:568), Na^+ retention with hypertension, mental status changes, rash, platelet dysfunction for 1 d. $2/d generic, $22/mo trade name

Ketoprofen (Orudis) (Med Let 1993;35:15) 50–75 mg po t-qid. Adverse effects: the usual NSAID ones. $38/mo generic, $140/mo trade

Naproxen (Naprosyn) 250 mg po qd to 500 mg tid, 13-h half-life; potentiated effects when used with ASA; for all arthritis except septic. Adverse effects: usual + tinnitus, mental status changes, hepatitis, platelet dysfunction for 1 d. $2/mo generic, $52/mo trade

Oxaprosin (Daypro) (Med Let 1993;35:15) 600–1800 mg po qd. Adverse effects: the usual NSAID ones. $44/mo

ACETIC ACIDS

Indomethacin (Indocin) 25–50 mg po t-qid, 3-h half-life, 75 mg bid for slow-release type, which is better tolerated; for all arthritis except septic, may be especially good for hip DJD, shoulder tendonitis, and gout. Adverse effects: usual + headache, dizziness, mental status changes/confusion, rash, pancytopenia, visual changes, acute oliguric renal failure especially when used with triamterene (Nejm 1984;310: 565), coronary artery constriction (Nejm 1981;305:471), platelet dysfunction for 1 d. $17/mo generic, $60/mo as Indocin

Sulindac (Clinoril) 100–200 mg po tid, 13-h half-life; for all arthritis except septic. Adverse effects: usual + headache, mental status changes/confusion, hepatotoxic, rash, pancytopenia. $50/mo

Tolmetin (Tolectin) 400 mg po 3–5× qd, 1-h half-life; for all arthritis especially Reiter's and ankylosing spondylitis but not septic, as effective as indomethacin but less toxic hence use in elderly. Adverse effects: usual + headache, mental status changes/confusion, hepatotoxicity, rash, depressed white counts, false-positive proteinuria even with 24-h urine but not in all patients, platelet dysfunction for 1 d. $40/mo as generic, $75/mo as Tolectin

ENOLIC ACIDS

Phenylbutazone (Butazolidin), no longer used

Oxyphenylbutazone (Tandearil), similar to phenylbutazone, no longer used

Piroxicam (Feldene) 10–20 mg qd, takes 11 d until reach steady state w 44-h half-life; for all arthritis except septic, better in elderly than many other NSAIDs. Adverse effects: usual + photosensitivity rash, tinnitus, platelet dysfunction for 2–4 d, confusion in elderly complicated by long half-life. $32/mo generic, $83/mo as Feldene

Meloxicam (Mobic) (Med Let 2000;42:47) 7.5–15 mg po qd; for DJD. Adverse effects: diarrhea, N+V, no platelet effect, incr lithium levels, may incr warfarin levels. $2/pill

FENAMIC ACIDS

Meclofenamate (Meclomen) 100 mg po t-qid, 5-h half-life; "hardly ever works." Adverse effects: usual + headache, rash, tinnitus, platelet dysfunction for 1 d. $65/mo as generic, $90/mo trade

NAPHTHYLALKANONES

Nabumetone (Relafen) (Med Let 1992;34:38) 1000–2000 mg po qd. Adverse effects: usual NSAID-type but gi toxicity only 0.02–0.9% compared to 2–4% ulcers/yr for other NSAIDs in aggregate. $71/mo

PYRANOCARBOXYLIC ACIDS

Diclofenac (Voltaren) 50–75 mg po bi-qid; or w 200 μgm misoprostol as Arthrotec (Rx Let 1998;5:7); $46/mo generic, $88/mo as Voltaren

Etodolac (Lodine) (Med Let 1991;33:79; J Intern Med 1991;229:5)
300 mg po b-qid; less gastric irritation than naproxen but 3× as
expensive as ibuprofen; $50/mo generic, $90/mo trade for tid

COX-2 SPECIFIC DRUGS
(Nejm 2001;345:433; Ann IM 2000;132:134; Rx Let 1999;6:32): Only
over age 18; for DJD and RA; compared to other NSAIDs, less gi
irritation (Jama 2000;284;1247) and no anti-platelet effects, similar
renal and allergic effects and celecoxib cross-reaction w sulfas. Both
may incr ASHD by 2.5× (Jama 2001;286;954)

Celecoxib (Celebrex) (Med Let 1999;41:11) 100–200 mg po qd-bid.
Adverse effects: sulfa-based unlike rofecoxib and may induce sulfa
allergies; drug interactions w warfarin, zafirlukast, fluconazole,
fluvastatin, and w some βblockers, antidepressants and antipsychotics;
100 mg bid costs $86/mo
Rofecoxib (Vioxx) (Med Let 1999;41:59) 12.5–50 mg po qd; 17 hr half
life; levels decr by antacids and rifampin; levels incr by methotrexate
and warfarin. Adverse effects: diarrhea, nausea and vomiting, edema;
$2.50/pill

OTHER PAIN MEDICATIONS

PYRROLES
Ketorolac (Toradol) (Med Let 1990;32:79) 10–30 mg im q 6 h; used as a
short-term pain med, not as an anti-inflammatory; as effective as 12 mg
morphine without respiratory depression, gi constipation, or addiction.
Adverse effects: usual NSAID ones including gi bleed esp if
>90 mg/d ×5d (Jama 1996;275:376), anaphylaxis in ASA-sensitive pt,
and especially renal failure more frequent if used >5d (Ann IM 1997;
126:193). $5 per dose vs $0.50 for morphine

NARCOTICS
All have addiction potential and cause respiratory depression and
constipation (hence should prophylact for constipation); iv
patient-controlled devices work well, cost $40–1500 (Med Let
1989;31:104); selective blocking of gi motility inhibition w
experimental drug may be possible (Nejm 2001;345:935)

Buprenorphine (Med Let 1986;28:56) 0.3 mg iv/im q 6 h; partial antagonist like butorphanol and pentazocine

Butorphanol (Stadol) (Med Let 1993;35:105; Nejm 1980;302:381) 1.5–2.5 mg im, similar nasal doses as good and last longer; as strong as 10 mg im morphine, less respiratory depression. Adverse effects: a narcotic antagonist so can precipitate withdrawal in addicted pts, addiction in migraine pts

Codeine 30–60 mg po q 3–6 h w ASA (Empirin Cmpd) or acetaminophen (Tylenol 3); analgesia inhibited by cimetidine, fluoxetine (Prozac), and quinidine

Dezocine (Dalgan) 11–30 mg iv/im; like pentazocine (Med Let 1990; 32:95)

Dihydromorphone (Dilaudid) 1–2 mg po q 3–4 h

Fentanyl (Duragesic) transdermal patch 25, 50, or 100 μgm/h, lasts 72 h (Med Let 1992;34:97), or as lozenge lollipop (Actig) (Med Let 1994;36:24) 200–1600 μgm, esp if can't take po; or as fast-acting lozenge (Actig) 100+ mg up to tid (Rx Let 1999;6:5); dangerously long-acting in elderly and fatal to children if mistake for lollypop

Levorphanol po for cancer pain, long (16 hr) half-life

Meperidine (Demerol) 50–150 mg iv/im, 3 h duration; irritating im/sc; beware fatal encephalopathy and serotoninergic syndromes when used w MAO inhibitors or SSRIs; toxic metabolite w 20 hr half-life esp in renal failure can cause dysphoria and even seizures

Methadone (Dolophine) 10–20 mg po and LAAM (methadol) both used for rx of heroin addicts and available only through federal clinics (Med Let 1994;36:52)

Morphine SO_4 (MS) 5–15 mg iv/im, or 1 mg intra-articular, eg, postarthroscopy (Nejm 1991;325:1123), or po 20 mg/cc w 4 h duration or 15+ mg bid if give po as long-acting form (MS Contin et al.) supplemented w immediate release prn breakthrough pain at 1/3 the single long acting dose q 2 hr prn, readjust long-acting dose q 24 hr by total MS past 24 hr and give 1/2 that dose bid as LA and immediate release 1/3 that dose q 2 hr; twice as effective if given with 5–10 mg amphetamine (Nejm 1977;296:712) but rarely done; cheap

Oxycodone 5–10 mg po q 3–6 h w ASA (Percodan) or acetaminophen (Tylox, Percocet)

Pentazocine (Talwin) 40–60 mg iv, im, po q 3–4 h. Adverse effects: depresses respirations, morphine antagonist like nalorphine

Propoxyphene (Darvon) (Nejm 1972;286:813) 30–65 mg po q 4–6 h.
  Adverse effects: abuse and death (Jama 1973;223:1125), rx OD with
  nalorphine (Med Let 1973;15:61)
Tramadol (Ultram) (Med Let 1995;37:59) 50–100 mg po q 6 h prn pain;
  as good as codeine + ASA, hepatic/renal excretion, unscheduled.
  Adverse effects: seizures and serotonin syndromes, esp w concomitant
  MAO inhibitors, antipsychotics or antidepressants (Rx Let 1999;6:27).
  $60/100 tabs

ANALGESIC ENHANCERS
  Caffeine 65–200 mg po, used w NSAIDs
  Hydroxyzine (Vistaril) 50–100 mg im, used w parenteral narcotics

IMMUNOSUPPRESSIVE DRUGS
  (Med Let 2000;42:57)

Azathioprine (Imuran) (p 330)
D-penicillamine (Depen) (Nejm 1979;300:274) 125–1000 mg po qd
  divided; "go low, go slow"; used in RA, decreases immune complex
  disease. Adverse effects: rash, itch, nephrosis, depresses polys and
  platelets. $62/mo generic, $123/mo as Depen
Gold compounds (p 779)
Hydroxychloroquine (Plaquenil) (J Clin Rheum 1997;3:1, Rheum Dis
  Clin N Am 1994;20:243), <3.5 mg/lb; used for discoid lupus, SLE,
  RA; stabilizes lysozymal membranes and decr interleukin-2 and
  macrophage production of TNF. Adverse effects: depigmentation of
  skin and hair; retinopathy with bull's-eye red patch, irreversible,
  dose-related (Nejm 1967;276:1168), prevent w q 6 mo ophthalmology
  visits; reversible cataracts, $25/mo generic, $40/mo as Plaquenil
Methotrexate (Rheumatrex) 2.5 to 25 mg po q 1 wk. Adverse effects:
  nausea and vomiting, hepatitis; rarely marrow suppression, pulmonary
  fibrosis, and hepatic fibrosis. $50/mo
Steroids, like prednisone 5 mg qd is physiologic unstressed replacement,
  up to 120 mg qd to rx arthritis and other diseases (steroid equivalents
  in order of diminishing mineralocorticoid component: hydrocortisone
  20 mg, prednisone 5 mg, methylprednisolone 4 mg, dexamethasone
  0.75 mg). Adverse effects (even w 10 mg prednisone qd): subcapsular
  cataracts, osteoporosis so pts on long-term rx even low dose (5 mg/d)

should get at least $CaCO_3$ + vit D (Ann IM 1996;125:964) and probably bisphosphonates, infections because inhibits polymorpho-leukocyte diapodesis, aseptic necrosis of hip, peptic ulcers if used with NSAIDs (Ann IM 1991;114:735)

Tumor necrosis factor agents (Nejm 2001;344:907; 1999;340:310; 1997; 337:141); all about equal clinically (Nejm 2000;343:1640) so choose by frequency, route of administration, and insurance coverage (iv forms covered by Medicare); check IPPD for latent tbc first (Nejm 2001;345:1098)

- Leflunomide (Arava) (Med Let 1998;40:110) 100 mg po qd × 3, then 10–20 mg po qd; as good or better than mtx. Adverse effects: incr NSAID and oral hypoglycemic levels, diarrhea, rash, hepatotoxicity and elevated LFTs, teratogenic in both men and women, must use cholestyramine to clear body levels. $240/mo

- Etanercept (Enbrel) (Ann IM 1999;130:478; Nejm 2000;342:763; 1999;340:253; Med Let 1998;40:110) 0.4 mg/kg up to 25 mg sc biw for up to 3 mos; recombinant TNF blocker/binder; for disease resistant to mtx, and may be marginally more effective and therefore better choice than mtx (Nejm 2000;343:1586). Adverse effects: local irritation, serious infection (Rx Let 1999;6:32), theoretical incr in autoimmune disease. $1100/mo

- Infliximab (Remicade) (Med Let 1999;41:19; 1998;40:110) 3–10 mg/kg iv q 4–12 wk; anti-TNF monoclonal antibody; used for Crohn's disease and RA. Adverse effects: hypersensitivity reactions including fever and urticaria, incr in autoimmune antibodies. $1100–3300/dose

ACTH, rarely indicated; maybe in children, acute gout, myasthenia, or in diagnostic testing

21.2 COLLAGEN VASCULAR DISEASES

ANKYLOSING SPONDYLITIS (Marie-Strümpell Disease)
Bull Rheum Dis 1987;37(1):1

Cause: Genetic, HLA association suggests close link to primary gene or immune interaction between antigen and agent, eg, *Klebsiella* antigens (Bull Rheum Dis 1989;39(2):1)

Epidem: Male:female = 3:1; 0.1–0.2% prevalence in whites; associated with HLA B27

Pathophys: Tendonitis, periostitis, and ligamentous inflammation and calcification lead to bony hyperplasia and ankylosis

Sx: Hip and foot arthritic sx, though can involve any joint; onset age 15–35 yr, or in late childhood

Back pain that improves with exercise, worsens with inactivity, unlike chronic low-back syndrome; sacroiliitis early and constant

Anorexia and weight loss, fever, sciatica (10% have it when first present)

Si: 10-cm mark on LS spine stretches on flexion only to <15 cm; chest expansion ≤2.5 cm (Ann IM 1976;84:1)

Painful SI joints on palpation

Crs: Relatively benign, rarely die of disease, but overall mortality is 4× normal (Nejm 1977;297:572)

Cmplc: Iridocyclitis (25%); aortic insufficiency (5%); mitral insufficiency (Nejm 1978;299:1448) and abnormal cardiac conduction including heart block (8%); kyphosis, fracture of cervical spine (Ann IM 1978; 88:546); pneumonitis (1%) that can look like old tbc; amyloidosis (4%)

r/o other seronegative spondyloarthropathies all with similar HLA B27 association and clinical syndromes, eg, Reiter's, regional enteritis, ulcerative colitis, psoriatic arthritis, post-*Yersinia* colitis (Nejm 1989;321:16)

Lab:

Hem: ESR increased (80%)

Serol: HLA B27-positive; 10% false negative, 8% false positive. 20% (Bull Rheum Dis 1981;31:35) of positive people with positive family hx get ankylosing spondylitis; of those who are HLA B27-positive but with negative family hx, only 2% get the disease

Xray: Bilaterally symmetric sacroiliitis with subchondral sclerosis (100%), osteitis of symphysis pubis, anterior spinal ligament calcification, late "bamboo spine" with bony fusion of spine and osteophytes are parallel not perpendicular to spine. Calcification of tendons and heels (cf Reiter's)

Rx: (Bull Rheum Dis 1981;31:35)

Exercise program most important to prevent fusion in kyphosis

NSAIDs, first indomethacin up to 200 mg po qd; then tolmetin, sulindac, or naproxen

Sulfasalazine (Br J Rheum 1990;29:2)

Steroids only for eye cmplc

DERMATOMYOSITIS (DM), POLYMYOSITIS (PM), AND INCLUSION BODY MYOSITIS (IBM)

IBM—Nejm 1991;325:1026; DM/PM—Nejm 1991;325:1487; Ann IM 1995;122:715; 1989;111:143

Cause: Multiple autoimmune, usually involving CD8 killer T cells (Nejm 1991;324:877); plastic surgical bovine collagen injections (Ann IM 1993;118:920)

Epidem: Incidence of all 3 about 1/100,000/yr

Dermatomyositis (DM): Females > males in both children and adults

Polymyositis (PM): Adults only

Inclusion body myositis (IBM): Male:female = 3:1; whites > blacks; most pts are > age 50 yr

Pathophys: Perhaps autoimmunity to own muscle protein. In DM, immune complex activation and vessel damage via complement (Nejm 1986;314:329); in PM and IBM, autoimmunity is T cell-mediated

Sx: Fever for weeks; proximal muscle weakness manifest by falling, trouble standing up, or with stair climbing, gradually progressive over weeks to months, occasionally pseudohypertrophic; painless (if painful, r/o polymyalgia rheumatica); dysphagia and regurgitation in 50%; never eye muscle involvement; Raynaud's syndrome. IBM may affect fine distal motor early as well; finger flexor or toe extensors impaired in 50%

Si: Proximal > distal muscle weakness, palatal paralysis; periungual hyperemia and telangiectasias, r/o hot water; minimal joint involvement; reflexes preserved unless muscle totally gone as often is the case with quadriceps in IBM

In DM, above plus facial edema and dusky erythema especially in sun-exposed areas; heliotrope (purplish) eyelid, periorbital, and facial coloring; rash w macular scaling plaques, especially in exposed areas and knuckles; scalp involvement (Jama 1994; 272:1939)

Crs: Weeks to months usually. IBM may be very slow over years and mimic limb-girdle muscular dystrophy

Cmplc: Respiratory failure from muscle weakness; amyloidosis; 10% get interstitial pneumonitis and fibrosis (Am Rev Respir Dis 1990;141: 727); myocardiopathy; heart block (Ann IM 1981;94:41). Cancer associated in 10% of PM and 15% of DM patients (Nejm 1992; 326:363) vs 20% and 40% (Ann IM 2001;134:1087). DM appears in overlap syndromes with other connective tissue diseases

r/o other causes of muscle weakness including inflammatory myopathies, colchicine myo/neuropathy (Nejm 1987;316:1562); drug-induced myopathies (Semin Arth Rheum 1990;19:259) from penicillamine, AZT, ipecac, cimetidine, chloroquine, steroids, lovistatin; and infectious myopathies from parasitic diseases, Lyme, and *Legionella*

Lab:

Chem: AST (SGOT), LDH, aldolase, and CPK increased (r/o muscular dystrophy)

Noninv: EMG, diagnostic small-amplitude action potentials and fibrillations

Path: Muscle bx is positive in 75+% (Am J Med 1963;35:646); segmental necrosis, enlarged central nuclei, regeneration (myoblasts, myocytes, basophilic myofibrils), focal inflammation especially around vessels

Serol: ANAs positive (83%); anti-Jo-1 in 40% polymyalgia (Bull Rheum Dis 1985;35:6) and if positive, >50% have interstitial lung disease; anti-KJ; anti-Mi-2, etc (Ann IM 1995;122:715)

Rx: (Ann IM 1995;122:715)

Steroids, eg, 60 mg prednisone qd × 3 mo, then taper to 5–10 mg q 1 mo as muscle strength increases and enzymes decrease; helps 80% (D. Dawson, HMS 3/85)

Azathioprine if steroids fail; also chlorambucil and cyclophosphamide

Methotrexate if lungs will tolerate it

Colchicine po may help inflammation with calcinosis in childhood type (Sci Am Text Med 1983)

Immunologic w immune globulin 2 gm/kg iv q 1 mo; expensive but clearly helps DM and may help PM and IBM (Nejm 1993;329:

1993); plasma exchange and leukophoresis no help (Nejm 1992; 326:1380)

POLYARTERITIS NODOSA (PAN) (Systemic Necrotizing Vasculitis)

Rheum Dis Clin N Am 1990;16:251

Cause: Idiopathic autoimmune

Epidem: Associated with hypertension, hepatitis B (Nejm 1997;337: 1739), and other medical diseases; males >> females

Pathophys: Immune complex deposition leads to fibrinoid necrosis of vessel wall and thrombosis. An acute necrotizing vasculitis of small and medium-sized vessels; focal lesions may lead to thrombosis or aneurysmal dilatation at site (Arth Rheum 1990;33:1065)

Less acute renal disease and more chronic renal disease and/or amyloidosis as go in the spectrum of disease from PAN to SLE to RA to SS to dermato/polymyositis (Petersdorf 11/68)

Sx: Fever, weight loss, arthralgias/arthritis, abdominal pain, headache, smoky urine, blindness

Si: Myalgias and myositis (39%), splenomegaly (34%), petechiae and purpura (20%), skin necrosis, urticaria, hypertension, mononeuritis multiplex, fever, fundal vessel damage, cutaneous and visceral nodular aneurysms, ulcers of corneal limbus

Crs: 1/3 die in <1 yr; in hep B surface antigen-associated type, disease burns out in 1 yr if survive

Cmplc: Renal involvement or failure (85%), infections, infarcts, and hypertension in 50%; hepatic infarcts and cirrhosis (66%); cardiac (76%) infarcts and conduction abnormalities; pancreatic (35%) cysts and hemorrhage, blindness from retinal artery occlusion; gi tract (51%) ulcers, hemorrhage, and perforations; aneurysms of mesenteric vessels (25%); asthma (29%); Kogan's syndrome (bilateral 8th cranial nerve palsies and eye keratitis)

Lab:

Hem: ESR elevated, eosinophilia (20%)

Path: Biopsies (pos if show involvement of nutrient vessels) of: kidney (also shows GN); sural nerve, especially if slowed nerve conduction velocities; liver; gastrocnemius or other muscle; testicular; skin

Polyarteritis Nodosa, continued

   Serol: Complement levels depressed; rheumatoid titers elevated;
     antineutrophil cytoplasmic autoantibodies, r/o Wegener's (Ann IM
     1990;113:656)
Xray: Diagnostic microfusiform aneurysms on renal and hepatic
     angiography (Nejm 1970;282:1024)
Rx: (Ann IM 1992;116:488)
     Steroids perhaps qod + cyclophosphamide or azathioprine

RAYNAUD'S DISEASE/SYNDROME
   Ann IM 1970;72:17

Cause: Primary, 15% have positive family hx in which case are almost
     never associated with a collagen vascular disease
     Prodrome or concomitant w other collagen vascular disease; systemic
     sclerosis (especially CREST syndrome types) more often than SLE
     which is more common than RA
     Cmplc of chemotherapy in testicular cancer (Ann IM 1981;95:288)
     Occupational (most common), 125 cps vibrations, noise, and cold;
     smoking doesn't worsen?!
Epidem: Males ≫ females for vibration-induced type; incr incidence w
     estrogen replacement rx, but not w estrogen/progesterone combo
     HRT (Ann IM 1998;129:208)
Pathophys: Autonomic dysfunction causes small vessel spasm with later
     development of permanent vessel impairment?; hand small vessels
     shown to have diminished constrictive and dilating response to
     normal cold and warm stimuli; may be because vessels respond
     abnormally to normal levels of sympathetic discharge; may be due to
     platelet receptor abnormalities (Rheum Dis Clin N Am 1993;19:53)
Sx: Idiopathic or cold-induced finger tip blanching, painful
Si: White fingers
Crs: May precede si and sx of associated collagen vascular disease by up
     to 10 yr
Cmplc: Fingertip ulcers, no gangrene, migraine headaches (61%—Ann IM
     1992;117:985)
     r/o systemic sclerosis (scleroderma) and SLE which are distinguished by
     their dilated nail capillaries and associated sx of other organ systems

Lab:

Xray: Ba swallow shows motility changes in many patients, rarely do they have sx. Arteriography of hand vessels normal after si and sx return to normal in contrast to what happens in collagen vascular diseases

Rx: (Curr Opinion Rheum 1997;9:544):

Decrease noise, vibration, and cold exposure by mitten use

Biofeedback; centrifugal arm swing

Plasmapheresis q 1 wk × 4 wk may yield long remissions

Meds:

Calcium channel blockers like amlodipine or nifedipine 20–60$^+$ mg po qd (Nejm 1983;308:880)

Prazosin 1 mg po bid (Ann IM 1982;97:67), then increase

Nitrate skin patches or paste

Reserpine 0.25–1.5 mg po qd? (Nejm 1979;300:713; 1979;285:259)

Iloprost (a prostacyclin) iv × 5 d? (experimental—Ann IM 1994;120:199)

ACUTE RHEUMATIC FEVER

Nejm 1968;278:183

Cause: Group A hemolytic streptococcus (rarely group A nonhemolytic—Nejm 1971;284:750), type irrelevant but presence of m-protein probably key, eg, nephrogenic strains especially skin ones, lack m-protein and never lead to ARF (Nejm 1970;283:561). Poststrep infection × 2–3 wk, though bacteria must still be present. Genetic susceptibility in some populations? (Bull Rheum Dis 1993;42:5)

Epidem: (Nejm 1991;325:783) Children, peak incidence age 5–15 yr; female:male = 3:1; incidence = 61/100,000/yr in NYC (Jama 1973;224:1593), marked decrease since use of penicillin (Nejm 1988;318:280), increased × 3 among the poor. Recent outbreak in Rocky Mt states (Nejm 1987;316:421)

Pathophys: Autoimmune theories, like strep A and humans share antigens, or at least haptens, so strep infections develop cross-reacting antibodies. But not the complete explanation, as L. Weinstein points out, because only strep pharyngitis causes ARF, not strep infections elsewhere in body unlike AGN

Sx: Jones criteria to make the dx (Alto—Am Fam Phys 1992;45:613) requires 2 major criteria, or 1 major + 2 minor, + positive ASO titer or culture or h/o scarlet fever; major criteria = carditis, polyarthritis, erythema marginatum, subcutaneous nodules, chorea; minor criteria = fever, arthralgias, distant h/o ARF, elevated wbc ESR or CRP, long PR interval or other EKG abnormalities. Members of same family tend to have same major sx (Nejm 1968;278:183)

Arthralgias, transitory; Sydenham's chorea, may follow other si and sx by weeks or months

Si:

- Erythema marginatum, associated with carditis
- Murmurs, valvular or mid-diastolic nonvalvular, associated with pericarditis
- Subcutaneous nodules at bony prominences, associated with carditis (94%)
- Pneumonitis
- Serositis
- Polyarthritis of large joints, may be only si (Ann IM 1978;89:917)

Crs: <10–12 wk in 80–90%. Murmurs all (95%) appear by 2 wk of sx onset

Cmplc: Chronic cardiac valve disease; mitral regurgitation with Jaccoud's arthritis (ulnar deviation which pt can voluntarily correct—Ann IM 1972;77:949); transient glomerulonephritis (Ann IM 1981;94:322)

Lab:

Hem: Elevated ESR

Noninv: EKG: PR interval increased

Serol: Streptozyme test (Med Let 1974;16:41); ASO (antistreptolysin O) >400 Todd U, means had β-strep, <125 U means didn't, 80% sensitivity; anti-DNAase titer; antistreptodornase titer

Xray: Chest shows interstitial, nonbacterial pneumonitis

Rx: Preventive: penicillin as pen V 250 mg po bid in adults or qd in children; or sulfasoxazole, or benzathine penicillin im q 1 mo most effective (Nejm 1971;285:646)

Acute, see Table 21.2.1:

Table 21.2.1

Rx Choice	If No Murmur	If Severe Carditis	If Sick/No Murmur
Penicillin	Yes	Yes + yrs of prophylaxis	Yes
ASA	Yes	Yes	Yes
Steroids	No	Yes	Optional unless has pneumonia then should rx (Weinstein)

RHEUMATOID ARTHRITIS

Nejm 1990;322:1277

Cause: Genetic, associated w HLA DRB$_1$, DR$_1$, and DR$_4$ (Ann IM 1992;117:801,869)

Epidem: (Epidem Rev 1990;12:247)

Adult female:male = 3:1, onset age 25–50 yr

Pathophys: Collagenase produced by granulation tissue (Nejm 1977; 296:1017)

Suppressor T-cell defect; don't suppress EBV antibody production normally, leads to chronic EBV antibody production? (Nejm 1981; 305:1238; rv of all theories including EBV ones—Ann IM 1984; 101:810)

Diagnostic criteria (Bull Rheum Dis 1988;38(5):1) have 90% sensitivity and specificity if have ≥4 of following criteria: (1) early morning stiffness >6 wk; (2) arthritis involving 3 or more joints >6 wk; (3) wrist mcp or pip joint involvement; (4) symmetric arthritis; (5) rheumatoid nodules; (6) positive rheumatoid titer; (7) bony xray changes

Sx: Fever >102°F (>38.9°C), erratic (1%); joint pain (100%), monoarticular arthritis (8%); insidious onset

Si: Subcutaneous (rheumatoid) nodules over pressure points; evanescent rash (6%); arthritis and thick synovium

Crs: Chronic over decades; often improves during pregnancy (Nejm 1993; 329:466)

Cmplc:

- Peptic ulcers in 75% (Ann IM 1979;91:517)
- Septic arthritis, subtle (Ann IM 1969;70:147)
- Scleral malacia perforans and uveitis
- Pulmonary interstitial pneumonitis and fibrosis (r/o gold-induced—Nejm 1976;294:919), empyema, pleuritis

- Pericarditis and aortic valvulitis (Nejm 1973;289:597)
- Sjögren's syndrome (p 801)
- Felty's syndrome (J Rheum 1989;16:864) (depressed white counts (p 364), frequent infections, sometimes splenomegaly, skin ulcers)
- Odontoid ligament rupture (Rheum Dis Clin N Am 1991;17:757; J Rheum 1990;17:134) (10%) (if on xray have >4 mm separation should have surgery) and other tendon/ligamentous rupture

Lab:

Joint fluid: Wbc ∼ 40,000, poor mucin clot, protein = 4–5 gm%, C′ decreased

Pleural fluid: Low glucose (<30 mg%); elevated LDH, protein >4 gm%, C′ decreased (distinguishes from cancer)

Serol: Rheumatoid factor titers

Rx: (Nejm 1994;330:1368; Med Let 1994;36:101; Bull Rheum Dis 1982;32:1)

Start w NSAID + gold, chloraquine, or methotrexate (Ann IM 1996; 124:699); follow with buttoning or shoe-tying time, and BP cuff grip strength test with cuff starting at 30 mm Hg (Ann IM 1994;120:26)

Medications (Ann IM 2001;134:695; Med Let 2000;42:57):

1st: Methotrexate 5–20 mg po q 1 wk (Med Let 1994;36:101; Ann IM 1991;114:999; Nejm 1985;312:818) w 1 mg folate po qd helps toxicity w/o decr efficacy (Ann IM 1995;122:833); no cancer risk (Ann IM 1987;107:358; Bull Rheum Dis 1986;36:4). Adverse effects: nausea and vomiting, pulmonary fibrosis, 10% get liver disease (Am J Med 1991;90:711)

2nd: Mtx sc

3rd: Mtx w chloroquine 200 mg bid + sulfasalazine 500 mg bid (72% improved vs 50% at 1 yr—Nejm 1996;334:1287)

4th: Mtx w tumor necrosis factor antagonists (p 789)

5th: Other older agents:
- Hydroxychloroquine (Am J Med 1995;98:156) 200–400 mg po qd, retinopathy unlikely at <7.7 mg/kg
- Sulfasalazine (Azulfidine) to 2–3 gm qd as good as gold or penicillamine (BMJ 1983;287:1099, 1102)
- ASA to blood levels of ∼25 mg%, or Na salicylate or other NSAID
- Steroids, into joints and po low-dose 5–10 mg only; 7.5 mg po qd × 2 yr causes fewer osteoporotic changes (Nejm 1995;333:142)

- D-penicillamine (Ann IM 1986;105:528) <1 gm qd, start at 250 mg qd, increase q 3 mo (Bull Rheum Dis 1988;28:948). Adverse effects: rashes, depressed wbc and platelets, proteinuria, Goodpasture's syndrome
- Gold, 10 mg im, then 50 mg im q 1 wk × 20 wk, then decrease gradually to q 1 mo (50 mg q 2 wk to 1500 mg, q 3 wk to 1800 mg, then q 4 wk). Doubts now re efficacy (Ann IM 1991;114:437). Adverse effects: rash, depressed wbc and/or platelets (Ann IM 1981;95:778), proteinuria (10%), pulmonary infiltrates (Br J Rheum 1991;30:214). Or po auranofin (Ridaura) 3 mg bid or 6 mg qd to 3 mg tid after 6 mo (Ann IM 1986;105:528); less effective than injectable (Arth Rheum 1990;33:1449). Adverse effects: bowel sx especially diarrhea (50%), reversible proteinuria (3%) which usually doesn't recur when resume. $100/mo for 3 mg bid
- Cyclosporine ~3 mg/kg/d po divided into bid doses (Nejm 1995; 333:137) w mtx
- Azathioprine, 6MP, cyclophosphamide

Experimental: γ-linolenic acid (converts to prostaglandin E_1) (Ann IM 1993;119:867); tetracyclines like minocycline or doxycycline 100 mg po bid (Rx Let 1999;6:58; Ann IM 1995;122:81); plasmapheresis over a protein A column (Prosorba) (Med Let 1999; 41:69) to absorb antibodies

JUVENILE RHEUMATOID ARTHRITIS (Juvenile Chronic Arthritis)

Nejm 1989;321:34; 1986;314:1269,1312; Bull Rheum Dis 1988;38(6):1

Cause:

Epidem: Incidence = 1.4/10,000 children/yr; prevalence = 1/1000 children in US

Pathophys: (J Rheum 1990; suppl 21:1)
Rubella virus present in 1/3 cases (Nejm 1985;313:1217)

Sx + Si: Polyarticular type (45%): onset at later age, occasionally rheumatoid factor positive; arthritis in ≥5 joints; no systemic sx or si
Pauci-articular type (30%); arthritis in <4 joints; often ANA positive; iridocyclitis leads to blindness often even when arthritis is inactive;

eye disease often asx (Clin Exp Rheum 1990;8:499; Bull Rheum Dis 1985;35(5):1)

Systemic type (25%): intermittent fever <103°F (<39.4°C), no arthritis; Still's disease variant: diurnal fevers, salmon-colored reticular rash, high ESR, pleuropericarditis, but rare or late arthritis

Crs: 20% still crippled at 10 yr

Cmplc: Growth impairment (Clin Orthop 1990;259:46)

r/o (Rheum Rev 1991;1:13) juvenile ankylosing spondylitis with positive HLA B27 (Bull Rheum Dis 1987;37(1):1); child abuse; neoplasms; infections (viral, endocarditis, Lyme disease); granulomatous disorders (Crohn's, sarcoid); connective tissue diseases like PAN, SS, giant cell arteritis, rheumatic fever, and SLE

Lab: No good diagnostic test

Hem: Anemia and leukocytosis

Serol: ANA often positive in pauci-articular type. HLA studies 90% positive for B27, cf Reiter's and ankylosing spondylitis (Nejm 1974;290:892); DRW2 and 3, when present, correlate with incr gold and penicillamine rx toxicity (Nejm 1980;302:300)

Rx: (Clin Orthop 1990;259:60; Bull Rheum Dis 1982;32:21)

Physical therapy (Rheum Dis Clin N Am 1991;17:1001) and NSAIDs like ASA or tolmetin; these alone enough in 50–60%, mostly the pauciarticular type

Methotrexate up to 1 mg/kg/wk

Tumor necrosis factor antagonists (p 789)

Gold (p 799)

OH-chloroquine or D-penicillamine? (both ineffective—Nejm 1986; 314:1269)

REITER'S SYNDROME

Bull Rheum Dis 1987;37(1):1; Ann IM 1984;100:207; Nejm 1983; 309:1606

Cause: Autoimmune

Epidem: Triggered by chlamydial urethritis and enteric pathogens like *Shigella, Salmonella, Yersinia, Campylobacter,* and HIV infection

(Bull Rheum Dis 1990;39(5):1). Associated with HLA B27-like ankylosing spondylitis (Ann IM 1976;84:8). Male:female = 9:1

Pathophys:

Sx: 2–4 wk incubation period after trigger (see above). First urethritis (85%), cervicitis, and/or prostatitis; then red eye (conjunctivitis); then weeks later, arthritis and arthralgias (99%), especially peripheral and in lower extremities, especially heels, knees, ankles, low back

Si: Peripheral arthritis and purulent urethral discharge (95%); red eye from conjunctivitis (40%) or uveitis (8%); fever (37%); painless skin or mucous membrane lesions (32%) especially circinate balanitis and keratodermia blennorrhagia (looks like pustular psoriasis)

Crs: 80% resolve after 4–12 mo, 20% go on to be chronic

Cmplc: Aortitis (1%); heart block (1%)

r/o chronic Lyme arthritis, gonorrhea, erythema multiforme variants, Behçet's syndrome, psoriasis, ankylosing spondylitis

Lab:

Joint fluid: WBC = 5000–50,000, mostly polys but lower % than gonorrhea with more monos, occasionally with ingested polys (LE phenomenon—Ann IM 1967;66:677)

Serol: RA titer negative; HLA B27 positive in 60–75%, but only 8% of people with pos titer have Reiter's (Ann IM 1982;96:70)

Xray: Periosteal new bone formation along shafts, eg, of phalanges

Rx: Tetracycline rx of presumed chlamydia of patient and partner (Bull Rheum Dis 1992;40(6):1)

NSAIDs as in ankylosing spondylitis (p 789)

SJÖGREN'S (Sicca) SYNDROME

Rheum Dis Clin N Am 1992;18(3); Bull Rheum Dis 1988;30:1046; Ann IM 1980;92:212

Cause: Autoimmune?; a retrovirus?; impaired response to cholinergic stimuli (Ann Rheum Dis 2000;59:48); primary, or secondary to scleroderma, rheumatoid arthritis, SLE, primary biliary cirrhosis, vasculitis, thyroiditis, hepatitis C (J Hepatol 1999;31:210), etc

Epidem: Females ≫ males; 2nd most common collagen vascular disease after RA. Associated with HLA B8 (54%) and HLA DRW3 (75%)

Pathophys: Lymphocyte-mediated destruction of exocrine glands leads to mucosal dryness; an immune complex small vessel vasculitis

Sx: Primary type: Raynaud's (20%); sicca syndrome with dry eyes and mouth and secondary caries, thirst; dry cough with frequent upper and lower respiratory infections; dysphagia; dyspareunia

Secondary type: other collagen vascular disease present

Si: Primary type: parotid enlargement (80%); pseudolymphoma; caries; positive Schirmer test (<5 mm/5 min filter paper ascent from eyelid) but many false positives and negatives, and hence not worth doing (Br J Rheum 1993;32:231)

Crs:

Cmplc: Primary type: obstructive and restrictive lung disease; gastric atrophy; pancreatitis; interstitial renal disease and Fanconi's syndrome; B-cell lymphomas (Nejm 1987;316:1118) and perhaps other cancers; staph conjunctivitis; blindness (Bull Rheum Dis 1985;35:5), and other MS-like syndromes in 20% (Ann IM 1986;104:322)

r/o other causes of sicca syndrome (Cornea 1999;18:625): type IV and V hyperlipidemia, sarcoid, hemachromatosis, amyloid, local irradiation, HIV infection which can be associated with as well as cause secondary *Sjögren's* (Bull Rheum Dis 1992;40(6):6)

Lab:

Hem: ESR elevated (Semin Arth Rheum 1992;22:114)

Path: Lip salivary gland bx shows lymphocytic infiltration (94%) (Nejm 1987;316:1118)

Serol: Positive RA titer (90%), ANA (50–80%), SSA, SSB (p 829)

Rx: Methylcellulose eye gtts and mouth wash, or "Lacrisert" methylcellulose lid insert q 12 h (Med Let 1981;23:104)

Steroids if marked parotid swelling or other life-threatening complications

of aphthous ulcers: tetracycline oral rinse

of dry mouth (Med Let 2000;42:70):

- Methylcellulose mouth wash, frequent sips of water, sugar free gum, hard candy
- Pilocarpine (Salagen) 5 mg po qid; helps xerostomia, at least radiation-induced type (Nejm 1993;329:390); $160/mo
- Cevimeline (Evoxac) 30 mg po tid; similar to pilocarpine, a cholinergic agonist. Adverse effects: sweating, N + V + D, rhinitis, worsens asthma, decr night vision. $120/mo

SCLERODERMA (Progressive Systemic Sclerosis) AND CREST* SYNDROME

Bull Rheum Dis 1981;31:7; Ann IM 1972;77:458

Cause: Genetic? Autoimmune?

Epidem: (Ann IM 1971;74:714)

Predominant in middle age, peak age 65 yr; 2.7 new patients/ million/yr; female:male = 8:1; recently rising incidence (Arth Rheum 1989;32:998)

Pathophys: Fetal Y chromosomes found in some skin lesions suggesting it may be a fetal graft vs host disease at least in some women (Nejm 1998;338:1186)

Collagen deposition in skin and muscles, especially smooth muscle, associated w incr mast cells (Ann IM 1985;102:182); debate if fibrosis or vascular disease is primary (J Rheumatol 1999;26:938)

Progressive sclerosis of skin, esophagus and rest of gut, lung, heart. Cardiac sx due to microvascular changes causing fibrosis (Nejm 1986;314:1397) which can be cold-induced (Ann IM 1986;105: 661). GI cmplc all due to bacterial overgrowth from diminished large and small bowel motility (Ann IM 1981;94:749)

Sx: Dx criteria (Bull Rheum Dis 1981;31:1): major = proximal scleroderma (proximal to mcp joints), 91% sens, 99% specif; minor = sclerodactyly,* digital pitting, basilar pulmonary fibrosis (30% false neg, 2% false pos)

Raynaud's* (86%); esophageal* reflux, dysphagia (75% gi involvement) w eventual nonmotile esophagus, pulmonary sx especially cough (50%), cardiovascular sx (20%), polymyositis, arthritis

Si: Pitting edema early, brawny nonpitting later, then thin mummy-like skin with incr pigmentation; periungual telangiectasias* (r/o constant hot water exposure); subcutaneous calcinosis*

Crs: 5-yr survival 68%, worse if renal > heart > lung involvement (Ann IM 1993;118:602)

Cmplc: Renal disease, progressive but reversible (60%—Ann IM 2000; 133:600), 76% 1-yr survival with ACE inhibitor (Ann IM 1990; 113:352); amyloid; malabsorp/digestion; Sjögren's (17%—Ann IM 1977;87:535); progressive acute and chronic pulmonary failure and HT (Arth + Rheum 1999;42:2638); primary hypothyroidism (Ann IM 1981;95:431); heart block and arrhythmias (Ann IM 1981;94: 38); MIs and microcirculatory changes (J Rheumatol 2000;27:155); impotence (Ann IM 1981;95:150) r/o sclerodactyly from air hammer use or ergot; porphyria cutanea tarda; **eosinophilic fasciitis** (Ann IM 1980;92:507) w "peau d'orange" skin and flexion contractures esp of upper extremities and complicated by carpal tunnel syndrome (Arth Rheum 1995;38:1707); and **eosinophilic/myalgia syndrome** caused by contaminated tryptophan, spares hands and feet, no Raynaud's (Nejm 1990;323:357; Ann IM 1990;113:124); similar syndrome related to incr 5-HT with pyridoxine, tryptophan, and carbidopa rx—Nejm 1980;303:782)

Lab:
  Path: Skin bx shows incr collagen, epidermal degeneration
  Serol: C' normal, SPEP shows incr IgG, rheumatoid titer elevated (25%), cryoglobulins, false positive serologic tests for syphilis. ANA (Bull Rheum Dis 1985;35(6):1) positive, especially speckled (centromere-staining antibodies) type, which is present in 70% of CREST; antinucleolar antibodies positive in 54% but 26% of SLE pos and 10% of RA (patterns, Nejm 1970;282:1174). Scl-70 specific but nonsensitive, positive in only 20%

Xray: Hand films show distal phalanx tuft resorption (cf. psoriasis) with periarticular calcification. UGIS shows esophageal dysmotility and reflux. BE shows "wide mouth" diverticula

Rx: (Semin Arth Rheum 1993;23:22; 1989;18:181)
  Physical therapy
  Steroids
  Relaxin, human recombinant type (Ann IM 2000;132:871) 25 μgm/kg sc qd; slows skin thickening and perhaps lung fibrosis
  D-penicillamine 500–1500 mg po qd (Bull Rheum Dis 1978;28:948), helps skin, organs, and survival (Ann IM 1982;97:652) but 1/3 can't tolerate (Ann IM 1986;104:699) and is falling out of favor in the 1990s
  Captopril po or other ACE blocker, prevents renal failure if BP elevated (Ann IM 1990;113:352; Nejm 1979;300:1417)
  Nifedipine for cardiac changes (Nejm 1986;314:1397) and Raynaud's
  Octreotide, a somatostatin analog, po helps gi motility (Nejm 1991; 325:1461)
  Minocycline (Lancet 1998;352:1755)
  Colchicine perhaps

of GERD: proton pump inhibitors (p 253)
of pulmonary fibrosis: cyclophosphamide (Ann IM 2000;132:946)

SYSTEMIC LUPUS ERYTHEMATOSUS

Ann IM 1995;123:42; Nejm 1994;330:1871

Cause: Idiopathic type is multifactorial in etiology but clearly there is a genetic predisposition, which has several HLA type linkages (Ann IM 1991;115:548)

Drug-induced type (Bull Rheum Dis 1991;40:4): procainamide (40% of pts become ANA-positive but a much smaller % develop SLE) especially slow-release preparation (Ann IM 1984;100:197); hydralazine (10% become ANA-positive—Ann IM 1972;76:365); INH (20% become ANA-pos); rarely quinidine (Ann IM 1984;100:840), methyldopa, chlorpromazine, penicillamine (Ann IM 1982;97:659); etc. Occurs sooner in slow acetylators (autosomal recessive) than rapids (Nejm 1978;298:1157)

Epidem: Female:male = 9:1 in idiopathic types; equal in drug-induced type. Black:white ratio = 3–4:1; prevalence = 40/100,000; seen especially in women during childbearing years

Pathophys: Tissue damage is from immune complex vasculitis, thrombocytopenia, and antiphospholipid antibody-induced thrombosis. The autoantibodies are from abnormally intolerant B and T cells (Nejm 1991;115:548). Associated with genetically decr suppressor T-cell function (Nejm 1985;312:1671). Renal disease occurs in idiopathic types only, not drug-induced types (Nejm 1972;286:908)

Sx: H/o stress, eg, UV exposure, pregnancy (rv—Ann IM 1981;94:666); facial rash; fever; visual sx; oligoarthritis (95%), episodic, pain > objective findings

Si: Rash, facial butterfly rash (33%), sun-sensitive, and unlike discoid lupus scarred delineated rash especially on ears, and differs from seborrheic rash in same area by spanning nasolabial folds; periungual atrophy; corneal staining (88% by fluorescein—Nejm 1967;276:1168); rheumatoid nodules (Ann IM 1970;72:49); lymphadenopathy (30%), especially with suppressed T-cell type (Nejm 1985;312:1671)

Crs: 90% 10-yr survival, worse w hypertension and/or nephritis; peripheral neuropathy usually regresses; renal progression depends on presenting sediment (Ann IM 1968;69:441)

Cmplc:

- Infections, the most common cause of death
- Nephritis, with nephrotic syndrome (prognosis no worse if have—Nejm 1983;308:187), and renal failure
- Serositis with pleuritis, pericarditis, and effusions
- Hemolytic anemia (Am J Med 2000;108:198), agranulocytosis (Ann IM 1984;100:197) and thrombocytopenia
- Neurologic vasculitis (Curr Concepts Cerebro Dis 1977;12:17), peripheral neuropathy, visual cortex (Ann IM 1975;83:163) and diffuse CNS involvement often causes seizures (Ann IM 1974;81:763), transverse myelopathy (Ann IM 1976;84:46), chorea
- Nasal septum ulceration and perforation (Nejm 1969;281:722)
- Liebman-Sachs endocarditis (Nejm 1988;319:817) with AI and MR; present in >50%? and assoc w 22% incidence of cmplc's (Nejm 1996;335:1424)
- Newborn heart block (Nejm 1983;309:209), fetal distress and loss (yes—Bull Rheum Dis 1992;40(6):3; Nejm 1985;313:152; no—Nejm 1991;325:1063), from lupus anticoagulant
- Thromboses, venous and arterial, from lupus anticoagulant, an antiphospholipid or anticardiolipin antibody (p 112)
- Sjögren's
- Bleeding from factor IX and XI inhibition (Ann IM 1972;77:543)
- Pneumonitis and fibrosis from immune complexes (Ann IM 1979;91:30)
- Cystitis (Ann IM 1983;98:323)
- Tendon rupture

Lab:

Hem: Thrombocytopenia, leukopenia, hemolytic and ncnc anemia (Ann IM 1977;86:220); ESR elevated

Path: Skin bx shows specific IgG immunofluorescence at epidermal-dermal junction in all skin, in contrast to only affected skin in discoid lupus (Ann IM 1969;71:753)

Renal bx (Nejm 1974;291:693; Ann IM 1970;73:929) may show:

- Benign focal proliferative glomerulonephritis (may progress to b)

- Diffuse proliferative GN with elevated BUN and nephrotic syndrome
- Membranous GN with nephrotic syndrome

Serol (Bull Rheum Dis 1985;35:6):

ANAs:

- Total ANA >1/64 in 95% over time, especially peripheral pattern; in drug-induced types, diffuse/homogeneous patterns most common
- Anti-Sm, very specific but not sensitive (present in 20–35%)
- Anti-Ro
- Anti-RNP (soluble nuclear antigen antibodies) (elevated in 50%) but also elevated in mixed connective tissue disease, levels correlate with SLE psychosis (Nejm 1987;317:265)
- Antihistones positive in many drug-induced SLE, 50% of other SLE, 20% in RA
- Anti-DNA antibodies against double-stranded (natural) DNA, specific, but not sensitive (misses half), associated with renal disease
- Anti-DNA against single-stranded DNA is nonspecific

STSs: VDRL falsely positive; FTA falsely positive, beaded (in 15%) (Nejm 1970;282:1287)

Complement levels decr, C'3 <100 mg% and CH_{50} < 50 U, especially with renal disease

Rx: (Bull Rheum Dis 1982;32:35)

Flu shots, don't cause flare (Ann IM 1978;88:729)

ASA (or indomethacin) to tinnitus-producing levels, though NSAID may itself induce renal failure (Nejm 1977;296:418)

OH-chloroquine 250 mg qd, <3.5 mg/lb relatively safe (p 788)

Total lymphoid irradiation (Ann IM 1985;102:450); doubtful worth it (Ann IM 1986;105:58)

of renal disease: systemic steroids with azathioprine, mycophenolate mofetil (Nejm 2000;343:1156), or cyclophosphamide (Ann IM 1995;122:940; 1992;116:114; Nejm 1986;314:614; 1984;311:491, 1528); or cyclophosphamide alone iv q 1 mo (Lancet 1992;340: 741; Ann IM 1990;112:674); renal transplant, rarely recurs in transplant (Ann IM 1991;114:183); plasmapheresis no help (Nejm 1992;326:1373)

of rare bullous eruption: dapsone (Ann IM 1982;97:165)

TEMPORAL ARTERITIS (Giant Cell Arteritis) AND POLYMYALGIA RHEUMATICA

Ann IM 1994;121:484; Arth Rheum 1988;31:745; Ann IM 1978;88:162; 1978;97:672

Cause: Autoimmune

Epidem: TA = 133/100,000; female:male = 5–17:1; usually in patients > age 60 yr, peaks in age 70–80. Cyclic incidence w 10 yr peaks (Ann IM 1995;123:192). Occasionally associated w HLA DR4 (J Rheum 1983;10:659)

Pathophys: A large-vessel vasculitis (r/o Takayasu's arteritis—Ann IM 1985;103:121); a spectrum from a little patchy involvement of medium vessels with arteritis in PMR to much more w TA. Muscle pain is probably claudication

Sx: Fever; polymyalgia syndrome w muscle aches and weakness esp in quads (33%) (Ann IM 1995;123:192); headache (77%) and scalp pain; sore throat and cough (Ann IM 1984;101:594); leg, tongue, and jaw claudication; weakness, malaise, and weight loss; synovitis, shoulder and hip pain

Si: Fever (27%) up to 103°F (39.4°C); mild muscle tenderness, asx knee effusions (8/18), tender indurated temporal arteries (53%), cherry red macular spot of retinal artery occlusion

Am Coll Rheum criteria (Arth Rheum 1990;33:1122) 3/5 of following findings:
- Age > 50
- New localized headache
- Temporal artery tender or diminished pulse
- ESR > 50 mm/hr
- Biopsy pathology positive

Crs: PMR and TA resolve in ±2 yr. No incr mortality with PMR (Ann IM 1978;88:162)

Cmplc: Sudden cranial nerve defects (17%), especially blindness, preventable with steroids and occurs in first 12 weeks if going to; psychosis; MI and CVA are the most common causes of death; aortic dissections and aneurysms (Ann IM 1995;122:502); hypothyroidism (5%) (Brit J Rheum 1991;30:349)

Lab:

Chem: Normal muscle enzymes, negative rheumatoid titer; liver function tests often slightly elevated

Hem: ESR elevated (incr α_2-globulin > 40 mg% [97%]), usually > 100, often only abnormal test; crit = 30–40% in 14/18, hgb < 11 gm % (23%)

Path: Muscle bx normal; temporal artery bx (take 3–4 cm) shows patchy (easily missed) giant cell arteritis that remain positive even after 14 d of prednisone rx (Ann IM 1994;120:987)

Urine: UA usually normal

Xray: Color duplex US of temporal arteries shows hypoechogenic edema around arteries (73% sens,? 100% specif) (Nejm 1997;337:1336, 1385)

Rx: Prednisone 40–60 mg (10–15 mg for PMR) po qd × 12 wk, then decrease to control sx's; keep up at least for 2 yr (Ann IM 1972; 77:845); qod doesn't work (Ann IM 1975;82:613)

Methotrexate 10 mg po q 1 wk allows lower steroid doses (Ann IM 2001;134:106; Arth + Rheum 1991;345:A43)

WEGENER'S GRANULOMATOSIS

Nejm 1997;337:1512; Ann IM 1992;116:488

Cause: Infectious agent? (Ann IM 1987;106:840); *Staphylococcus aureus* nasal carriage associated w relapses, possibly through induction of autoimmunity (Ann IM 1994;120:12)

Epidem: Rare but all forms of ANCA associated small vessel vasculitis are the most common type of vasculitis in adults

Pathophys: ANCA associated necrotizing granulomatous vasculitis of the small blood vessels of the upper and lower respiratory tract (90%) and kidney (80%, though <20% on presentation)

Sx: Purulent rhinitis; sinusitis; insidious onset; fever; arthralgias, pneumonitis

Si: Pneumonitis, sinusitis, otitis media, rhinitis, peripheral neuropathies, purpura, arthritis

Crs: Fatal in 80% at 1 yr, and 93% at 2 yr without rx; 95% survival with rx (Ann IM 1983;98:76)

Cmplc: Pulmonary insufficiency (20% of fatalities), massive pulmonary hemorrhage, tracheal sclerosis w stridor (15% adults, 50% children); renal failure (80% of fatalities)

r/o **midline granuloma** with local facial erosion, rx with xray (Ann IM 1976;84:140); malignant or benign **lymphomatoid angiitis**

and granulomatosis, unresponsive to chemotherapy (Ann IM 1978;89:691); other ANCA-associated vasculitis (see below)

Lab:

Chem: Creatinine elevated, IgA incr in blood and secretions, normal IgG and IgM

Hem: ESR elevated, eosinophilia

Path: Bx of nose, throat, and lung show focal angiitis with granulomas; bx of kidney shows GN

Serol: IgG antineutrophil cytoplasmic antibodies (p-ANCA or c-ANCA) elevated, 66% sens, 98% specif (Ann IM 1995;123:925), can use to follow rx; but as many as 1/3 of the positives may be polyarteritis or idiopathic renal vasculitis? (Ann IM 1990;113:656); r/o other ANCA associated small vessel vasculitis: microscopic angiitis, Churg-Strauss syndrome, and drug-induced type

Urine: Red cell casts

Xray: Cavitating pulmonary nodule

Rx: Rapid rx, crucial to survival, w cyclophosphamide ~2 mg/kg/d to keep poly count ≥3000 + prednisone iv at 7 mg/kg/d at first tapering to 1 mg/kg/d then change to qod over 3–4 mo; 93% complete remission, 30% cure? with good long-term survival (Ann IM 1983;98:76)

Tm/S DS given bid as prophylaxis decr recurrences by preventing immune stimulating infections (Nejm 1996;335:16) esp by staph, helps 90%? (Ann IM 1987;106:840); decr *Pneumocystis* infections in pts on cyclophosphamide

---

21.3 CRYSTAL DISEASES

GOUT

Bull Rheum Dis 1984;34(6):1; Ann IM 1979;90:812; Nejm 1979; 300:1459

Cause: Hyperuricemia, with pain due to wbc ingestion of crystals? Primary type is due to a transferase deficiency (normally salvages urate); may be genetic, sporadic. Secondary type due to tissue breakdown or decr renal tubular excretion or urate

Epidem: Primary type more common in higher social classes; male:female = 20:1; peak onset in males age ~30 yr and postmenopausally in women

Secondary type seen w leukemia especially when being rx'd, polycythemia, hemolytic anemia, starvation even in obese, diuretic rx, moonshine drinkers due to lead in alcohol (Nejm 1969;280:1199), alcoholics because incr urate production and perhaps decr excretion (Nejm 1982;307:1598)

Pathophys: In kidneys, uric acid is normally 100% filtered, 100% resorbed, 100% excreted in distal tubule but may be competitively inhibited by lactate, ETOH, ketone bodies (Nejm 1971;284:1193). Podagra from traumatically incr synovial fluid from which water resorbed at night faster than urate leading to a gouty attack (Ann IM 1977;86:230,234)

Sx: Family hx (50%); podagra (inflammation/swelling of 1st mp joint of big toe) (84%) or other severely painful arthritis; low-dose ASA (<4 gm) precipitates and/or worsens

Si: Arthritis including podagra, tophi (ear > elbow > finger > foot)

Crs: Acute attacks last 1–14 d, sx free between attacks but increasing frequency over years; without rx, permanent damage ensues

Cmplc: DJD; no increase in pseudogout; renal stones, but the nephropathy is only associated with lead-related gout (Nejm 1981;304:520)

r/o sarcoid arthritis which also improves with colchicine (Nejm 1971;285:1503); Reiter's; septic joint; RA; pseudogout; DJD; rare hyperuricemic X-linked recessive **Lesch-Nyhan syndrome,** characterized by choreoathetosis, dystonic spasticity and self-mutilation (Nejm 1996;334:1568; 1981;305:1106)

Lab:

Chem: Uric acid >10 mg%, r/o other causes including
- Idiopathic without gout (10% of Framingham population have)
- Hemolysis
- Leukemia
- Diuretics
- Psoriasis
- Fanconi's syndrome
- Chronic beryllium disease
- Down syndrome (never get gout)
- Starvation
- Lead poisoning
- Alcoholism

Gout, continued

False depressions of uric acid from uricosurics, eg, ASA, allopurinol, xray dyes (Ann IM 1971;74:845); false increases from methyldopa, L-dopa

Joint fluid: With polarizing scope, long thin urate crystals, some inside wbc's, negatively birefringent (yellow parallel to red filter axis, blue when perpendicular)

Urine: 24-h urine acid ≥ 1 gm; urate/creat ratio > 0.75;
Urate$_u$/Creat$_u$ × Creat$_s$/Creat$_u$ > 0.7 = high excretor on AM spot urine (Ann IM 1979;91:44)

Xray: Soft tissue swelling; in chronic type, DJD and punched-out areas of bone

Rx: (Nejm 1996;334:445; Ann IM 1979;90:812):

Prevention: no need to rx asx increases in uric acid (Nejm 1981; 304:535)
- Colchicine 1–2 mg po qd
- Probenecid 1–3 gm po qd divided, start with 0.5 gm or
- Sulfinpyrazone 800 mg po qd divided; both prevent 100% resorption, use especially if 24-h urine urate <600 mg
- Allopurinol 200–400 mg po qd if 24-h urate >600 mg, or renal disease (decrease dose to 100 mg qd in anuria to prevent rash/fever/hepatitis syndrome, or tophi; can precipitate an attack)

Acute: if attack <10 d old,
- Colchicine 0.6 mg po q 1 h up to 7 mg; renal excretion, inhibits microtubular (actin) formation hence decreases lysozymes which cause inflammation. Adverse effects: NV + D, B$_{12}$ malabsorption from ileum (Nejm 1968;279:845), alopecia, decr wbc's; myo- and neuropathies (Nejm 1987;316:1562), or
- Indomethacin 50 mg po t-qid until relief then rapid taper over a week, or
- Steroids intra-articularly or systemically; or ACTH 80 IU im/iv, then 40 mg 12 h later (Arth Rheum 1988;31:803) especially if sx >10 d

PSEUDOGOUT

Bull Rheum Dis 1985;25:804; Ann IM 1977;87:241

Cause: Calcium pyrophosphate crystals

Epidem: Increased incidence in neuropathic joints (Ann IM 1973;79:341), hemochromatosis, hypothyroidism, hypo Mg^{2+}, hyperparathyroidism, gout, RA, DJD (Bull Rheum Dis 1984; 34(6):1)

Pathophys: Poly ingestion of crystals results in enzyme release in the joint and subsequent inflammation

Sx: Acute arthritis

Si: Knee > mcp > wrist > shoulder

Crs:

Cmplc: r/o calcium oxalate deposition in renal failure (Ann IM 1982; 97:36)

Lab:

Joint fluid: With a polarizing scope, calcium pyrophosphate crystals (rhomboid, positively birefringent in red filter) (p 812), may be small and require oil immersion lens to see

Xray: Semilunar calcifications of joint cartilages

Rx: Indomethacin; local steroid joint injections or systemic steroids

21.4 INHERITED AND OTHER RHEUMATOLOGIC DISEASES

AMYLOIDOSIS

Nejm 1997;337:902; 1990;323:508; 1980;302:1283; Bull Rheum Dis 1991;40(2):1

Cause: Deposition of short-chain proteins in many parts of the body; several proteins are responsible for such deposition: AL, AA, AF, AH, AP

AL, an immunoglobulin light chain, amyloidosis (primary type): patients with B- or plasma cell disorders like multiple myeloma or Waldenström's; idiopathic

AF, abnormal familial protein subunit found in affected families, usually present in middle or late life as myocardiopathy or neuropathy (Nejm 1997;336:466)

AA, amyloidosis (secondary type) associated w SAA protein, an acute phase reactant: collagen vascular diseases, Crohn's disease, cystic fibrosis, iv drug use, chronic infections (tbc, familial Mediterranean fever, osteomyelitis, etc.)

AH, a β_2-microglobulin accumulated in serum of dialysis pts

AP, normal serum protein

Epidem:

Pathophys: Infiltration of organs by protein; in all types: kidney, liver, spleen, gi tract, skin; in AL type, predominantly: vessels, heart, marrow, lung infiltration with hemoptysis, joints (synovium), peripheral nerves, factor X deficiency, pancreatic islets (in myeloma, light chains taken up by macrophages, then excreted into interstitium where polymerized—Nejm 1982;307:1689)

Sx: Exertional muscle pain (due to arteriole infiltration and ischemia—Ann IM 1969;70:1167); fatigue; carpal tunnel syndrome

Si: Hepatosplenomegaly; raised skin plaques, if rubbed results in purpura, "greasy nose syndrome" (amyloid infiltration); "shoulder pad" deposition associated with arthropathy (Nejm 1973;288:354); RA-like acute arthritis; "scalloped pupils" in familial type (Nejm 1975;293:914); macroglossia (AL type only; sensory and autonomic neuropathy)

Crs: AA type amyloidosis may revert, especially the nephrotic syndrome, with rx of the primary disease (Nejm 1970;282:128)

Cmplc: Functional asplenia, nephrotic syndrome, CHF, water-losing nephropathy (r/o DI and postobstructive syndrome), factor X deficiency which rx with splenectomy (Nejm 1981;304:827; 1979; 301:1050; 1977;297:81); peripheral or polyneuropathy (Nejm 1991;325:1482); atrial thrombi and embolization (Nejm 1992; 327:1570)

Lab:

Path: Rectal or other tissue bx shows protein infiltration with green birefringence on polarizing scope exam with Congo red staining; in AA type, Congo red affinity can be leached out by K-permanganate unlike AL type. Normal-appearing skin will be positive in ~ half of all patients with either type

Urine: 24-h protein >3 gm and thus nephrotic

Xray: Chest shows cardiomegaly if cardiac infiltration. Serum amyloid P scan (Nejm 1990;323:508)

Rx: AA type, rx primary disease

AL and other types (Nejm 1997;336;1202), rx with melphalan + prednisone (Nejm 1987;316:1133), or as 2nd choice, colchicine (Ann IM 1977;87:568); plasma exchange helps neuropathies (Nejm 1991;325:1482)

AF type, liver transplant (Ann IM 1997;127:618)

in cardiomyopathy, avoid calcium channel blockers and digoxin (Am J Cardiol 1985;55:1645; Circ 1981;63:1285)

MARFAN'S SYNDROME

Bull Rheum Dis 1980;30:1016 (rv of all connective tissue disorders); Nejm 1979;300:772

Cause: Genetic, autosomal dominant on chromosome #15 (Nejm 1994; 331:148; 1992;326:905; 1990;323:935); however, 15% of cases are sporadic

Epidem:

Pathophys: Defect in elastic collagen (Nejm 1981;305:989), caused by a defect in microfibrillar fibers on which elastin is laid (Nejm 1990; 323:152); cystic medical necrosis of thoracic aorta (95%)

Sx: Pos family hx; tall; frequent joint dislocations with minor trauma

Si: Arachnodactyly, arm span > height; hernias; lenticular dislocations (80%), upward, unlike downward in homocystinuria; aortic insufficiency (60%) with click, also mitral insufficiency due to posterior leaflet prolapse; arched palate

Crs: Average age at death is 32 yr, most from aortic root dilatation causes such as dissection, rupture, and aortic and mitral insufficiencies (Nejm 1972;286:804)

Cmplc: Aortic dissection (12%), accounts for 90% of deaths (Nejm 1986;314:1070); SBE; vascular rupture during pregnancy (Ann IM 1995;123:117)

r/o homocystinuria (p 241); **Ehlers-Danlos** syndrome (Nejm 2001; 345:1167; 2000;342:675,730) due to genetic collagen defects; all types have skin fragility, bruising, DJD; type IVs die from aortic, arterial, bowel or uterine rupture; not usually assoc w hyperextensibility types

Lab:

Xray: Chest; echocardiogram

Rx: of scoliosis (p 653)

of ascending aortic aneurysm: propranolol qid po or other β blocker to keep exercise P <100, slows progression of aortic disease (Nejm 1994;330:1335); or surgical when 6⁺ cm gives good result (Nejm 1986;314:1070)

OSTEOARTHRITIS

Cause:
  Endogenous factors:
- Changes in articular cartilage like incr brittleness, decr water binding, decr chrondroitin sulfate, perhaps incr protein/polysaccharide ratio
- Lubrication and viscosity failure
- Genetic defects in procollagen (Nejm 1990;322:526) which are autosomal dominant

  Exogenous factors:
- Trauma, including injuries decades before (Ann IM 2000;133:321)
- Congenital anomalies
- Metabolic diseases like gout and ochronosis
- Endocrine diseases like acromegaly
- Inflammatory joint diseases
- Obesity, increases knee DJD especially (Am J Med 1999;107:542; Bull Rheum Dis 1992;41(2):6)

Epidem: Older patients

Pathophys: (rv of pathophys—Nejm 1989;320:1322) See Fig. 21.4.1
  Quadriceps weakness may precede and somehow cause knee arthritis (Ann IM 1997;127:97)
  Pain due to adjacent marrow space edema (Ann IM 2001;134:541,591)

Sx: Post-rest stiffness, pain on motion. Joints most frequently involved are great toe and thumb mcp's, knee, hip, sacral and cervical spine

Si: Motion preserved but local tenderness. Bony enlargement at dip joints called Heberden's nodes, or at pip joints called Bouchard's nodes. Local inflammation occasionally, especially in erosive osteoarthritis variant with hot joints seen in middle-aged women

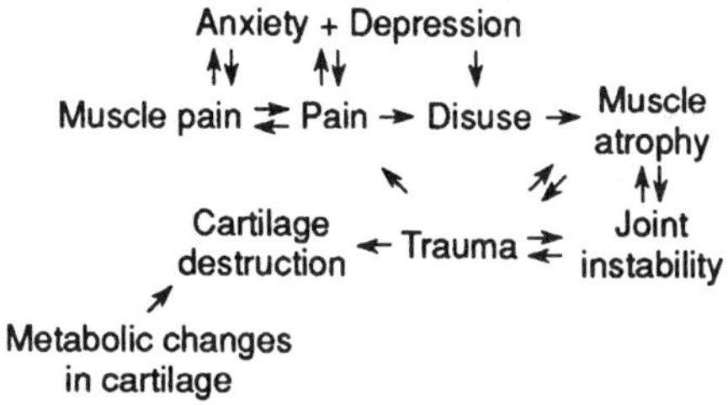

Figure 21.4.1

Crs:

Cmplc: CNS sx's from cord or vertebral artery compression (**cervical spondylosis**) occasionally causing paraplegia; but neck, head, and shoulder pain all common

r/o avascular necrosis: of femoral head, especially in patients on steroids, alcoholics, or with sickle cell disease; of knee, medial femoral condyle or tibia in elderly (Bull Rheum Dis 1985;35:42)

Lab:

Path: Synovial bx shows fibrous cartilaginous degeneration especially at points of stress

Xray: Hypertrophic changes, eg, osteophytes, sclerosis, and bone cysts without cortical bone changes unlike RA

Rx: (Ann IM 2000;133:726)

Braces, exercise (Ann IM 2000;132:173), weight reduction, psychiatric rx

Calcium + vit D po to prevent osteoporosis and slow progression (Ann IM 1996;125:353)

NSAIDs including acetaminophen which does help pain (Nejm 1991; 325:87)

Glucosamine sulfate 500 mg po tid OTC dietary supplement may help (Med Let 2001;43:111), but may worsen diabetic control (Rx Let 1999;6:58) and variable purity w OTC products a problem

Chondroitin sulfate may also help (Jama 2000;283:1469) but studies not rigorous, as w glucosamine

Intra-articular

• Steroid injection may help as long as joint is stable (Med Let 1968; 10:31)

• Hyaluronan (Hyalgan, Synvisc) (Rheumatol 1999;38:602; Med Let 1998;40:69; J Rheumatol 1996;23:1579) weekly × 3–5; $700

21.4 Inherited and Other Rheumatologic Diseases **817**

Surgical arthroplasties, joint replacements (hip—Nejm 1990;323:725; knee—Nejm 1990;323:801), etc.

OSTEOMYELITIS
Nejm 1997;336:999

Cause: *S. aureus* (60%), tuberculosis, group A strep, *Haemophilus, Pneumococcus, Salmonella,* gonorrhea, enterobacter group, fungal; in neonates, group B strep, *E. coli; Pseudomonas* in drug addicts, in sneaker wearers who step on nails
- Hematogenous via bacteremia, especially in children with open epiphyses, starts in metaphysis
- Compound fractures and other open injury with bone contamination, eg, surgery
- Direct extension from adjacent infected tissue, eg, joint

Epidem: 85% of cases are children; *Salmonella* osteomyelitis very frequent in sickle disease; also common in diabetics w foot ulcers (Nejm 1994;331:854) and pts w decubitus ulcers (Arch IM 1983;143:683)

Pathophys: Bacteremia results in bacteria picked up by slow blood flow area of metaphysis; infection can't penetrate epiphysis so moves down bone via haversian and Volkmann's canals; may rupture through thin metaphyseal cortical bone; sequestration of dead bone prolongs recovery. Persistence may be a result of intracellular survival especially w tuberculosis

Sx: Localized pain; antalgic use of limb; fever

Si: Often nothing besides fever; may have local redness, swelling, drainage

Crs: 20% mortality without antibiotics; chronicity in 15% even with rx

Cmplc: Altered (incr or decr) epiphyseal growth of one limb due to changes in blood supply, Brodie's abscess, sequestration and reactivation years later, acute glomerulonephritis (Ann IM 1969;71:335), amyloidosis, local epidermoid carcinoma in 0.5%

Lab:
Bact: Blood cultures; if neg, bone aspiration positive in 60%, bone biopsy positive in 90%. Culture of draining sinus unreliable
Hem: ESR elevated (but not always—Nejm 1987;316:763)

Table 21.4.1 Antibiotic Treatment of Osteomyelitis in Adults.*

Microorganisms Isolated	Treatment of Choice	Alternatives
S. aureus		
Penicillin-sensitive	Penicillin G (4 million units every 6 hr)	First-generation cephalosporin (e.g., cefazolin, 2 g every 6 hr), clindamycin (600 mg every 6 hr),or vancomycin (1 g every 12 hr)
Penicillin-resistant	Nafcillin (2 g every 6 hr)[†]	First-generation cephalosporin, clindamycin (as above), or vancomycin (as above)
Methicillin-resistant	Vancomycin (1 g every 12 hr)	Teicoplanin (400 mg every 24 hr; first day, every 12 hr intravenously or intramuscularly)[‡]
Various streptococci (group A or B β-hemolytic or *Streptococcus pneumoniae*)	Penicillin G (4 million units every 6 hr)	Clindamycin (as above), erythromycin (500 mg every 6 hr), vancomycin (as above), or ceftriaxone (2 g once a day)
Enteric gram-negative rods	Quinolone (ciprofloxacin, 750 mg every 12 hr orally)	Third generation cephalosporin (eg, ceftriaxone, 2 g every 24 hr)
Serratia or *Pseudomonas aeruginosa*	Ceftazidime (2 g every 8 hr) (with aminoglycosides for at least the first 2 wk)[§]	Imipenem (500 mg every 6 hr), piperacillintazobactam (4 g and 0.5 g, respectively, every 8 hr), or cefepime (2 g every 12 hr) (with aminoglycosides for at least the first 2 wk)[§]
Anaerobes	Clindamycin (600 mg every 6 hr intravenously or orally)	Amoxicillin–clavulanic acid (2.0 and 0.2 g, respectively, every 8 hr) or metronidazole for gram-negative anaerobes (500 mg every 8 hr)
Mixed aerobic and anaerobic microorganisms	Amoxicillin–clavulanic acid (2.0 and 0.2 g, respectively, every 8 hr)	Imipenem (500 mg every 6 hr)[¶]

*All antibiotic treatments are given intravenously unless otherwise stated.
[†]In Europe, flucloxacillin is the treatment of choice.
[‡]Teicoplanin is currently available only in Europe.
[§]Aminoglycosides may be given once a day or in multiple doses.
[¶]Imipenem should be given when infection is due to aerobic gram-negative microorganisms resistant to amoxicillin–clavulanic acid.
Reproduced with permission from Lew. Current Concepts: Osteomyelitis. Nejm 1997;336: 999. Copyright 1997, Mass. Medical Society. All rights reserved.

21.4 Inherited and Other Rheumatologic Diseases **819**

RHEUMATOLOGY/ORTHOPEDICS

Xray: MRI or CT very sensitive, esp early before changes on plain films
Plain films may show gross deformities with lytic and blastic activity
after 2–4 wk
Bone scan positive within weeks, 50–75% false pos, 70–90% sens
(J Gen Intern Med 1992;7:158)
Rx: Appropriate long-term parenteral antibiotics (Nejm 1997;336:1004)
and surgical removal of sequestrum (refer to Table 21.4.1)

PAGET'S DISEASE
Nejm 1997;336:558

Cause: Benign neoplasia of bone remodeling unit? (Nejm 1973;289:25)
Epidem: 3% of population will develop it sometime in lifetime, although
severe disease much less common
Pathophys: Excessive formation and destruction of bone constantly;
normally sequence is incr osteoclast followed by incr osteoblast
activities; but in Paget's the rate of this progression is markedly incr
(Nejm 1973;289:15). High blood flow due to idiopathic shunting at
a capillary level, no true arteriovenous shunts (Nejm 1972;287:686).
Increased vertebral size leads to neural compression syndromes
Sx: Fractures; knee, hip, and other joint arthritis; bone pain
Si: Angioid streaking of retina (r/o sickle cell disease and pseudoxanthoma
elasticum); deformed long bones; head enlargement
Crs:
Cmplc: CNS compression syndromes including deafness from calvarial
deformities (eg, Beethoven), pathologic fractures, high-output CHF,
osteogenic sarcoma (2%), renal stones especially with
immobilization, heart block due to bundle calcifications
Lab:
Chem: Alkaline phosphatase incr markedly, highest values of any
disease, r/o osteomalacia (Am J Med 2000;108;296)
Urine: Calcium and phosphate levels elevated
Xray: Sclerotic bone, expanded bone size (only Paget's will do this); bone
scan hot spots correlate with pain sx better than plain film changes
(Ann IM 1973;79:348)

Rx:

1st: Bisphosphonates (p 311)
- Alendronate (Fosamax) 40 mg po qd, $120/mo
- Etidronate (Didronel) 5–20 mg/kg/d po × 6 mo (see Nejm 1990;323:73 for use in osteoporosis), can cause fractures at high doses (Ann IM 1982;96:619; Med Let 1978;20:78)
- Pamidronate (Aredia) 60 mg iv over 24 h q 1–3 yr (Med Let 1992;34:1)
- Risedronate (Actonel) (Med Let 1998;40:89) 30 mg po qd × 2 mo; $763
- Tiladronate (Skelid) (Med Let 1997;39:65) 400 mg po qd; $450/mo

2nd:
- Calcitonin, human 0.5 mg sc, $177/mo (Med Let 1987;29:47); or salmon calcitonin (Calcimar) (Jama 1972;221:1127) 50 U sc qd until asx, then tiw, $81/mo. Both inhibit osteocyte progenitor duplication and speed conversion of clasts to blasts (Ann IM 1981; 95:192; Nejm 1973;289:25)

Others:
- Plicamycin (formerly mithramycin) (Nejm 1970;283:1171) 15–25 μgm/kg iv qd × 10 d, but toxic and not FDA approved
- Gallium nitrate? iv/sc × weeks (Ann IM 1991;114:846)

SARCOIDOSIS

Nejm 1997;336:1224; Ann IM 1981;94:73

Cause:

Epidem: 10–50/100,000/yr in US; black:white = 1:6; associated with regional enteritis, perhaps shared etiology (Nejm 1971;285:1259)

Pathophys: Activated T cells (also seen in Crohn's disease, perhaps same pathophysiology—Ann IM 1986;104:17) and macrophages, unclear why activated. Diminished cellular immunity due to incr suppressor cell prostaglandin synthesis (Ann IM 1979;90:169). Granuloma formation without necrosis or inflammation, often involves lung, skin, and RES; occasionally bone, kidney, eye, gi tract. Hypercalcemia due to incr vit D sensitivity; PTH levels very low, in immeasurable hypoparathyroid range (Nejm 1972;286:395)

Sx: Fatigue, weight loss, fever/malaise

Sarcoidosis, continued

Si: Dyspnea, cough, rales; neurologic (Ann IM 1977;87:336); uveitis, anterior chamber tissue masses, corneal precipitant and band keratopathy; splenomegaly, lymphadenopathy; skin lesions blanch with pressure, residual brown pigment, erythema nodosum on shins without scarring

Crs: 75–90% spontaneous resolution without rx in 2 yr

Cmplc: Restrictive lung disease (r/o chronic berylliosis—Ann IM 1988;108:687); pulmonary cavities with *Aspergillus;* pleuritis occasionally with exudative lymphocytic effusions (Ann IM 1974;81:190); hypercalcemia and hypercalciuria with renal stones; meningitis with low sugar; pituitary tumors with thirst and diabetes insipidus (Nejm 1980;303:1078); Bell's palsy; arthritis especially of knees and ankles

r/o primary biliary cirrhosis overlap syndrome (Nejm 1983;308:572); berylliosis; Wegener's granulomatosis; tuberculosis; histoplasmosis; and **Löfgren's syndrome,** a sarcoid variant in young person w erythema nodosum, bilateral hilar adenopathy and bilateral ankle arthritis, which is self-limited in 6 mo w no residua (Am J Med 1999;107:240)

Lab:

Chem: Elevated angiotensin converting enzyme, but very nonspecific; elevated Ca^{2+}

Noninv: PFTs show decr volumes, decr diffusion capacity, pO_2 often ok at rest but decreases w exercise

Path: Bx of minor salivary gland, supraclavicular node, or transbronchial (95% positive) shows noncaseating granuloma

Xray: Hilar adenopathy and interstitial pattern (one or both present in 90%)

Gallium scan positive over lung (macrophages) and nodes; very nonspecific

Rx: Steroids, eg, prednisone 30–40 mg po qd × 8–12 wk, then taper to 10–20 mg qod over 6–12 mo; possibly anti-TNF meds like infliximab (Ann IM 2001;135:27)

of skin: chloroquine 250 mg po bid

of elevated calcium and/or renal calcium stones: steroids, decrease vit D intake, chloroquine as above (Nejm 1986;315:727)

21.5 ENTRAPMENT SYNDROMES

ANTERIOR COMPARTMENT SYNDROME, CHRONIC

Cause: Genetic predisposition? or trauma

Epidem: Males in their 20s; trauma to anterior legs

Pathophys: Anterior tibial compartment claudication from congenitally or traumatically edematous small compartment that prevents normal vascular engorgement of exercising muscles

Sx: Anterior shin pain especially if walking on heels, usually bilateral. Relief by walking on toes or resting; can run ok

Si: BP can be auscultated after exercise over dorsalis pedis pulse without BP cuff. Muscle hernias through anterior fascial compartment

Crs:

Cmplc: Ischemic necrosis of anterior tibial muscles possible even without pain

    r/o **Shin splints** caused by periostitis and microfractures of bone; bone scan is positive; more frequent in osteoporotic athletes (Ann IM 1990;113:754); rx by discontinuation of running trauma

    Acute anterior compartment syndrome after trauma, w acute swelling which, if not relieved surgically can lead to ischemic death of anterior compartment muscles

Lab:

    NIL: Measurement of compartment pressures during exercise

Rx: Fasciotomies of anterior tibial compartments rarely indicated

LOW-BACK SYNDROMES

    Nejm 2001;344:363; Ann IM 1990;112:598

Cause: Ruptured herniated intervertebral disc; musculoligamentous strains/trauma; osteoarthritis of facet joints; perhaps leg length discrepancies; in elderly, vertebral compression fractures

Epidem: 65% of the population have low-back sx sometime in their lives; M = F, onset age 30–50

Pathophys: Myofascial, skeletal, disc, and/or ligamentous entrapment/
compression of nerve conduction/vascular flow causing secondary
edema, spasm and contracture and/or neurosensory
hyperstimulation or deficits

Sx: Focal (segmental) pain distal radiation of burning/shooting pain
and/or parestheisas, often worsened by cough; decr range of motion
due to pain and/or muscular restriction

Si: Rv of exam—Bull Rheum Dis 1983;33:4

Straight leg raising (SLR) <60° on affected side induces sx; if SLR on
opposite side induces, this positive "crossed leg sign" is highly
specific for central disc rupture

Levels: depression/loss of knee jerk = L_{3-4} (L_4 root); ankle jerk =
L_5–S_1 (S_1 root); toe extensors especially extensor hallucis longus
(big toe extensor) and sensation loss in medial foot especially
between first and second toes = L_{4-5} (L_5 root)

Crs: Most (>90%) improve with conservative rx over several days-weeks
and no workup is required unless motor loss present and does not
improve or worsens over this time period. 2/3 recur within 1 yr,
pain lasts 2 mo on average (Spine 1993;18:1388)

Cmplc: Workman's compensation (Ann IM 1978;89:992); cauda equina
syndrome w rectal or bladder dysfunction

r/o **spinal stenosis:** pain, pseudoclaudication, numbness, worse with
hips extended, eg, walking downhill; bilateral in 2/3 (Ann IM
1985;103:271)

Lab:

Xray: MRI/CT good if observed abnormality correlates with sx and si,
but 1/3 of CTs interpreted as abnormal (Spine 1984;9:549); and, in
normal asx people, bulges (50%) and protrusions (25%) are present
on MRI (Nejm 1994;301:69)

Scanograms for leg length are the only way to measure but rarely
needed; tapes are inaccurate (Spine 1983;8:643)

Rx:

Prevention: exercise programs w aerobic conditioning and leg/back
strenghthening helps; back belts no help (Jama 2000;284:2727)

Primary care strategy (Ann IM 1994;121:187), 70% better by 1 mo:
• Educate re chronic/recurrent nature but that severe flareups are
time-limited

- Pain rx only as time-limited, scheduled regimens, not prn; limited (<2 d) bedrest
- Referral for surgical evaluation only for abnormal neurologic findings
- Graded increasing activity even if pain not better/resolved

Education and/or lumbar supports of questionable value (Jama 1998;279:1789)

Bedrest: even 2 d bedrest slows recovery as do exercises, best strategy is cont'd normal activity as tolerated (Nejm 1995;332:351), true even if have sciatic sx (Nejm 1999;340:418); hard bed/bed board.

NSAIDs; heat; massage; muscle strengthening and flexibility exercises as well as a progressive fitness program (BMJ 1995;310:151); manipulation probably speeds recovery of acute and subacute types by 10–20% (RAND meta-analysis—Ann IM 1992;117:590). But exercise rx of acute pain is no help (Spine 1993;18:1388) but is helpful when chronic (>4 wk) (Bmj 1999;319:279). Steroid injections no help (Nejm 1997;336:1634; 1991;325:1002)

Manipulative techiques if not better in 3 wk, including high velocity low amplitude, strain/counter strain, and craniosacral; chiropractic or PT care of acute low back pain is more expensive though more satisfying for pt w same result as primary care doc care (Nejm 1998;339:1021; 1995;333:913)

Surgery if worsening motor weakness after 2 wk; better than chymopapain injection (Spine 1992;17:381) or microsurgery, but long term the latter comes out the same if combined with medical rx (J Gen Intern Med 1993;8:487)

of chronic low back pain: percutaneous electrical nerve stimulator (PENS) 30 min tiw × 3 wk helps (Jama 1999;281:818); magnets no help (Jama 2000;283:1322); multi-disciplinary pain center referral; opioids not that helpful

CARPAL TUNNEL SYNDROME

Jama 2000;283;3110; Nejm 1993;329:2013; Ann IM 1990;112:321

Cause: Local swelling and entrapment of median nerve at wrist

Epidem: Associated with occupational repetitive hand movements in 2/3, also pregnancy, myxedema, amyloidosis, tumor, rheumatoid arthritis, tenosynovitis, acromegaly, diabetes, wrist fracture, gout, myeloma, ganglia, renal failure with chronic dialysis

Female:male = 2:1 usually but in an occupational setting ratio is equal (Am J Pub Hlth 1991;81:741). Prevalence = 125–500/100,000 adults; but up to 1.5% in high-risk occupations; perhaps as high as 2^+% (Jama 1999;282:153,186)

Pathophys: Swelling within the carpal tunnel formed by the transverse carpal ligament impairs blood flow to median nerve

Similar entrapment syndromes can occur elsewhere but are very rare, eg, very similar **tarsal tunnel syndrome** in lateral foot; in the pronator teres (Nejm 1970;282:858); or of the ulnar nerve at the wrist, usually sx there only after sx's in median nerve distribution first

Sx: Numbness in median nerve distribution of the hand; worse at night (77%), shaking and/or hanging improves; pain and paresthesias often radiate proximally to elbow and shoulder; later, weakness of pincer grip, eg, holding a cup

Si: No pain, position or touch loss objectively, but often hypesthesia in median nerve distribution. Thenar wasting (15%) from loss of all but short thumb flexor

Tinel's sign (60% sens, 67% specif) = paresthesias when tap over median nerve at wrist; or Phalen's sign (75% sens, 47% specif) = paresthesias with forced wrist flexion for 60 s; or median nerve paresthesias with 1 min of BP cuff pumped up above systolic pressure

Crs: Slowly progressive, or may wax and wane

Cmplc: Permanent loss of thenar median nerve function, weakness and/or numbness

r/o other causes of similar sx including Raynaud's, cervical arthritis w radiculopathy, bursitis of shoulder, thoracic outlet syndrome, and ulnar neuropathy from elbow entrapment which is less easily helped by local measures (Nejm 1993;329:2016)

Lab:

Noninv: EMG nerve conduction velocities markedly decr (90% sens, ?% specif)

Rx: NSAIDs; steroids (Bmj 1999;319:884) 4 mg of methylprednisolone or 25 mg hydrocortisone locally injected proximally improves 80% at

1 mo, 50% at 1 yr; diuretics; splinting; change jobs; yoga program ×
8 wk helps more than splint (Jama 1998;280:1601)
Surgical, especially if thenar wasting present, or if patient plans to
continue heavy work, or when conservative rx has failed

THORACIC OUTLET SYNDROME

Nejm 1993;329:2017; 1972;286:1140

Cause: See pathophys

Epidem: Associated with cervical ribs and malformations of first rib

Pathophys: Compression of vessels or nerves between first rib and
clavicle, cervical rib, bony anomalies, muscles, etc. Vascular
compression: of subclavian vein causes edema and venous
distension leading to thrombosis; of subclavian artery results in loss
of pulse, claudication, and arterial thrombosis; of sympathetic
nerves causes Raynaud's; of peripheral nerves causes pain,
paresthesias, and weakness

Sx: Arm edema, claudication, Raynaud's, pain, paresthesias, weakness

Si: Loss of pulse at "attention" or with other maneuvers no longer felt
helpful (Jama 1966;196:109) because also found in 15% of normal
persons; motor nerve impairments, especially of intrinsic hand
muscles plus ulnar sensory losses

Crs:

Cmplc: r/o carpal tunnel (p 825)

Lab:

Noninv: EMG shows impaired nerve conduction velocities subclavian
fossa to hand (normal = 68–75 m/s); maybe not (Nejm
1984;310:1052)

Rx: Passive range of motion, physiotherapy, posture changes,
occupational health evaluation, and/or manipulation techniques
(J Am Osteop Assoc 1990;90:686,810; 1989;89:1046), alone if
NCVs >60 m/s; if less, then consider surgical decompression, eg,
resect first rib

21.6 MISCELLANEOUS

Ankle and foot injuries
Si: Distinguish sprain vs fx and need for xray (see Fig. 21.6.1; "Ottawa ankle rules"—Jama 1994;271:827) only if (1) can't bear weight; (2) bone tenderness over edge or tip of medial or lateral malleolus (ankle); or (3) bone tenderness over base of 5th metatarsal laterally or over navicular medially (foot). When applied, this protocol decr xrays × 25% and misses no significant fx's (Jama 1997;278:1935)

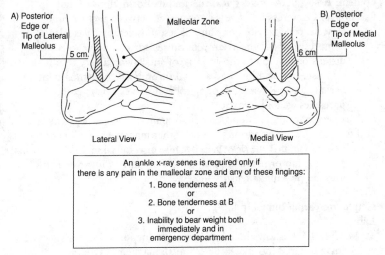

Figure 21.6.1 Ottawa Ankle Rules. Reprinted with permission, Journal of the American Medical Association, 2000;284:80. Copyrighted 2000, American Medical Association.

Autoantibodies and clinical disease correlates (M. Duston 10/94); see Table 21.6.1

Calcium levels, corrected in serum
Normal = total: 8.6–10.4 mg %; or 2.15–2.60 mEq/L; unbound: 4.5–6.0 mg %. Corrections for protein levels: at normal protein levels (4 gm % albumin), 47% is free and is the level by which parathormone adjusts feedback to parathyroids and bone. To correct, increase or decrease by 0.8 mg % (total)/gm of albumin; or corrected Ca = total

measured Ca (0.6) + total measured Ca (0.4) × total protein/7.4
(Nejm 1969;281:55); or corrected $Ca^{2+} = Ca^{2+} - (albumin) + 4$

Table 21.6.1

Autoantibody	Clinical Disease Correlate
Antinuclear antibody (ANA)	Nonspecific
Anti-dsDNA (double stranded DNA)	High specif for SLE
Anti-ds and ss (single stranded) DNA	Active SLE, especially renal
Antihistones	Drug-induced SLE and RA
Anti-Sm	High specif for SLE, no correlation w disease activity; also seen in other causes of autoimmune hepatitis
Anti-Ro/SSA	Neonatal lupus (w anti-La/SSB); photosensitivity; subacute cutaneous lupus
Anti-La/SSB	Neonatal lupus (w anti-Ro/SSA); Sjögren's
Anti-phospholipids	Inhibition of in vitro coagulation tests; thrombosis; recurrent fetal abortion/wastage; focal neurologic deficits; thrombocytopenia
Anticentromere	Limited cutaneous scleroderma (CREST)
Scl_{70} (antitopoisomerase)	Diffuse scleroderma
$Anti-Jo_1$ (antitransfer RNA)	Polymyositis

Hallux valgus
Cause: Shoes
Epidem: 33% adult prevalence though most mild
Si: Lateral deviation of 1st MP joint of foot
Rx: Chevron ostotomy, 90% successful and better than orthotics (Jama 2001;285:2475)

Joint fluid (use heparin for cell counts) (rv—Nejm 1993;329:1013); see Table 21.6.2 (p 830)

Knee injuries and rx (Nejm 1988;318:950): In acute injury, xray only if age >55, tender head of fibula, isolated patellar tenderness, can't flex $\geq 90°$, or can't bear weight; 100% sens (Ottawa knee rules: Jama 1997;278:2075, 1996;275:611). See Fig. 21.6.2 (p 831)
- Anterior cruciate tear; caused by anterior subluxation injuries usually involving forward motion on planted foot with a twisting motion; sx = "trick knee." Test by (1) anterior drawer si at 30° flexion + (2) pivot/ shift si = 20° flexion, relaxed quad, then axial or valgus force on knee

Table 21.6.2

Dx	Viscosity	Mucin Clot	WBC/mm^3	% Polys	Other
Traumatic	high	good	<200	<25%	Fat in joint
Osteoarthritis	high	good	<2K	<25%	Red cells often
Lupus	high	good	~5K	10%	LE cells in joint fluid
Rheumatic fever	low	good	10–12K	50%	
Pseudogout	low	good to poor	1–5K	25%–50%	Positively birefringent crystals
Gout	low	poor	10–12K	60%–70%	Negatively birefringent crystals
RA and HLA B27 disease incld Reiter's	low	poor	15–20K	50%–60%	Occasional cholesterol crystal
Tuberculosis	low	poor	25K	75$^+$%	AFB positive
Septic (Nejm 1985;312:764)	low	poor	80–200K (95% >20K)	75$^+$%	Gram stain + and culture; glucose low in 50%

Reproduced with permission from McCarly DJ, ed. Arthritis and allied conditions: a textbook of rheumatology. 12th ed. Baltimore: Williams & Wilkins, 1992:72.

and knee is flexed + extended, if cruciate deficient will go in and out of subluxation. 1/3 resolve, 1/3 are functional though sx, 1/3 go on to progressive damage. Repair early if young or avulsed insertion on lateral tibial condyle apparent on xray

- Meniscal injury may occur acutely or later when they are trapped because anterior cruciate doesn't keep femur and tibia aligned; 60% incidence w ACL tear. Sx = "locked knee," pain, "popping." Test for by Apley compression test prone, McMurray test, and lateral medial/lateral grind test. Repair or partial resection better than total resection
- Medial collateral tear. Test: knee opens medially when extended. Rx: conservative with immobilization and ROM and strengthening exercises × 3–6 wk; or if severe, hinged brace locked at 30° × 3 wk then full ROM × 3–5 wk additional
- Posterior cruciate tear; caused by posterior subluxation injuries, eg, dashboard or fall on flexed knee. Leads to early DJD, especially of medial femoral condyle, and damage to medial meniscus. No good rx

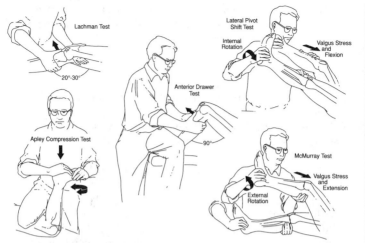

Figure 21.6.2 Right knee shown. Examination maneuvers include the Lachman, anterior drawer, lateral pivot shift, Apley compression, and McMurray tests. Lachman test, performed to detect anterior cruciate ligament (ACL) injuries, is conducted with the patient supine and the knee flexed 20° to 30°. The anterior drawer test detects ACL injuries and is performed with the patient supine and the knee in 90° of flexion. The lateral pivot shift test is performed with the patient supine, the hip flexed 45°, and the knee in full extension. Internal rotation is applied to the tibia while the knee is flexed to 40° under a valgus stress (pushing the outside of the knee medially). The Apley compression test, used to assess meniscal integrity, is performed with the patient prone and the examiner's knee over the patient's posterior thigh. The tibia is externally rotated while a downward compressive force is applied over the tibia. The McMurray test, used to assess meniscal integrity, is performed with the patient supine and the examiner standing on the side of the affected knee. Reprinted with permission from Jama 2001;286:1614

yet available; conservative rx if isolated, surgical if associated w multiple ligamentous injuries

Anterior knee pain syndromes

- Lateral facet compression syndrome; rx w patellofemoral rehab or arthroscopic lateral release
- Chronic patellar subluxation in patients with valgus knees or lateral tracking of patella; rx w rehab or quadriceps realignment
- Inflamed synovial plica; rx w NSAIDs, steroid injections, rehab, or arthroscopic plicectomy

- Patellar tendonitis, "jumper's knee" (Nejm 1988;318:950); rx'd with NSAIDs and rehab; r/o **Osgood-Schlatter disease,** inflammation of anterior tibial tubercle apophysis in adolescent
- Anterior fat pad impingement; rx w rehab, steroids

Lymphedema
Cause: Mastectomy, filariasis, inflammation, lymphatic agenesis, idiopathic
Rx: Conservative measures like PT and compressive stockings
Benzopyrone 400 mg po qd (Nejm 1993;329:1158)

Polyarthritis with fever; differential dx (Nejm 1994;330:769)
- Infectious
    Bacterial: septic arthritis (gc/staph), SBE, Lyme, tbc, fungal
    Viral: hep B, parvovirus, rubella, HIV
- Reactive: Enteric infection, Reiter's, rheumatic fever, IBD, Whipple's
- RA/Still's
- Vasculitis
- SLE
- Crystal diseases
- FMF
- Acute leukemias/lymphomas
- Dermatomyositis
- Behçet's
- Henoch-Schönlein purpura
- Kawasaki's
- Erythema nodosum
- Erythema multiforme
- Pyoderma gangrenosum
- Pustular psoriasis
- Sarcoid

Scaphoid fractures (Phys and Sportsmed 1996;24(8):60)
Sx: Fall on outstretched hand
Si: Tender snuff box w thumb extended; pain w axial compression and w resisted wrist pronation
Cmplc: Avascular necrosis
Xray: Fracture, distal, waist or proximal types

Rx: if no fx but has pain, thumb spica × 2 wk, then re-xray; if still neg but still sx and suspicious, then CT or bone scan

Surgery for waist or proximal types

Thumb spica × 6–8 wk for distal types

Tendonitis/bursitis syndromes

- Injecting the functional structure causing pain with steroids and lidocaine much better than pain trigger points (75% vs 20% success—BMJ 1983;287:1339)
- Shoulder tendonitis (Nejm 1999;340:1582), rx w NSAIDs, steroid injections, or if that fails, ultrasound (Nejm 1999;340:1533)
- Prepatellar and olecranon bursitis occasionally infected with staph and may need tap, I + D, and antibiotics (Ann IM 1978;89:21), but rarely
- Tennis elbow, rx w steroid injection, NSAIDs, or pain meds; all w equal outcome at 1 yr (Bmj 1999;319:964)
- Greater trochanteric bursitis

Vasculitis etiologies (Jama 1997;278:1962, Nejm 1997;337:1512)

Large vessel: giant cell and Takayasu's arteritis

Medium sized vessels: polyarteritis and Kawasaki's disease

Small vessel:

ANCA (antineutrophil cytoplasmic autoantibodies)-associated types: microscopic polyangiitis, Wegener's Churg-Strauss, drug induced

Immune complex types: Henoch-Schönlein purpura, cryoglobulinemic vasculitis, SLE, RA, Sjögren's, Behçet's, Goodpasture's, serum sickness, drug induced, infection induced

Paraneoplastic

Inflammatory bowel disease

Whiplash injury of neck

Cmplc: Chronic cervical pain from zygapophyseal joints

Rx: Hourly range of motion exercises, started w/i 4 d of injury helps diminish long-term sx (Spine 2000;25:1782). Rarely, w needle radiofrequency neurotomy (Nejm 1996;335:1721)

FUNCTIONAL SOMATIC SYNDROMES (Medically Unexplained Physical Sx [MUPS])

Ann IM 1999;130:910

Multiple manifestations some of which may have some physiologic basis like: chemical sensitivities, sick building synrome, chronic whiplash, silicone breast implant syndrome, chronic irritable bowel syndrome, chronic food allergies, mitral valve prolapse, chronic mononucleosis, etc. (see somatization d/o p 705). Overall strategy (Am Fam Phys 2000;61:1073,1423) is to r/o organic disease, look for depression and panic disorder especially to rx, set functional not curative goals, apply cognitive behavioral rx and/or antidepressants (J Fam Pract 1999;48:980), see regularly and avoid repetitive w/u's

Chronic fatigue syndrome

Jama 1998;280:1094; 1997;278:1179; Ann IM 1994;121:953, 1988;108:387

Cause: Biologic vs psych causes debated; lots of circumstantial evidence for biologic connections (T. Kamaroff—Am J Med 2000;108:169, 172). Assoc w neurally mediated hypotension always (70% have abnormal tilt table test w/o pharmacologic precipitation); thus rx for that may help (p 562, 120) (Jama 1995;274:961)

May be equivalent to old dx of "neurasthenia," but unlikely that caused by EBV, and more likely that the EBV antibodies are the result not the cause of the syndrome. Acyclovir rx no help (Nejm 1988;319:1692). Other purported causes: *Candida* (Nejm 1990; 323:1165, 1717), hypoglycemia, fibrositis, depression, Lyme disease (Ann IM 1993;119:503, 518), human herpesvirus type 6 (Ann IM 1992;116:103); no evidence of a retrovirus (Ann IM 1993;118:241)

Sx: Fatigue ≥6 mo, normal labs (Chem 20, CBC, ESR, TSH, UA) and ≥4 of the following sx: impaired memory/concentration, sore throat, tender cervical/axillary nodes, myalgias, arthralgias, headache, poor sleep, postexertion malaise

Cmplc: r/o depressions; fibromyalgia overlaps; alcoholism

Lab: Chem panel, CBC, ESR, UA; optionally ANA, cortisol, RA titer, SPEP, IPPD, Lyme titer, HIV serology

Rx: (Jama 1995;274:961)

Cognitive behavioral therapy (Lancet 2001;357:841) and graded exercise programs (Bmj 2001;322:387) help

Avoid salt restriction, diuretics, vasodilators, tricyclics; incr salt in diet; fludrocortisone (Florinef), but RCT doesn't confirm efficacy (Jama 2001;285:52); β blockers; anticholinergics like disopyramide (Norpace) all in that order. Avoid low-dose steroids, which are of minimal help but cause adrenal suppression (Jama 1998;280:1061)

Gulf War syndrome

No incr hospitalization or medical illness but incr accidental death, ? related to depression or greater risk taking (Nejm 1996;335:1498, 1505); may be caused by organophosphate poisoning and/or DEET exposure, causing chronic measurable neuropsych dysfunction (Jama 1997;277:215,223,231,238,259); but other studies find no such correlations (Am J Med 2000;108:695; Jama 1998;280:981)

Fibromyalgia syndrome (Ann IM 1999;131:850; Post Grad Med 1996;100:153)

Cause: Unknown, possibly related to chronic fatigue syndrome
Epidem: F >>> M
Pathophys: Increased sensitivity to pain; otherwise not understood
Sx: Musculoskeletal pains and stiffness, sleep disturbances, headache, fatigue
Si: Multiple tender areas/points
Cmplc: r/o spondyloarthropathy (Am J Med 1997;103:44)
Lab: r/o other diseases w CBC, chemistry panel, TSH, ESR, CPK
Rx: (Rx Let 2000;7:67) Exercise, education, biofeedback, hypnotherapy, acupuncture
  Amitriptyline 10–75 mg po hs qd; or cyclobenzaprine (Flexeril) 10–20 mg po bid (Arth Rheum 1994;37:32); or SSRIs like sertraline (Zoloft) which probably just help latent depression unlike TCAs
  Pain meds like tramadol (Ultram), Lidocaine injections of trigger points; clonazepam (Klonopin) for sleep; perhaps gabapentin (Neurontin)

Index

INDEX

INDEX

INDEX

INDEX

Kogan's syndrome, 793
Konyne, 351
Koplik's spots, 516
Korsakoff's psychosis, 240
Krukenberg's ovarian tumor, 256
Krukenberg's tumors, 600
Kussmaul's respirations, 201
Kussmaul's si, 57
Kussmaul's sign in pericarditis, 91
Kwell, 463

Labetalol, 41
Labor and delivery, 610
Labor, premature, 610
Labor, premature rx, 613
Labyrinthitis, 582
Lacerations, 161
LaCrosse viral encephalitis, 513
Lactase deficiency, 286
Lacunar stroke, 531
Laënnec's cirrhosis, 268
Lamictal, 543
Lamisil, oral, 130
Lamisil, topical, 128
Lamivudine, 488
Lamotrigine (Lamictal), 543
Lampit, 464
Lansoprazole (Prevacid), 253
Lantus, 196
Lanugo hair, 701
Large bowel diseases, 293
Lariam, 464
Larval migrans, visceral/cutaneous, 481
Laryngeal carcinoma, 178
Laryngeal papillomas from HPV, 147
Lasix, 44
Latanoprost (Xalatan), 635
Lateral medullary plate syndrome, 532
Lateral sinus thrombosis in otitis media, 167
Latex allergy, 135
Lathyrism, 105
Laxatives, 304
L-dopa, 552
Lead pipe colon, 296
Lead pipe hypertonia, 526
Lead poisoning, 30

Lead screening, 32, 684
Leflunomide (Arava), 789
Left ventricular enlargment w/o LVH, 119
Left ventricular hypertrophy
    by physical exam, 119
    by xray, 119
Legg-Perthes' Disease, 652
Legionella pneumophilia, 410
Legionellosis, 410
Legionnaires' disease, 410
Leiden mutation, 111
Leiomyoma of uterus, 594
Lennox-Gastaut syndrome, 545
Lentigo maligna, 152
Lepirudin, 38
Leprosy, 436
Lesch-Nyhan syndrome, 811
Lescol, 211
letrozole (Femara), 588
Leukemia
    acute lymphocytic (blastic), 366
    acute nonlymphocytic, 365
    chronic lymphocytic, 367
    monoblastic, 365
    myeloblastic, 365
Leukemia, chronic myelogenous, 362
Leukeran, 330
Leukocytoclastic vasculitis, 357
Leukoencephalopathy, multifocal
        progressive, 495
Leukoplakia, 162
Leukoplakia, hairy, 518
Leukotriene receptor antagonists, 715
Leuprolide (Lupron), 593
Levaquin, 387
Levatol, 40
Levetiracetum (Keppra), 543
Levocabastine (Livostin), 640
Levofloxacin (Levaquin), 387
Levonorgestrel implant, 621
Levorphanol, 787
Lhermitte's si, 557
Librium, 688
Lice, body/head, 486
Lichen planus, 156
Lichen sclerosis of vulva, 162
Licorice ingestion, 185

Moraxella catarrhalis, 411
Morgan-Dennie fold, 136
Moricizine, 38
Morning after BCP contraception, 622
Morphine SO$_4$, 787
Morphine, cardiac use, 47
Motion sickness, 305
Motrin, 784
Mountain sickness, acute, 725
Movement disorders, 549
M-protein disease, 374
Mucomyst, 723
Mucor infections, 461
Mucorales spp, 461
Mucosa associated lypnoid tissue
    (MALT), 256
Mucoviscidosis, 721
Multicystic dysplasia of kidney, 761
Multicystic renal disease, 761
Multifocal atrial tachycardia, 70
Multifocal leukoencephalopathy,
    progressive, 495
Multiple endocrine neoplasia, 216
Multiple endocrine neoplasias, 238
Multiple myeloma, 374
Multiple personality disorder, 703
Multiple sclerosis, 557
Mumps, 519
Mupirocin (Bactroban), 390
Mural thrombi in MI, 59
Murmur
    basal ejection, 668
    physiologic, 668
    Still's, 668
Murmur mimics, 119
Murmurs, benign pediatric, 667
Murphy's si, 263
Muscle spasms, rx, 559
Muscle weakness, causes, 792
Muscle weakness, differential dx, 578
Muscular dystrophy, Becker's, 565
Muscular dystrophy, Duchenne's, 564
Muscular dystrophy, Emery-Dreifuss,
    565
Muscular dystrophy,
    pseudohypertrophic, 564
MUSE, 780
Mushroom picker's disease, 717

Mustard, nitrogen, 330
Mycelex, 144
Mycobacterium marinum, 435
Mycobacterium avium/intracellulare,
    434
Mycobacterium fortuitum, 434
Mycobacterium leprae, 436
Mycobacterium scrofulaceum/kansasii,
    434
Mycobacterium tuberculosis and bovis,
    431
mycophenolate (CellCept), 752
Mycophenolate mofetil (CellCept), 333
Mycoplasma pneumonia, 445
Mycosis fungoides, 153
Mycostatin, 128
Myelofibrosis, 361
Myeloid Metaplasia, 361
Myeloma, multiple, 374
Myelomeningocele, 663
Myeloproliferative disorders, 359
Myesthenia gravis, 555
Mylanta, 253
Myleran, 330
Mylotarg, 334
Myocardial infarct
    emergent rx, 11
Myocardial infarction, 56
Myocardiopathies, 93
Myocarditis, 92
Myoclonic seizures, 543
Myoclonus, differential dx and rx, 577
Myoglobinuria causing ATN, 754
Myotonia, 566
Myotonia, cold, 566
Myotonia, excitement, 566
Myotonic dystrophy, 566
Myotonic syndromes, 566
Mysoline, 542
Myxedema, 226
Myxoma, atrial, 90

N$_3$ fatty acids, in rx of ASHD, 52
Nabumetone (Relafen), 785
Naegleria gruberi, 469
Nafarelin, 593
Nafcillin, 384
Naftifine, 128

INDEX

Porcelain gallbladders, 264
Porphyria Cutanea Tarda, 344
Porphyria, acute Intermittent, 344
Porphyria, variegate, 344
Porphyrias, 344
Port wine stains, 133
Positive airway pressure ventilation, 734
Positive end expiratory pressure, 734
Positive predictive value, 672
Postabortal syndrome, 602
Postcholecystectomy pain syndrome, 264
Postcoital contraception, 622
Posterior inferior cerebellar artery occlusion, 532
Postpartum bleeding, 611
Postphlebitic syndrome, 112
Posttraumatic stress disorder, 699
Post-tubal syndrome, 623
Postural hypotension, 120
Postural hypotension rx, 562
postural tachycardia syndrome, 562
Postvoid residuum measurement, 326
Potassium sparing diuretics, 44
Pott's disease, 432
Powassan encephalitis, 501
Power-of-attorney, for elderly, 324
Pramipexole (Mivapex), 552
Pravachol, 211
Pravastatin (Pravachol), 211
prayer si in diabetes, 192
Praziquantel (Biltricide), 464
Prazosin, 47
Predictive values, neg/pos, calculation, 672
Prednisone, 788
Preeclampsia, 613
Prefest, 625
Pregnancy, 603
Pregnancy in diabetes, management, 200
Pregnancy induced hypertension, 613
Pregnancy Rashes, 158
Pregnancy, ectopic, 595
Premarin, 624
Premature infant, 661

Premature labor, 610
Premature labor, rx, 613
Premature rupture of membranes, 604
Premature rupture of membranes (PROM), 610
Premature rupture of membranes, rx, 612
Premature ventricular contractions, 76
Premenstrual syndrome, 630
Prempro, 625
Prenatal labs, 605
Prepartum bleeding in 3rd trimester, 611
Presbycusis, 171
Pressure sores, 159
Prevacid, 253
Preven, 622
Prevention, 671
in adults, 674
Preveon, 489
PrevPac, 252
Prickle cell antibody, 154
Priftin, 433
Prilosec, 253
Primaquine, 465
Primary Adrenal Insufficiency, 186
Primary atypical pneumonia, 445
Primary biliary cirrhosis, 264
Primary sclerosing cholangitis, 266
Primaxin, 386
Primidone (Mysoline), 542
Prinivil, 46
Pro-Banthine, 253
Procainamide, 38
Procarbazine (Matulane), 333
Procardia, 43
Prochlorperazine (Compazine), 305
Proctitis, ulcerative, 296
Pro-Gest, 630
Progesterones, 625
Progressive multifocal leukoencephalopathy, 495
Progressive supranuclear palsy, 551
Progressive Systemic Sclerosis, 803
Promethazine (Phenergan), 305
Prometrium, 625
Pronestyl, 38

Propafenone, 39
Propantheline (Pro-Banthine), 253
Propecia, 159
Prophylactic antibiotics, 451
Propoxyphene (Darvon), 788
Propranolol, 40
Proptosis of eyes, 229
Propulsid in esophagitis, 247
Propylthiouracil, 230
Proscar, 771
ProSom, 689
Prostaglandin E, 780
Prostaglandin E$_2$, to induce abortion, 603
Prostate cancer, screening, 681
Prostate specific antigen testing, 774
Prostatic carcinoma, 773
Prostatic hypertrophy, benign, 769
Prostigmin, 556
Protatitis, 767
Protease inhibitors, 489
Protective isolation, 364, 452
Protein C deficiency, 111
Protein S deficiency, 111
Proteinuria, 781
Proteinuria, diabetic, 194
Prothrombin time, 349
Protist infections, 466
Proton pump inhibitors, 253
Protonix, 253
Protozoan infections, 466
Protriptyline (Vivactil), 693
Proventil, 713
Provera, 625
Provigil, 559
Prozac, 694
Pruritic urticarial papules and plaques of pregnancy, 158
Pruritus differential dx, 163
Pseudocyst, pancreatic, 257
Pseudogout, 813
Pseudohemophilia, 351
Pseudohermaphroditism, female, 188
Pseudohypertrophic muscular dystrophy, 564
Pseudohypoparathyroidism, 218
Pseudomembranous colitis, 426

Pseudomonas aeruginosa, 419
Pseudomonas cepacia, 420
Pseudomonas mallei, 420
Pseudoseizures, 545
Pseudotubercular thyroiditis, 232
Pseudotumor cerebri, 568
Psoriasis, 138
Psoriasis, guttate, 138
Psychedelic Drug Use/OD, 23
Psychiatric medications, 688
Psychiatry, 688
Psychogenic water drinker, 747
Psychosis, 703
Puberty, precocious, 188
Pulmicort, 714
Pulmonary diseases, 708
Pulmonary edema, acute mountain type, 725
Pulmonary edema, emergent rx, 9
Pulmonary edema, high altitude, 725
Pulmonary embolus, 726
Pulmonary function tests, 735
Pulmonary hypertension, 723
Pulmonic stenosis, congenital, 103
Pulse pressure, wide, 121
Pulseless electrical activity, 2
Pulsus paradoxus, 91
Pupillary abnormalities, 580
Purpura and platelet disorders, 352
Purpura fulminans, in meningococcal infection, 414
Purpura fulminans, neonatal, 111
Purpura, anaphylactoid, 356
Purpura, Henoch-Schönlein, 356
Purpura, idiopathic thrombocytopenic, 357
Purpura, palpable, 157
Purpura, thrombotic thrombocytopenic, 353
Purpuric rashes, 157
PUVA rx of psoriasis, 139
Pyelonephritis
    acute, 765
    chronic, 766
Pyloric stenosis, 650
Pyoderma gangrenosum, 289, 296
Pyrantel pamoate (Antiminth), 465
Pyrazinamide, 434

INDEX